CW01186941

THE RENAISSANCE HOSPITAL

The Renaissance Hospital
HEALING THE BODY AND HEALING THE SOUL

JOHN HENDERSON

YALE UNIVERSITY PRESS
NEW HAVEN AND LONDON

Copyright © 2006 by John Henderson

All rights reserved. This book may not be reproduced in whole or in part, in any form (beyond that copying permitted by Sections 107 and 108 of the U.S. Copyright Law and except by reviewers for the public press) without written permission from the publishers.

For information about this and other Yale University Press publications, please contact:
U.S. Office: sales.press@yale.edu   www.yalebooks.com
Europe Office: sales@yaleup.co.uk   www. yaleup. co.uk

Publication of this book has been assisted by a grant from the Lila Acheson Wallace – Reader's Digest Special Grants Subsidy.

Set in Minion by Northern Phototypesetting Co. Ltd, Bolton
Printed in Great Britain by St Edmundsbury Press Ltd, Bury St Edmunds

ISBN 0 300 10995 4

Library of Congress Control Number: 2006927747

A catalogue record for this book is available from the British Library.

10 9 8 7 6 5 4 3 2 1

Published with assistance from the foundation established in memory of Oliver Baty Cunningham of the Class of 1917, Yale College.

TO JULIAN, YVETTE, AND ROSETTE

Contents

List of Plates	xi
List of Figures	xvii
List of Maps	xviii
List of Tables	xix
Acknowledgements	xxi
A Note on Currency, Weights and Measurements	xxiii
INTRODUCTION	
The Renaissance Hospital in Italy	xxv

PART I
HOSPITALS AND THE BODY OF THE CITY

CHAPTER 1
Before the Black Death: The Birth of the Clinic		3
Introduction		3
1.1	Early Foundations: 'Patients in sordid and fetid beds, where many die from fetor and corruption of the air'	7
1.2	Towards Specialisation	14
1.3	The Growth of Medicine	25
1.4	The Common Good: Between Church and State	28
Conclusion		31

CHAPTER 2
The Early Renaissance: Medicine for the Body and Medicine for the Soul		34
Introduction: The Black Death and its Aftermath		34
2.1	'The Hospital is a Great Charity': S. Maria Nuova and the Impact of the Black Death	36

2.2	'For the poor of Christ of both sexes who languish and are sick': New Foundations in the Early Renaissance	38
2.3	Balancing the Books at S. Maria Nuova: 'It is believed it would today have owned most of the property of Florence through bequests left by diverse people at different times if…'	54
2.4	'Do not marvel that our expenditure exceeds our income': Hospital Finance	60
Conclusion		67

CHAPTER 3
The Late Renaissance: Beauty, Sickness and the Poor — 70

Introduction		70
3.1	'Our city above all others is copiously provided with hospitals, which are beautiful'	71
3.2	Behind the Façade: 'capacious and adapted and organised to receive any sick or healthy person who is wretched'	81
3.3	The 'System of Care'	88
3.4	Hospitals and 'the multitude of those sick from plague'	93
3.5	'The Boils of the French Disease' and the Incurabili Hospital	97
3.6	Crisis and Reform: 'to keep open the hospital for the benefit of the poor of Christ'	101
Conclusion		109

PART II
HEALING THE SOUL

CHAPTER 4
'To the Almighty Physician no infirmity is incurable': The Role of the Hospital Church — 113

Introduction		113
4.1	Christus Medicus	113
4.2	The Hospital Church: Devotion, Decoration and the Cure of the Soul	117
4.3	'For the salvation of his soul and of his successors': Hospital Churches and Commemoration	135
4.4	Tranquillity and Transition: The Hospital Cloister	140
Conclusion		146

CHAPTER 5
'Splendid houses of treatment built at vast expense': Wards and the Care of the Body and Soul   147
Introduction   147
5.1 Wards Seen from the Outside   149
5.2 Ward Interiors: 'Beautiful and sufficient and suitable to receive any sick or well person who is wretched'   151
5.3 The Care of the Sick and the Material Culture of Health   161
5.4 Wards and the Cure of the Soul: 'When he is dead they clothe him in linen, and place him on a bier in the middle of the ward where the chapel is'   168
Conclusion   184

CHAPTER 6
Serving the Poor: The Nursing Community   186
Introduction   186
6.1 Entering the New Life   187
6.2 'For the health and tranquillity of his soul'   192
6.3 'Patience, dedication and hard work'   197
6.4 Living and Working for the Community   200
6.5 Identity: 'men and women of a saintly life'?   210
Conclusion   221

PART III
HEALING THE BODY

CHAPTER 7
Treating the Poor: Doctors and their Duties   225
Introduction   225
7.1 From Physicians to Eye Doctors to Women 'skilled in surgery'   226
7.2 'To recognise the variety of the sick and to know the qualities of urine': The Physician's Task   230
7.3 To Shave, Let Blood, Cut and Medicate: Surgeons and their Surgeries   235
7.4 Hospital Doctors: 'Always the best in the city'?   241
7.5 Professional Networks   244
Conclusion   249

CHAPTER 8
'Antechambers of Death'? 251
Introduction 251
8.1 'Almost like Christ in their persons': Admitting the Poor 253
8.2 Death and Disease 256
8.3 'He could only speak like a wolf': Patients and their Ailments 262
8.4 The Different Faces of Poverty 267
8.5 *Cittadini* and *Contadini* 272
Conclusion 279
Appendix 8.1   S. Maria Nuova's Patients with Surnames 282
Appendix 8.2   Provenance of Patients from S. Maria Nuova: Florence and *Contado* 283

CHAPTER 9
Treating the Poor: Apothecaries, Pills and Potions 286
Introduction 286
9.1 'To make the medicines and syrups that need to be made up for our patients': Apothecaries and Pharmacies 286
9.2 'A universal book of many things, all recipes tried and tested': S. Maria Nuova's Medical Recipes and their Authors 297
9.3 'We begin first of all with the ailments of the head, descending as far as the feet' 304
9.4 Plagues, Pestilences and Fevers 306
9.5 'The head of our body is made like the chimney of the house' 309
9.6 Digestion, Excretion and Sex 323
Conclusion 334

CONCLUSION 336

Appendix
Provisional List of Hospitals Founded in Florence, 1000–1550 341
Notes 356
Bibliography 423
Index 441

Plates

I	Bicci di Lorenzo, *Martin V Confirming the Consecration of S. Egidio*, 1424–5, Salone di Martino V, Ospedale di S. Maria Nuova	xxvii
1.1	Pietro del Massaio, *Veduta di Firenze*, 1472, from Ptolemy's *Geografia* (Rome, Vatican Library, Codices Urbinates Latini, no. 277)	3
1.2	Domenico di Bartolo, 'A Pilgrim', detail of *Feeding the Poor*, 1440–4, Pellegrinaio ward, S. Maria della Scala, Siena	10
1.3	Francesco Rosselli, *Veduta di Firenze detta 'della Catena'*, c.1471–80: detail of Hospital of S. Gallo	12
1.4	Church of the Spedale di Gesù Pellegrino, Via S. Gallo	16
1.5	Hospital of the Pigeon, Via Romana: a. View towards Porta Romana; b. Detail of façade	18
1.6	Hospital of S. Niccolò della Misericordia dei Fantoni, Via Romana: a. View of façade; b. Detail showing symbol of the Confraternity of the Bigallo	19
1.7	Symbol of the Cross from the Spedale di S. Spirito, Via Romana	20
1.8	Hospital of S. Maria della Scala, Via della Scala	20
1.9	Ground plan of the Hospital of S. Maria Nuova, c.1500 (adapted from an original design by Patrick Sweeney)	22
1.10	Codice Rustici, *Hospital of S. Maria Nuova*, c.1445	24
2.1	Spedale di S. Piero Novello dei Ridolfi, Via Romana: a. Façade; b. Architrave with inscription and Ridolfi family coat of arms	41
2.2	Spedale di S. Giovanni Battista della Calza, Piazza della Calza	42
2.3	Spedale di S. Giuliano a Colombaia, Via Senese	42
2.4	Codice Rustici, *Spedale di S. Antonio*, c.1445	48
2.5	The leprosarium of S. Eusebio at Campoluccio, 1709–10 (ASF, Arte di Calimala 146)	48
2.6	Ground plan of the Ospedale di S. Maria Nuova, 1780 (ASF, Ospedale di S. Maria Nuova 24: Plan 2)	59

3.1	Façade of the Ospedale degli Innocenti, Piazza SS. Annunziata	73
3.2	Cosimo Zocchi, *Veduta dell'Ospedale di Messer Bonifazio*, 1744	74
3.3	Façade of the Ospedale di S. Matteo, Piazza S. Marco	74
3.4	Façade of the Ospedale di S. Paolo, Piazza S. Maria Novella	74
3.5	Cosimo Zocchi, *Veduta della Piazza di S. Maria Nuova*, 1744	75
3.6	Loggia of the Ospedale di S. Matteo, Piazza S. Marco	76
3.7	Loggia of the company of the Bigallo, Piazza S. Giovanni	76
3.8	Ospedale di S. Paolo, Piazza S. Maria Novella: Andrea della Robbia, c.1498: a. Church portal lunette, *The Meeting of SS. Francis and Dominic*; b. Loggia half-roundel, *Portrait of the Hospital Director Bonino Bonini*	78
3.9	Ospedale degli Innocenti: Andrea della Robbia, roundel of foundling, 1487	78
3.10	Façade of the Ospedale del Ceppo, Piazza S. Lorenzo, Pistoia, with glazed terracotta frieze by Giovanni di Andrea della Robbia's workshop, 1525–9	79
3.11	Gherardo and Monte di Giovanni di Miniato: a. *Arrival of Martin V at S. Egidio*; b. *Martin V Greeted by the Spedalingo of S. Maria Nuova*; c. *Departure of Martin V* from S. Maria Nuova (S. Egidio, Breviary, 1474: Museo Nazionale del Bargello MS A68, f. 161v)	81
3.12	Ground plan of the Ospedale di S. Matteo in 1780 (ASF, Ospedale di S. Maria Nuova 24: Plan 5)	83
3.13	Francesco Rosselli, *Veduta di Firenze detta 'della Catena'*: detail of the Ospedale di S. Matteo, 1471–80 (Museo di Firenze Com'era)	84
3.14	Ospedale di S. Matteo, Piazza S. Marco: male cloister	84
3.15	Ground plan of the Ospedale di Messer Bonifazio in 1780 (ASF, Ospedale di S. Maria Nuova 24: Plan 9)	87
3.16	Ground plan of the Ospedale di S. Paolo in 1780 (ASF, Ospedale di S. Maria Nuova 24: Plan 7)	87
3.17	*Beggar with the French Disease Seated on a Handcart*, incised marble plaque, outside Church of S. Maria in Porta Paradisi, Hospital of S. Giacomo, Rome	99
4.1	'Man of Sorrows', detail of Bicci di Lorenzo, *Martin V Confirming the Consecration of S. Egidio*, 1424–5, Salone di Martino V, Hospital of S. Maria Nuova	114
4.2	Florentine School, *Christ Showing His Wound*, c.1420–5 (Victoria and Albert Museum, London)	114
4.3	*Coronation of the Virgin*, attributed to Dello Delli, c.1424: detail of Bicci di Lorenzo, *Martin V Confirming the Consecration of S. Egidio*, Salone di Martino V, Hospital of S. Maria Nuova	116

4.4	Gherardo and Monte di Giovanni di Miniato, *Celebration of Mass*, 1474 (S. Egidio, Missal: Museo Nazionale del Bargello MS 67, f. 151r)	116
4.5	Interior of S. Egidio today	122
4.6	Gherardo and Monte di Giovanni di Miniato, *Pope Martin V Blessing the Altar of S. Egidio in 1420* (S. Egidio, Missal, 1474: Museo Nazionale del Bargello MS 67, f. 285r)	122
4.7	Lorenzo Monaco, *Adoration of the Magi*, 1420–2 (Galleria degli Uffizi)	124
4.8	Fra Angelico, *Coronation of the Virgin*, c.1435–43 (Galleria degli Uffizi)	124
4.9	Hugo van der Goes, *Adoration of the Shepherds*, 1475–83 (Galleria degli Uffizi)	129
4.10	Hugo van der Goes, *Annunciation*, exterior of the *Adoration of the Shepherds*, 1475–83 (Galleria degli Uffizi)	129
4.11	Gherardo and Monte di Giovanni di Miniato, *Annunciation of the Virgin* (S. Egidio, Missal, 1474: Museo Nazionale del Bargello MS 67, f. 5r)	134
4.12	Master of S. Verdiana (Tommaso del Mazza), *SS. John the Baptist and Anthony of Padua with Bonifazio Lupi* and *SS. John the Evangelist and Louis of Toulouse with Caterina dei Franzesi*, c.1386 (Musée du Petit Palais, Avignon)	134
4.13	Andrea di Cione, 'Orcagna', and Jacopo di Cione, *S. Matteo*, 1368: a. Detail of head; b. S. Matteo in his counting-house (Galleria degli Uffizi)	139
4.14	Gherardo and Monte di Giovanni di Miniato, *Annunciation of the Virgin Mary*, showing view of hospital cloister (S. Egidio, Missal, 1474: Museo Nazionale del Bargello MS 67, f. 220r)	141
4.15	S. Maria Nuova: Chiostro delle Medicherie	141
4.16	S. Matteo, Piazza S. Marco: male cloister, ledge at base of plinth	141
4.17	S. Maria Nuova: female cloister	143
4.18	Fra Bartolommeo and Mariotto Albertinelli, *The Last Judgement*, 1499–1500 (Museo di S. Marco, Florence)	143
5.1	*The Corsia Sistina, Hospital of S. Spirito, Rome: View from the Crossing*, from P. Saulnier, *De capite sacri ordinis* (Rome, 1649)	148
5.2	S. Maria Nuova: Entrance to female ward today, Piazza S. Maria Nuova (now the Archivio Notarile)	150
5.3	Stefano Bonsignori, *Plan of City of Florence*: detail of S. Maria Nuova, 1584 (Museo di Firenze Com'era)	150
5.4	S. Maria Nuova: Interior of the female ward today (Archivio Notarile, Florence)	155

5.5	Domenico di Bartolo, 'Sala di S. Piero' (detail of *Care of the Sick*, 1440–4, Pellegrinaio ward, Hospital of S. Maria della Scala, Siena	155
5.6	Domenico di Bartolo, *Care of the Sick*, 1440–4, Pellegrinaio ward, Hospital of S. Maria della Scala, Siena	162
5.7	Circle of the Master of the S. Giorgio Codex, *Chaplains Confess Patients*, Hospital of S. Spirito, Rome, *Liber regulae Sancti Spiritus*, c.1350 (ASR, Ospedale di S. Spirito 3193, f. 49r)	163
5.8	Circle of the Master of the S. Giorgio Codex, *Nurses Delouse Patients and Wash their Feet*, Hospital of S. Spirito, Rome, *Liber regulae Sancti Spiritus*, c.1350 (ASR, Ospedale di S. Spirito 3193, f. 128v)	163
5.9	Giovanni di Andrea della Robbia's workshop, *Care of the Sick*, 1525–9, Ospedale del Ceppo, Pistoia (detail showing bed numbers)	165
5.10	Domenico di Bartolo, 'Confession of a Dying Patient', detail from *Care of the Sick*, 1440–4, Pellegrinaio ward, Hospital of S. Maria della Scala, Siena	165
5.11	Hospital bed from the Ospedale del Ceppo, now in the church of S. Maria del Letto, Pistoia, 1336–7: a. View of whole bed; b. Detail of painted headboard	167
5.12	Giovanni Ortolani, *View of the North Arm of the Corsia del Sacramento*, showing Buontalenti's Chapel, male ward, S. Maria Nuova, 1849 (ASF, Ospedale di S. Maria Nuova 717, c. 32)	169
5.13	Arch of Buontalenti's Chapel, male ward, 1575 S. Maria Nuova	170
5.14	Giambologna, altar for male ward, S. Maria Nuova, 1591 (now in S. Stefano al Ponte)	170
5.15	Niccolò di Pietro Gerini: *The Last Judgement* and *The Adoration of the Magi*: fragments of fresco cycle, 1414, female ward, S. Maria Nuova, Florence (Archivio Notarile)	171
5.16	Mariotto di Cristofano, 1445–7 (Galleria dell'Accademia, Florence): a. *Mystical Marriage of St Catherine of Alexandria with Saints*; b. *Resurrection of Christ*	174
5.17	Gherardo and Monte di Giovanni di Miniato, *Friar Preaching to S. Maria Nuova's Commesse* (S. Egidio, Missal, 1474: Museo Nazionale del Bargello MS 68, f. 17r)	177
5.18	a. Bernardo Rossellino and Lorenzo Ghiberti, tabernacle from women's ward, Hospital of S. Maria Nuova, 1450 (now in S. Egidio); b. Lorenzo Ghiberti, *Sportello* (detail)	178
5.19	Circle of the Master of the S. Giorgio Codex,*Corpse of a Patient in Front of Ward Chapel*, S. Maria Nuova, Florence (Archivio Notarile) *Liber regulae Sancti Spiritus*, c.1350 (ASR, Ospedale di S. Spirito 3193, f. 162v)	180
5.20	Circle of the Master of the S. Giorgio Codex, *Death and Burial of a*	

PLATES

	Patient, Hospital of S. Spirito, Rome, *Liber regulae Sancti Spiritus*, c.1350 (ASR, Ospedale di S. Spirito 3193, f. 162v)	180
5.21	a. Tomb of Folco di Ricovero Portinari, 1289 (S. Egidio); b. Detail of the Portinari coat of arms, 1289 (S. Egidio)	181
6.1	Gherardo and Monte di Giovanni di Miniato, *A Crutch*, symbol of the Hospital of S. Maria Nuova, *with Two Putti* (S. Egidio, Breviary, 1477: Museo Nazionale del Bargello MS A68, f. 116v)	190
6.2	Tomb slab of Monna Tessa, Hospital of S. Maria Nuova	190
6.3	Mariano del Buono, *St Elizabeth Visits a Patient in Bed* (S. Egidio, Breviary, 1477: Museo Nazionale del Bargello MS A68, c. 148)	191
6.4	a. Gherardo and Monte di Giovanni di Miniato, *Commesse Praying* (S. Egidio, Breviary, 1477: Museo Nazionale del Bargello MS A68, f. 137r); b: Nuns' grille, in S. Egidio	193
6.5	Gherardo and Monte di Giovanni di Miniato, *The Funeral of S. Egidio* (S. Egidio, Breviary, 1477: Museo Nazionale del Bargello MS A68, f. 28v)	197
6.6	Jacopo Pontormo, *Scenes in a Ward*, 1513–14 (Galleria dell'Accademia, Florence)	198
6.7	Plan of first floor of S. Matteo, c.1780 (ASF, Ospedale di S. Maria Nuova 24: Plan 6)	202
6.8	Plan of the cellars, Hospital of S. Maria Nuova, c.1780 (ASF, Ospedale di S. Maria Nuova 24: Plan 1)	202
6.9	Stefano Bonsignori, *Plan of City of Florence*, 1584: detail of Via S. Gallo (Museo Firenze Com'era)	208
6.10	Upper terrace of women's hospital, S. Maria Nuova	208
7.1	Giovanni di Andrea della Robbia's workshop, *Care of the Sick*, 1525–8, façade, Ospedale del Ceppo, Pistoia	227
7.2	Domenico di Bartolo, 'The Physician', detail of *Care of the Sick*, 1440–4, Pellegrinaio ward, Hospital of S. Maria della Scala, Siena	232
7.3	Domenico di Bartolo, 'Surgeon with Pincers', detail of *Care of the Sick*, 1440–4, Pellegrinaio ward, Hospital of S. Maria della Scala, Siena	232
7.4	Domenico di Bartolo, 'Wounded Male Patient', detail of *Care of the Sick*, 1440–4, Pellegrinaio ward, Hospital of S. Maria della Scala, Siena	235
7.5	'The Medicheria', frontispiece, Peter of Spain, *Thesaurus pauperum* (Florence, 1497) (Wellcome Institute Library, London)	235
8.1	Circle of the Master of the S. Giorgio Codex, *Receiving the Poor at the Hospital Door*, Hospital of S. Spirito, Rome, *Liber regulae Sancti Spiritus*, c.1350 (ASR, Ospedale di S. Spirito 3193, f. 131v)	252
8.2	Domenico di Bartolo a. 'A Semi-Clad Man'; b. 'A Crippled Beggar'	

		details of *Care of the Sick*, 1440–4, Pellegrinaio ward, Hospital of S. Maria della Scala, Siena	252
9.1		Anon., *Interior of a Pharmacy*, c.1500, Castle of Issogne, Valle d'Aosta	292
9.2		Late sixteenth-century Tuscan albarello from Montelupo (private collection)	292
9.3		A two-handled pharmacy jar from S. Maria Nuova (Fitzwilliam Museum, Cambridge)	292
9.4		Andrea Mattioli, 'The First Furnace', from *Dei discorsi di M. Pietro Andrea Mattioli Sanese* (Venice, 1585) (University Library, Cambridge)	296

I am grateful to the institutions listed here for supplying me with photographs for the plates and granting me permission to reproduce them here:

Archivio di Stato di Firenze: su concessione del Ministero per i Beni e le Attività Culturali (n. protoc. 3018/XI): 2.5, 2.6, 3.11, 3.14, 3.15, 5.12, 6.6, 6.8, 6.9
Archivio di Stato di Roma: su concessione del Ministero per i Beni e le Attività Culturali (n. ASR, 37/2005): 5.7, 5.8, 5.19, 5.20, 8.1 (ASR, Fondo Ospedale di S. Spirito 3193)
Biblioteca Lancisiana, Rome: 5.1
Brigata del Leoncino, Pistoia, and Carlo Quartieri: 5.9, 7.1
Fondazione Michelucci: I, 2.4, 4.1, 4.2, 4.3, 5.18 (b)
Foto Oto Alpina, gennaio 1978: Archivio fotografico della Soprintendenza per i Beni e le Attività Culturali, su concessione della Regione Autonoma Valle d'Aosta: 9.1
Kunsthistorisches Institut Florenz: 1.1, 1.3, 1.9, 3.2, 5.6
Ministero per i Beni e le Attività Culturali: Soprintendenza Speciale per il Polo Museale Fiorentino: 3.11 (a–c), 4.4, 4.6, 4.7, 4.8, 4.9, 4.10, 4.11, 4.13 (a) and (b), 4.14, 4.18, 5.14, 5.16 (a) and (b), 5.17, 6.1, 6.3, 6.4 (a) and (b), 6.5, 6.6, 6.7
Musée du Petit Palais, Avignon: 4.12 (a) and (b)
Museo Firenze Com'era: 3.12, 5.3, 6.11
Santuario of the Madonna del Letto, Pistoia: Padre Natale and the administration of the Ospedale del Ceppo: 5.11
Soprintendenza per i Beni Artistici e Storici di Siena (S.B.A.S. – Siena): 1.2, 5.5, 5.10, 7.2, 7.3, 7.4, 8.2 (a) and (b)
Syndics of the Fitzwilliam Museum, Cambridge: 9.3
Syndics of the University Library, Cambridge: 9.4
Victoria and Albert Museum, London: 4.2
Wellcome Institute Library, London: 7.5

Figures

8.1 Hospital of the Misericordia, Prato: admissions and deaths, 1402–78 — 255
8.2 Hospital of S. Matteo: male and female deaths, 1413–56 — 257
8.3 Hospital of S. Maria Nuova: deaths per month: a. Male, 1513–30; b. Female, 1518–30 — 259
8.4 Hospital of S. Maria Nuova: deaths per month, 1525–30: a. Male; b. Female. — 260

Maps

1.1	Hospitals founded in Florence, 1000–1550	4
1.2	Hospitals founded in Florence, 1000–1249	8
1.3	Hospitals founded in Florence, 1250–1349	15
2.1	Hospitals founded in Florence, 1350–1449	40
8.1	Provenance of patients who died at S. Maria Nuova, 1513–30: Tuscany	274
8.2	Provenance of patients who died at S. Maria Nuova, 1513–30: Florentine *contado*	277

Tables

1.1	Hospitals founded in Florence, 1000–1550: (a) by date of foundation or (b) by first mention	6
1.2	Typology of hospitals founded in Florence, 1000–1349	14
2.1	Typology of hospitals founded in Florence, 1350–1449 and 1250–1349	39
2.2	Income and expenditure of S. Maria Nuova, 1373–4 in (*lire di piccioli*)	55
2.3	Hospital expenditure in 1428: S. Matteo, Messer Bonifazio, S. Eusebio, S. Maria Nuova (in *fiorini d'oro*)	64
6.1	Hospital of S. Maria Nuova: occupations of *commessi* and male relatives of *commesse*, 1541–6	213
7.1	Medical practitioners at the main medical hospitals in Florence, 1320–1500	228
7.2	Geographical origins of doctors in the Guild (1409–44) and of hospital doctors in the Quattrocento (where known)	241
7.3	Geographical origins of hospital physicians, doctors and surgeons in the Quattrocento (where known)	242
8.1	Hospital of S. Maria Nuova: male patients: admissions and mortality, 1513–28	256
8.2	Hospital of S. Maria Nuova: length of stay of patients who died: male, 1513–28; female, 1518–27	262
8.3	Hospital of S. Paolo: diagnoses of male patients, 1567–8	266
8.4	Hospital of S. Maria Nuova: occupational data for male patients who died, 1513–30	270
8.5	Hospital of S. Maria Nuova: patients with surnames, 1513–30	271
8.6	Hospital of S. Maria Nuova: marital status of female patients who died, 1518–30	272
8.7	Hospital of S. Maria Nuova: provenance of all patients who died, 1513–30	273

8.8	Provenance of S. Maria Nuova's patients in the *contado* with over fifty patients and within 40 km of Florence, 1513–30	278
9.1	S. Maria Nuova's *Ricettario*, 1515: recipes and their authors	299
9.2	S. Maria Nuova's *Ricettario*, 1515: recipes of Diotifeci d'Agnolo Ficino	302
9.3	S. Maria Nuova's *Ricettario*, 1515: body parts and symptoms	305
9.4	S. Maria Nuova's *Ricettario*, 1515: general symptoms associated with the head	310
9.5	S. Maria Nuova's *Ricettario*, 1515: specific symptoms associated with the head	310
9.6	S. Maria Nuova's *Ricettario*, 1515: symptoms associated with the eyes	319
9.7	S. Maria Nuova's *Ricettario*, 1515: symptoms associated with the mouth	320
9.8	S. Maria Nuova's *Ricettario*, 1515: recipes for the abdomen	323
9.9	S. Maria Nuova's *Ricettario*, 1515: recipes for the liver and spleen	325
9.10	S. Maria Nuova's *Ricettario*, 1515: recipes for female urogenital conditions	327
9.11	S. Maria Nuova's *Ricettario*, 1515: recipes for male urogenital conditions	332
9.12	S. Maria Nuova's *Ricettario*, 1515: recipes for the bladder and kidneys	333

Acknowledgements

This book is the fruit of a long gestation and I am grateful to all who have wittingly and unwittingly participated in its birth. I have undertaken research and incurred numerous obligations to friends and colleagues in two countries, England and Italy. First and foremost I should like to express my gratitude to the Wellcome Trust for their financial support, and to Robert Baldock of Yale University Press for his faith in this longstanding project. During this period my main institutional bases were in Cambridge: first as Wellcome Trust Senior Research Fellow at the Wellcome Unit for the History of Medicine, where I should like to thank above all the late Roger French for his generous friendship, and then in the stimulating atmosphere of the 'family' of the Cambridge Group for the History of Population and Social Structure under the directorship of Richard Smith, to whom I owe much for his unstinting support and friendship over the years, and to Jim Oeppen for his invaluable advice on statistical matters. Furthermore, I have continued to benefit enormously from the marvellous service provided by the Literary and Linguistic Computing Centre and above all from the unstinting help and advice of John Dawson and Beatrix Bown, whose patient and meticulous assistance in the preparation of two major databases made possible the publication of detailed analyses of patient records and medical recipes.

In the wider Cambridge environment I have benefited from numerous enjoyable lunchtime conversations with Peter Jones at King's College and from congenial and stimulating friendships among the Fellowship of Wolfson College. I wish to record my particular debt to two friends and fellow medieval medical historians, Carole Rawcliffe and Peregrine Horden, who have unfailingly stimulated me into thinking in new ways about medieval and Renaissance medicine. And last but far from least I wish to thank Christianne Heal, who has provided constant support over the years while this book has taken shape.

In Florence I have been very fortunate in a wide circle of friends who have provided help and advice over the years. Many work for institutions where I have done research: the Sala di Studio of the Archivio di Stato di Firenze has proved an enormously friendly and efficient place to work, especially as a result of the ever-helpful presence of Irene Cotta. Lucia Sandri has both helped me in research at the archive of the Ospedale degli Innocenti and generously shared with me her knowledge of Florentine hospital history. I also owe a debt to the Centro di Documentazione per la Storia della Sanità Fiorentina and particularly to Marco Geddes da Filicaia and Esther Diana for their help in obtaining photographs and permissions. In Pistoia my thanks go to Sandro Pagnini for his introduction to the Brigata del Leoncino and for its members' generosity in commissioning the photograph by Carlo Quartieri of the Della Robbia terracotta frieze from the façade of the Ospedale del Ceppo as well as to Padre Natale and the administration of the Ceppo for permission to reproduce an image of the fourteenth-century bed from S. Maria del Letto. In Florence I have benefited from the delightful and ever-stimulating ambience of Villa I Tatti, Harvard University's Center for Renaissance Studies, both as Visiting Professor and on many subsequent visits. Most recently I have been fortunate to be a Visiting Fellow of the Department of History and Civilisation of the European University Institute where this book was completed.

A number of people have read individual chapters and made extremely useful suggestions which have improved the book enormously, and I should like to thank them all; of course, any mistakes which remain are my own. On questions of art and architectural history: Georgia Clark, Megan Holmes, Crista Gardner von Teuffel, Julia DeLancey, Sharon Strocchia, Ludovica Sebregondi and Tim Wilson. I am very grateful to Francesca Carrara, who generously made available to me her unpublished reconstructed plans of the phases of the architectural development of S. Maria Nuova. For advice on the world of medical doctors and also their relationship with the Studio and College of Physicians: Jonathan Davies and especially Katy Park. For help over medical recipes: Teresa Huguet-Termes and James Shaw. For help with the complex question of the geographical origins of patients: thanks also to Sam Cohn and above all to Paolo Pirillo, who also provided invaluable help in checking translations of documents. My thanks to Dagmar Stiebral for inputting the data, to Daniela Rizzi for preparing the maps, and to the members of the University of Cambridge's Anatomy visual media group for their friendly and efficient service in the preparation of the visual material. Finally I should like to thank Candida Brazil and Stephen Kent for their extraordinary care in editing and designing this book.

A Note on Currency, Weights and Measurements

Currency

£1 = 1 lira = 20 soldi
s1 = 1 soldo = 12 denari = 12d
1 scudo = 7 lire
The exchange rate between the lira and florin varied constantly, for which see: Goldthwaite, *The Building of Renaissance Florence*, Appendix 1.

Weights and Measurements in Florence

lb = libbra
oz = oncia
dr = dramma
s = scrupolo
gr = grano
1 braccio fiorentino: 0.587626 metres
1 moggio = 24 staia
1 staio = 24 litri

INTRODUCTION

The Renaisssance Hospital in Italy

> In Tuscany, in keeping with the long-standing local tradition for religious piety, wonderful hospitals are to be found, built at vast expense, where any citizen or stranger would feel there to be nothing amiss to ensure his well-being.
> Leon Battista Alberti, *L'Architettura* (*De re aedificatoria*), ed. G. Orlandi and P. Portoghesi (Milan, 1966), Vol. 1, pp. 367–8

This passage, written in the mid-1450s by the Florentine humanist architect Leon Battista Alberti, is one of a series of contemporary eulogistic comments about the appearance and services of hospitals in Renaissance Italy. Two centuries earlier another Tuscan, the rhetorician Boncompagno da Signa, presented a more negative view. He described one of Florence's largest hospitals, S. Giovanni Evangelista, as a depressing place full of impoverished old men, who were given disgusting food and vinegary wine and were kept awake at night in their fetid beds by the sighs and laments of their companions.[1] It is the second image that is conjured up in traditional books on medical history and even by today's press, which tend to use the expression 'medieval hospital' to signify institutions that were insanitary in the extreme and to which the poor were sent to die rather than to recover.

This book is part of a new movement in the historiography of medieval and Renaissance hospitals which seeks to get away from both traditional prejudices and uncritical eulogies, recognising that the writings of Alberti, Boncompagno and present-day journalists all contain elements of exaggeration. Tuscany will lie at the centre of this enquiry. Hospitals in this region have long been seen as providing the example to cities and rulers in other parts of Italy and Europe who were engaged in planning the foundation and design of institutions for the sick poor. For example, the appearance and plans of S. Maria Nuova in Florence and S. Maria della Scala in Siena were examined when rulers in northern Italy were considering the establishment of S. Matteo in Pavia and the new Ospedale Maggiore, or Great Hospital, in Milan.[2] Then in 1513 the Medici pope Leo X, as a good Florentine son, thought that the physicians of even the world-famous S. Spirito hospital of Rome could benefit from the advice of those who ran S. Maria Nuova, the leading hospital of his native city.[3]

In the sixteenth century and beyond, information and favourable comments about Italian hospitals were carried north of the Alps by travellers from Martin Luther and Michel de Montaigne to Thomas Hoby and Fynes Morrison.[4] Many of these gentlemen on their tours through Italy praised the magnificent appearance and services of these large civic institutions, which they viewed as important both as monuments and as examples of relief to the poor. The rulers of states in other parts of Europe were often so impressed by these reports that they sent for copies of their statutes and architectural designs to use as the basis of hospitals they planned to establish themselves, as when King Henry VII founded the Savoy Hospital in London. Its rules were based on the 'Ordinances' of S. Maria Nuova in Florence, provided by the papal protonotary at the English court, Francesco Portinari, whose family had founded the Florentine hospital.[5] According to the prefatory letter, the Savoy Hospital's aim was to provide 'a place of residence and succour for the sick poor', a far cry from the role of the hotel that much later was to take its place on the Strand.[6]

The aim of this book is to unpick the various elements that make up the reputation of the Renaissance hospital in relation to the themes and debates in two fields, Renaissance studies and the history of medicine. Very broadly, this reputation is based on three main features which themselves underlie the organisation of this book. The first is that they were civic institutions and played a vital role in the preservation of the health of the city. The second is their appearance: their *bellezza* was in line with contemporary architectural principles of the relationship of beauty and function, reflected in both their graceful façades and in the series of devotional images they commissioned from leading painters and sculptors. The third element is their medical role: they had a large staff trained in the latest techniques of Renaissance medicine for the treatment of a wide range of sicknesses. In this way the Renaissance hospital combined the cure of the body with the cure of the soul.

Some of these themes of the Renaissance hospital are represented graphically in the impressive fresco by Bicci di Lorenzo, *Pope Martin V Confirming the Consecration of S. Egidio*, painted between 1424 and 1425 on the façade of Florence's largest medical hospital, S. Maria Nuova (Plate I). The fresco recorded a public ceremony on 9 September 1420[7] at which Pope Martin V confirmed the consecration of the hospital church of S. Egidio and its rededication to the Virgin following a two-year programme of enlargement of the original church.[8] The placing of the fresco on the façade rather than in the

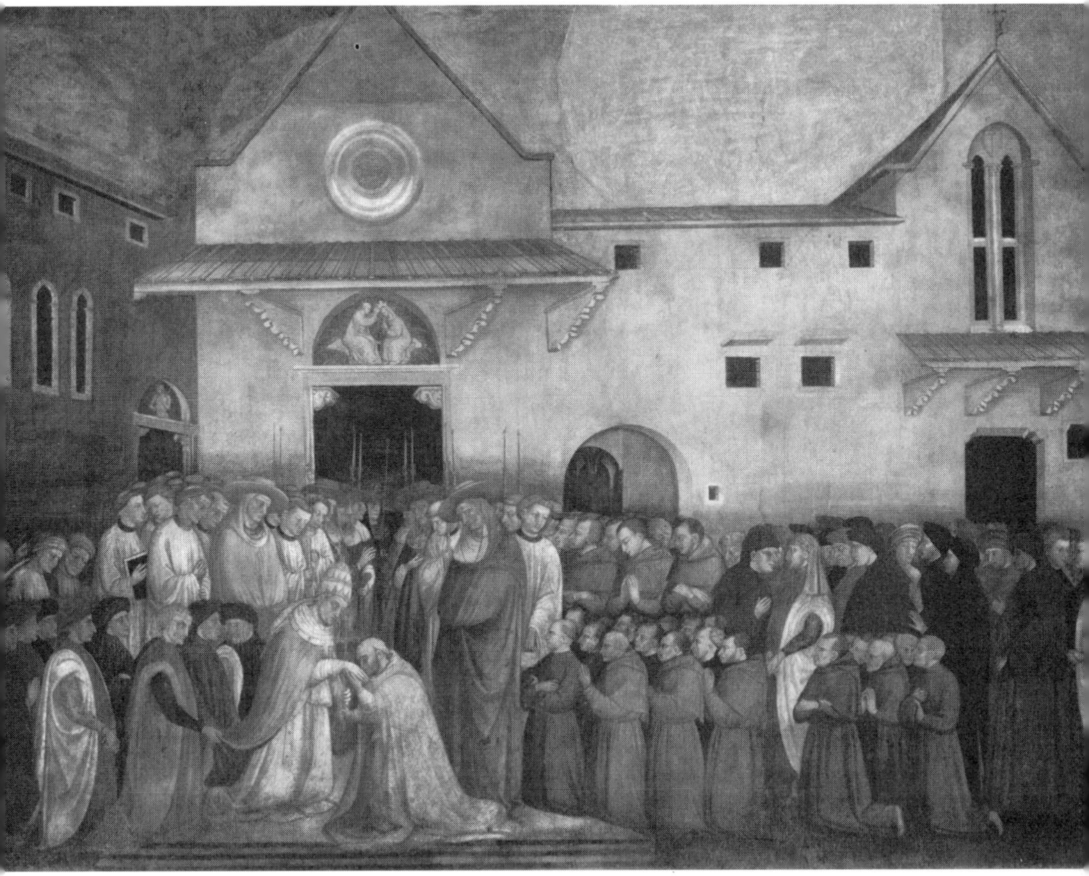

Plate I: Bicci di Lorenzo, *Pope Martin V Confirming the Consecration of S. Egidio*, 1424–5, Salone di Martino V, Ospedale di S. Maria Nuova

interior was a very public declaration of the significance of the ceremony for this major charitable institution and the city it served.

In the fresco two of the main functions of the Renaissance hospital are intertwined; its civic and religious roles. The inclusion of S. Egidio as part of the pope's processional route on his exit from Florence emphasised the centrality of the hospital as one of the city's major monuments. Bicci di Lorenzo's contemporary view underlines the importance of the event for Florence, reflected in the size of the crowd in the piazza and the presence of leading members of the secular and ecclesiastical establishments.[9] According to a contemporary eyewitness, Bartolommeo di Michele del Corazza, this splendid procession included members of the executive or Signoria and the legislative colleges and a large group of patricians, as well as 'many bishops and archbishops'.[10] Following tradition, Bicci di Lorenzo distinguished different strata of society by their clothing: Martin V in his red cloak and papal tiara receiving the obeisance of Messer Michele di Fruosino da Panzano, the rector of the hospital in his embroidered white and gold robes, the cardinals in their red hats, simply dressed tonsured clergy and, on the right, members of the patriciate in their brightly coloured clothes.[11] In the centre, in contrast, is a soberly dressed kneeling group of *conversi* or male members of staff in grey tunics, who with the *converse* nursed the sick and gave the hospital its reputation for excellent care.

Although Bicci di Lorenzo took pains to represent individual members of the crowd, the central actor in the drama was the building itself, which made concrete the main themes of the Renaissance hospital. Even seen from the outside, it is evident that the building was on a very substantial scale, underlined by the fact it faced a piazza sufficient to provide enough space for a large crowd. On the far right, and reflecting the hospital's medical role, was the main door to the men's ward surmounted by a small roof under a mullioned window with two lights (*bifore*), the height of which emphasised the loftiness of the internal space; above this was a sculpted representation of a crutch, the symbol of S. Maria Nuova. If the ward reflected medicine in action, the door to the left under another small roof led to the main religious centre, the church of S. Egidio. The two other doorways to the right and left of S. Egidio both led into cloisters. To the right was the Chiostro delle Medicherie, a transitional space between the cure of the soul in the church and the cure of the body in the ward. On the left of the fresco was the entrance to the so-called Chiostro delle Ossa, or Cloister of Bones, a graphic name for the hospital's cemetery.

The importance of this ceremony in the life of the hospital cannot be exaggerated; S. Maria Nuova became thereafter an increasingly important centre for artistic patronage. This was a very public expression of the honour of the patrons, the Portinari, and of their pious and charitable motivations in establishing and maintaining their hospital. In this way Bicci di Lorenzo's fresco encapsulates many of the features of Renaissance hospitals identified by contemporaries and subsequent historians. While the design of their buildings can be seen as an expression of Renaissance magnificence, they also achieved their local, national and international reputation through the adoption of rational administrative models and serving the ideal city to promote the health of the people through physical and spiritual medicine.

The hospital was thus emblematic of some of the cultural, political and socio-economic developments and achievements of the Florentine Renaissance, and its study is as relevant to the historiography of that field as to the history of medicine. Just as Jacob Burckhardt saw the Renaissance as representing the origins of the modern world, so the grand narratives of medical history have seen the developments in hospitals in this period as forming important stepping stones in the medicalisation, and therefore modernisation, of medicine, leading to the hospitals we know today. However attractive these broad ideas may appear, they now sound overly simplistic after the developments in the historiography of both fields over the past half-century.[12] Some of the old certainties have been challenged and modified and the tendency in both fields has been to blur excessively rigid distinctions. No longer is there a widespread belief that the Renaissance represented an abrupt break with the Middle Ages, whether in terms of political thought and organisation, social and economic realities, or artistic developments. Nor is it accepted any more that the dominant Christian ethos was questioned and replaced by new secular ideas under the influence of the revival of classical studies.[13]

Just as continuity, rather than a radical fissure from the past, is now broadly stressed in the history of the period, the same story is true of hospitals in the three hundred years covered by this book.[14] Those features identified above as characteristic of the hospital in this period stemmed not just from the artistic, political and architectural ideas and achievements of the Renaissance, but also grew out of pre-existing features. Nowhere was this combination of continuity and innovation more evident in the history of the hospital than in the role of religion, which remained central to its main function, the cure of the soul reinforcing the cure of the body. The intermingling and interdependence of secular and spiritual medicine are also reflected in recent trends in medical history, whether in relation to late medieval England or early modern Europe.[15] This new approach can also be seen in studies of hospitals in the period, such as the innovative work of Carole Rawcliffe on late medieval Norwich or of André Hayum on Grünewald's *Isenheim Altarpiece*.[16]

Study of medieval and Renaissance hospitals has also been influenced by wider trends in the history of medicine which have sought to blur some of the traditional distinctions between care and cure, between licensed and unofficial medical practitioners, between the roles of doctors and the nursing staff, and between servants and patients.[17] At the same time a more active role has been assigned to the patient in the choice of practitioner and more attention has been paid specifically to how the hospital patient was 'constructed'.[18] What is now emphasised, then, is that both practitioners and patients shared the same Galenic world-view based on humoral theory, according to which disease was seen in terms of an imbalance of certain qualities within the body, such as hot and cold, and of the humours themselves. It was therefore the aim of medicine to restore the body to its proper balance both through preventative medicine and intervention by doctors, surgeons and apothecaries. However, also vital was the regulation of the so-called 'non-naturals', those physical and environmental factors that affected health, such as exercise, food and drink, sleep and emotion. In this sense the hospital itself can be seen as a 'non-natural environment' in which all the various personnel made important contributions to help return the patient to health by the administration of physical and spiritual medicine, providing the right diet and also adjusting the temperature and air supply of his or her physical surroundings.[19]

In this way the traditional image of pre-modern hospitals as hell-holes where people were taken to die has been overturned and the entry of a patient into hospital is now seen as one among a number of options depending on his or her financial means, including the physician, surgeon, apothecary, wise woman and miraculous shrine. Hospitals are therefore now seen in much more nuanced terms as part of the broader medical marketplace and as providing a very distinctive form of social, religious and medical support. At the same time they were important elements of the renewed fabric of the Renaissance city, employing leading architects to design their buildings and leading artists and sculptors to provide devotional programmes to adorn their internal spaces.[20]

In order to explore these topics I have adopted a thematic approach so that the main sections of the book coincide broadly with the main features of the Renaissance hospital. Thus Part I (Chapters 1–3), 'Hospitals and the Body of the City', traces the evolving civic role of the Florentine hospital over the course of three centuries, from 1250 to 1550. Hospitals became a vital element in society's strategies to cope with the sick poor, the diseased organs of the body of the city, in response to changing socio-economic and demographic pressures. This was achieved by their growing specialisation, reflecting the general move in charity away from broadly defined poor relief, providing shelter to pilgrims and helping the 'poor of Christ', towards concentration on specific categories, such as widows and orphans, and above all on the sick poor.[21] Hospitals also played a central role in the state's campaign against plague, which from the mid-fourteenth century returned almost every ten to fifteen years. Indeed, it is argued that the whole process of the 'medicalisation' of hospitals, with the employment of larger numbers of trained medical experts, was in part a reaction to society's growing awareness of the threat of epidemic disease, which increasingly hit the poorer members of society who formed the vast bulk of hospital patients.[22] The last fifty years of the period saw the emergence of a frightening new epidemic, the Mal Francese or Great Pox, whose hideously diseased victims sharpened public intolerance towards the poor. Public opinion was shaped by the policies of a new type of specialised hospital, the Incurabili, which provided the highly expensive wonder drug of Guaiacum, and by the moralistic, muscular Christianity of the Counter-Reformation.[23]

These strategies may smack of social control, but it will be argued that they were a long way from Foucaultian ideas of the 'confinement of the poor'. Although there was a general hardening of official policies towards the poor in early modern Europe, this was a much more complex matter than the Foucaultian model suggests. Measures and institutions created during periods of emergency should not be confused with the general tenor of attitudes that underlay society's mechanisms to deal with the poor. This is exemplified by two major institutions typical of early modern Italy: the lazzarettos for plague victims and beggars' hostels. If isolation hospitals were employed for other purposes after an epidemic, the Ospedali dei Mendicanti were only used to 'confine' the poor at times of heightened poverty caused by famine and disease and had little in common with nineteenth-century workhouses as was once believed.[24] This reassessment is also part of a more general tendency to examine the history of hospitals in a wider perspective. Charitable institutions are no longer simply studied from a top-down point of new, but are seen as part of the whole intermeshing network of support for the poor and marginalised groups of society, from state welfare to the 'economy of makeshifts' of informal and familial networks.[25]

An underlying theme also addressed in Part I is the much-debated question of the relative roles of Church and State in the provision of poor relief. The traditional picture of a shift towards lay control is too simplistic, reflecting as it does the cliché of the 'secularisation' of Italian society during the Renaissance.[26] Recent studies have shown that both Church and State were involved in new charitable initiatives.[27] Greater emphasis now tends to be placed on the role of religion and Christianity in many aspects of contemporary life and, as I have shown elsewhere, even welfare programmes during emergencies were fuelled by both a desire for social control and Christian piety.[28]

Part II will take this theme further by examining a fundamental function of the Renaissance hospital, the cure of the soul in the treatment of sickness. Though there already exist studies of the religious origins of Italian hospitals and their relationship with the Church, much work remains to be done on the therapeutic role of spiritual medicine and of devotional imagery. Chapters 4 and 5 will examine the two main religious spaces within the hospital: the church and ward chapel. Here, the intervention of Christ, the Virgin Mary and a series of healing saints was invoked through the liturgy of the divine office to provide spiritual comfort to patients and staff and commemorative Masses and festivals for patrons, guild members and the public. The importance of these devotional roles helps to explain why hospitals became significant centres of artistic patronage in the Renaissance city, leading to the commissioning of major artists to produce the altarpieces and sculptural and fresco cycles necessary for the proper medico-spiritual functioning of these spaces. The function of hospital art has been discussed in more detail for other Italian cities, such as at S. Maria della Scala in Siena and S. Spirito in Rome,[29] but this remains a topic to be explored properly for Florence. Existing studies of some of the major painters and sculptors who worked in the city will form a fundamental basis for the exploration of this theme in relation to the *bellezza* of the Renaissance hospitals of Florence.[30]

The religio-medical role of the hospital was also reflected in its physical structure. Drawing on studies of hospital architecture in Florence and elsewhere, I shall discuss how the way they were built gave physical expression to the belief of Renaissance writers in the relationship of beauty and utility.[31] Chapter 5 will reconstruct the appearance and design of ward chapels and examine how these enormous spaces were used for the care and treatment of patients. Chapter 6 will extend this analysis to other sections of the hospital, such as refectories, dormitories and kitchens, to discuss the role of the nursing staff, who, in contrast to countries such as England, France and Spain, have received only patchy attention from historians in Italy. Though these areas were more associated with satisfying physical appetites, many contained reminders of the spiritual role of the hospital through the presence of frescoes and panel paintings. A combination of religious and material considerations also underlay the motivation of the staff. An analysis of their contracts and socio-economic backgrounds will suggest that an important part of the appeal of being a nurse was that the hospital provided a secure physical environment and free board and lodging, particularly attractive to poor widows without family support. Indeed this institutional arrangement was familiar throughout medieval Europe, in both monasteries and hospitals. These members of staff were known by a bewildering variety of titles including brothers and sisters, corrodians, oblates, and, in Italian as *converse* or *conversi*, *commesse* or *commessi*, *devote* and *devoti*, all implying a devout commitment to services to the poor sick.[32]

The chapters that constitute Part II are, then, as much about the functional flexibility of these spaces as they are about the overlap and complementary roles of their staff in the spiritual and physical treatment of the sick poor. I shall argue that, just as convents and monasteries gave wealthy lay patrons exciting opportunities to demonstrate their piety, so the hospital provided the physical space within which the individual or corporate patron could exercise a religious and charitable role, whether in support of architectural projects or in the commissioning of devotional programmes within church, ward and cloister. Indeed, it was this patronage that created the *bellezza*, the second distinguishing feature of the Renaissance hospital.

If Part II examines medicine for the soul, Part III concentrates on 'Healing the Body'. The three final chapters focus on the role and range of medical staff and the types of medicines prescribed as well as on the diseases, fates and identities of patients. Doctors and medical treatment formed the third element of the reputation of the Renaissance hospital, and indeed struck outsiders such as

INTRODUCTION   xxxiii

Luther as unusual.[33] By tracing the backgrounds and careers of the medical personnel, Chapter 7 argues that not only did the Renaissance hospital achieve its reputation through them, but that these posts became a significant part in the professional portfolio of some of the leading practitioners in the city. This mutually beneficial relationship lent prestige to hospitals, which thereby became important centres for the practice of the latest techniques of Renaissance medicine and where young doctors were trained in the treatment of a wide variety of medical conditions.

In Chapter 8 the patient finally comes into focus. Building on existing studies of Tuscan patient registers,[34] I shall present an in-depth analysis of over eight thousand patients who died at S. Maria Nuova between 1512 and 1530. Here the body of the patient takes centre stage through an analysis of conditions treated, and of survival and mortality rates within the wider demographic context. This was a dramatic period for the city: it experienced two major outbreaks of plague and a lengthy siege with associated severe food shortages and epidemic disease. A reconstruction of patients' social backgrounds, marital status and lengths of stay also helps to place their entry into hospital within a wider context of their own life-cycle and changes in society and the economy. A more nuanced view of the hospital patient thus emerges, also reflecting the results of recent studies of foundlings, which have shown that parents, in common with patients of medical hospitals, often saw institutionalisation as a temporary expedient in response to periods of poverty.[35]

The final chapter will take this theme further by examining in depth one of the main appeals to the poor of the new large-scale Renaissance hospital: the free provision of a wide range of specialised medical treatments which the average patient could not have afforded. Indeed, the way that medicine was practised and how medical prescriptions or recipes were used are among the most neglected areas of the history of pre-industrial hospitals and are only just beginning to be examined, principally by Spanish historians.[36] Vital to this discussion is the role of the apothecary and his pharmacy, which provides the link between doctor and patient. Though evidence will be drawn from all the major medical hospitals of Renaissance Florence, the unique feature of Chapter 9 is its analysis of a major collection of over eight hundred recipes 'prescribed and tested' at S. Maria Nuova, one of the largest hospitals in Europe. Only through a detailed examination of the simple and compound substances prescribed for its patients can one really understand the practice of medicine within a Renaissance hospital and its relationship to medical theory. This analysis will also underline one of the major themes of this book, the holistic approach of the Renaissance hospital in the treatment of body and soul through the combination of natural and supernatural medicines.

Parts I–III therefore examine the three main characteristics of the Italian

Renaissance hospital, which fused many elements of Renaissance culture. Hospitals thus played a significant role in realising the contemporary concept of the ideal city with its emphasis on health and hygiene, rational organisation and the relationship between beauty and function.[37] Many of these features were underlined by Alberti, with whom I began, and give added importance to the examination of the physical context of the functions and activities of the hospital. Above all, Alberti's treatise *De re aedificatoria* is infused with the belief that the design of a building is an expression of civic and familial pride, reflecting honour and magnificence on patrons and city alike. Alberti's characterisation of hospitals as 'wonderful buildings built at vast expense' demonstrated both his pride as a Florentine citizen and the honour accorded to those who paid for their construction. Such ideas can be seen as part of a long tradition of Florentine patronage, but Alberti gave them extra intellectual credibility by justifying them in terms of the humanist rediscovery of the classics and the Ancients providing *the* model for architecture. Despite his tendency to link churches to pre-Christian temples, he does not undervalue the Christian motivation behind the construction of Tuscan hospitals, which he saw as stemming from the 'long-standing tradition of religious piety'. If the Renaissance is sometimes still seen as an opposition between classical and Christian views of society, to Alberti hospitals were a vehicle to reconcile the secular and sacred.

Of course, if the Renaissance hospital fused the secular and sacred for contemporaries, today by extension it offers an immensely fertile ground for interdisciplinary study. Although scholars from a wide variety of disciplines have examined aspects of the hospital, rarely has there been an attempt to reconstruct the experience in its full richness and complexity. It has thus been necessary to bring together not just medical and socio-economic studies, but also approaches taken from religious, art and architectural history. In this way this book provides a new and dynamic multi-disciplinary model for studying the hospital as a microcosm of the city itself.

PART I

HOSPITALS AND THE BODY OF THE CITY

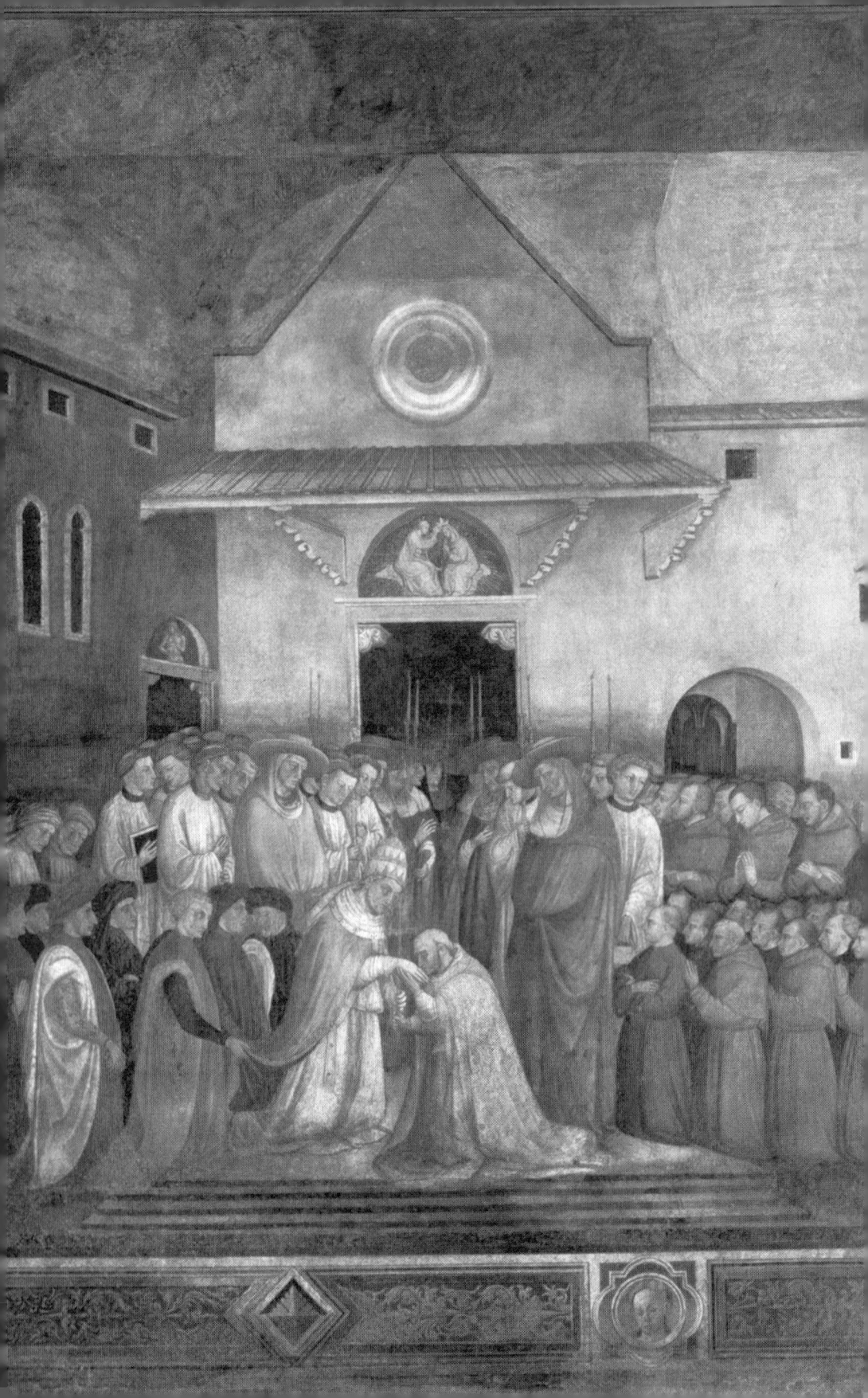

CHAPTER 1

BEFORE THE BLACK DEATH:
THE BIRTH OF THE CLINIC

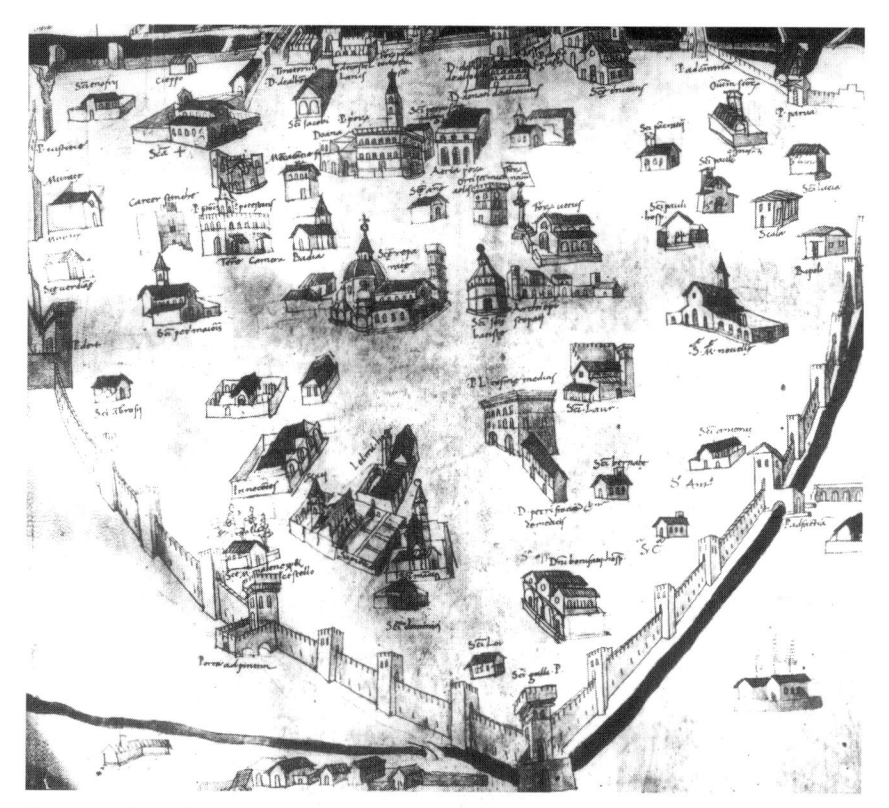

Plate 1.1 Pietro del Massaio, *Veduta di Firenze*, 1472, from Ptolemy's *Geografia*

Introduction

The pride of Florentines in their hospitals is graphically reflected in contemporary views and plans of the city, one of the earliest of which is the view by Pietro del Massaio in Ptolemy's *Geografia* of 1472 (Plate 1.1). In this, the larger and better-known hospitals took pride of place alongside the major secular and ecclesiastical monuments of the city, all of which were exaggerated in scale to create greater visual impact.[1] Twelve of the city's main hospitals were shown. These included many that had been built or expanded over the previous century,[2] such as the main medical hospitals of Messer Bonifazio, S. Matteo and S. Paolo, while the largest of all, S. Maria Nuova, was present but not labelled. Other smaller hospitals included S. Antonio for those sick from St Anthony's Fire, S. Gallo for the sick and orphans, dating from the early thirteenth century, and the two orphanages of the Scala in Via della Scala and the Innocenti in Piazza SS. Annunziata.

Massaio's view of Florence serves to underline a number of important points: first, the very evident pride of Florentines in their hospitals, both as important charities and as significant architectural monuments. This explains the partiality of this view with its concentration on the larger institutions, just over a fifth of the total number of hospitals in the city by the mid-fifteenth

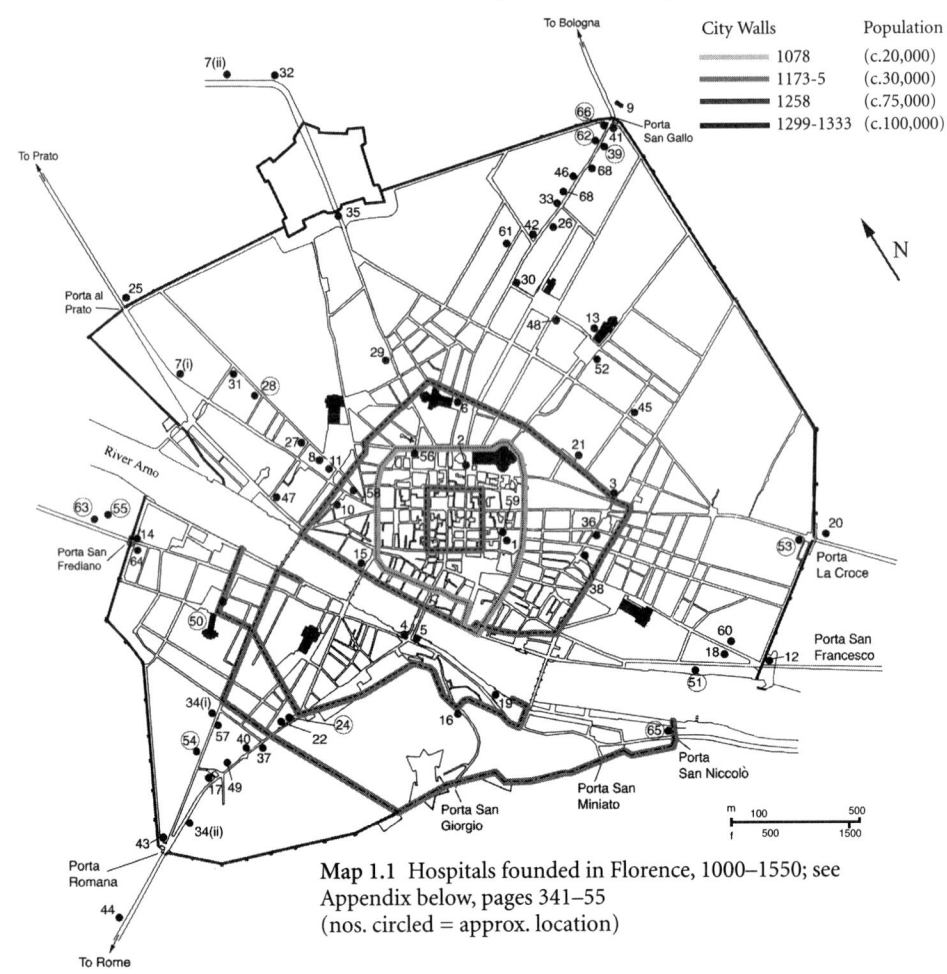

Map 1.1 Hospitals founded in Florence, 1000–1550; see Appendix below, pages 341–55 (nos. circled = approx. location)

century. Furthermore, most represented were situated north of the Arno. The only two charitable institutions shown to the south are the house of the Convertite, the hostel for reformed prostitutes, and the hospital of the Calza for pilgrims and travellers.

The selectivity of Massaio's view can be appreciated from Map 1.1, which shows the topographical distribution of all the main hospitals known to have been founded in medieval and Renaissance Florence. There was a minimum of sixty-eight different hospitals founded in the city in the period from about 1000 to 1550 (see Appendix). Though future research may well reveal the existence of others, those will probably prove to have been small-scale institutions founded in the eleventh and twelfth centuries, which, in common with smaller confraternities, tended to have more fragile and limited life-spans.[3] What is remarkable is the longevity of the average hospital. Thus, over half (thirty-eight) existing during these 550 years survived well into the sixteenth century. Even more striking when compared with countries such as England, with the rupture of charitable provision caused by the Reformation, was that twenty-four of these sixty-eight hospitals survived into the second half of the eighteenth century, when they were suppressed either by the Enlightenment policies of the grand duke Pietro Leopoldo or the Napoleonic regime. Still others survived these anti-clerical policies well into the nineteenth century and some of the largest, such as S. Maria Nuova and the foundling home of the Innocenti, into the twenty-first century (see Appendix).

Table 1.1 examines when these hospitals were founded over this 550-year period, a distinction having been made between those with a known date of foundation (a) and those with only an earliest documented reference (b). The dramatic contrast between the period 1000 to 1200 and the subsequent 350 years partly reflects a lack of surviving documentation from the first period. Even so, many of these early institutions were associated with monastic foundations and were therefore more orientated towards their own community than outsiders. What is striking is the extraordinary proliferation from the mid-thirteenth to the mid-fourteenth centuries, which saw the foundation of 43 per cent of all the hospitals established in Florence during the whole period. This surge in foundations came in response to demand and corresponded to a period of substantial demographic expansion. In c.1200 Florence counted some fifty thousand inhabitants, which had grown to about 110,000 by the end of the century, a level not achieved again until the early nineteenth century.[4]

The relevance of hospital foundations to this background hardly needs stressing: the growth of the city's population can be put down partly to natural increase, but much of it came from large-scale immigration from the surrounding countryside.[5] Inevitably immigrants would have left behind the

Table 1.1 Hospitals founded in Florence, 1000–1550: a. by date of foundation; or b. by first mention

	a.	b.	Tot.	%
1000–49	2	–	2	2.9
1050–99	1	2	3	4.4
1100–49	–	1	1	1.5
1150–99	1	–	1	1.5
1200–49	2	3	5	7.4
1250–99	6	9	15	22.1
1300–49	11	3	14	20.6
1350–99	7	1	8	11.8
1400–49	5	4	9	13.2
1450–99	2	4	6	8.8
1500–49	3	1	4	5.9
Total	40	28	68	100

Source: see Appendix below, pages 341–55

kin and neighbourhood networks that would normally have provided them with support in adversity and sickness. Although in time they would have developed their own informal methods of support, institutional charity remained a significant alternative. Hospitals would have been part of this solution, as would membership of religious confraternities, which provided these new arrivals with social and spiritual insurance in times of personal insecurity or general crisis.[6]

Even though Florence's demographic expansion began to slow down after 1300, a considerable number of new hospitals continued to appear. On the eve of the Black Death it is likely that the city contained about 90,000–95,000 people and about forty-one hospitals, fourteen of which had been founded since 1300.[7] Thus, while there was a definite link between population size and the rate of hospital foundation, other elements have to be taken into account. Among the most important were fluctuations in standards of living caused by economic crises and natural disasters such as famine and epidemic disease. Indeed, Florence and its territory shared in this period with other parts of Europe the effects of a series of crises, which gradually pushed up the cost of living, including subsistence crises in 1311, 1322–3, 1328–30, 1339–41, 1343 and 1346–7. These were exacerbated by a gradual cooling down of the Florentine economy, culminating in what has been characterised as 'the decade of disaster', 1338 to 1348.[8] This period saw a severe economic recession owing to a number of local and international factors, the most significant effect of which was the crash of two of the city's major banks, the Bardi and Peruzzi, the collapse of seven other major companies and the subsequent bankruptcy of the businesses of a number of small shopkeepers and craftsmen. All these periods of economic fluctuation and crisis led to high unemployment and high prices, exacerbated by the recurrence of dearth and a series of epidemics, some related to food shortages, as in 1328–30, and others, such as those of 1340 and 1348, to exogenous disease.[9]

Two important related features of Florentine society thus help to explain the foundation pattern of hospitals in the 150 years leading up the Black Death: in the first hundred years there was a general rise in demand for temporary accommodation, hand-outs and medical treatment from the poor in general, and in particular from the new immigrants who had flooded into the city in search of work. Then, as economic conditions worsened after 1300, especially during periods of famine, dearth and epidemic disease, those at the lower levels of society were driven increasingly to seek institutional support. It is no accident that this period also saw an increase in the number of confraternities, those lay brotherhoods so common throughout late medieval Europe which provided a charitable and spiritual assurance to their members. While hospitals gave free accommodation and medical help to the poor, confraternities provided subsidies in cash and kind.[10] In addition, the government stepped in at times of real dearth to ensure the availability of basic foodstuffs such as grain and bread at subsidised prices.[11] This combination of institutional arrangements was part of an integrated policy to help the poor through a kind of public-private partnership.

1.1 Early Foundations: 'Patients in Sordid and Fetid Beds, where Many Die from Fetor and Corruption of the Air'[12]

The close relationship between the evolution of hospital foundations and population growth was reflected in the topographical distribution of these institutions (see Map 1.1). As in many medieval towns and cities, demographic expansion was mirrored in the various phases of the construction programme of the city walls. In c.800 the population of the city, which may have been as low as 2,000–2,500, occupied the central area enclosed by the sixth-century walls, represented by the small square in the city centre. The eleventh century saw the beginning of Florence's economic and demographic revival, which eventually led it to become one of the largest cities in Italy. At the time of the building of the walls in 1078 the population had expanded to c.20,000, and to c.30,000 by 1173–5, when for the first time a part of the city to the south of the river, the Oltrarno, was enclosed; this was extended eighty years later when Florence's population had grown to 75,000. As this upward trend continued in the last quarter of the thirteenth century the government initiated a truly massive building programme of city walls; between 1299 and 1333 the intramural area was enlarged from 200 to 1,500 acres or nearly two-and-a-half square miles.[13] The length of time taken to build these walls is explained partly by the expense and size of the project and partly by the fact that the population rise had begun to slow down and with it the urgency of the project had diminished.

The demographic development of Florence and the related construction programmes of walls provide the necessary background to understand the topographical distribution of hospitals. Just as the population expanded out from the centre, so did hospital foundations. For example, between 1000 and the mid-twelfth century most of the six new hospitals were situated within or near the walls completed in 1173–5 (Map 1.2, nos 1–6). This is hardly surprising given their close association with churches and monasteries established in the centre in the eleventh century, including S. Niccolò at the Badia Fiorentina, S. Giovanni Evangelista between S. Reparata and the Baptistery, and S. Paolo a Pinti associated with S. Pier Maggiore. These hospitals were

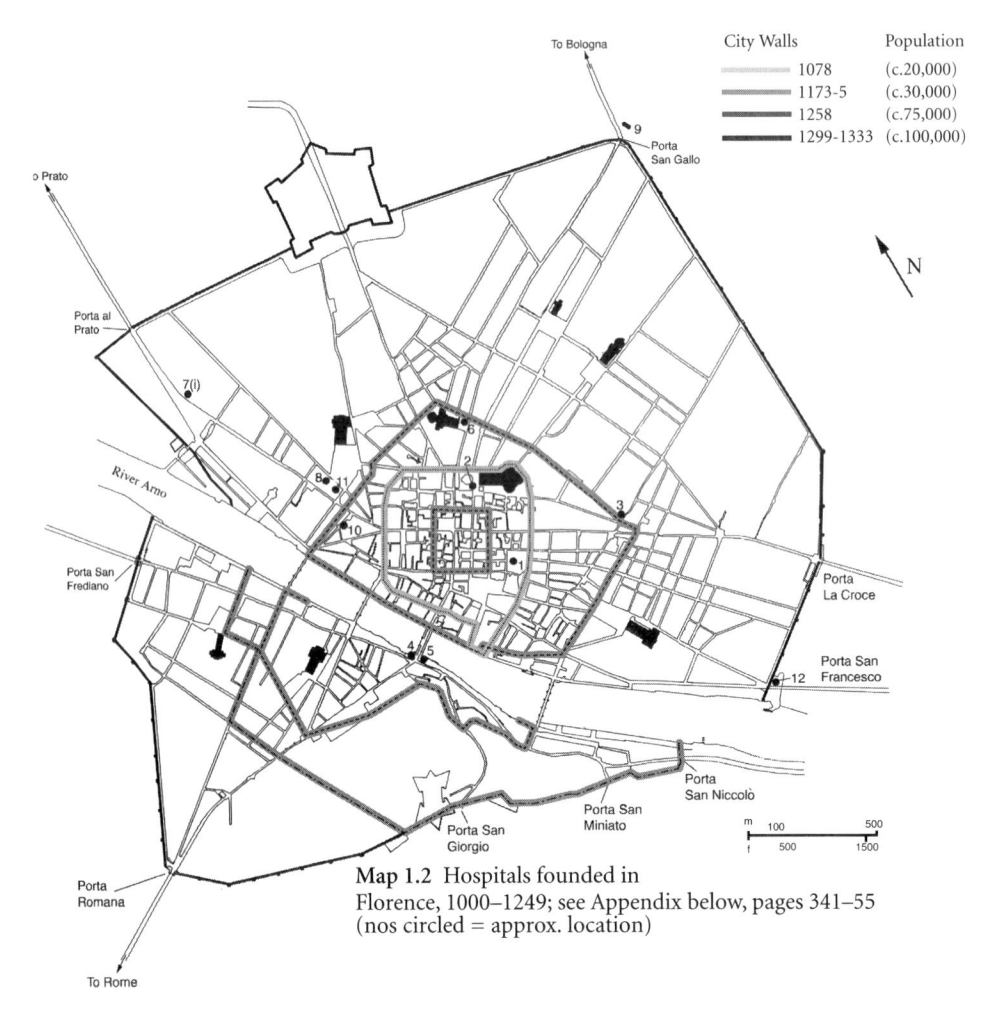

Map 1.2 Hospitals founded in Florence, 1000–1249; see Appendix below, pages 341–55 (nos circled = approx. location)

designed by the communities of monks or canons to care for their own personnel, providing infirmaries and sanatoria for sick and elderly monks and nuns, whose charitable activities deserve further investigation.

Some monastic hospitals may, as in southern Italy at this time, have been centres of medical care,[14] but the majority would just have provided hostels for travellers and regular doles of food to the local poor, as with the Spedale di S. Miniato (5) run by the Benedictine monks of S. Miniato al Monte.[15] This was also the declared intention of those hospitals established by the crusading orders throughout Christendom, though none could match the proportions of the Knights Hospitallers' foundation in Jerusalem which by the late twelfth century consisted of eleven wards with a capacity of up to a thousand people.[16] When they established a small hospital in Florence, S. Sepolcro next to the south end of the Ponte Vecchio (4), it formed part of a Europe-wide programme providing short-term accommodation to pilgrims rather than the type of medical treatment developed by the order's hospital in the small town of Altopascio near Lucca, which by 1239 employed four physicians, two surgeons and an apothecary.[17]

By the period 1173 to 1258, when the Oltrarno walls were further extended, the city's population had more than doubled, and Florence had become the fastest growing urban centre in Tuscany. During these years nine more hospitals were founded in the city (Map 1.2). Although two, S. Pancrazio and S. Trinita, were within the mid-thirteenth-century walls, the others were outside on one of the axial routes leading out of the city. S. Paolo and S. Niccolò were in the suburban area to the west being developed by the Dominican Order as the site for its new church of S. Maria Novella on the road to Prato (7),[18] while S. Gallo and Buonamico were just outside the city gates to the north (9) and west (14), respectively.

Historians usually provide a rather negative view of the activities of hospitals founded in Florence before the mid-thirteenth century, citing, for example, evidence of court cases against their personnel. Thus, the Spedale de' Pinti, the hospice belonging to the convent of S. Pier Maggiore, came to the attention of the Church court in 1300. Its director, Giunta Bencivenni, had attended the Jubilee in Rome and was later discovered to have funded his journey with an unauthorised sale of property, the income from which had been intended for the maintenance of the old and sick.[19] But this type of evidence gives more information about the misdeeds of administrators than about the services provided by hospitals. A more detailed account cited briefly above in the Introduction was Buoncompagno da Signa's description of the conditions in c.1230 at the large Spedale di S. Giovanni Evangelista, in the very centre of Florence. He recounts that elderly sick men were fed poor-quality food and wine and housed in fetid beds.[20] Although this is a highly coloured account of the *spedale*, it is significant because it confirms that by the 1230s it was best known for caring for the sick poor rather than pilgrims.

The other seven hospitals built during these hundred years tended to concentrate on providing temporary accommodation for travellers and pilgrims, for Florence was on one of the main routes for trade and travellers from northern to southern Italy. This role as hospice for pilgrims can be even better appreciated in the case of other major cities on pilgrimage routes, such as Siena and Rome. S. Maria della Scala in Siena was an important stopping-off point for pilgrims on their way to Rome and it can be no accident that the hospital was placed opposite the cathedral to which pilgrims would have made their way on their arrival in the city. In Rome itself S. Spirito was literally a few hundred yards from St Peter's Basilica, the focal point for all pilgrims in western Europe. In the case of both of those hospitals there is iconographic evidence for their continued importance as hospices for pilgrims well into the fifteenth century. In Domenico di Bartolo's frescoes in the Scala's Pellegrinaio or pilgrims' ward a bearded pilgrim can be seen among the crowd in the piazza at the entrance to the hospital; he can be identified as a pilgrim because attached to his hat is the distinctive emblem of the shell from Compostela as well as the image of Christ from Turin (Plate 1.2).

The emphasis on hospices for pilgrims or poor travellers is too prescriptive a view of all hospitals founded in the central Middle Ages; even the admission

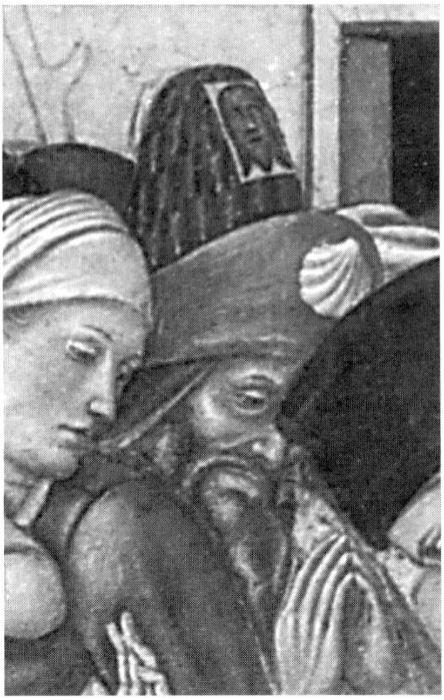

Plate 1.2 Domenico di Bartolo, 'A Pilgrim', detail of *Feeding the Poor*, 1440–4, Pellegrinaio ward, S. Maria della Scala, Siena

records of the more 'medicalised' hospitals of the fifteenth century used the terms 'poor' and 'sick' interchangeably.[21] Furthermore, generalisations about earlier medieval foundations usually fail to take into account their adaptability in the face of changing conditions in society and the economy. For example, when in 1218 Guidalotto di Volto dall'Orco refounded the hospital of S. Gallo, outside the city gates on the road to Bologna (Map 1.2, no.: 9), he defined its function as 'for the sustenance of the poor and of male and female pilgrims'. But in the late thirteenth century Pope Boniface VIII recorded in a papal privilege that it now received a 'multitude of sick and poor [people]'.[22] This was confirmed by a comment by the preacher Giordano da Rivalto of the same period. Speaking of the spiritual benefits of a visit, he invited his audience to 'Go also to the hospitals, or there to S. Gallo; [among] the sick you will see those who lack a nose or a hand or a foot; he who is deaf or blind or dumb, he who has cancer or fever or pains, he who is mad, and thousands of sicknesses and thousands of ailments.'[23]

Even if the comments about the incredible variety of chronic conditions are exaggerated, Giordano does underline the medical role of S. Gallo. A better idea of the scale of its activities and site is provided within a few decades by an inventory of the hospital's possessions:[24]

> First of all a little old church with an altar and a sacristy next to the said church and a bell-tower with four large bells. And a house partly on one floor and partly on two floors next to the said church halfway along the side of the church called the church of Sancta Maria…
>
> Item another new church near to the old church with the piazza in between…
>
> Item a house which is called the old hospital, which was built at the beginning with other houses added to the said hospital, which houses male patients and where [the place they store] the barrels is called the cellar, and on the western side is the house in which the sisters of the hospital live with land behind…
>
> Item a piece of land between the said hospital and the Mugnone river: on this said land is a large house built from stone and lime in which the clergy and laymen stay and where the grain is stored.

Francesco Rosselli's 'Catena' view of the city – so-called because it is framed by a chain – enables one to identify these buildings as they would have appeared in the last quarter of the fifteenth century before they were demolished during the preparations for the siege of Florence in 1529 (Plate 1.3). It shows a small complex immediately outside the Porta S. Gallo with the buildings grouped around a piazza through which the road from Bologna passes. The 'little old

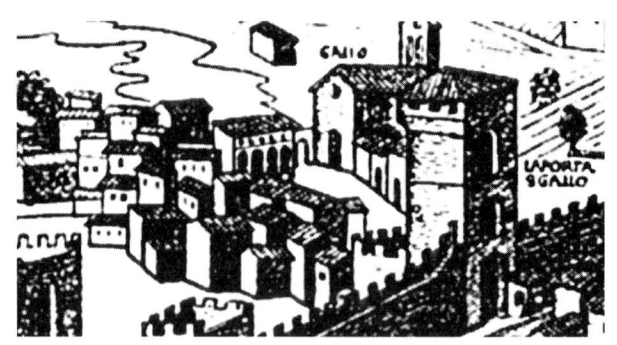

Plate 1.3 Francesco Rosselli, *Veduta di Firenze detta 'della Catena'*, c.1471–80: detail of Hospital of S. Gallo

church' with its bell-tower is clearly visible to the right and next to it and between the gate is the house 'partly on one floor and partly on two floors'. The new church, built by Guidalotto dall'Orco, is presumably the building with a portico facing the viewer, while the other houses for the sick, the sisters and short-term visitors would have been those to the north and west of the piazza. The combination of ecclesiastical and secular buildings on this site made concrete the dual role of the medieval hospital to cure the body and soul. The link between physical and spiritual sickness is underlined by Giordano da Rivalto in another sermon in which he portrays mortal sin as equivalent to the worst fever:[25]

> And these fevers come from disordered heat, which is in the body, in the same way as mortal sin is in the soul and takes away its essence and makes it fall. Also the heat of the corrupt soul creates the conditions to make the soul fall, making it so weak that it falls, like bad humour and the bad heat in the body … Hence the mortal sins are like the effects of the fevers of the soul.

In this way Giordano explains sin in terms readily understandable not just to a medical audience, but to a medieval congregation familiar with the idea of heat corrupting the humours and generating disease.

The same combination of physical and spiritual treatment lay behind the basic ethos of another medical hospital founded in the late twelfth century, the leprosarium of S. Eusebio, though one could be forgiven for assuming the supremacy of temporal interests from the tribulations it suffered towards the end of the century. Established on the road to Prato just outside the mid-twelfth-century walls (Map 1.1, no. 7), the hospital came to the attention of the city governent in 1278 when the lepers rebelled against the merchants' guild, the Arte di Calimala, that had administered it since 1192.[26] The lepers accused the guild of maltreating them and elected both a new rector and administrator from among their company. The government then stepped in, but without the guiding hand of the Calimala there developed 'ceaseless, intolerable, and terrible enmities' among the personnel and especially between the rector, Ser Bartolo di Vita, and one of the oblates, another priest called Ser Boninsegna di Boninsegna da Montauto.[27] Accusations were exchanged concerning the reason for the lack of sufficient income to support the lepers. This lack was exacerbated by the fact that various magnate families, including the Tornaquinci and Tosinghi, had taken control of hospital property through rental agreements; indeed, the chronicler Giovanni Villani says that S. Eusebio had been 'occupied by these "grandi uomini" '.[28] The status quo was restored in 1293 by a further intervention from the Florentine republic, which elected three independent arbitrators to reinstate the position of the Calimala. This episode should also be understood within the wider political context: 1293 saw the republican victory over the magnates, codified in the 'Ordinances of Justice'. The republic was now able to force the magnates out of the property belonging to both S. Eusebio and S. Gallo, the other Florentine hospital that had built up considerable wealth in real estate.[29]

The motivations behind this official intervention appear to have been mixed. First and foremost there was concern about the fate of the considerable amount of property owned by the hospital, as reflected in the high amount of tax paid under the papal Decima of 1276–7.[30] Second, it was done to ensure that the male and female lepers were properly fed so that they did not have to suffer more than necessary. Third, the offences for which people could be expelled were established, as in the cases of the lepers Caterina and Spinello, who were removed 'for having committed many scandals and dishonest [acts] and because their madness was a threat to the tranquillity of the other sick people'.[31] In this instance more details than usual are recorded and the patients appear to have had their say; indeed, discontent must have reached a very high level to have led them to 'bloody rebellion'.

Another decision taken by the republic in 1293 was to arrange for the removal of the hospital further from the city centre.[32] The area in which it was sited was being developed to include an open green space, which came to be known as the Prato, where markets were to be held. The Calimala guild was therefore asked in 1293 to remove the lepers within fifteen days, and within three months to build a new hospital at a place outside the projected walls at a spot called Campoluccio beyond the Mugnone river. Though part of the reason for the proposed move was to protect the city from disease generated by the 'infecti et infecte',[33] their removal was not achieved until 1338, almost a decade after the appointment of two magistrates specifically to 'expel these infected people from the city, *borgi* and suburbs' of Florence.[34]

This mixture of factors relating to the location of S. Eusebio, including the political ambitions of individuals, guilds and governments, and contemporary projects for urban expansion, is linked to a growing awareness of the necessity of implementing sanitary legislation. Concern for public health came increasingly to characterise official policies during subsequent centuries, especially with the repeated epidemics of plague after the Black Death. This preoccupation was also behind the growing awareness of the relationship between poverty and disease and thus the growing 'medicalisation' of hospitals in Renaissance Florence.

1.2 Towards Specialisation

If detailed information about the activities of hospitals in Florence until the mid-thirteenth century is scant and most appear to have been on a relatively small scale, the subsequent hundred years present a complete contrast. As has been seen from Table 1.1, hospital foundations soared: twenty-nine new ones appeared between 1250 and 1349, a full 43 per cent of all those known between 1000 and 1550. The contrast was not just a question of numbers: many were on a much larger scale than previous foundations. This period also saw the growth in the scope and capacity of existing hospitals, such as S. Gallo and S. Paolo, and the establishment in 1286 of S. Maria Nuova, which within forty years became the most substantial medical hospital in the city.

Table 1.2 Typology of hospitals founded in Florence, 1000–1349

	1000–1249	1250–1349
1. Pilgrims and travellers	8	6
2. Poor	1	5
3. Sick	1	6
4. Old	–	–
5. Foundlings	–	1
6. Women	–	–
7. Artisans	–	3
8. Religious	1	2
9. Unknown	1	6
Total	12	29

Source: Appendix below, pages 341–55

The contrast between the types of hospitals founded in this period compared with the previous 250 years can be appreciated from Table 1.2.

Although the process of categorisation leads to simplification,[35] especially with the overlap of hospitality and charity to travellers and the 'poor', the records do reflect a shift towards greater specialisation. The new six hospitals for the sick rather than for the professional poor – monks, nuns or friars – represents a deliberate choice on the part of testators and a departure from practices in earlier centuries.[36] Also new were the three small hospices established by groups of artisans to provide sickness benefit and almshouses for themselves necessary for immigrants with shared skills from the same area, and for the porters from Norcia. The policy of providing relief to artisans was shared by the professional guilds, which were established in precisely this period in Florence and in all the major Italian cities.[37]

These new foundations represented a response to the growing needs of the poorer members of society in a period characterised by strong demographic growth followed by a series of dearths and epidemics and a substantial rise in the cost of living. The location of these new hospitals also clearly reflects this

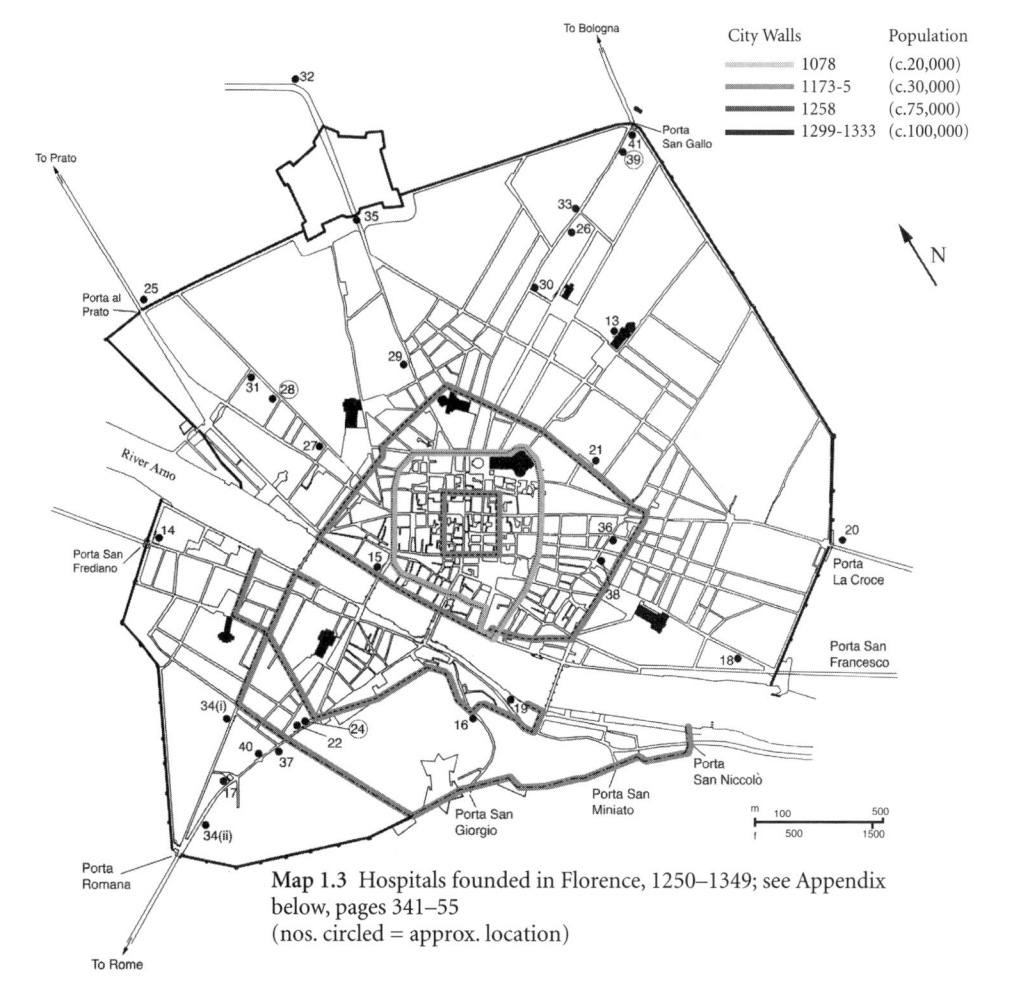

Map 1.3 Hospitals founded in Florence, 1250–1349; see Appendix below, pages 341–55
(nos. circled = approx. location)

response to demand, as is made immediately obvious by comparing Maps 1.2 and 1.3. Many of the earlier foundations were within or near Dante's 'cerchia antica' – the 'old circle' [of walls] – of 1173–5, while in the period 1258–1348 they were established principally in the areas that came to be contained by the final circle of 1299–1333. It was precisely these suburban zones that had seen recent settlement by immigrants, in particular in areas parallel to the city walls and along the main streets leading from the four main gates to the city centre.[38] This was a pattern shared by the distribution of hospitals in other contemporary cities, such as Valencia, Arles, Lyon and Paris.[39] However, one difference from many other cities was that fewer large hospitals were sited in proximity to the river. The explanation for this is largely that the Florentine water-table is very high and hospitals were able simply to sink wells in order to provide an adequate supply of water (see Plates 2.6, 3.12, 3.15 and 3.16).

In Via S. Gallo to the north there were four new hospitals (Map 1.2, nos 26, 30, 33, 39),[40] including S. Giovanni Decollato (26), founded by the company of porters from Norcia in c.1297 for 'the service of the poor of Christ' but in practice for their own old and infirm members,[41] and Gesù Pellegrino (30),

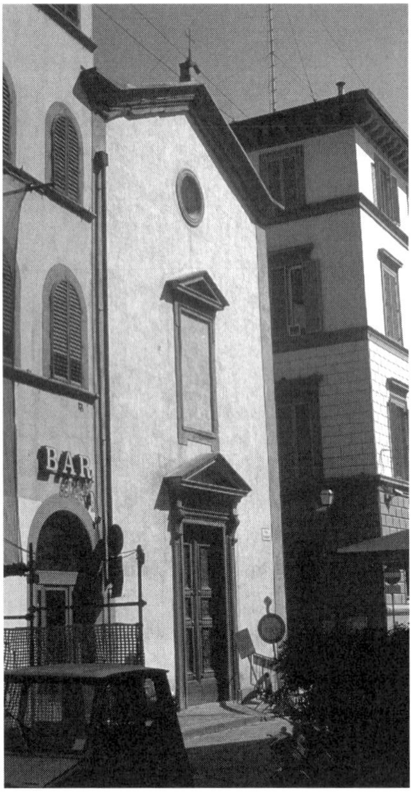

Plate 1.4 Church of the Spedale di Gesù Pellegrino, Via S. Gallo

founded in 1312 to provide accommodation for elderly priests and travelling clerics.[42] Though suppressed by Grand Duke Pietro Leopoldo in 1785, the church still stands in Via S. Gallo (Plate 1.4). Its façade retains the simplicity of its original early Trecento design with a plain door surmounted by a *pietra serena* pediment, a small oculus and a large glazed window which is now bricked up.[43]

To the south of the River Arno there was another clustering of new foundations on Via S. Pier Gattolino (now Via dei Serragli) and Via Romana, the two streets leading to Porta Romana and along which travelled those arriving from southern Tuscany and Rome. This pattern was in complete contrast to the years leading up to 1258, when no hospitals had appeared in this area (cf. Map 1.2). The new foundations included a *spedale* in Via S. Pier Gattolini which was nicknamed the 'Pigeon' after the dove symbol of the *laudesi* company of S. Spirito which had established it in 1332 (34). An inscription reading 'Hospitale S. Marie de Laudibus' still remains on the cornice over the grey *pietra serena* surround to the entrance to the house in Via Romana which the hospital came to occupy when it moved there in 1460 (Plate 1.5).

The four new hospitals in Via Romana (17, 22, 24, 37) were situated on a short stretch of road to the south of the church of S. Felice in Piazza and included S. Niccolò della Misericordia, founded by Lapo Fantoni in 1338 to provide short-term lodging (37). As Plate 1.6 shows, the hospital was one of a series of terraced houses, its façade distinguished by a bas-relief of a cock, the symbol of the confraternity of the Bigallo which came to act as its administrator. Another, the Spedale di S. Spirito in Via Romana, was linked to the famous Roman hospital (22); the symbol of the cross still marks its original site on the wall of the house (Plate 1.7).[44]

There were also three new *spedali* to the west (31, 27, 28), the largest of which, S. Maria della Scala (31) in Via della Scala, was named after the Sienese hospital of the same name and to which it was linked. It was established in 1316 by a Florentine carpenter, Cione di Lapo di Gherardo Pollini, for pilgrims and travellers, which was appropriate given its position on the new street, completed only seventeen years previously, which led from Piazza S. Maria Novella towards the city walls.[45] Because of its importance the silk guild of Por S. Maria took over the administration of the Scala in 1351. By this stage the hospital not only provided accommodation for poor travellers, but had also become an orphanage: the abandonment of children was a characteristic feature of periods of dearth, high prices and financial hardship, as in the mid-Trecento.[46] The foundation thus shared the mixed functions of its parent organisation in Siena.[47] The Florentine hospital had two wards and, according to an inventory of 1362, there were fourteen beds for wet-nurses in the 'children's ward' and another twenty-two beds for the poor.[48] Furthermore, as

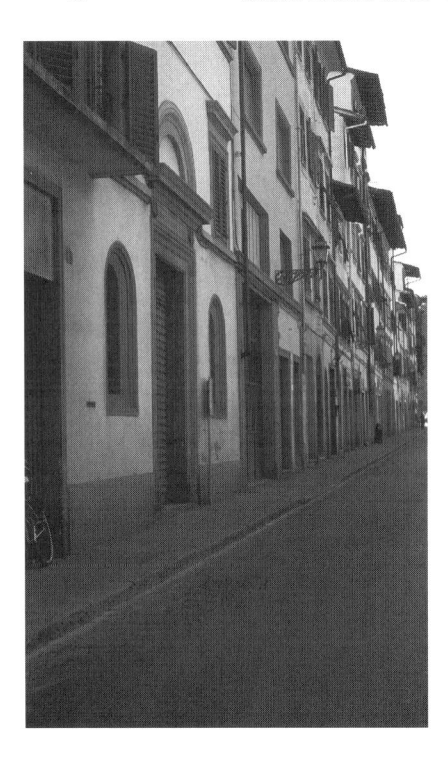

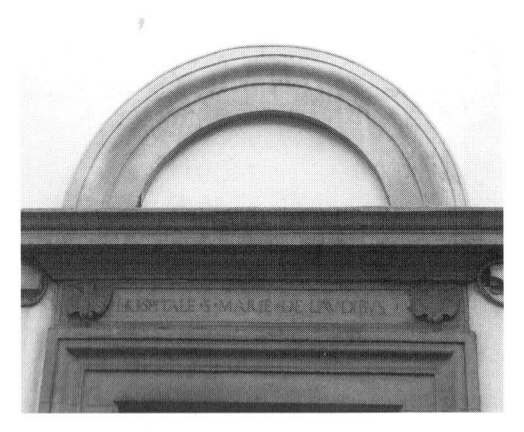

Plate 1.5 Hospital of the Pigeon, Via Romana: a. View towards Porta Romana; b. Detail of façade

at the Innocenti, it had a turning box or wheel set in the exterior wall where abandoned babies could be left and the parents retain their anonymity. The church was also fronted by a loggia, the remains of which can still be made out; the columns form part of the external walls of the building on the corner of Via della Scala and Via degli Orti Oricellari (Plate 1.8).

Hospitallers were another type of outside agency that led to the foundation of hospitals, as in the case of S. Sepolcro at the Ponte Vecchio (4) and Buonamico in Borgo S. Frediano (14), either directly founded or taken over by the Knights of St John of Jerusalem.[49] In 1317 the order established another hospital north of the River Arno to receive the sick, both male and female. This was the Spedale di S. Giovanni fra l'Arcora, so called because it was built outside Porta al Prato near the remains of the arches of the Roman aqueduct which had brought water into the city from Monte Morello (32).[50] Although it was destroyed during the siege of Florence in 1529, Vasari records that it had contained a series of pictures by Buonamico Buffalmacco, including a scene appropriate to the role of the hospital: 'On the same façade [there were] depicted Sant'Ivo of Brittany, who had at his feet many widows and children; it was a good image and there were also two angels hovering in the air who crowned him; they were done in the sweetest fashion.'[51]

The Antonites also established a hospital for the poor sick in this period, the

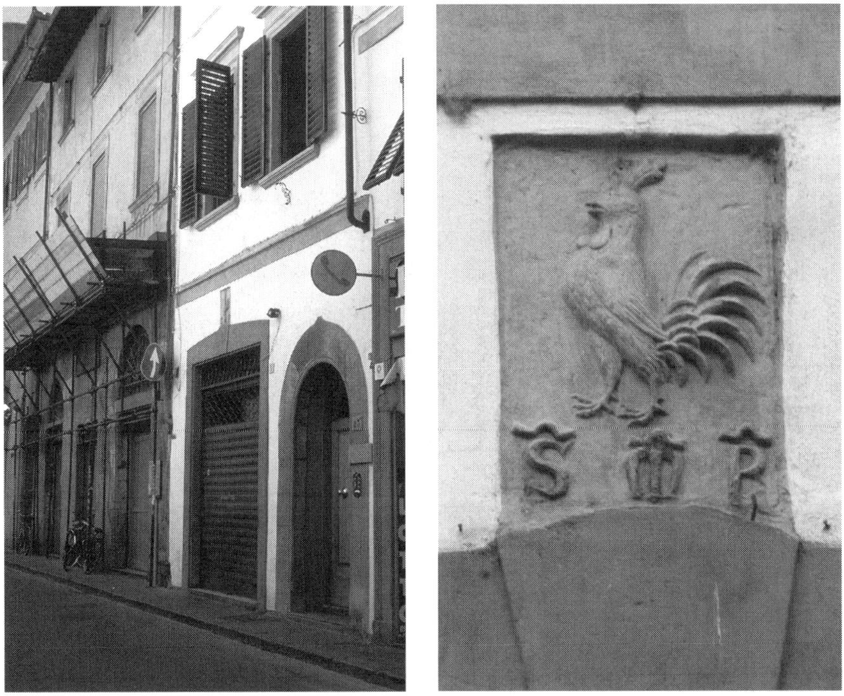

Plate 1.6 Hospital of S. Niccolò della Misericordia dei Fantoni, Via Romana a. View of façade; b. Detail showing symbol of the confraternity of the Bigallo

Spedale di S. Antonio in 1333 (35). This order, also known as the Canons Regular of S. Antonio, though dating back to the late eleventh century, had only achieved a properly independent status in 1297 following Pope Boniface VIII's intervention. They looked after those suffering from St Anthony's Fire or the 'Mal Persiano', a gangrenous disease characterised by sharp burning pains and associated with eating mouldy rye bread infected with the ergot fungus, hence 'ergotism'.[52] Once again, the hospital was built in an area on the outskirts of Florence, just inside the recently completed city walls and close to the new gates of Porta a Faenza; construction work was begun in 1358.[53]

Another important reason for the establishment of hospitals at the edge of the city was availability of land,[54] as in the example of two hospitals which became major medical institutions in the city centre, S. Paolo and S. Maria Nuova.[55] The first, founded in 1208 near Porta di S. Paolo just outside the 1173–5 walls, was located between Piazza S. Maria Novella and Via Palazzuolo (28).[56] Its beginnings apparently stemmed from a confraternity, but its expansion was due to the influence of a movement that led to many charitable and pious enterprises in Italy: the Third Orders associated with the Mendicant friars. S. Paolo, which was run by the Franciscan Penitenti, was at first a hospice

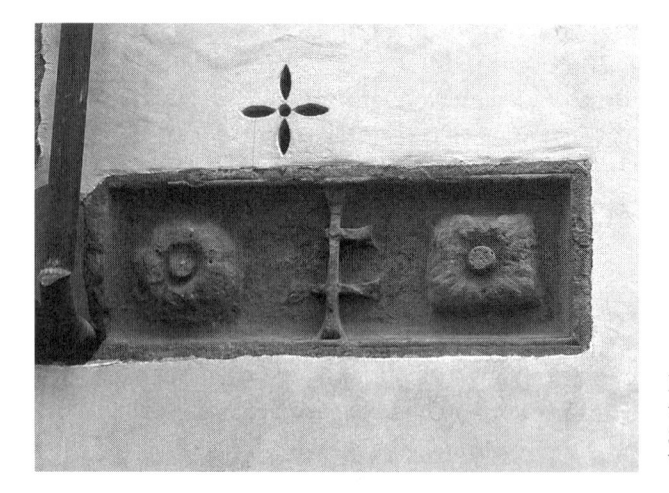

Plate 1.7 Symbol of the Cross from the Spedale di S. Spirito, Via Romana

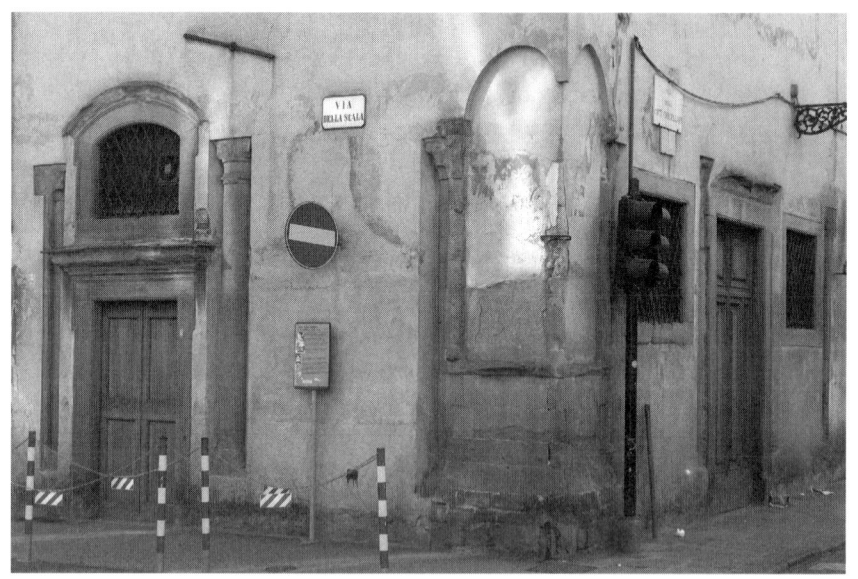

Plate 1.8 Hospital of S. Maria della Scala, Via della Scala

that provided short-term accommodation for pilgrims and the poor.[57] In the late Duecento it expanded its premises and functions, facilitated no doubt by the demolition of the old city walls, and in the early Trecento built a number of houses on the piazza.[58] In a 1313 inventory the Penitenti described the centre of their premises as 'Two hospitals in Borgo S. Paolo, one to accommodate men and the other women',[59] many of whom had settled in the area around S. Maria Novella.[60]

S. Maria Nuova, sited directly to the east of the cathedral (21), began as a relatively modest affair. It was founded in 1285 by Folco di Ricovero Portinari, the father of Dante's Beatrice, 'for the hospitality and sustenance of the poor and needy',[61] for whom he supplied 'seventeen beds furnished with straw mattresses, blankets, sheets, covers, feather pillows and bedsteads, which have already been put in place in the said hospital for the use of the poor'.[62] The opportunity to found a new hospital in the city centre was created by two events: the first was that land was being made available through the demolition of the northern perimeter of the late twelfth-century city walls, and the second was that the convent of the Frati Saccati, who ran the nearby small church of S. Egidio, had been suppressed by Pope Gregory X in 1274 and gradually their land and premises were acquired by Portinari and the *spedalingo*, or hospital director.[63]

The original complex of the Frati Saccati was at the centre of the site (Plate 1.9) and would have comprised S. Egidio (2) with probably a small cloister to the right of the church (3). The conventual buildings would have included a refectory, which may have formed the nucleus for what was to become the hospital's refectory (7), a room for the prior, which may have become the office of the *spedalingo* (5), and a dormitory above on the first floor. Then a cemetery known as the Cloister of Bones (4) was created, apparently in the second decade of the Trecento, probably to expand a pre-existing burial site.[64]

While some existing spaces could be adapted for the uses of the hospital, others needed to be newly built. The most significant was the ward to the right of the cloister (1a), which initially housed male and female patients. But by the early years of the Trecento it treated only men. Then by 1313/15, when it was enlarged into a hall-like form typical of many medieval hospitals, it concentrated on men, the women having already moved south of the piazza.[65] One of the main sources for this early period is an unpublished history of S. Maria Nuova written in 1662 which may very well be based on documentation now lost, but which may also be only partially accurate, given the laudatory intentions of this type of institutional history.[66]

The development of the women's ward to the south of the piazza had also been made possible by the availability of land.[67] The sources were twofold: the first was the commune, which had sold off the late twelfth-century walls and the contiguous public spaces to the south of the piazza, the second was the owners of the adjoining land which had housed the workshops of a number of kiln-makers.[68] Much of the construction on the site was carried out under the long tenure of the *spedalingo*, Messer Lorenzo di Jacopo da Bibbiena (1308–32).[69] This new complex came to consist of a substantial ward running alongside Via delle Pappe, the initial phase being completed between c.1308 and 1322 (10): the refectory and kitchen to the right of the ward (12, 13) as well

Key

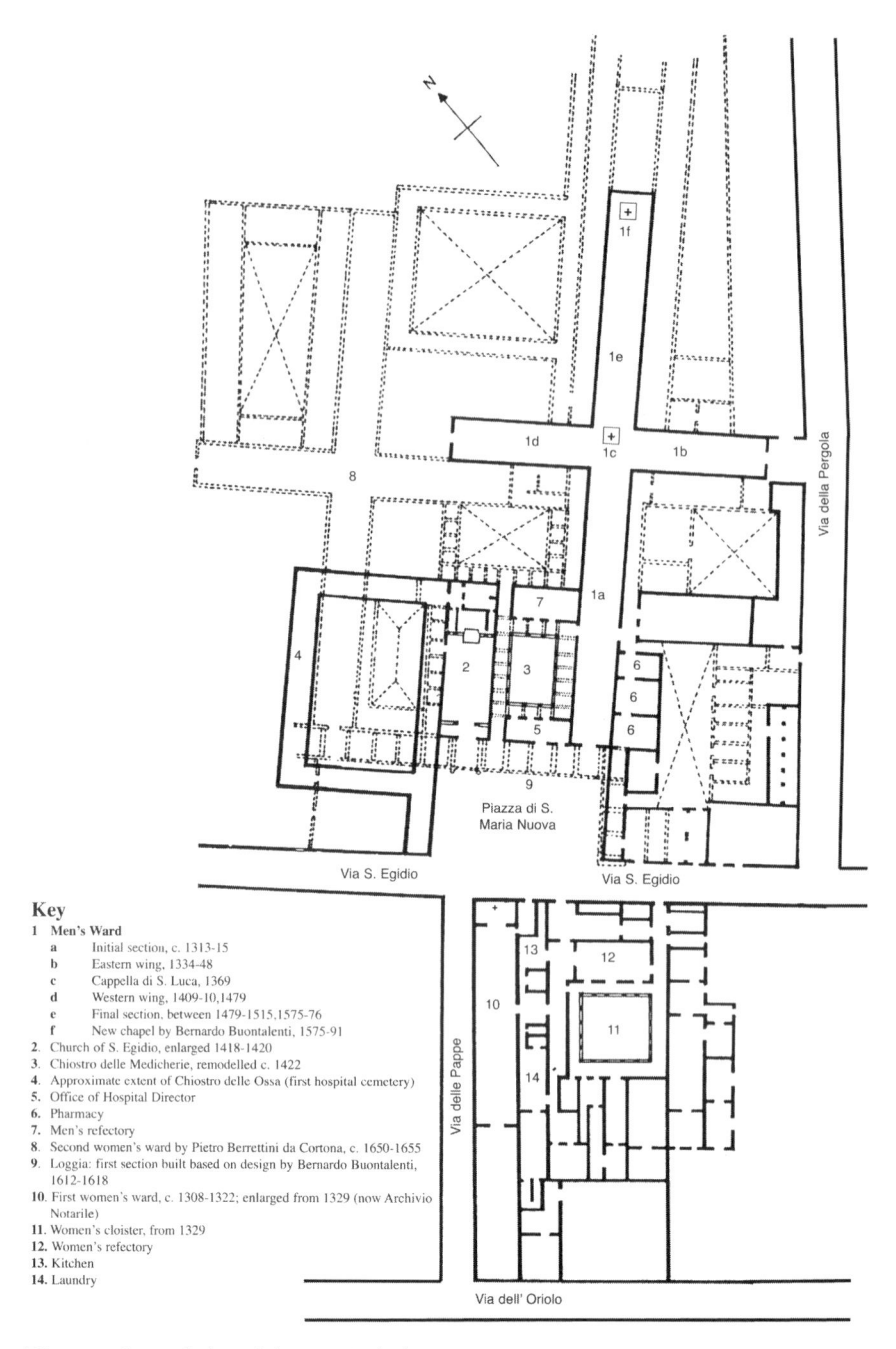

1 **Men's Ward**
   a   Initial section, c. 1313-15
   b   Eastern wing, 1334-48
   c   Cappella di S. Luca, 1369
   d   Western wing, 1409-10,1479
   e   Final section, between 1479-1515,1575-76
   f   New chapel by Bernardo Buontalenti, 1575-91
2. Church of S. Egidio, enlarged 1418-1420
3. Chiostro delle Medicherie, remodelled c. 1422
4. Approximate extent of Chiostro delle Ossa (first hospital cemetery)
5. Office of Hospital Director
6. Pharmacy
7. Men's refectory
8. Second women's ward by Pietro Berrettini da Cortona, c. 1650-1655
9. Loggia: first section built based on design by Bernardo Buontalenti, 1612-1618
10. First women's ward, c. 1308-1322; enlarged from 1329 (now Archivio Notarile)
11. Women's cloister, from 1329
12. Women's refectory
13. Kitchen
14. Laundry

Plate 1.9 Ground plan of the Hospital of S. Maria Nuova, c.1500 (dotted lines represent later phases of construction; adapted from an original design by Patrick Sweeney)

as the laundry (14) and other associated service areas; a cloister known as the Chiostro delle Oblate (11); and the living areas on the first floor for the staff.[70] Payments to builders and suppliers in 1325–7 for the 'new hospital for women' suggest that the ward and ward chapel were nearing completion.[71]

In 1334 attention was turned to the men's ward. According to the seventeenth-century history, the second *spedalingo*, Orlando Pierozzi (1332–48), 'increased the size of the hospital of the men in a marvellous way, but did not finish the construction: he lengthened the hospital as far as the crossing that one sees today constructing the right-hand arm towards the east which goes as far as Via della Pergola so that the hospital was in the form of a seven'. Thus, the ward, now shaped like a reversed figure 7 (1b), reached the point that later became the crossing of the cruciform shape.[72] In fact, it is unlikely this additional work would have been completed in that year, as is usually suggested; even a cursory glance at the hospitals' surviving account books shows that building continued through the 1330s and 1340s.[73]

On completion of the first phase of expansion in 1313–15 the men's ward would have conformed to the design of a medieval open ward typical of hospitals throughout Europe in this period. The addition of the shorter eastern extension in 1334 increased capacity and the design meant that patients in both arms could still be seen by the medical and nursing staff standing where the wards met. This was also important from the perspective of spiritual care for this was the location of the chapel dedicated to St Luke, which took its final form in May 1369.[74] According to the seventeenth-century hospital historian, it was 'placed under a small cupola, however, covered with timber and tiles'.[75] This formed the focal point so that patients and staff alike could participate in the daily celebration of Mass.

Some idea of the hospital's appearance can be gained from the view of S. Maria Nuova by Marco di Bartolommeo Rustici (Plate 1.10). Although dating from over a hundred years later, and therefore including further additions, the drawing shows the body of the church of S. Egidio as it would have appeared in the fourteenth century, with its pitched roof and oculus. The men's ward is shown parallel to the east, though in a schematic and partial view. More idea is provided of the height than the depth of the male ward building, although we know that it projected beyond the far wall of the cloister and came to measure almost double the length of the church of S. Egidio. The other features shown include the cloister, which separated the two main building structures – though it would have been smaller than the design represented here – and the green area to the north-west, the site of the cemetery and garden.

The development of S. Maria Nuova into the largest medical hospital in the city centre by the time of the Black Death was partly facilitated by the availability of land in the late thirteenth and early fourteenth centuries and partly

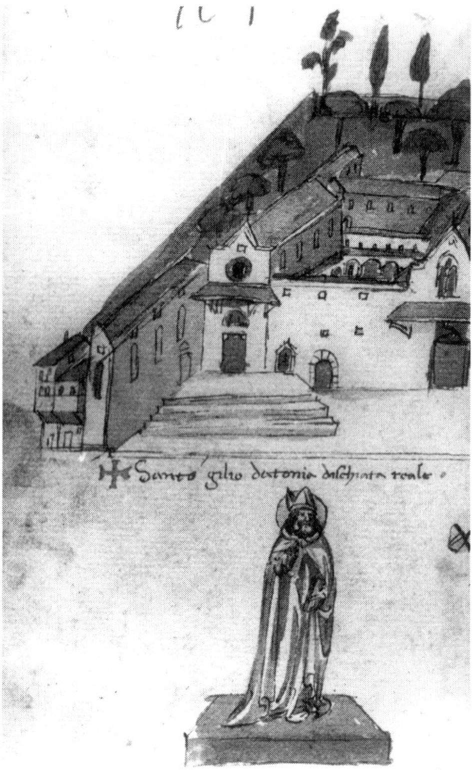

Plate 1.10 Codice Rustici, *Hospital of S. Maria Nuova*, c.1445

by government policy. As the chronicler Giovanni Villani recorded, 'it is from the need for money, and so not to impose more taxes that they [government officials] sold the old walls and the land inside and outside [them] to neighbouring property owners'.[76] Another aspect of urban planning to benefit S. Maria Nuova was the decision in 1296 to pull down the Spedale di S. Giovanni Evangelista, which lay between the Baptistery and S. Reparata, in order to improve the circulation of people and goods in the area.[77] S. Maria Nuova now became the only substantial hospital in the city centre and would have experienced increased demand for its services.

In this rapid survey of hospitals established in Florence between the mid-thirteenth and mid-fourteenth centuries a number of factors have been seen as leading to and facilitating their foundation. On the one hand, this explosion of new charitable institutions can be interpreted as a response to demand, for these ninety years, and especially the first half of the Trecento, were characterised by rising living costs and periods of financial crisis for the poorer levels of society caused by epidemic disease and dearth. Florence, which depended on immigrant labour for its expanding commercial and industrial base, was thus going some way to help those who had come to the city in search of employment, but in the process had left behind their social and economic support networks. It was no accident that the suburban areas in which most of the new hospitals were established were the zones of the city where land was also available to provide new housing for immigrants.

Furthermore, the men who provided the largest benefactions to establish new hospitals were all men of the world, who because they worked in the local commercial or industrial sectors would have been only too aware of the demands of the poorer levels of society in the late thirteenth and early fourteenth centuries. For example, Folco di Ricovero Portinari, the founder of S. Maria Nuova, was a member of the Cerchi bank and also of the silk guild of Por S. Maria, while the family of Lippo Forese del Soldato, the founder of the hospital of S. Jacopo in Campo Corbolini in 1311, was not only of noble lineage and a leading merchant, but had also been elected as prior, the highest office in the republic. Others, such as the family of the founder of the hospital of S. Spirito in Via Romana, Messer Gianni degli Amidei, were merchants and bankers who had been declared manifest usurers, as were various relatives of Bennuccio Senni del Bene, who had founded the Spedale di S. Bartolomeo in 1295.[78] This is a theme that will recur in the following chapters since some of the patrons of major Florentine hospitals had been declared usurers; the foundation of these institutions was one way they could return some of their ill-gotten gains and at the same time make a very public declaration of their charity.

1.3 The Growth of Medicine

One of the significant new features of hospitals in this period was their increasing 'medicalisation', concentrating on looking after the poor sick and having them treated by professional medical staff.[79] Table 1.2 shows that a fifth of the new foundations specifically described themselves as for the 'sick poor'. Some of these specialised in conditions such as leprosy or St Anthony's Fire, while others like S. Paolo and S. Maria Nuova treated a wide range of acute diseases.

The process of 'medicalisation' is well illustrated by the development of the hospitals of S. Paolo and S. Maria Nuova in the first half of the Trecento.[80] S. Paolo's physical expansion meant it could house a growing community of Tertiaries who had the right to pass from being a nurse to a patient as they grew old and infirm, underlining the elasticity of the line between care and cure.[81] Though few substantive records survive before the 1320s, the statutes and account books of 1325–6 reflect the existence of a complex outdoor system of relief, distributing alms to the needy poor in their own houses.[82] Emphasis was placed on providing alms to family units and in particular to households with larger than the average number of children. The Tertiaries also showed a particular sensitivity towards mothers since they specialised in providing alms to 'donne in parto', women in childbirth, reflecting a contemporary recognition of the risks to the health of women and infants associated with birth.

Over the following decade the hospital made a conscious decision to concentrate even more clearly on the sick poor, a shift that was evident in the increase in the number of subsidies to people with physical ailments from 1325 to 1338. The scale of its operation had also increased massively; from 707 in 1324–5, the number receiving out-relief subsidies grew to 3,729. Then in 1345 it made a decisive switch to in-house treatment of the sick poor, as recorded by the Penitents: 'on 24 November in the said year we began to house the sick in the hospital of the poor, which was completed in the said month of November at the time of the said friars Piero Bindi and Giovanni Lozzi, ministers [of the poor].'[83] Account books from two years later indicate that the new system was in operation. The long lists of subsidies to the poor disappeared, to be replaced by expenses specifically to buy clothes for the patients and materials, such as bedclothes, to equip the hospital to receive the sick poor.[84] Further expansion took place when two more houses were bought in the parish of S. Paolo for 150 gold florins, 'which are very useful and necessary to the said friars for the poor of Christ'.[85] For the first time salaried medical staff appear on the hospital's books, fulfilling one of the main definitions of a 'medicalised' hospital. A certain Maestro Ambrogio was now employed as a surgeon with an annual salary, the barber Sennuccio was employed to cut hair and to bleed the inmates, and Bonaiuto di Michele, apothecary of the parish of S. Simone, was paid the very considerable sum of 133 lire for 'confectionery and medicines and wax for the sick and the dead of the hospital'.[86]

The same process of 'medicalisation' was apparent at S. Maria Nuova, though on a much bigger scale. The development was much more rapid and took place during the fifty years after its foundation. While the act of foundation had spoken simply of an institution 'designated for the hospitality and sustenance of the poor and needy',[87] by 1330, when the hospital's statutes were revised, its function was now said to be for the 'good service of the poor sick of the said hospital'.[88] Furthermore, narrowing down those whom it could accept, the statutes declared that 'it is not possible to receive in the said hospital any person, male or female, a member of the regular or secular clergy, who is not sick, for more than three consecutive days without the knowledge of the patrons'.[89] Clearly, whatever changes in function had been made received the full consent and knowledge of the Portinari family, who retained a tight control over the hospital.

S. Maria Nuova's 1330 statutes only broadly define the hospital's function as being for the 'poor sick',[90] but contemporary financial records add more detail. Thus, from 1325 to 1331 the hospital retained the services of seven different medical specialists on a wide range of contracts. The most stable employee was Maestro Silvestro, who received a regular salary and was employed as 'nostro medico', 'our physician'.[91] Others were brought in on a more ad hoc basis as consultants, like Ser Cione, who specialised in external lesions such as wounds, ulcers or sores,[92] and Maestro Filippo, 'who treats eyes'.[93] The latter's job was probably the removal of cataracts, a complex operation that involved using a needle to lower the lens behind the pupil.[94] The other doctors mentioned in the records were paid to supply 'medicines and syrups' for the treatment of patients for at this stage S. Maria Nuova did not possess a full-time live-in pharmacist.[95]

Of our main practitioners, Maestro Silvestro should be distinguished from Cione and Filippo; the former was a physician, while the latter were surgeons. But there was a less rigid social and professional distinction between the two than in northern Europe, where a surgeon was usually on a par with a barber.[96] In Italy surgery was a university discipline, which required both theoretical knowledge and practical skills, and while few surgeons may actually have had this lengthy university training its very existence conferred status on the profession, underlined by the necessity for practitioners to be members of the Guild of Physicians and Apothecaries.[97] Indeed, S. Maria Nuova employed a barber on a separate contract to cut the hair of the patients and staff.[98]

The examples of the hospitals of S. Maria Nuova and S. Paolo have shown how in the fifty years before the Black Death two major charitable institutions transformed themselves both in scale and function. S. Maria Nuova, which had begun with only seventeen beds for the 'poor of Christ', by 1347 catered for over 220 'sick poor'.[99] S. Paolo, on the other hand, moved from a system based on out-relief, with a marked bias towards numerous families and women in childbed, to a self-consciously new policy based on the treatment of the sick poor.

This shift in emphasis, which I have called the 'medicalisation' of charity, is easier to chronicle than to explain. Internal records simply document the changes without providing the reasons for them. At its most general one can see this change as being part of a move in charity towards greater specialisation in Italy in the later Middle Ages. This is a process that has often been linked to the Black Death, but, in common with other demographic and economic trends, the great plague merely accelerated an existing tendency.[100] Indeed, it is the demographic and economic context that probably provides the most convincing explanation for these shifts in charity. For the first half of the fourteenth century saw a continuation of high population levels combined with falling standards of living caused by, among other economic factors, a series of epidemics and subsistence crises. In this situation levels of both endemic and epidemic poverty rose not just for traditional categories of the indigent (widows, orphans, etc.), but also for artisans and shopkeepers who would normally have been able to keep their heads above the financial water line.[101]

If the expansion of hospitals can be seen as due partly to increased demand, this still does not explain why the institutional response should have assumed a medical character at that time. Part of the explanation must lie in the development of the medical profession itself and the wider process through which it achieved autonomy from the Church.[102] It is no coincidence that it was precisely in the early Trecento that the profession was beginning to assert its newly found corporate identity. The Arte dei Medici e Speziali had been established in 1266 and then reconfirmed by the 'Ordinances of Justice' in 1293 as one of the seven major guilds of the city.[103] In this way physicians were able to close professional ranks against practitioners without proper qualifications and in the process insist on entry requirements based on a university degree or on passing the Arte's own examination.[104] The hospital played an important part in the process by which medical practitioners made their professional presence felt. Since these institutions inspired considerable local pride, prestige accrued to physicians and surgeons who worked in them, especially if it were known that they provided their services at relatively low rates as an expression of their Christian charity to the poor.[105] Furthermore, working in hospitals enlarged their practice and gave them experience of a much wider range of conditions than they would normally have encountered.

The 'medicalisation' of hospitals in the first half of the Trecento cannot, however, simply be attributed to the urgings of the medical profession. It was also part of a more general growing belief in the efficacy and importance of medical practitioners in public health. The waves of severe dearths and epidemics led to a heightened perception of the link between disease, 'mal' aria (bad air) and the domestic and industrial effluence generated by crowded living and working conditions in one of Europe's largest and most prosperous industrial and commercial centres. This awareness of the problems of public health was also reflected in the growing body of sanitary legislation in Italian cities and the appointment of doctors by Italian communes to provide free medical treatment for the sick poor.[106]

1.4 *The Common Good: Between Church and State*

Growing contemporary perception of the importance of the services provided by hospitals for the poor and sick was also expressed through the Florentine government's continued support for the rights of these institutions. Thus, in 1255 a commission was set up to investigate the hospitals of the city and the *contado* – the rural area surrounding Florence and under the control of the commune – in order to establish how far their rights to property might have been usurped by individuals and how far they were fulfilling the roles for which they had been founded. The following year the commission was given full powers to force anybody who had taken over property to return it to the institutions concerned and to make sure that the hospitals now served the poor according to their founders' original intentions.[107] This policy has already been seen in action in relation to communal intervention over the property rights of the hospital of S. Eusebio in 1293 (see above, pages 12–13). Another aspect of government policy was reflected in the 1316 decision to exempt from tax liability all goods left to the hospital of S. Maria della Scala.[108] Even more significant was the series of legal privileges granted from 1329 to S. Maria Nuova to enable it to defend itself against heirs who disputed the hospital's right to inherit, the most important of which was the freedom to elect a legally recognised procurator.[109] This privilege had been granted nineteen years earlier to the wealthy charitable Company of Orsanmichele and is some sign of official recognition of the importance of the role played by S. Maria Nuova in looking after the poor and sick, especially during the 1329 famine.[110] Then, in 1347, during the next particularly severe famine to affect the city, the hospital director petitioned the commune on 29 April for financial help, emphasising the precariousness of its finances given the strain of housing 220 sick people, a number that, the *spedalingo* lamented, was increasing daily.[111]

The Church too had a long tradition of defending the rights and property of hospitals, usually against laymen. The seventeenth clause of the Council of Vienne of 1311–12 expresses almost identical concerns as those of the Florentine commune:[112]

> It happens that now and then those in charge of hospices, leper-houses, almshouses or hospitals disregard the care of such places and fail to loosen the hold of those who have usurped the goods, possessions and rights of these places. They indeed permit them to slip and be lost completely and the buildings to fall into ruin.
>
> They have no care that these places were founded and endowed by the faithful so that the poor and lepers might find a home and be supported by their revenues. They have the barbarity to refuse this charity, criminally turning the revenues to their own use.

Indeed, given the affluence of hospitals, local and international ecclesiastical and secular politics could become involved in their affairs, as can be seen in the history of S. Gallo in the thirteenth century. When Giudalotto di Volta dall'Orco refounded and enlarged the hospital in 1218 he made a point of placing it under the protection of the Church.[113] On 4 October Cardinal Ugolino Ostiense took possession of it in a ceremony that culminated in his saying to the *spedalingo*: 'Take this hospital for me and for the Church of Rome, and do not give it to anybody else except for the Church itself.' This privileged status served the patronal family well and meant that the hospital could bypass the power of the local bishop, demonstrated in 1249–50 when Innocent IV quashed a bid by the friars of the hospital, who with episcopal support had tried to remove the *spedalingo*.[114]

Hospital founders and patrons could not ignore the bishop. Although these institutions were positioned somewhat ambiguously between secular and ecclesiastical authorities, episcopal intervention was required to consecrate the altars in hospital churches and wards. Thus, in 1288, when Folco di Ricovero Portinari petitioned the bishop for permission for a priest and minister to live at S. Maria Nuova, he mentioned that 'in one of those houses he had erected an altar which the Bishop had blessed … and then granted an indulgence of a year and forty days to all who were present'.[115] In the same petition Folco asked the bishop for 'immunity and full liberty, as have other hospitals subject to his jurisdiction'.[116] In addition to these privileges, the bishop also granted others including the right of burial at S. Maria Nuova for the rector and his staff and any patient who had died there. This was extended to Portinari and his descendants, who retained the right to hear the Divine Office there and to confess to the rector of the church.[117]

In some cases, the very fact that Church and State had a shared policy with regard to the rights and property of hospitals led to conflict as the former attempted to impose taxes and the latter sought to provide protection against what it interpreted as ecclesiastical depredation.[118] This could also give rise to conflict over rights to the presentation of a hospital director, who was in a powerful position to control the finances of his institution, even given the checks and balances provided by the patronal family and administrative bodies such as guilds, as in the case of S. Gallo (Plate 1.2). In 1294 the Florentine commune took the hospital under its jurisdiction on the pretext of preserving and increasing the services offered by the hospital, for, as the accompanying law says in an excess of patriotic fervour: 'This hospital shines above other hospitals and is most useful for the souls of not only the Florentines and the Tuscans, but also those of other Italian provinces; it is very important for providing the means of avoiding many infanticides and for feeding many poor people whom they support.'[119] The solution here, as in the case of the leper-house of S. Eusebio, was to place S. Gallo under the administrative control of a guild, the Arte della Seta, an expedient that came to be ever more widely adopted in Florence in the fourteenth and fifteenth centuries to protect and to guarantee the safe running of hospitals. But even this did not always provide a resolution to the conflict.[120] Thus, in 1330 the consuls of the Calimala guild were excommunicated by the vicar of the Florentine bishop when they defended their right to administer the property of the leper hospital of S. Eusebio. The situation became dramatic, when the consuls barricaded themselves into the hospital and used soldiers to stop the pope's favourite from taking over.[121]

This history of conflict over temporal possessions between Church and State, locally and internationally, should not lead us to forget the important religious dimension of these institutions. Despite the traditional belief of 'laicisation', a theme that remains important in much historiography of the Renaissance period, the idea of the *bene comune*, or 'common good', underlay not just an enterprise such as a hospital or charitable confraternity, but also more generally the government of the city-state.[122] Indeed, public ceremonies involving hospitals were an expression of *caritas* and civic religiosity, as with the consecration of the church of the priests' hospital of Gesù Pellegrino in 1312, when the bishop of Florence processed from the cathedral to Via S. Gallo accompanied by members of the clergy and the Florentine public.[123] Celebratory occasions could also become regular commemorative events, as with S. Eusebio, which Florentines visited annually on May Day when they gave alms to church and hospital.[124] Indulgences were offered in perpetuity to anyone visiting an altar in the hospital church or ward on the anniversary of the day of its consecration and helped to swell its income by encouraging gifts.[125]

At the individual level the religious influence remained as vital an inspiration for those people who founded and ran hospitals in Italy as in other parts of late medieval and Renaissance Europe. The hospital remained, like the confraternity, the physical embodiment of the concept of Charity. It fulfilled a social role in looking after the bodies and souls of the poor and at the same time provided spiritual benefits to benefactors. The importance of the role of these charitable institutions was evidently well understood by the wealthier classes, who left them an ever-increasing number of legacies to finance the construction programmes. This reflected a deliberate choice by patrons and testators alike to channel their funds into institutions to help the increasing number of poor people in Italian cities rather than the professional poor, the monastic orders and the newer mendicant friars.[126]

Conclusion

Hospitals founded in Florence up to the mid-thirteenth century, with the possible exception of S. Eusebio and S. Gallo, ostensibly fulfilled fairly traditional roles, providing hospitality to the clergy, whether resident or passing through the city, and temporary accommodation to lay men and women, including both locals and pilgrims.

When, however, this picture is compared with developments in other major Italian cities in this period, the activities of Florentine hospitals seem rather unadventurous and small in scale. To the north, in Milan, the Brolo, which had become one of the largest hospitals in the city, exercised a variety of functions right from its foundation in 1158. Its statutes declared that its purpose was to look after the 'poor sick' and 'abandoned children' and that it was to distribute alms to the poor of the city.[127] The same picture was also true to the south in Rome, where in the late twelfth century Pope Innocent III had founded the hospital of S. Spirito. From the outset its rule or *Regola* envisaged that the hospital should exercise a wide range of functions, including feeding and giving hospitality and clothes to the poor, looking after and housing the sick, pregnant women and abandoned children, and helping prisoners.[128]

Even in Siena, Florence's nearest rival city-state, the late tenth-century foundation of S. Maria della Scala was another example of an early large-scale multi-functional hospital. In the early thirteenth century S. Maria della Scala provided a number of services, including looking after abandoned babies, giving alms in cash and kind to the poor and beggars, and housing pilgrims, all on a much larger scale than in Florence's earliest hospitals.[129] Then in Altopascio, near Lucca, a recent study has shown that from 1239 the hospital employed four leading physicians and two surgeons and a pharmacy for the preparation of the recipes prescribed by the medical experts.[130]

The reasons for different patterns of development of hospital provision are manifold and perhaps somewhat illusory given our lack of knowledge about the activities of the earliest Florentine hospitals. However, in both Siena and Rome, the close links with pilgrim routes help to explain these precocious developments. Siena was on the main pilgrimage route through Italy, the Via Francigena, while Rome was obviously the centre of devotion and Innocent III's hospital of S. Spirito was in close physical proximity to St Peter's itself. The popularity of these hospitals among pilgrims led to their enrichment through gifts and bequests, allowing them to develop their more general role as providers of charity. Even so, in the case of S. Maria della Scala in Siena the process of its 'medicalisation' took place at much the same time as in Florence, that is, in the first two decades of the fourteenth century.[131] The early development of Altopascio can be explained by the influence of an international crusading order, the Knights of St John of Jerusalem, rather than by a precocious medical demand from this small Tuscan town.[132]

As will be seen in the next chapter, from the Trecento Florence's provision of hospitals and hospital facilities was on a par with many of the other large cities in northern and central Italy, even if each developed in slightly different ways according to local political and economic conditions. Despite these differences, the expansion of the medical role of Italian hospitals meant they had more in common with each other than they did with, for example, hospitals in France, where they tended to be smaller, with a few notable exceptions such as the Hôtel-Dieu in Paris, and only developed a medical function somewhat later.[133]

CHAPTER 2

The Early Renaissance: Medicine for the Body and Medicine for the Soul

Introduction: The Black Death and its Aftermath

In our city of Florence there occurred a marvellous thing in the year of the said mortality: that people when they were dying … without any human precedent, left … to the captains of that Company [of the Madonna S. Maria d'Orto San Michele] to distribute to the poor more than 350,000 gold florins … And … the Company of the Misericordia was left property and possessions to a value of more than 25,000 gold florins … And the hospital of S. Maria Nuova of S. Gilio was also left in that mortality [goods to] the value of 25,000 gold florins…

When the mortality ceased in Florence … the poor beggars were almost all dead, and every young woman was now well fed and had an abundance of goods, so that they did not need to seek alms.

Matteo Villani, *Cronica*, I.7

These observations by the chronicler Matteo Villani reflect contemporary perceptions that the Black Death had a profound impact on both the institutions that provided charity and on the poor themselves. Here Villani suggests that those members of the lower levels of society who survived and charitable institutions benefited from the crisis.

How far his words can be regarded as generally applicable must remain questionable. Certainly the picture that is normally painted of the fortunes of hospitals following the Black Death in many parts of northern Europe (England, for example),[1] sharing a decline in finances and services, does not conform to Villani's vision of great institutional affluence. More recently it has been argued that, as with the economy in general, those hospitals suffering financially after 1348 had already been in decline since the early fourteenth century.[2] Villani's implication that the two confraternities and the hospital no longer had the same relevance since the poor 'had an abundance of goods' is an oversimplification of the economic impact of the Black Death on the lower levels of society.

There is no denying that the scale of poverty had been reduced by massive mortality, but this did not eradicate the problem or the need for poor relief.[3] Instead particular categories of the poor assumed greater prominence and charitable institutions became more specialised to cope with their demands. Those who benefited most were widows, orphans and the sick.[4] The first two categories were the immediate living casualties of the Black Death and a number of Italian city-states passed legislation protecting them. Many widows and orphans had at worst been left disinherited or at best had to fight for their rights in an unfair battle, since theoretically in law they were unable to defend themselves personally in court. Greater emphasis on these groups can also be seen among Florence's confraternities. The most striking example was the great Company of Orsanmichele, which during the decade following the Black Death became the most affluent charity in the city and directed very considerable sums towards poor girls in need of dowries. Indeed, I have argued elsewhere that this confraternity may have subsidised the dowries of up to 20 per cent of girls getting married in Florence during the years immediately following the Black Death.[5] Interest in Florence in these two vulnerable sections of society did not decline once the immediate charitable funds made available as a result of the Black Death had been exhausted, but was institutionalised. In 1376 the hospice of the Orbatello opened with room to accommodate up to two hundred poor women, mostly widows, and in 1419 the hospital of the Innocenti was established for foundlings.[6]

The fifty years following the Black Death also saw a notable expansion of the city's institutional services for the sick poor through the growth of S. Maria Nuova and S. Paolo and the foundation of the two major hospitals of S. Matteo and Messer Bonifazio Lupi.[7] This chapter will examine the growth of the hospitals for the sick in relation to the development of the other thirty or so charitable institutions calling themselves *spedale*. In this way it will be possible to understand how their medical role fitted into their wider social and religious functions in the community, underlining the theme of this book: the complementary relationship between medicine for the body and medicine for the soul.

Nowhere is the closeness of the relationship between the religious and medico-social roles of hospitals more evident than in the period of the Black Death and the following century. On the one hand, hospitals became the recipient of bequests left for the benefit of the souls of their benefactors and, on the other hand, with the plague they suffered the severest challenge to their medical services they had yet encountered. Indeed, I shall argue that it was the Black Death and the subsequent recurrence of epidemics almost every ten years that led to the increased medicalisation of charity. More generally, this was part of a growing awareness of and response to the problems of urban disease, reflected in the expanding authority of the medical profession and an increase in public-health legislation and plague measures in many Italian cities.[8]

2.1 'The Hospital is a Great Charity': S. Maria Nuova and the Impact of the Black Death

All the major new institutions for the sick poor, widows and orphans dating from between the Black Death and 1450 were founded by single bequests of affluent individuals. As Messer Bonifazio Lupi said in his testament of 1377, he had established his hospital for 'the salvation of his soul and those of his ancestors',[9] an endowment that was increased subsequently through further legacies. Although the Black Death obviously did not initiate the process,[10] it did make a considerable impact on the fortunes of a series of charitable institutions of which S. Maria Nuova was a leading beneficiary. In his *Cronica*, Matteo Villani explains why the hospital was so favoured:

> And the hospital of S. Maria Nuova of S. Gilio was also left in that mortality [goods to] the value of 25,000 gold florins ... These bequests were distributed by the hospital very well, since the hospital is a great charity and always full of male and female patients, who are served and treated with much diligence and [given] an abundance of good food ... and looked after by men and women who lead a saintly life.[11]

This passage contains a similar eulogy of S. Maria Nuova as offered by commentators in later periods. Emphasis was placed on the hospital's size and reputation. The latter was based on the excellence of the care provided by 'saintly' nurses and the treatment prescribed by the physicians. Although the Black Death impacted considerably on S. Maria Nuova in terms of deaths among its personnel, the hospital continued to serve the sick during the Summer of 1348. Exactly what level of medical care was provided at the height of the plague is difficult to judge from surviving documentation, but the hospital took on new medical personnel to replace those who died. From 1 September 1348 the barber-surgeon Jachopo was contracted to 'come to cut the hair of the *famiglia* [resident staff] of S. Maria Nuova' and 'to let the blood of the *famiglia* and of the sick of the hospital'.[12] Then in the following May a physician, Maestro Francesco Noli, was employed to 'treat the sick of the hospital, the men and the women', and was soon joined by Maestro Tone.[13] Other entries in the account book provide a glimpse of the patients' diet, which was based heavily on poultry products, especially the chicken soup for which the hospital became so well known.[14]

S. Maria Nuova should not be allowed to dominate the picture of the provision of medical care in Florence. Those hospitals treating the sick poor well before 1348 continued to do so following the Black Death, as is evident at S. Paolo.[15] In February 1349 the hospital purchased a guide to treatment, 'un libro medicinale per sanità de' poveri', and its barber Sanuccio had evidently survived the plague.[16] Within ten years S. Paolo was employing two medical practitioners, the physician Maestro Fruosino at 6 gold florins a year and the surgeon Maestro Francescho di Ser Niccolò, at 10 gold florins.[17]

The excellence of S. Maria Nuova's services was clearly appreciated widely given the substantial sum of 25,000 gold florins bequeathed by testators during the Black Death.[18] Unfortunately the records of legacies to S. Maria Nuova are not complete, so it is not possible to test the accuracy of Villani's claim any more than it is for Orsanmichele and, anyway, the real value of legacies can only be assessed by taking into account payments of debts and beneficiaries.[19]

When Villani recorded the amounts left to Orsanmichele and S. Maria Nuova he was at pains to contrast the honesty and probity of the officials who ran the hospital with the dishonesty of those who administered the confraternity, whom he alleged diverted the funds for their own ends.[20] As I have discussed elsewhere, assessing the accusations of corruption levelled against the captains of Orsanmichele is not straightforward. While they may have been lining their own pockets, the commune also wanted an excuse for facilitating the process of diverting its monies into its own coffers. Even if the republic did not attempt to influence the election of the *spedalingo*, as it had in the case of Orsanmichele's captains, the priors were still evidently interested in the hospital's finances. In 1351 the *spedalingo*, Ser Guido di Baldese da Fronzola, was imprisoned by them in the debtors' prison of the Stinche, as recorded by the hospital's notary: 'Item we paid [10 lire] on 5 August when Ser Guido was arrested by the priors and was put for twelve days into the Stinche for not having wanted to give the money from the poor to the Priors and then he did not pay them anything. God be praised.'[21]

Apart from this cryptic note there is little evidence of the commune's success in siphoning off money left for the poor. The experience of the Black Death must have put severe strains on the hospital's finances, particularly if, as Villani claims, on the eve of the plague it was 'always full of male and female patients'. Conditions in S. Maria Nuova must have been appalling: there is no evidence that the hospital was spared the high mortality suffered by other institutions.[22] Indeed, in the following autumn its notary recorded that the plague had caused the death of the 'majority of the hospital's staff'.[23] Administrative order was restored gradually after the appointment of a new treasurer on 10 September 1348 and of more staff to run the hospital and look after the patients. In fact, one of those who had died during the Black Death was the *spedalingo* himself, the priest Orlando di Pierozzo da S. Casciano.[24] He was replaced on 29 June 1348 by another *spedalingo*, and even though, as recorded by the notary, 'the said Ser Guido [di Baldese da Fronzola] was sick for much of the time',[25] he survived in office for another twenty-two years.[26]

As Orsanmichele had found in the same period, it could prove difficult to obtain the promised funds from bequests to pay for the services required by the testators, leaving the hospital in debt. This is reflected in a letter addressed by the *spedalingo* to the captains of Orsanmichele in 1355–6 asking for alms for the sick, who were 'in much need':

> To you, Lord Captains of the Company of the Virgin Mary of Orsanmichele, the hospital director and those that serve the sick of the hospital of S. Maria Nuova send you many greetings and pray for the love of God and of the Virgin Mary that you help to give alms to them in order to satisfy the needs of the said patients who have many sicknesses and are in much need and may the Holy Spirit illuminate you in as much as you can do. Amen.[27]

The financial needs of the hospital as it expanded remained a constant theme over the following fifty years. The commune also retained its interest in what was perceived as being a potentially useful source of income. In August 1363, for example, a law was passed that gave the priors access to monies received through inheritance by S. Maria Nuova along with the hospitals of S. Gallo and S. Maria della Scala, adding to the list of confraternities that also fell into this category: Orsanmichele, the Misericordia, the Bigallo and the company of S. Zanobi. The commune could now borrow from these corporations all revenues accruing from bequests received since 1345 as well as property inherited during the following twelve months. These sums were to be used to pay the creditors of the commune and provision was made to repay these 'loans' within a period of ten years.[28] A major reason that the commune remained interested in S. Maria Nuova was, as Samuel Cohn has argued, because hospitals in general and S. Maria Nuova in particular came to receive an increasing proportion of legacies left to pious causes in Florence.[29] Indeed, as will be seen in the following section, new hospitals appeared during the century following the Black Death, a reflection of the general belief in the efficacy of their role in a period characterised by a heightened awareness of the problems of epidemic disease.

2.2 'For the Poor of Christ of Both Sexes Who Languish and Are Sick': New Foundations in the Early Renaissance[30]

In contrast to the pattern in some countries north of the Alps, hospitals continued to be founded in Florence during the century following the Black

Death: 25 per cent of the total for the whole period (1000–1550), or seventeen new ones, appeared between 1350 and 1449 (Table 2.1).[31] Though this was fewer than during the previous hundred years, it was more than made up for by the very substantial scale of some of these new foundations. This was part and parcel of the wider process of charitable specialisation. For example, five of the new hospitals were designed specifically for women. This, as discussed above, was part of a wider awareness of the vulnerability of women during this period, in particular of the unmarried and widows.[32] Another increasingly obvious feature was the greater specialisation of the larger institutions in contrast to the smaller ones, which remained more general in their scope. These smaller hospitals remain particularly difficult to categorise since contemporary descriptions are often vague, compounded by the fact that different records often refer to them as having different functions. This is particularly true of the first two categories in Table 2.1, 'pilgrims and travellers' and the 'poor'. The way in which these functions overlapped is well expressed by Benedetto Varchi in his brief account of the city's hospitals in the 1520s: 'The other type of hospital is that which receives and gives lodging not only to travellers and other healthy people, but also to the poor of the city, who for a night or two receive food and lodging without paying anything.'[33] Evidently little distinction was made between local inhabitants and those from outside the city when offering temporary accommodation, in contrast to many early modern relief systems which emphasised the obligation to the local poor and tended to send away those from elsewhere.

Table 2.1 Typology of hospitals founded in Florence, 1350–1449 and 1250–1349

	1250–1349	1350–1449
1. Pilgrims and travellers	6	6
2. Poor	5	1
3. Sick	6	3
4. Old	–	–
5. Foundlings	1	1
6. Women	–	5
7. Artisans	3	1
8. Religious	2	–
9. Unknown	6	1
Total	29	18

Source: Appendix, pages 341–55

If there was a detectable change in the typology of hospitals founded in Florence in the century following the Black Death, their topographical distribution largely extended the pattern of the previous century (Map 2.1). In this period the vast majority of hospitals were established in the suburban areas where land was more readily available. One of the immediate effects of the high mortality of the Black Death and the epidemics that hit Florence almost every decade was that the population remained at a much lower level than in the first half of the Trecento: 1351: 42,000; 1362: 65,000; 1401: 60,000; 1427: 37,000; 1480: 40,000.[34] There was less demand for new streets of the small-scale domestic terraced housing typical of Florence's construction industry before 1348. Instead the fifteenth-century city saw the erection of new large-scale patrician palaces.[35]

These two themes are also reflected in the construction programmes of hospitals in the second half of the fourteenth century. Many of the smaller foundations were established in pre-existing houses bequeathed to an organisation like a confraternity for conversion to charitable uses. This period was also typified by ambitious new building programmes, as with the enlargement of S. Maria Nuova and S. Paolo. Completely new large-scale hospital

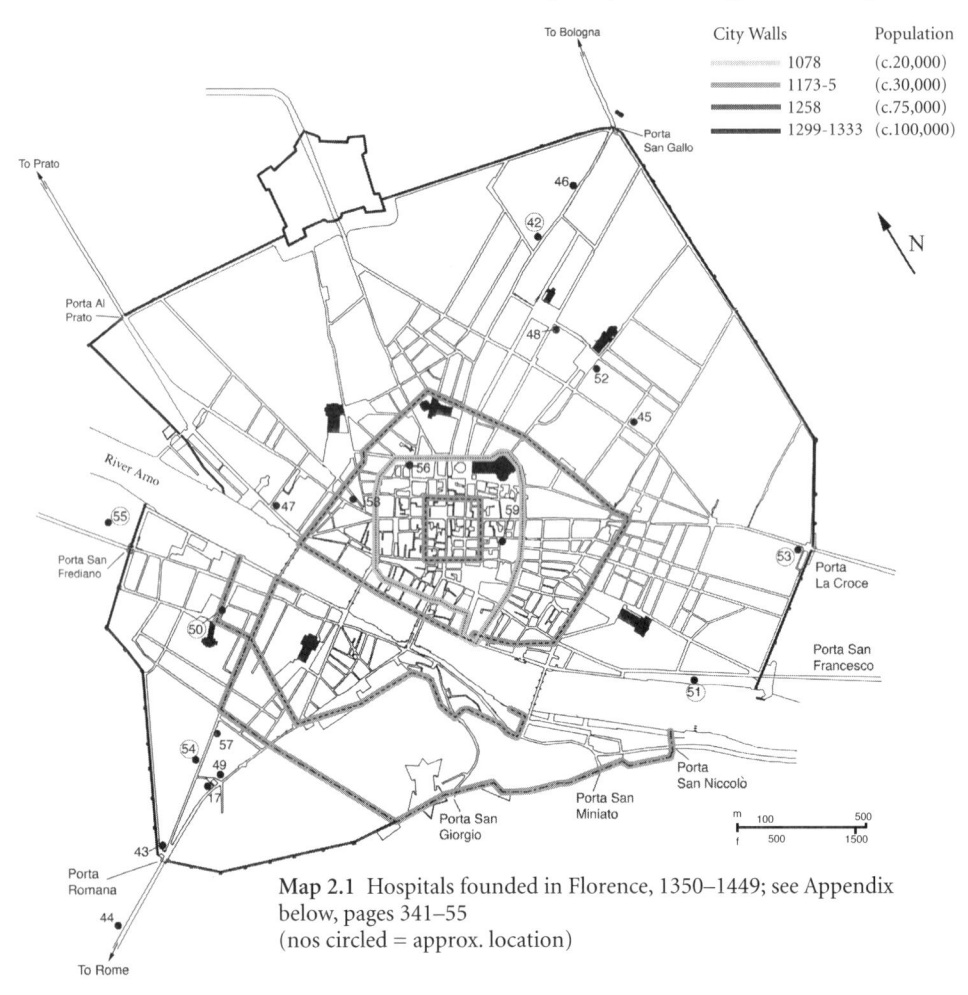

Map 2.1 Hospitals founded in Florence, 1350–1449; see Appendix below, pages 341–55
(nos circled = approx. location)

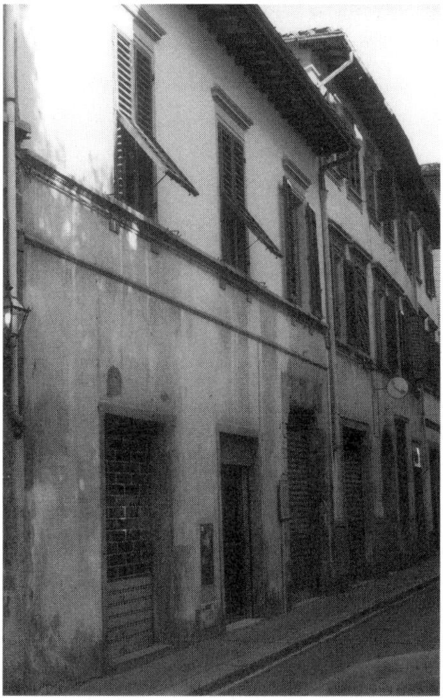

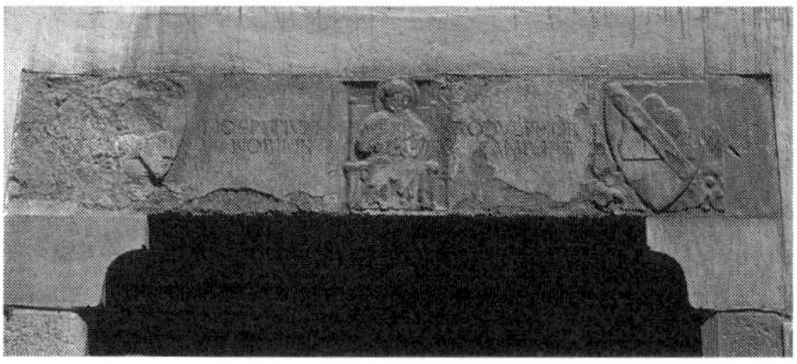

Plate 2.1 Spedale di S. Piero Novello dei Ridolfi, Via Romana
a. Façade; b. Architrave with inscription and Ridolfi family coat of arms

complexes were also constructed, most notably Messer Bonifazio in Via S. Gallo, S. Matteo on Piazza S. Marco, and Brunelleschi's famous foundling home of the Innocenti on Piazza SS. Annunziata, which has become synonymous with the graceful elegance of Renaissance architecture.

The location of these new hospitals depended on the availability of land, and the tendency was to build on the edge of built-up areas; the Innocenti looked out over a series of gardens and fields towards the city walls. When Messer Bonifazio was established on Via S. Gallo, the street was still surrounded by fields and gardens, though the area was rapidly built up as it developed into the largest concentration of religious and charitable institutions in the city.[36] Only S. Matteo was founded on a site that had already been developed (as part of the convent of S. Niccolò).

As in the previous hundred years the main arterial roads of the city proved particularly popular as a location for hospital foundations (Map 2.1). In the south of the city seven new hospitals were founded on one of the two main streets leading to Porta Romana. The hospital of S. Pier Novello, for example, was established in Via Romana the year after the Black Death. It contained ten beds to provide overnight accommodation for the poor (40).[37] As can be seen from Plate 2.1a, this was a simple two-storey terraced house, typical of artisan dwellings in this area. The founder, Piero di Cione Ridolfi, was a member of a

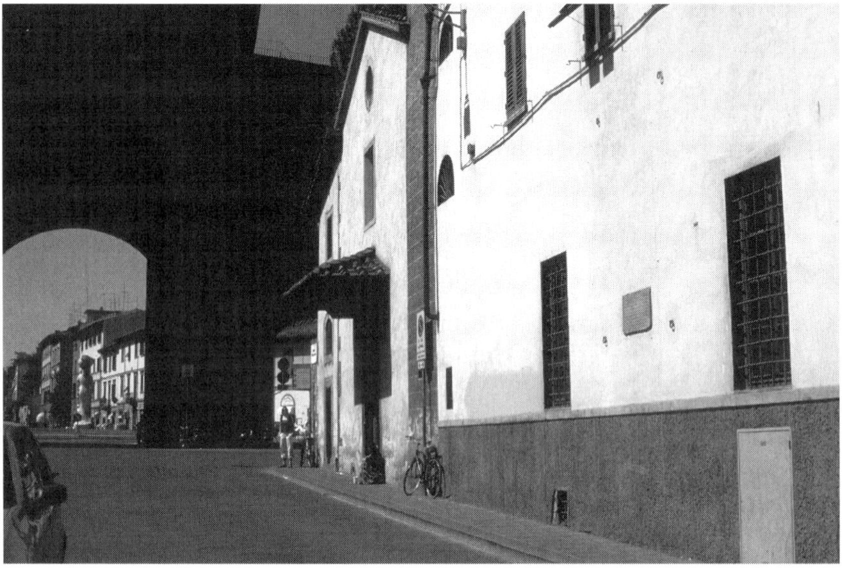

Plate 2.2 Spedale di S. Giovanni Battista della Calza, Piazza della Calza

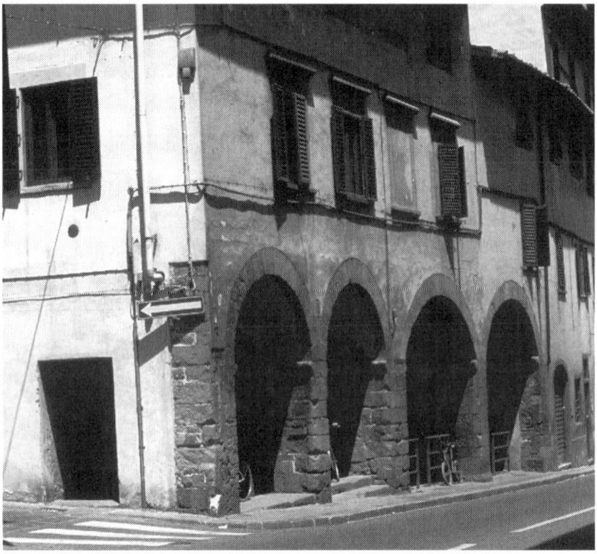

Plate 2.3 Spedale di S. Giuliano a Colombaia, Via Senese

major patrician family, whose coat of arms can still be seen above the main door leading into the hospital, as well as a rather worn inscription reading 'Hospitalium Nobilis Rodolphus Familiae' (Plate 2.1b).

Next to Porta Romana was the hospital of S. Giovanni Battista della Calza, founded in 1362 by the Knights of St John of Jerusalem (43), the second hospital associated with the order in the Oltrarno.[38] The first had been

S. Sepolcro to the south of the Ponte Vecchio, which had passed to the order in 1311 after the dissolution of the Knights Templar (4) and which was badly damaged in the 1333 flood.[39] The role of the Calza was to look after the poor and sick, and its proximity to Porta Romana (Plate 2.2) suggests it would also have provided accommodation to travellers. Significantly, though, its function was not linked to pilgrims, reflecting a more general decline in this as a declared role of new foundations. One exception in this part of town was the Spedale di S. Giuliano a Colombaia (44) on the Via Senese, established in 1363 by another patrician, Messer Pagholo Boccucci dei Vettori. The hospital declared in its tax return in 1428 that its function was specifically to 'lodge poor pilgrims passing through the city' for whom it provided twenty-four beds.[40] The reason for adopting this role may very well be linked to its position outside the city walls on the road leading south towards the convent of S. Gaggio and the village of Galluzzo (Plate 2.3). Much of the original structure still survives and, as can be seen from the view of its façade, the ground floor consists of a loggia, which would have acted as a reception area for pilgrims and travellers where they could rest and be refreshed, in much the same way as the loggia in front of the company of the Bigallo in Piazza S. Giovanni was used to receive abandoned children.

New hospitals also appeared to the eastern and western parts of the city (Map 2.1). S. Maria dell'Umiltà, for example, was established in 1380 to the west in Borgo Ognissanti (47). The founder was an affluent silk merchant called Simone di Piero Vespucci, who intended the hospital for poor sick men and women who were to be treated with both secular and spiritual medicine. He provided eighteen beds and petitioned the pope to allow him to erect two altars in the hospital.[41]

The archives of many of these hospitals, especially the smallest, have vanished. Therefore the survival of the 1427/30 direct tax returns of the Catasto provide an invaluable source of information to supplement our knowledge of their activities, capacity, personnel and finances.[42] Even if hospitals, in common with other religious institutions, such as convents, confraternities and churches, were tax-exempt, they still had to make a declaration of their assets and expenses. The Catasto officials appear, with a few exceptions, to have been surprisingly successful in obtaining compliance in submission of returns, even in the countryside.[43] The following section will explore further the activities of some of the thirty-five hospitals listed in Table 2.1, though the major medical hospitals will be examined separately.

The Catasto returns of the hospitals categorised as for 'pilgrims and travellers' and the 'poor' contain variable types of information, from a description of their function (S. Giuliano a Colombaia) to the salaries of the *spedalingo* and his wife, who at S. Lucia de'Magnoli 'maintain the [twenty-one] beds of the said hospital'.[44] The presence of permanent staff was essential, for these institutions were not all small and obscure, as seen in the case of S. Giuliano a Colombaia, with its twenty-four beds, and S. Maria dell'Umiltà, with eighteen.[45] Sometimes their returns contain no information about function, as with the Spedale della Cappella di S. Maria del Fiore, which simply recorded that 30 florins were paid to a chaplain to officiate in the chapel and 10 florins were spent on the maintenance of its property.[46]

Although the Catasto returns of hospitals in this general category give little indication of how their clientele were defined, there was some variation in terminology, as between S. Giuliano in Verzaia's 'poor of God', S. Salvadore's 'poor people' and the Ceppo's 'spiritual poor'.[47] Even if all basically meant indigents without a roof over their heads, these terms did distinguish the institutions from the other hospices whose declared function was to put up travellers and pilgrims, as with the Broccardi's male and female hospices for 'men and women travellers' and the so-called 'Spedaluzzo delle Donnucce' for female pilgrims from Spain.[48] However, these hostels for pilgrims and travellers were self-defining in that they restricted the length of stay of their guests. The Spedale di S. Lò, founded in 1361 to provide 'six beds for pilgrims' ruled that no guest was allowed to remain for longer than three days. Restrictions on the length of stay also became more widespread among the larger medical hospitals, such as at S. Maria Nuova by 1330 and at Messer Bonifazio in the following century.[49]

Some of the new *spedali* were designed for men who worked in the same profession, although traditionally these had been rather few.[50] Each of the four represented in the Catasto of 1427–30 appears to have been a simple affair, consisting of a house for the *spedalingo*, a small chapel and a room where poor members of their trade could sleep. Some idea of the state of the accommodation can be gained from the contents of an inventory of the Spedale di S. Giovanni Battista in Via S. Gallo which was run by the porters from Norcia:

28 old bedsteads and 28 used straw mattresses
8 cloth bed coverings, good and bad
8 mattresses in bad condition
5 pairs of used sheets
1 pair of sheets in good condition and three old chests[15]

Underlining its spiritual role, the *spedale* had a humble chapel which contained a wooden image of its patron saint, St John the Baptist, and a table with two trestles, probably to serve as an altar when Mass was celebrated.

Even if these artisans' hospices were small-scale – containing between six and thirteen beds – they did provide necessary accommodation for members of their trade from outside Florence. They would also have provided accommodation for elderly fellow tradesmen, as did the single largest category of hospital in the period 1349–1450, those for women.

The emphasis on women points both to the general movement towards the specialisation of charity and to an increasing awareness of the plight of women in post-Black Death Florence. The wide age-gap between spouses, with men marrying on average at thirty and women at eighteen, led to a growing pool of single women, exacerbated by the tendency of men to predecease their partners. Widowers also tended to remarry younger women, underlined by the relatively low rate of remarriage for women. All these factors led to the establishment of houses providing either temporary or permanent accommodation for women. These facilities may not have been lavish when compared with potential demand – three out of five had space for fewer than ten women – but they did nevertheless provide a solution for the fortunate few.

Hospitals in this group were distinguished from the majority of *spedali* because they tended to be for long- rather than short-term residents. The exception was 'the Spedaluzzo delle Donnucce' for Spanish women pilgrims (56).[52] The specific nature of its calling probably reflects that it was founded under the terms of a bequest of a Spanish resident. The same was true of many of the other small hospices for poor women; for instance, Lisa di Ranieri Paganelli's foundation in 1430 for four widows of honest life of at least fifty-five years of age (57).[53] Inevitably, given the nature of tax returns little information is provided about the residents of these institutions. One exception was the Spedale delle Devote della Vergine Maria on the Piazza di S. Maria del Carmine (50). This was run under the terms of a bequest of 1403 by the Laudesi confraternity of S. Agnese, which met in the nearby Carmelite church. There were seven women present, varying in their declared age from twenty-five up to eighty, with an average age of over forty-four. Sickness and old age were given as reasons for support. One, Monna Maria, widow of Andrea d'Antonio da Firenze, who was allegedly eighty, was described as 'ill and does not leave bed', while another, Monna Sandra, orphan of Maso da Firenze, who was only twenty-five, was clearly beyond help: '[she] has been sick for a year or more and from this illness will not ever recover except when she dies from it [sic].'[54] These women suffered from chronic conditions or disabilities such as blindness rather than the acute sicknesses that were more typical of the patients of the large medical hospitals. Whether sick or not, their main claim to the charity of the confraternity was that they were unable to support themselves. Only one was stated to be a widow, while the others were described as being daughters of deceased fathers, as in the case of 'Monna Nicholosa, daughter of Giovanni da Casentino deceased, aged fifty, crippled and sick'.[55] In both instances they evidently lacked adequate support from male relatives.

All these hospices were on a relatively modest scale and served the needs of no more than a few women who were handpicked by the board of a guild or confraternity. The need to fulfil certain requirements of respectability would also have lain behind the selection of the residents of the largest women's hostel, the Orbatello (45). This *ospizio* was established in 1372 by Niccolò di Jacopo Alberti, a leading member of the post-Black Death city government. He died in 1377 and left the patronage of the Orbatello to his family. However, two years later the Alberti were exiled and patronage devolved to the Captains of the Parte Guelfa, the body responsible for administering the goods of exiles. When finished, the Orbatello was remarkable for its size. It had two hundred separate rooms and housed a hundred women, mostly widows, each of whom was allocated two rooms and a shared kitchen with her neighbour.[56] Though granted free accommodation, they were not provided with food, which had to be earned through their own work or from alms.

If institutions for poor women were differentiated from the vast majority of charitable institutions in Florence by the provision of long- rather than short-term assistance, the same was true of another type of *spedale*, the foundling hospital. There were three in Florence: the earliest was S. Gallo; the second, S. Maria della Scala, dated from the early fourteenth century; and the third, the Innocenti, was in the process of being built in 1428 as it recorded in its Catasto return: 'Also the said guild, Arte di Por S. Maria, is having built a hospital on the Piazza de' Servi of Florence to receive poor abandoned children.'[57] Another feature serving to distinguish these orphanages from the average *spedale* was their size. In 1428 S. Maria della Scala had 152 children in its care, in 1448 S. Gallo had 150, and the Innocenti 700 by 1469.[58] By the middle of the fifteenth century these three institutions together would have catered for about a thousand abandoned children.

The Catasto return of S. Maria della Scala provides us with a snapshot of the overall activities of a foundling hospital in the early fifteenth century,[59] and is particularly useful as a counterbalance to the normal discussion of the subject which tends to be dominated by the Innocenti.[60] S. Maria della Scala had developed into a fairly large-scale operation during the hundred years since its foundation. The 152 children in its care required different kinds of treatment depending on their age and sex. Thus, for instance, abandoned babies were sent out to wet-nurses in the countryside. The hospital had 106 women on its books who acted as *balie*, although evidently they were not all employed in 1428 because only sixty-seven babies are recorded as being at a wet-nurse. The average age of these infants was one year and eight months and, in common with the sex ratio discovered at other foundling hospitals, more female children were abandoned than male: fifty-one compared with sixteen.[61] While the majority were infants, the *balia* usually retained a child until three years old. If they survived, they were then returned to S. Maria della Scala. In 1428 there were fifty-eight girls and twenty-seven boys living in the hospital with an average age of six years and eight months. Thus, the vast majority of children were under ten, although again there was a bias in the sex distribution; only one of the twenty-seven boys was over the age of eight, compared with twenty-six of the fifty-eight girls.

Sex differences in abandonment practices and the subsequent treatment of the foundlings reflect differences in contemporary attitudes towards male and female children. The higher value placed on males explains both the smaller number who were abandoned and why they were removed at an earlier age, either to apprenticeship schemes or as a result of being reclaimed by their parents. The girls remained longer at S. Maria della Scala. Two women were employed to 'teach the boys of the house to read', while a third, one of the hospital's nurses, was paid an annual salary of 4 gold florins to teach the girls of the house to 'cut [cloth] and to cook'.[62] In this way the foundlings were taught a series of skills to turn them into useful members of society; the boys were given a modicum of education and the girls were prepared for marriage and employment in the city's textile industry.

One of the features of both of these last two categories of *spedale*, for poor widows and children, was an interest in sickness, reflecting the fact that these two stages of the life-cycle were the most susceptible to disease. Hence the employment by S. Maria della Scala of Maestro Benedetto as house doctor and barber, and the presence of the sick women in the Spedale delle Devote della Vergine Maria.[63] When the Innocenti opened its doors in 1445 it employed three well-known physicians as well as a barber, who was contracted to 'shave, draw blood, and treat the *famiglia*'.[64] S. Gallo had even more medical staff: a physician, a surgeon and two barbers; now it looked after foundlings, and also received and treated the sick poor. In 1427 S. Gallo declared that it had 'thirty beds where they put up the poor'; some, if not all, of these were unwell, a fact reflected in the amount of money spent 'buying linen and woollen covers for the sick'.[65]

These examples of hospitals for women and foundlings indicate that many types of hospital became more medicalised during the century following the Black Death. This process was not simply a function of their acceptance of the sick poor, since the dividing line between care and cure had always been very fluid, but more overtly of their increased employment of trained medical staff. The shift was most evident in those large hospitals designated as being for the sick poor which became such a feature of Florence from the late Trecento. However, before examining in more detail the foundation of the new, more general medical hospitals and the expansion of existing ones, I shall first return to examine the fate of the two small-scale medical hospitals discussed above in

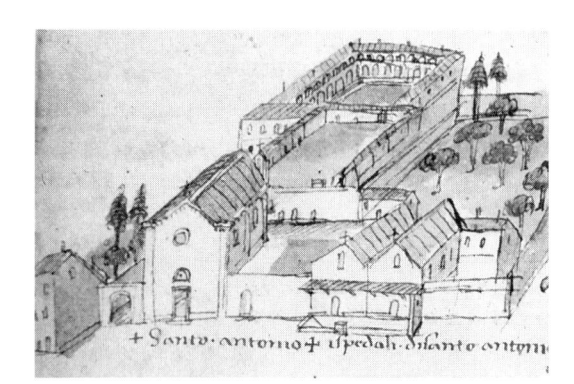

Plate 2.4 Codice Rustici, *Spedale di S. Antonio*, c.1445

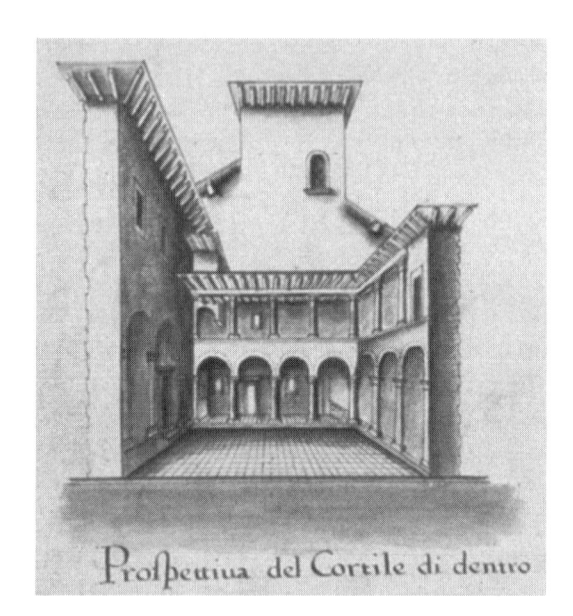

Plate 2.5 The leprosarium of S. Eusebio at Campoluccio (1709–10)

Chapter 1, which dealt with victims of two chronic epidemic diseases, S. Antonio and S. Jacopo a S. Eusebio (Appendix, nos 35 and 7).

S. Antonio was run by the Order of St Anthony of Vienne for those suffering from St Anthony's Fire.[66] By 1428 its premises were described in its Catasto return as 'the church, hospital and house of Antonio of Florence with the orchard or indeed garden and two small houses all linked together in the parish of S. Lorenzo of Florence, the place called S. Antonio'.[67] This description can be supplemented by the mid-fifteenth-century view from the Codice Rustici (Plate 2.4). S. Antonio occupied quite a large site, which contained the original church of S. Antonio, two parallel buildings at the front, probably the male and female wards, three linked cloisters, which grew larger the further they were from the street, a garden and a series of hospital buildings.

Even if this property suggests self-sufficiency in material and spiritual terms, no further information survives to flesh out the details of the treatments available to the occupants. It is known, however, that S. Antonio was held in esteem by the republic. In 1446 a special law was passed ordering the leading officials of the city's guilds to process to the church and make offerings there on 19 January, the feast day of S. Antonio, a procession that was joined after 1450 by the leading members of government.[68]

The Catasto return of the leprosarium of S. Eusebio was considerably better documented than that of S. Antonio.[69] As has been seen in Chapter 1, S. Eusebio had been founded in the late twelfth century on the road to Prato.[70] This whole area, which came to be known as the Prato d'Ognissanti, was enclosed by the new city walls of the early Trecento and led to the creation of a split site. The hospital director continued to live at the intramural site, but in 1338 a new leprosarium was created outside the new city walls at Campoluccio, where by 1428 the *spedale* catered for seven lepers. A hundred years later this number had been reduced to just two.[71] According to an inventory of the hospital's possessions of 1410, the main site of S. Eusebio consisted of 'the house of the hospital director of the said hospital with church, courtyard, basement and the main room, bedroom, well, orchard and garden in Florence in the parish of S. Lucia d'Ognissanti on the Prato'.[72] Like other hospitals it had a main administrator, called the guardian, who in 1428 was paid an annual salary of 36 florins plus his board and lodging.

The 1410 inventory provides a basic description of the extramural site at Campoluccio: 'A building for a hospital with houses and living area for the hospital director and the church in phase of construction, where the patients live and are treated outside of the city of Florence.'[73] This complex can be seen in an eighteenth-century view (Plate 2.5), which shows the courtyard, two-storey loggia and surrounding buildings. Once again both the physical and the spiritual health of the patients was catered for in ward and church. Though this hospital was not large it was staffed by a number of full- and part-time men and women who tended to the needs of the lepers. In 1410 the Campoluccio hospital was run by a man and wife, Piero di Giunta and Monna Francesca. The leprosarium employed a doctor, though it is not clear from the records whether the *medico* was a physician or a surgeon. Other expenses included clothing and 'necessary things' for the lepers as well as food for patients and staff alike. Purchases included wheat for making bread, meat, salt, oil, wine, and wood for cooking and heating the houses and hospital, while other consumables, such as fruit and vegetables, would have come from the *spedale*'s garden or its other properties.[74]

Despite the fact that there were few inmates, maintenance of the leprosarium was expensive. However, because the *spedale* was not full there was surplus income generated by their property to distribute to the poor. In addition, it owned some houses contiguous to the site which were either let out cheaply or rented free to 'povere persone'. It also owned a small house outside Florence in the parish of S. Piero a Sieve in the Mugello, which was used as a hospice to provide accommodation to 'poor travellers for the love of God'.[75]

By the mid-fifteenth century, then, Florence contained a wide variety of hospitals of diverse functions and sizes. Over the previous 450 years some fifty-eight *spedali* had been established and, even if not all survived for the whole period, at least forty-two were active in 1450, underlining the longevity of these institutions. Of these, almost half were founded during the hundred years after the Black Death, many of them by patricians or wealthy merchants. Their motivation, like that of the personnel who subsequently ran their foundations and tended to the needs of the sick and poor, was a mixture of the social and religious. The hospitals met a very specific need and there was no lack of demand for their services, despite the improvement in standards of living over these hundred years. Also, as underlined above, these institutions fulfilled an important religious role not just in the 'cure of the soul' of patients, but also in the spiritual health of the personnel and benefactors.

It is just as necessary to avoid losing sight of the wider social and religious context when discussing the two substantial new hospitals for the sick poor, those founded by Messer Bonifazio Lupi and Lemmo Balducci (S. Matteo), which opened in 1388 and 1410 respectively (Map 2.1 nos 46 and 48).[76] Both men came from outside Florence, as did Francesco di Marco Datini, the merchant who established the Innocenti. In this way the establishment of all three institutions symbolised the acceptance of three *stranieri* in Florence. In the process of building substantial new complexes, they also contributed to the magnificence of the Renaissance city.

Where Balducci and Datini were nouveaux-riches Tuscans, Messer Bonifazio Lupi came from further afield, Parma, and from a noble lineage. Lupi, who had been employed by the Florentine republic as a *condottiere* or mercenary, was, according to Matteo Villani, 'a solitary man of few words, but with a generous heart and known for his wisdom'.[77] He was made a citizen in 1370 and, wishing to commemorate his connection with Florence, he founded the hospital in 1388 out of his 'special love that he had and has still towards the people and city of Florence',[78] and more personally 'for the salvation of his soul and those of his ancestors'.[79]

Lemmo Balducci came from Montecatini, a small town to the north-west of Florence renowned for its thermal baths. He was a self-made man who had amassed his fortune in banking, but because his methods were not entirely legitimate – or perhaps lacked the right contacts to cover his tracks – he was declared a manifest usurer in 1384 and forced by the bishop of Florence to make restitution to some of his victims and to provide 200 gold florins for the poor.[80] This episode apparently convinced Balducci to mend his ways and since he was no longer a young man – he died five years later – he began to think more seriously about the health of his soul. The following year he decided to establish a hospital for the poor,[81] more especially because, as was explained in Urban VI's bull of November 1389, a month before Lemmo's death:

> This Lemmo considering that everyone when he is dying and comes before Christ's tribunal will render account of what he has done in his life and that if he has considered the poor and those without goods during the pilgrimage of his life he will be liberated by God at this time and preserved and beatified during his earthly life and He will not deliver him into the hands of his enemies…[82]

The merchant of Prato, Francesco di Marco Datini, did not suffer the humiliation of being charged with usury, but he had made large amounts of money through a wide variety of enterprises including money-lending.[83] He was persuaded to found a hospital not through patriotism for his adopted city nor as restitution for wrongdoing, but rather owing to the prompting of a friend, the notary Ser Lapo Mazzei. The nub of Mazzei's argument was contained in a letter written to Datini the day after Christmas 1406, expressed in mercantile terms that would have been as familiar to his friend as to Lemmo Balducci: 'We have one chance to settle this account with Him … If for God's sake you could spare half an hour for Mass [so that] when God sees your alms, followed by your sacrifice, He will thank you heartily for not valuing false riches … God's love cancels out our multitude of sins.'[84] Another powerful argument employed by Mazzei a few years earlier was linked to the contemporary obsession with self-commemoration. He illustrated his point with a very specific example: 'Here [in Florence] is a large hospital that will always be known as the hospital of Messer Bonifazio.'[85] Certainly one or a combination of these arguments eventually led Datini to found first the Spedale del Ceppo in his native Prato and then the Innocenti in Florence in 1419.[86]

These three men founded their institutions from a mixture of motives familiar from other Renaissance patrons: from self-aggrandisement and self-commemoration to self-confessed affection for the city of Florence and above all out of concern for the health of their souls. If all of these were respectable motives from a contemporary perspective, they also reflect a specific desire to provide a service for 'the poor of Christ of both sexes who languish and are sick', whom their hospital wished as far as they could afford to 'receive, look after and take care of, retain and feed until they are cured or die'.[87] These sentiments express a new concern for the sick poor, which may stem from an increasing awareness of the causal link between sickness and poverty with the recurrence of plague every decade.[88] But, as suggested above, this was also part of a general move towards greater specialisation of charity during the 150 years following the Black Death. Datini, for example, was moved by both the penitential movement of the Bianchi and a plague epidemic, and made his will in summer 1400 in which he left half of his fortune to the foundling hospital of S. Maria della Scala in Florence.[89]

The hospitals of Messer Bonifazio and S. Matteo, in common with S. Maria Nuova and S. Paolo, represent a combination of the religious and the medical. Each was governed by a rector, who was normally a priest, and the sick were nursed by a community of pious lay men and women (*conversi* and *converse*), who together belonged to the *famiglia*.[90] A particular feature that came in time to distinguish these medical hospitals – with the exception of S. Maria Nuova – was that they were placed under the patronage and control of a professional guild. Both the leprosarium of S. Jacopo a S. Eusebio[91] and Messer Bonifazio were administered ultimately by the merchants' guild of the Calimala and S. Matteo by the bankers' guild of the Arte del Cambio.[92] Founders tended to choose the guilds of which they themselves were members, believing that by appointing these bodies they would ensure their wishes were maintained after their death. It was not long before S. Paolo followed suit, falling under the Arte dei Guidici e Notai in 1398. Patrons also placed their hospitals under the care of the silk guild of Por S. Maria; Pollini adopted this option for the Scala in 1351 in order to counter the influence of the Sienese parent hospital. Then, following the death of Francesco di Marco Datini, the executors of his estate assigned to the Arte della Seta the administration of the costly enterprise of building the Innocenti.[93]

The appointment of guild consuls as administrators appears to have ensured that the testators' wishes concerning the medical role of these hospitals were to a large extent fulfilled. Messer Bonifazio and S. Matteo employed two physicians and paid an annual salary to a barber to 'cut hair and let blood'.[94] Messer Bonifazio also paid a regular salary to an apothecary to work in its own *Spezieria* or pharmacy,[95] while S. Matteo sent out for its medicines in an already made-up form. The year before S. Matteo opened its doors in 1410 Maestro Giovanni da Radda placed a large order to stock its pharmacy with compounds and simples for the conditions he envisaged treating among its patients.[96] In common with S. Maria Nuova, all three institutions accommodated a good number of nursing staff: thirty-six in S. Matteo, twenty-six in Messer Bonifazio, and twelve tertiaries or *pinzochere* at S. Paolo.[97] In the case of the newer hospitals at least, there was a very favourable ratio between nurses and patients, with the latter receiving considerable personal attention.

The employment of trained medical experts, the purchase of medicines for the treatment of specific conditions and the existence of a substantial patient population all point to a process of 'medicalisation' in hospitals in Florence by the early Quattrocento. However, it is important to avoid drawing too linear a development. At S. Paolo, while the main emphasis may have been on the sick poor by 1370, a variety of functions was maintained. By this date it had revived the out-relief system even though the number of recipients had much diminished, a process paralleled at Orsanmichele;[98] it now made a monthly delivery of bread and sometimes wine to the debtors' prison of the Stinche; and later in the century it provided limited hospitality to poor pilgrims and the homeless.[99] Furthermore, just as the relationship between physical and spiritual medicine was close, so was that between care and cure: as the nursing staff of S. Paolo grew older and fell sick, so they too became patients.[100] These are subjects to which we shall return in more detail in later chapters. At this stage the important point to grasp is the scale of the activities of all these different hospitals and the significance of their contribution to the city's welfare.

There was considerable variation in size even among the medical hospitals. The smallest was probably that attached to the Stinche.[101] Although no information survives concerning the number of beds it contained, we do know that the commune paid an annual salary to a doctor to treat both those prisoners who fell ill and 'those who have a member amputated or removed at the Porta della Giustizia', the place of public execution where criminals were punished through death or amputation.[102]

As seen in the earlier sections of this chapter, the city's major medical hospitals were on a considerably larger scale than any other *spedali* in Florence, except those for foundlings. By the early fifteenth century S. Maria Nuova had 120 beds, S. Matteo 48, San Paolo 35 and Messer Bonifazio 31.[103] It should be remembered that to calculate the patient population one needs to double these figures, since it was normal practice to place two people in each bed. This would have meant that by the early fifteenth century these four hospitals alone would have provided in-house treatment for about 468 people at any one time,[104] and this is not taking into account either the many smaller *spedali* discussed above or their out-patient services. But this does not tell us anything about turnover; since patients stayed for only brief periods, the numbers treated each year could be very considerable. By the early sixteenth century S. Maria Nuova alone received on average 6,500 male and female patients per year, equivalent to about 10 per cent of the city's population.

It is less straightforward to assess the comparative significance of the number of hospitals in relation to the size of the population. In Florence, as Villani indicates, there were thirty hospitals in 1338 when the city's population stood at about 95,000. Comparison with contemporary Pisa, for example, where there were fifty-five hospitals for a population of less than half the number of citizens (40,000), would suggest that Florence was under-provisioned. But Milan in the same period had only ten hospitals for a population of 100,000.[105] These examples point to the difficulty in making a meaningful comparison, given the great discrepancies in sizes. To cite only the most extreme example: the Brolo in early Trecento Milan had a vast operation. It housed 500 patients, paid for 350 foundlings and gave out-relief to over five hundred poor people.[106] Even if this assessment of the Brolo's activities was exaggerated by the local chronicler Bonsevin de La Riva in his eulogistic description of the city, none of Florence's hospitals even approached this scale of operation in this period. But this is a complex question and will only be resolved with the publication of studies of comparable data about Italian hospitals where their capacity and turnover can be calculated in relation to the total population of the city.[107]

Though the scale and utility of Florentine hospitals seem to have been appreciated by contemporaries, the latter did not always comprehend the expense involved. Hospitals walked a thin line between debt and profit, often crossing over to the wrong side depending on the efficiency and probity of their administrative staff or being adversely affected by external epidemiological and economic factors. The final section of this chapter will examine the financial records of the larger hospitals in the late Trecento and early Quattrocento to provide a more detailed account of the more general changes presented so far.

2.3 Balancing the Books at S. Maria Nuova: 'It Is Believed It Would Today Have Owned Most of the Property of Florence through Bequests Left by Diverse People at Different Times If...'[108]

Economic historians have long recognised the importance of the financial records of late medieval and early modern hospitals in providing long-term data on the price of foodstuffs and wage levels, since these institutions played significant roles as employers, landholders and consumers. In Florence the account books of S. Maria Nuova present one of the most complete series of such records,[109] but they have never been analysed in detail to provide an overall picture of the hospital's budget. This section will first examine the main components of its budget in 1373–4, then compare them with those of fifty years before and after, and finally place them in the context of the finances of three other major medical hospitals in the late 1420s.

The main reason for choosing the mid-1370s for analysis is the survival of a new set of statutes and a detailed contemporary inventory of the hospital's possessions.[110] The hospital had become a very substantial financial operation (Table 2.2). Annual expenditure had increased, at least in nominal terms, by over seven times since the mid-1320s to over 20,000 lire.[111] Also, given that the hospital managed to balance its books in this year, income had also increased twenty-fold and indeed it was in the black by 1,786 lire, though most of this figure (1,526 lire) had been brought forward from profits of the previous financial year.

These substantial sums were a concrete reflection of Villani's statement about the income generated by the 'faith of the citizens' in the charity and integrity of those who ran the hospital. To gain some idea of the meaning of this figure in contemporary terms, 20,000 lire was equivalent to 25 per cent of the commune's receipts for the six-month period from November to April 1373–4 from one of the city's major sources of income, the 'gabelle' or indirect tax on wine sold retail.[112] In other words, S. Maria Nuova's operations were a significant contribution to the Florentine economy, helping to explain the commune's continued interest and support in its operation.

Table 2.2 Income and expenditure of S. Maria Nuova, 1373–4 (in *lire di piccioli*)

Income*	food/drink	wood	clothing	pharmacy	building	salaries	heirs	alms	Total expend	Total balance
22,137	6,728	613	1,727	1,053	1,651	3,947	4,394	238	20,351	1,786
	33%	3%	9%	5%	8%	19%	22%	1%	100%	

Source
Expenditure: SMN 4426; income: SMN 4427, ff 88v–104r
* Includes balance of 1,526 lire from previous financial year

The majority of S. Maria Nuova's income derived from bequests or property rental. Under the first category it received 8,334 lire; the size of the sum may have been swelled by that year's outbreak of plague between March and October, for charitable institutions usually benefited from periods of high mortality, also reflecting support for the hospital's role in housing plague victims since there was no separate lazzaretto.[113] Income from property was significant and can be divided into two sources: rent from houses in town and country (4,737 lire), and money from the sale of property and goods left to the hospital (7,062 lire). The hospital also derived a regular but smaller source of income from alms (1,036 lire). This consisted of first the 'cercha del denaro', the collection of alms by a hospital employee passing through the streets of the city, and amounted to little more than 5 lire a week. Second, there were receipts from the collection boxes on the hospital's premises at the entrances to the male cloister and the male and female wards.[114]

The greatly increased income compared with fifty years earlier also led to changes in the way that money was spent (Table 2.2). In the 1320s and 1370s the main preoccupation was the stomachs of patients and staff. Expenditure on food and drink can be divided into five categories: wheat and other grain for making bread (15 per cent), meat (26 per cent), poultry (14 per cent), eggs and fish (22 per cent), and finally wine (20 per cent). A distinction was made between different kinds of meat on the basis of the number of animals' feet: pork and beef were 'animals with four feet', while poultry such as chickens, pigeons and capons were described as 'flying animals with two feet'.[115] Only occasionally is it possible to determine from these account books purchases of specific food items intended for patients, as when they state 'fresh eggs for the sick'.[116] However, as one of the six non-naturals, diet was an important part of treatment and is a significant aspect of hospital life which needs much further investigation.[117]

Another significant item of expenditure shared by patients and staff was clothing and bed covers, which amounted to over £1,700, and included 'clothes made of linen and wool belonging to patients and to the members of the household and … cheap fur covers and nightcaps' – under- and over-clothes for both the sick and members of the community.[118] When patients entered hospital they put on clothes supplied by the personnel, reclaiming their normal clothes on exit. When patients died, their personal clothes were sold to second-hand clothes' dealers, whose inventories provide a guide to the financial health of their previous owners.[119]

The hospital now spent £1,053 on medicines, ten times the sum spent fifty years earlier. The vast majority of purchases were made from the company run by the apothecary Ugholino di Bonsi,[120] who also supplied materials for lighting the hospital, including large and small candles and tapers. Medicines purchased were for both internal and external use. The former included generic 'pills', ingredients for an electuary, aniseed as a cordial for the stomach and cassia to purge bile from the humours. Large quantities (88lb) of roses were bought for distillation into rose-water, which was used for its cooling properties and to disinfect wounds and lesions before they were covered with cotton, plasters and poultices.[121] The hospital inventory of two years later makes it clear that the medicines were now being prepared on site in contrast to the 1320s, when drugs prescribed had been ordered from an outside apothecary's workshop. Indeed, the size and contents of the pharmacy were impressive. Simple and compound medicines were kept in three separate areas: the pharmacy proper, the front room where an out-patient would have come with a prescription, and the separate upper and lower sections where medicines were stored in jars and containers.[122]

The emphasis on the medical side of the hospital's activities was reinforced by its contemporary statutes and the reiteration of the prohibition first enunciated in 1330 against anybody who was not sick staying longer than three days. Exception was only made for a member of the clergy who served in the hospital church of S. Egidio.[123] S. Maria Nuova also gave out alms to the poor. Some of the twenty-six individuals listed in this account book, who each received between 10 soldi and 3 gold florins, were evidently known personally to the staff, as in the case of the 'young daughter of Francesco, our servant for the love of God'. Others were paid to go on journeys for both their physical and spiritual health: 'Frate Franceschino, who is sick in the hospital and is paid 3 florins on 23 October [1373] to go to the baths', and Domenicho di Bartolo was paid on 2 April 1374, to go to 'S. Iachopo di Ghalizia for the love of God' as a pilgrim to Compostela.[124]

Salaries were another major expenditure underlying the development of the hospital's functions over the past fifty years (19 per cent). It employed a physician, Maestro Lucha di Cecho, and two barbers; by 1400 there were three physicians in addition to a surgeon and a full-time apothecary who lived on the premises.[125] The growth of S. Maria Nuova also included an expansion in its bureaucracy, with the employment of additional servants, notaries, clerks and lawyers (*advochati, prochuratori*), who were paid to represent them in court over disputed bequests or to provide advice (*consigli*), as did Messer Giovanni de' Ricci, who was a member of one of the main mercantile and ruling families of Florence.[126] Indeed, the continued importance of bequests is reflected in the hospital's budget. In this year 22 per cent of outgoings were associated with testamentary expenses, though skewed by payments from three testators who had made S. Maria Nuova their executor and heir.[127]

The amounts received and paid out under the terms of bequests underline the crucial importance of the hospital's dual religious role in providing commemorative Masses for patrons and spiritual succour for its patients. Many of the payments of 'money given for the love of God' were related to bequests and were to pay priests to say Mass for the souls of patrons and benefactors, above all those of the Portinari.[128] Commemorative Masses were held in both S. Egidio and the ward chapels where Folco di Ricovero Portinari and his sons Manetto and Accerito were buried.[129] Apart from benefactors, hospital directors also warranted splendid funerals, as in the case of Ser Piero Mini, who died on 20 October 1413. Filippo di Tomaso's company of apothecaries was paid the considerable sum of 30 gold florins on 16 November for the 'wax, sheets and drapes and benches for the burial of our father' and on 30 November the silk merchant Michele di Jacopo received 10 lire for four silk napkins for the cushions placed on the bier.[130]

The combined spiritual-medical role of the hospital was reflected in the rubric of the first chapter of the new statutes on 'How the poor must be received and looked after';[131] all the members of the hospital, including the *spedalingo, conversi* and servants, were admonished to take diligent care of the sick 'for the health of their souls'.[132] Religious imagery was central to the description of the hospital's patients, who were envisaged as 'almost like Christ in their persons'.[133] This was no pious throwaway line, but key to the very purpose of the hospital and the role of the staff who tended to the sick. Each patient was to be tended as though he or she were like the Son of God. This reflected the image of Christ the Pilgrim, popularised in Florence through the dedication of religious confraternities to this cult,[134] and in late medieval depictions of the reception and treatment of the sick, as in the illustrations to the *Liber regulae* of S. Spirito in Rome (see chapter 5).

The devotional life of S. Maria Nuova in the mid-1370s and its role in the 'cure of the soul' for patients and staff were reflected in the objects owned by the hospital.[135] The inventory of 1376 lists a long series of liturgical objects in S. Egidio, including vestments, choir books, small crucifixes, tabernacles and altarpieces, while account books record purchases for the ward chapels, such as a payment to the painter Andreuzza in 1374 for 'designing the altarpiece of S. Luca' in the male ward and to the smith Francesco Donati for two pairs of large iron candlesticks for the altars in both wards.[136]

The growth of all these religious, medical and administrative activities since the Black Death also led to developments in the hospital's physical structure. Even at the height of the epidemic in summer 1348 work continued on the roofs of the male and female wards and the main storeroom, and in the following months new projects were begun, including the hospital's infirmary,[137] and the projecting roof over the entrance to the men's ward as seen in Bicci di Lorenzo's fresco of 1424–5 (Plate I).[138] Further construction projects were pursued over subsequent decades.[139] In the autumn of 1368 work was begun on renovation of the chapel in the men's ward dedicated to S. Luca, who was also the patron saint of the painters' confraternity, which met regularly in front of the altar to celebrate Mass. Payments for building and decorative work were recorded until May 1369, when the 'new chapel' was finally consecrated.[140] New windows had been created in the chapel and mention was made of work on the tombs, presumably those of the Portinari family. The fact that it took some seven months to complete the restructuring of the chapel suggests a quite lengthy programme of expansion. This was followed by a burst of building activity on the women's side.[141]

As can be seen from Table 2.2, construction work was ongoing in 1373–4; 8 per cent of overall expenditure of £20,507 was devoted to building costs.[142] A convenient summary of the stage reached in the construction programme and how the spaces were used in the mid-1370s is provided by the 1376 inventory. The growth of the two wards over the previous forty years was reflected in their bed capacity (sixty-two: male; fifty-eight: female). An extra twenty beds were now provided for the nursing staff in their dormitories,[143] as were twenty

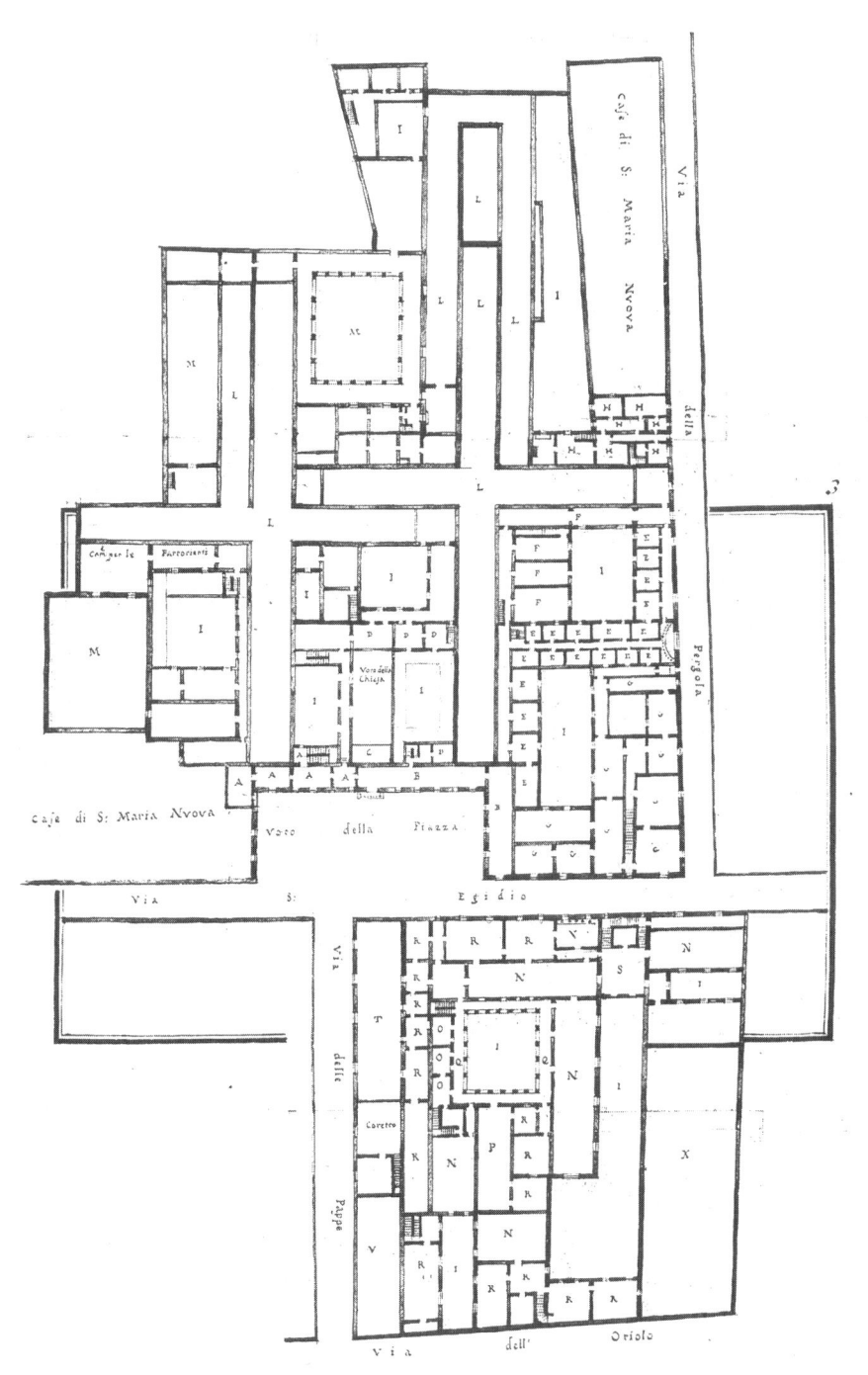

Plate 2.6 Ground plan of the Ospedale di S. Maria Nuova, 1780 (ASF, Ospedale di S. Maria Nuova 24: Plan 2)

bedrooms on the first floor for staff or reserved for members of affluent families and servants.

In addition to wards, refectories and cooking areas the ground floor also housed the offices of the administrative and ecclesiastical staff. The office of the *spedalingo*, for example, was placed at the front of the northern complex between the church and the male ward, reflecting a pattern common to hospital and monastic complexes (Plate 1.9, no. 5; cf. also Plate 2.6).[144] His living quarters on the first floor must also have been quite substantial and well furnished, judging by the number of objects listed in the 1376 inventory.[145]

The picture that has emerged of S. Maria Nuova in the late Trecento conforms to many of the characteristics of the Renaissance hospital identified by contemporaries. Discussion of the physical development of the other major medical hospitals will be pursued in later chapters, but at this point it is necessary to place S. Maria Nuova within a wider context by examining the finances and functions of other major institutions catering for the sick poor in Florence.

2.4 'Do Not Marvel That our Expenditure Exceeds our Income': Hospital Finance[146]

David Herlihy in his analysis of the Catasto returns of a series of religious institutions in nearby Pistoia concluded that hospitals were by far the richest corporations in the city. The budget of, for example, the Ceppo was nearly twice that of the very considerable budget of the bishop.[147] The same picture is true of Florence. In 1430 S. Maria Nuova's capital was calculated at 42,587 gold florins, which was 6,000 gold florins more than the very considerable wealth of the archbishop and the cathedral canons combined.[148] Although other hospitals did not approach the affluence of S. Maria Nuova, both S. Gallo and Messer Bonifazio (13,557 and 15,527 gold florins respectively) held substantial assets.[149] This placed the wealth of these hospitals at about the same level as the largest charitable confraternity of the city, Orsanmichele (14,947 gold florins), and not much below the combined assets of the now united Bigallo and Misericordia (18,085 gold florins).[150] The two other major medical hospitals, S. Paolo and S. Matteo, had capital of 10,430 gold florins (in 1438) and 8,186 gold florins, at much the same level as the largest and most affluent canonical church, S. Lorenzo, supported by the Medici family (9,359 gold florins).[151] As mentioned above, a hundred years later Benedetto Varchi stated that S. Maria Nuova would have owned most of the property in Florence 'if from time to time for the needs of the hospital and for other reasons the directors had not sold and alienated goods belonging to the hospital'.[152]

These hospitals were exceptional, for the majority were small, poor and, in common with many of the city's confraternities and parishes, had assets of under 300 gold florins in value. They ranged from hospices for pilgrims, such as SS. Jacopo e Filippo (249 gold florins) and the '*spedaluzzo*' of Spanish Donnucce (155 gold florins), to those for the poor in general, such as S. Salvadore (225 gold florins) and S. Lucia de' Magnoli (129 gold florins).[153] Evidently Florentines who patronised the city's hospitals – whether as founders or subsequent donors – chose to channel an increasing amount of their charitable funds into the larger-scale institutions dealing principally with the sick poor and foundlings. This dual mission came together in one of the city's oldest hospitals, S. Gallo, which provided thirty beds for the sick while fulfilling its principal role of looking after foundlings.

The main assets of most hospitals consisted of property in the city and the countryside, although the larger institutions tended to diversify their investment strategies. Property consisted of private houses, commercial shops and stalls in the marketplace, and farms, fields and vineyards in the Florentine *contado*.[154] The more enterprising directors of the larger hospitals managed their assets with a view to maximising their output. Giuliano Pinto has shown that S. Gallo, for example, adopted a deliberate policy to rationalise its landholdings over a number of years, mostly by selling off far-flung parcels of land and buying up farms in areas north of the city. In this way the land could be farmed more efficiently and fresh produce for patients procured more locally.[155]

Larger institutions such as S. Maria Nuova also became involved in a series of investment strategies, partly through inheritance and partly through the policies of individual directors. In common with the large charitable fraternities, hospitals were also left property and shares in the Monte Comune, the city's communal debt.[156] And from 1464, S. Maria Nuova itself offered a service to investors: interest of 5 per cent was paid to anybody who deposited money with the hospital.[157] This was an extension of a pre-existing role common to many ecclesiastical institutions, providing a safe-deposit box. The best-known example is when the Portinari themselves deposited in c.1480 the famous fleur-de-lys or crown jewels of Maximilian, archduke of Austria, weighing over 19lb.[158] More typical is the case of Curado the German:

> We record that Curado Tedescho from Nuremberg, a tall man with a red beard, gave on 12 April 1362 64 gold florins and said in the presence of Ser Jacopo from Arezzo and of Nastagio di Nino that if he did not return for these said 64 gold florins before 17 April 1362 that they should be given to the poor of the said hospital of S. Maria Nuova, and he left us also a gold groat which on one side had two saints and the other side one saint and he kept one which was the same. Curado reclaimed the said monies on 3 May 1362 in the presence of Nastagio and Ser Jacopo d'Arezzo.[159]

The surviving financial records of hospitals, such as the Ceppo in Prato or S. Maria Nuova, suggest that large sums passed through the hands of their treasurers. It has been calculated, for example, that between 1505 and 1515 Michelangelo deposited 11,252 large gold florins in S. Maria Nuova's account.[160] However, the provision of this service does not necessarily mean the hospital itself was enriched. As in the case of S. Maria della Scala in Siena,[161] it was quite possible for a hospital to be appointed as executor of substantial legacies, the proceeds of which were distributed to the relatives of the deceased or to other pious causes. In this way little might be left for the executing institution. Communal authorities recognised this as a problem and sought through legislation to protect both hospitals and religious confraternities so that they were able legally to refuse to act as executor for estates that were heavily in debt. During the first phase of the Black Death in April 1348, the Florentine commune had permitted the company of Orsanmichele to disclaim liability for debts exceeding assets by requiring an inventory to be taken before accepting any inheritance.[162] This and many other privileges were extended in August 1348 to both the company of the Misericordia and S. Maria Nuova, the other main charitable institutions to have benefited most from the largesse of testators during this and recent epidemics.[163]

This legal protection helped S. Maria Nuova to balance its books thirty years after the Black Death (Table 2.2), and continued to do so in the 1420s, by which time the hospital's income had more than doubled.[164] Although its complete tax returns have not survived, its contemporary account books enable one to calculate actual income and expenditure. As might be expected from such a venerable and affluent institution, annual expenditure was almost ten times that of even the other large medical hospitals, at 13,559 gold florins (Table 2.3). Remarkably enough its income was listed as 13,837 gold florins, leaving a positive balance of 278 gold florins, some achievement given the magnitude of the hospital's annual expenses. Thus, despite having been subjected to the same adverse economic and epidemiological factors as other hospitals, it was protected by a sufficiently large financial cushion. The balance had been achieved because it had brought forward its profit of 1,622 gold florins from the previous financial year.[165]

S. Maria Nuova was one of the notable exceptions to a general pattern of hospital indebtedness in the early fifteenth century. S. Matteo, for example, declared that it had a deficit, despite having been founded only forty-two years earlier. It had substantial holdings – 12 houses of various sizes, 19 farms, 4 vineyards and 3 shops – but was owed money by a large number of people. At the end of its tax return the administrator wrote: 'From all the above-listed debtors it is impossible to collect one penny either because [the person] is dead or has gone away or has gone bankrupt … so that we have to conclude that these debts are lost.'[166] While it would be easy to surmise from these laments that the hospital was exaggerating the parlous state of its finances to protect itself against the depredations of impecunious governments, this was a common complaint of hospitals in Florence and elsewhere. In the 1420s the Ceppo in Pistoia had a deficit of roughly 525 gold florins, while the Innocenti had incurred a debt of more than 1,000 gold florins owing to the expense of building. This pattern was also a feature of the smaller hospitals. The director of S. Maria in Via Chiara complained that it was always in debt because 'the alms and other income are always spent on the sheets and the hospital's other necessities', while the Spedale dei Preti told the Catasto officials 'not to marvel' that its expenditure exceeded income.[167]

If S. Matteo's negative balance was typical, was the way it spent its income typical too? The answer to this question can be addressed most systematically by comparing the returns of three other medical hospitals in the city: Messer Bonifazio, which was of comparable size; the smaller and more ancient leprosarium of S. Eusebio; and the largest of all, S. Maria Nuova (Table 2.3). Discussion of the expenditure of these four will be widened by drawing on the returns of other hospitals represented in the Catasto.

Although these four hospitals divided their budget along broadly similar lines, they did not all present their returns in the same way. Interpreting the significance of these differences is not straightforward. If one takes food, for example, S. Matteo and Messer Bonifazio devoted 76 and 61 per cent respectively of their total expenditure to this item, compared to just under 20 per cent at S. Eusebio and S. Maria Nuova. However, it is also important to look at the absolute figures: it is striking, for instance, that the amount spent on food by S. Maria Nuova was over 500 gold florins more than the combined expenditure of the two medium-sized hospitals.

The reasons S. Matteo declared such a high expenditure on food can be examined further because, unusually for Catasto returns, the administrators distinguished between food bought for the staff and that consumed by the sick. The first, the 'cost of providing food and drink to thirty-six mouths, including men and women who serve the sick and the gardener and priests and a cleric and a manager', was calculated at 12 gold florins a head per year,[168] while the second was estimated at 15 gold florins a head for forty-five patients. Part of the explanation for the large amount spent on food may lie in the small proportion it spent on salaries (5.5 per cent), especially compared with S. Eusebio (72.6 per cent). A proportion of S. Matteo's salary bill may therefore have been subsumed under the food budget, with many of its employees being paid partly in kind, including nurses, surgeons and apothecaries. Though if S. Matteo did not itemise its food bill, S. Gallo did. The latter declared that each year its 'forty-five mouths' consumed 40 *moggia* of grain, 50 *cognie* of wine, 24

Table 2.3 Hospital Expenditure in 1428: S. Matteo, Messer Bonifazio, S. Eusebio, S. Maria Nuova (in *fiorini d'oro*)

hospital	food	wood	clothes	pharmacy	building	salaries	heirs	alms	misc.	Total
SM	1,107	0	125	70	50	80	19	0	11	1,462
	75.7%		8.6%	4.8%	3.4%	5.5%	1.3%		0.8%	100%
BON	952	56	100	64	161	220	0	0	0	1,553
	61.3%	3.6%	6.4%	4.1%	10.4%	14.2%				100%
SE	19.5	1.9	0	0	0	72.1	0	5.8	0	99.3
	19.6%	1.9%				72.6%		5.8%		100%
SMN	2,520	255	739	587	1,666	301	7,491	*0	0	1,3559
	18.6%	1.9%	5.5%	4.3%	12.3%	2.2%	55.3%			100%

* alms subsumed under the building account

Source

SM: Catasto 185.II, ff. 601r–607r; **BON**: Catasto 291, ff. 25r–34r & 292, ff. 230v–232v

SE: Catasto 291, ff. 16v–23v

SMN 4476, ff. 34r–63v (income); SMN 4477, ff. LXr–CXVIr (expenditure)

cognie of oil, 2,000lb of *castrone*, 1,500lb of pork and 12 bushels of salt. Those fed at the hospital included three priests, a storekeeper, a cook, two clerics, a gardener, the hospital director and a wet nurse, as well as those who lived out, such as the physician, the surgeon and two barbers.[169]

The high proportion of income spent by S. Matteo on food (76 per cent) also underlines the important role of diet as one of the six non-naturals in the treatment of the sick and in maintaining the health of the staff. Many account books of the time record purchases of large numbers of chickens and eggs to produce the simple nourishing fare of broth for the sick. Along with the administration of drugs, this was regarded as an essential element in the overall regime of any patient, which helps to explain why medicines and other expenses associated with the pharmacy represented a relatively low proportion of the overall budget (a maximum of 5 per cent). However, as will be seen in Chapter 9, their importance in treatment should not be underestimated. Many of the simples used were plant-based and could either be bought cheaply or supplied from the hospital's own garden or property in the country. It should also be remembered that since this only represents a snapshot of their expenses in one year, these hospitals may have purchased more expensive medicines in previous years. Only S. Maria Nuova spent a considerable sum on refurbishing its large and well-developed pharmacy (587 florins), though the overall proportion of income was no higher than elsewhere.

Other expenses relating to both staff and patients were for the maintenance of beds and the purchase of clothes. Messer Bonifazio, for example, declared that it spent 50 gold florins each year on 'beds, nightshirts and blankets', and another 50 gold florins on 'clothes, socks, shoes for twenty-five people who serve the male and female sick'.[170] Inevitably the amount devoted to these items by S. Maria Nuova dwarfed that of even the other medical hospitals: it spent 739 gold florins to clothe and shoe staff and patients. At the smaller hospitals the maintenance of beds and washing of bedclothes was the largest annual expense after the *spedalingo*'s salary.[171] Indeed, some clearly did not have enough income to make proper repairs, judging by the description in the return of S. Maria del Bigallo: 'And in the said hospital there are thirty beds for the use of the poor and foreigners with small mattresses and old covers, old and torn, and split and ragged sheets.'[172]

The need to make repairs also explained why Messer Bonifazio devoted 10 per cent of its budget to its buildings. In this case it was the repair of roofs of both the hospital and its properties in town and countryside.[173] But it was S. Maria Nuova that spent most.[174] As mentioned in the Introduction, between 1418 and 1420 the hospital church of S. Egidio had been enlarged; from 1422 it expanded the cemetery (Chiostro delle Ossa), constructed the cloister known as the Chiostro delle Medicherie and then added a number of rooms for services including a grain store.[175] The expenses recorded in its account books of 1428 were thus part of an ongoing building campaign, which led it the next year to remodel its pharmacy and in 1437 to begin a five-year building programme on the women's ward.[176]

These Catasto returns also reflect the hospitals' important devotional roles, both in the cure of the souls of patients and staff and in the commemoration of the souls of patrons. To this end S. Matteo employed three priests and a cleric, Messer Bonifazio two chaplains and two clerics.[177] Other expenses included buying oil and wax for the candles and lamps lit in the church for the celebration of divine office. A hospital that had been in existence for some time might have accumulated quite substantial obligations: each year S. Eusebio paid out 140 gold florins and 158 bushels of wheat on 'ordinary expenses and obligations of testaments, commemorative meals and offices at certain churches and other expenses'.[178] Not surprisingly, the hospital for priests, Gesù Pellegrino in Via S. Gallo, was involved in extensive commemorative duties: each year it held 115 offices at 10 lire each.[179]

Again it was S. Maria Nuova that spent an inordinate amount, almost 7,500 gold florins, on heirs and testamentary obligations, a sum that had greatly increased since the mid-1370s, reflecting the growing importance of the hospital church of S. Egidio in the religious life of the city. The public celebration of festivals associated with their churches was also a feature of the smaller hospitals, for it was through the externalisation of their activities that they attracted public attention and sponsorship. The small dyers' hospital of S. Onofrio spent over 140 lire on its patronal festival, while the hospice run by the Laudesi confraternity of S. Spirito celebrated the Festa di Nostra Donna in March, with the performance of lauds in the vernacular by, among others, the *spedalingo*, Antonio di Pietro, who was described as a Laudesi singer.[180]

Though these Catasto returns provide a snapshot of the financial priorities in one year in the late 1420s, some presented the hospital's current financial position as representative of its recent history, especially when an institution wanted to emphasise that it was 'always in debt'. One aspect of this that was unlikely to be mentioned was the effect of periods of financial decline caused either by the negligence or even corruption of officials. A case in point is the alleged state of S. Paolo in 1425, which may help to explain the absence of its return among the Catasto records.[181] Over the previous century the hospital had gradually transformed itself from providing short-term accommodation and out-relief to concentrating on in-house treatment of the sick. But between the late fourteenth and early fifteenth centuries it went through periods of difficulty. The first of these was the result of a tug-of-war between the commune and bishop over the status of the hospital as a lay or ecclesiastical entity.[182] The Tertiaries resisted the Church's claim to the hospital, and therefore its property, and the squabble led to a full-scale investigation by Pope Martin V in 1425. According to the resulting Bull, the hospital was in a state of financial and moral disorder, although one must not forget the context for these statements. The findings were set out in passages of purple prose: 'that certain men of this order [Third Order of S. Francesco] and place have governed with the vice of ingratitude and have not feared to render bad for good, and have dissipated the goods and the houses of the said hospital and their privileges through which they have been honoured.'[183] These general accusations were then made more concrete:

> And the most important thing to consider is that these goods have been the subject of exquisite frauds and they were ashamed to put them into secular hands, and others were more seduced by a blind cupidity in using their dishonest hands to steal the goods and the rights of the said hospital; and if a solution cannot be found it will lead to the destruction of the hospital.[184]

It is quite probable that some financial misdealing had taken place in the recent past – the handling of large sums could obviously lead to abuses – but it is difficult to judge the truth of the papal allegations, given that these statements also provided a justification for the Church's plans to exercise greater control over the institution. The pope's reference to the 'exquisite frauds' of laymen may refer partly at least to the Church's dislike of the influence of the Guild of Judges and Notaries after it had become the hospital's patron in 1403.[185] Though no concrete evidence has survived to support the pope's accusations, this type of qualitative record does give a fresh dimension to the history of a hospital which is rarely provided in the drier financial records of the commune.

Conclusion

As this example relating to the history of S. Paolo reveals, the interest and intervention of outside authorities in the affairs of charitable institutions in the fourteenth and early fifteenth centuries were usually provoked by concern about money.[186] The priors of the republic provided protection against individuals who attempted to defraud charities of their inheritance, including administrators of these institutions accused of diverting funds into their own pockets or those of their friends. Whether official motivation was itself as pure as it was portrayed in legislation must remain questionable, especially when it was tempted by the rich pickings of a charity such as the company of Orsanmichele, which had become so affluent through inheritance during the Black Death.[187] Indeed, as has been seen, in 1351 the Priors had even thrown the *spedalingo* of S. Maria Nuova into prison because he had refused to hand over funds destined for the poor. In 1398 the hospital of Messer Bonifazio petitioned the commune for tax exemption and for the status of a 'locus pius' because it had been subjected to forced loans from the government. The petitioners declared that it was 'neither just nor fair that what belongs to the poor should be spent for other things'.[188]

It would be thus a mistake to assume that communal intervention in the affairs of hospitals was always motivated by predatory policies. Indeed, patrons petitioned the commune for help against outside agencies, as in 1351 when the Pollini family, patrons of the hospital of S. Maria della Scala, petitioned the Signoria for help, complaining that the foundlings were now looked after in a subhuman fashion because funds had been diverted to the Sienese hospital. In response the commune appointed a treasurer to take over the administration and placed the hospital under the control of the silk guild of Por S. Maria, an arrangement confirmed in an agreement with the Sienese hospital in 1371.[189] Protectionism remained one of the themes of public interest in hospitals over the following 150 years. Just as before the Black Death the major hospitals, especially S. Maria Nuova, received legal privileges to protect themselves against heirs who challenged the right of these institutions to inherit legacies, so many major hospitals received exemption from communal taxes, in particular from indirect taxes or gabelles.[190] Exemptions were usually obtained as a result of petitions by a hospital director, as when the *spedalingo* of S. Maria della Scala complained in 1395 about tax burdens exacerbating its general lack of funds and making it difficult to cope with the increasing number of foundlings.[191]

Money was not the only reason for Church and State becoming involved in the lives of hospitals. They also shared in the celebration of important events associated with these institutions, as is evident in the public ceremonies performed in front of the hospitals. These occasions played an important role not just in the life of a hospital, but also in that of the city itself, as with the reconsecration of the hospital church of S. Egidio by Pope Martin V in 1420. Public ceremonies involving the presence of secular and ecclesiastical leaders took place whenever a hospital was inaugurated, as at the Innocenti in 1445 and the consecration of its church in 1451 by Antoninus, archbishop of Florence.[192] Other hospital churches became the centre of guild and communal processions on their feastdays, as in the case of S. Antonio, where from 1446 offerings were made each year on 19 January by leading members of the guild community.[193] But none was quite on the scale of S. Maria della Scala in Siena where, following the hospital's acquisition of a large and important collection of relics from Constantinople, the commune voted that the hospital should henceforth be the centre of the city's celebration of the festival of the Annunciation, at which the communal magistrates were present.[194]

Public involvement in the ceremonial role of hospitals in city life reflected local pride in these institutions and led both citizens and visitors alike to write eulogistic descriptions of Florence's hospitals underlining the main characteristics of the Renaissance hospital, including the impressive scale of the buildings and conscientious medical treatment of the sick poor. These appreciative comments were part too of the priors' increasing concern for the health of the community, for hospitals such as S. Maria Nuova and S. Matteo bore the brunt of dealing with those sick from epidemic disease since there was no dedicated lazzaretto in the city until the late fifteenth century.[195]

Although for the purposes of this chapter I have mainly emphasised the medical side of their activities, Renaissance hospitals should not be viewed in anachronistic terms as secularised institutions run for and by the laity without reference to the very important religious tradition on which they were modelled. It was no coincidence that the sections on hospital architecture in the treatises of Filarete and Alberti appeared immediately after the discussions of monasteries. After all, the design of all the major hospitals was based on the monastic model of chapel, cloisters, refectory and infirmary. Furthermore, the personnel who staffed the hospitals as nurses were usually Tertiaries, and, as in all medieval cures, the *medico spirituale* remained as important as the *medico fisico*. These themes remain central to understanding the development of the Renaissance hospital in Florence over the next century.

CHAPTER 3

The Late Renaissance:
Beauty, Sickness and the Poor

> It is said that our city above all others is copiously provided with hospitals, which are beautiful and capacious and are adapted and organised to receive any sick or healthy person who is wretched and needs to be received for whatever reason, except [for] those who are sick from plague.
>
> ASF, Provv. Reg. 157, f. 58r: 12.vi.1464[1]

Introduction

This self-congratulatory statement by the city's priors in 1464 noted that the only defect of the hospital system was the lack of a lazzaretto for plague victims. The features identified here broadly reflect those identified in the Introduction to this book as characteristic of the Renaissance hospital. The first was their civic character. Florence is presented by the priors as having a fully integrated system of care, with a 'copious' number of hospitals sufficient to look after a wide range of poor and sick people. Second was the *bellezza* of their appearance, the 'wonderful buildings built at vast expense' of Alberti's *De re aedificatoria*. This aesthetic appreciation was also reflected in the comments of other Florentines writing in the fifteenth century and beyond; Gregorio Dati in his description of the monuments of the city saw hospitals as contributing to the sum of Florence's 'beautiful and ornate buildings'.[2] Furthermore, the Renaissance hospital was seen as being organised efficiently on a sufficiently large scale, both administratively and architecturally, to guarantee excellence of treatment. The religious character of hospitals in this period was another important point mentioned by Alberti and the 1464 law cited above, and indeed provided the motivation for the staff, from the nurses to the physicians. It is this combination of religious motivation, care and medical treatment that sums up the central function of the Renaissance hospital: the cure of the body and the cure of the soul.

In this chapter I shall explore two of the main features of Renaissance hospitals, beginning with a discussion of what contemporaries thought constituted their *bellezza*, and then examine the evolution of the various elements of the hospital 'system' in this period. In the second half of the chapter it will be seen that while the Renaissance hospital had taken form in a period of relative prosperity, after the mid-fifteenth century there were major challenges to this system from an expanding population and a gradual fall in standards of living. The period was characterised by repeated outbreaks of epidemic disease and shortages, especially in the 1490s and the 1520s, exacerbated by the disastrous siege of Florence, which in part led to an overhaul of the charitable system by the new Medici dukes of Tuscany. Following the theme developed in the preceding chapters, it will be argued that many of the reforms introduced in the city's welfare system stemmed from the increasing association of poverty with disease. This in turn contributed to the continued 'medicalisation' of the services provided by the city's hospitals and to the growing institutionalisation of reactions to threats to public health. These included creating systems for dealing with epidemics of plague and the new 'Mal Francese' with, on the one hand, the establishment of the lazzaretto or isolation hospital for plague victims, the associated Sanità or health board, and the revival of the fraternity of the Misericordia; and, on the other, the foundation of the Incurabili hospital for those suffering from the mysterious 'French Disease'.

Population growth, falling standards of living and epidemic disease were not unique to Florence, but common to many parts of Europe in this period, which led to shared reactions towards the poorer members of society north and south of the Alps. This theme of emergent poor-relief schemes is well known to students of welfare and included increased intolerance towards the poor, particularly beggars, and the making of distinctions between the 'worthy' and 'unworthy' poor. The new measures in turn led to the institutionalisation of what is perceived as the new character of relief in the early modern period, based on greater centralisation, underlain by a new moralistic attitude towards the more marginalised sections of society in both Catholic and Protestant Europe. However, as will be argued in this chapter, it is important not to forget the dependence of these reforms on the models and systems of care and treatment evolved in the later Middle Ages and the Renaissance. Furthermore, a fundamental element of this system was the hospital, whose role was made concrete and visible through the impressive new structures that became an increasingly visible part of the urban landscape.

3.1 'Our City above All Others Is Copiously Provided with Hospitals, Which Are Beautiful'

It was the exterior of hospitals that excited the aesthetic sense of Renaissance Florentines, their responses being reflected in contemporary literary descriptions and views of the city. Hospitals were presented as important monuments alongside the churches and secular buildings in such works as Pietro del Massaio's *Veduta di Firenze* (Plate 1.1), produced only five years after the law cited at the very beginning of this chapter, which highlighted a number of major hospitals for the sick, including Messer Bonifazio and S. Maria Nuova, and the new foundling hospital of the Innocenti. To determine those elements of design that came to be seen as typifying the appearance of a Renaissance hospital, I shall begin with S. Maria Nuova, usually regarded as the model for Florentine hospitals, and then go on to the other major hospitals in the city.

The best guide to the façade of S. Maria Nuova before the construction of the loggia in the late sixteenth century is Bicci di Lorenzo's fresco *Martin V Confirming the Consecration of S. Egidio* (Plate I). Even if one should resist 'reading' this picture as an accurate depiction, it nonetheless provides a guide to the main features regarded as important by those who commissioned the fresco, including the *spedalingo*, and by the artist. The view shortens the width of the hospital, but the number of main entrances and their relationship to one another can be verified from the ground plan of the site made in 1780 (Plate 2.6). The centre of attention is S. Egidio, shown with its plain façade surmounted by a pitched roof under which is a round glazed window, a low projecting tiled roof and lunette containing the terracotta group of the *Coronation of the Virgin*, sculpted by Dello Delli between 1420 and 1424 (Plate 4.3).[3] One can also see here, but more clearly in an illumination of some fifty years later by Gherardo and Monte di Giovanni di Miniato (Plate 3.11b: *Martin V Greeted by the Spedalingo of S. Maria Nuova*), that the church was raised above the level of the piazza, for there was a flight of steps which led up to the main door and on the right a small tabernacle on the wall.

To the right were the entrances to the main cloister for male patients, the Chiostro delle Medicherie, and the male ward, surmounted by a roof and tall mullioned window. On the left of the fresco was the entrance to the hospital's cemetery. In the lunette above the doorway to the cemetery can be seen a half-length figure of *Christ Showing His Wound* (Plates 4.1–2). In general terms this was a representation of the popular theme of the 'Man of Sorrows' and a more specific reference to the idea that the wound in Christ's side represented a door to salvation.[4]

The view of S. Maria Nuova in the Bicci di Lorenzo fresco shows, then, a hospital façade from the first half of the fourteenth century; the mullioned window of the male ward was a more typically 'Gothic' element. Although its exterior was not typically Renaissance, specific architectural details and interior plans were imitated by architects of fifteenth-century hospitals in Florence and elsewhere. Furthermore, it was very evidently regarded as one of the monuments that contributed to the sum of the city's *bellezza*.

Even if the front elevation of S. Maria Nuova did not become a model, the façades of hospitals built in Florence from the later fourteenth century onwards have been hailed by historians as part of the Renaissance aesthetic. The best known is Brunelleschi's graceful design for the Innocenti, which is often characterised as a milestone in the development of architecture and one of the major achievements of the early Renaissance. However, the loggia was not a new feature of either secular, ecclesiastical or hospital architecture. In the Trecento, the loggias constructed by patricians were often separate from the palaces themselves, as at the Rucellai Palace.[5] The loggia was also allegedly a feature of two of the oldest hospitals in the city, dating from the eleventh century: S. Lorenzo and S. Giovanni Evangelista.[6]

Brunelleschi's design for the façade of the Innocenti, built between 1419 and 1426 (Plate 3.1), made reference to three Trecento hospitals. The first was the

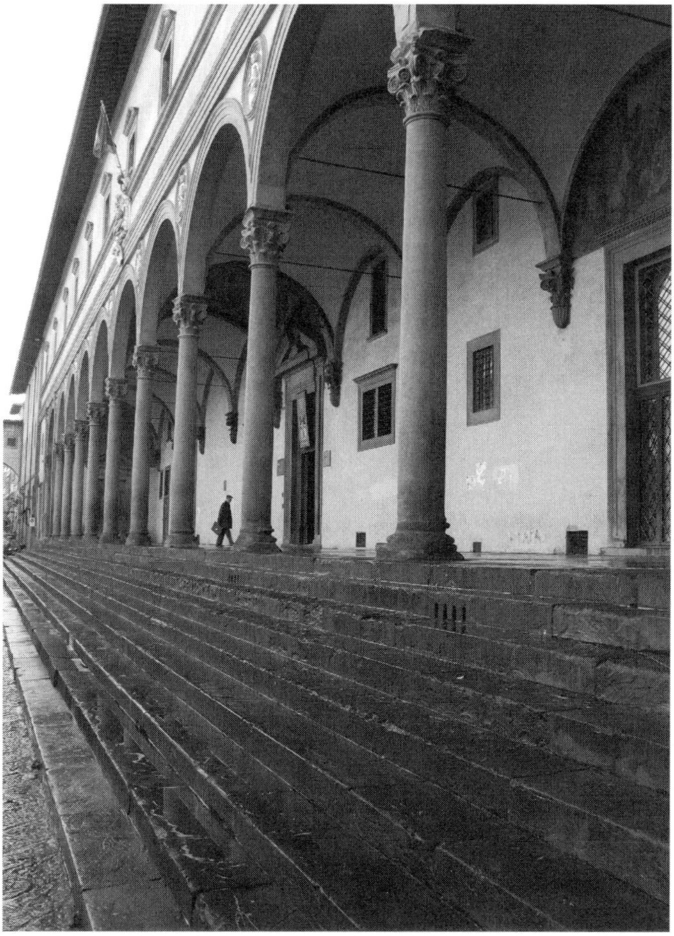

Plate 3.1 Façade of the Ospedale degli Innocenti, Piazza SS. Annunziata

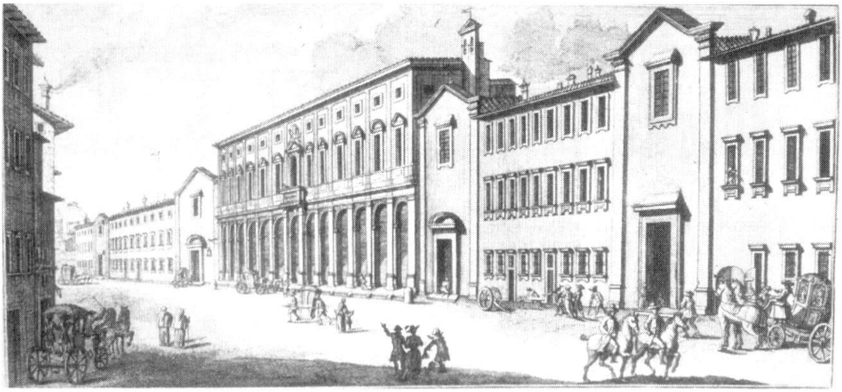

Plate 3.2 Cosimo Zocchi, *Veduta dell'Ospedale di Messer Bonifazio*, 1744

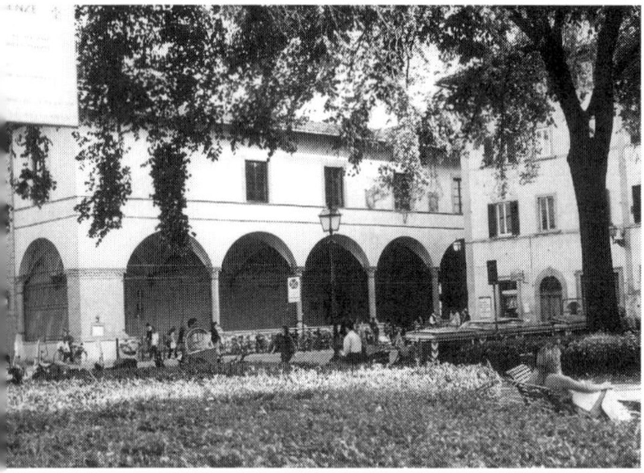

Plate 3.3 Façade of the Ospedale di S. Matteo, Piazza S. Marco

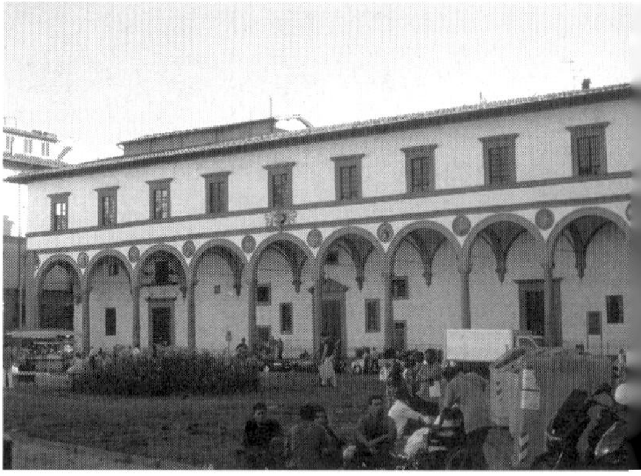

Plate 3.4 Façade of the Ospedale di S. Paolo, Piazza S. Maria Novella

foundling hospital of S. Maria della Scala; one can still see the outline of the loggia on the corner of Via della Scala and Via dell'Albero (Plate 1.8). The other two hospitals in the same part of the city as the Innocenti dated from the late Trecento and both were fronted by loggias:[7] Messer Bonifazio, completed by 1388 (Plate 3.2), and S. Matteo, begun in 1385 and completed by 1410 (Plate 3.3). Later in the century Michelozzo added a loggia to the façade of S. Paolo based on the Innocenti (Plate 3.4).[8] Finally, in the early seventeenth century S. Maria Nuova itself came to conform to this model: Giulio Parigi il Vecchio's design for the addition of the portico on the main façade of the hospital was realised between 1612 and 1616, as seen in Zocchi's mid-eighteenth-century view (Plate 3.5).[9]

The similarities between the exterior of these hospitals suggest a self-conscious policy of imitation, even given the existence of certain stylistic

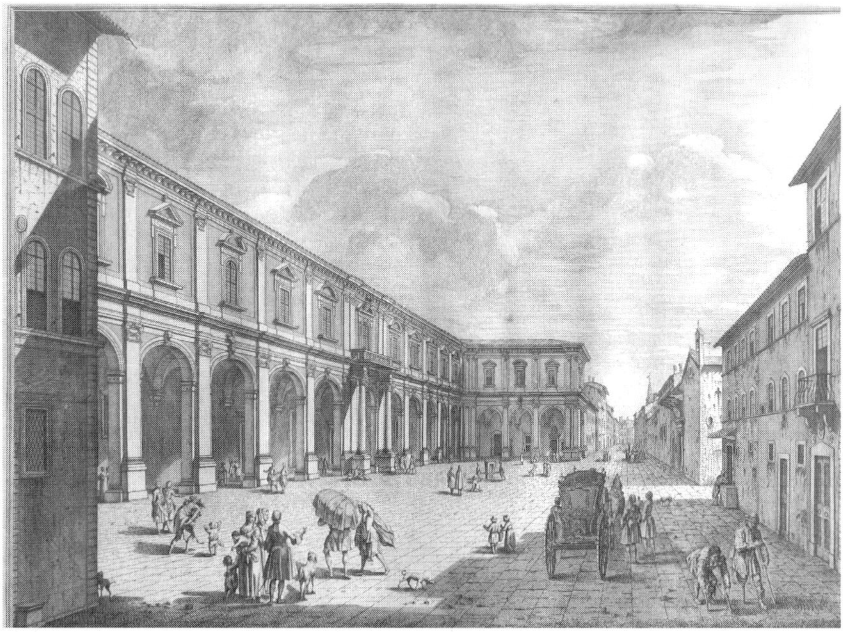

Plate 3.5 Cosimo Zocchi, *Veduta della Piazza di S. Maria Nuova*, 1744

differences. This hypothesis is confirmed at S. Matteo in the wording of the contract of 1388 between the founder, Lemmo Balducci, and two master masons, Romolo del Bandino and Sandro del Vinta. Lemmo stipulated that they should

> build a portico with columns in front of the doors of the two wards in imitation of the shape and form of the portico that is built with columns in front of the doors of the said wards of the hospital of Messer Bonifazio Lupi in Florence in Via S. Gallo, with a wall in front and a parapet as large as is necessary and as high as the parapet of the said portico of the above-mentioned hospital of Messer Bonifazio.[10]

Lemmo was sufficiently concerned that the appearance should match that of Messer Bonifazio that he even stipulated how the wall of the loggia should appear: 'as well and delicately plastered as it is plastered at the Spedale di Messer Bonifazio in Via S. Gallo' (Plate 3.2).[11]

S. Matteo itself provided a model for the façade attributed to Brunelleschi of the Spedale di S. Antonio in nearby Lastra a Signa.[12] S. Antonio was built between 1415 and 1422, precisely in the period when plans for the construction of the façade of the Innocenti were being put into effect.[13] Furthermore,

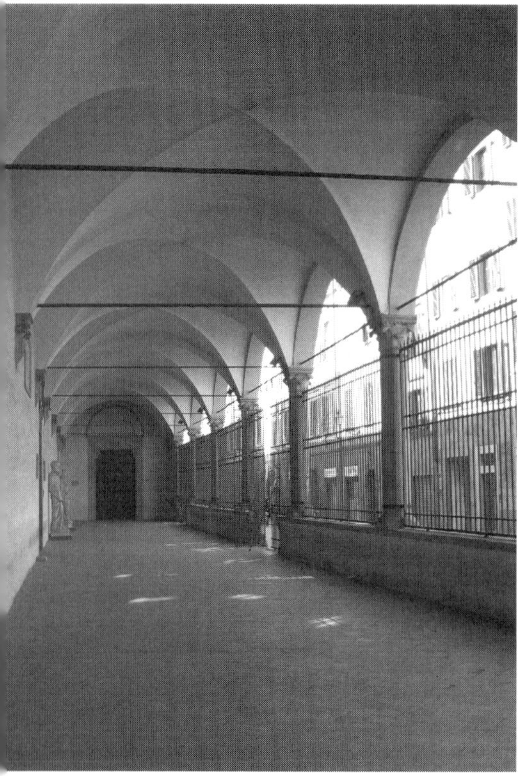

Plate 3.6 Loggia of the Ospedale di S. Matteo, Piazza S. Marco

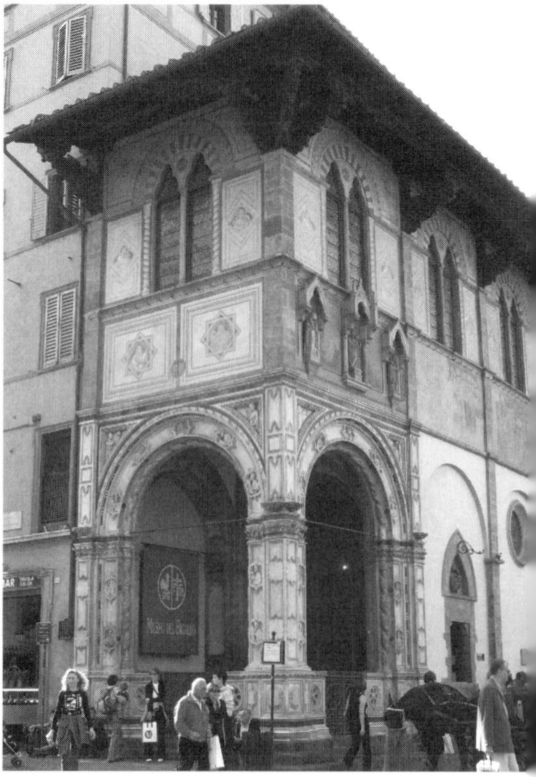

Plate 3.7 Loggia of the company of the Bigallo, Piazza S. Giovanni

both projects were under the direction of the Arte della Seta and, despite the officials involved changing frequently, the same group of people essentially dominated the silk guild throughout.[14]

The popularity of the loggia as part of a hospital façade suggests it was seen as having an important function. Even if contemporaries remained surprisingly reticent about its role, subsequent historians have not.[15] It has been suggested that it had an important aesthetic role in providing a uniform façade for a jumble of pre-existing buildings, for instance at S. Paolo (Plate 3.4). The loggia also distinguished the hospital from other public buildings, since it was neither a church nor a palace. Indeed, in Florence there was a venerable tradition for the association between loggias and charitable institutions, as in the case of the company of the Bigallo whose loggia fronts onto the Piazza di S. Giovanni opposite the Baptistery (Plate 3.7)

The loggia mediated between the public and private spaces of the street and institution, in this way reflecting the ambiguous nature of a charity that was run with the aid of private funds yet performed a public function. Perhaps its most obvious function – as Alberti mentions when discussing porticos in front of palaces – was in providing a waiting area for patients seeking admission or an appointment with a physician, buying prescriptions or attending outpatient clinics. Loggias also had a very practical function, to protect people against extremes of temperature – as Alberti says: 'In winter they receive the gentle sun, and in summer they offer grateful shade or any breeze there may be.'[16] This role as an antechamber to the main hospital can still be seen today at the ex-hospital of S. Matteo, where the loggia is used by students of the Accademia del Disegno as a shelter or as a place in which to meet and talk (Plate 3.6)

Brunelleschi at the Innocenti and then Michelozzo at S. Paolo (though not the architects of Messer Bonifazio and S. Matteo) took their plans one stage further by placing the loggia above street level. This is best seen at the Innocenti where the loggia is raised on a podium reached by a flight of stairs, thus elevating the entrance well above the level of the piazza. At S. Paolo the flight of six steps did raise the loggia, particularly at the northern end, though to nothing like the same height as at the Innocenti on Piazza SS. Annunziata. In contrast, Brunelleschi's compatriot Filarete outlined the virtues of not having stairs at the Ospedale Maggiore in Milan: 'It would have been a great expense and … it is not for spectacles nor for standing to watch games and parades.'[17]

It was, then, the desire of hospital patrons, directors and builders to provide a façade that combined functionality and beauty. This in turn contributed to the wider civic Renaissance aesthetic, as the magistracy of the Ufficiali di Torri acknowledged when they gave their approval to the Innocenti's planned loggia, which they saw as 'becoming to the beauty of the aforesaid city'.[18]

Another element to add to the *bellezza* of hospital façades and that helped to distinguish them from other civic buildings was the external decorative programmes which reflected both their religious and charitable functions. These could take the form of frescoes, as at S. Maria Nuova, S. Maria della Scala in Siena or the charitable confraternity of the Bigallo.[19] More common were the sculpted figures in lunettes over the main entrances, which from the fifteenth century were increasingly of glazed terracotta, particularly those from the famous Della Robbia workshop. These images might include references to the dedication of a chapel or hospital, or to a particular event or person associated with an institution. Many included the Virgin, as with the *Coronation* scene over the entrance to S. Egidio, the *Ascension* over the door leading into S. Matteo's male ward and the *Annunciation* over the church door at the Innocenti. The presence of Mary, the caring Mother of Christ, reflected her appropriateness to these institutions with their commitment to tending to the sick and other helpless members of society. More direct references to the function of a hospital can be seen in the most famous roundels, the Andrea della Robbia infants on the façade of the Innocenti commissioned in 1487 (Plate 3.9).[20]

The lunette above the church door of S. Paolo instead made direct reference to the founders of the mendicant orders with which the hospital was closely associated. The subject was the Meeting of SS. Francis and Dominic, an apposite choice since the Franciscan Third Order had for many years run the

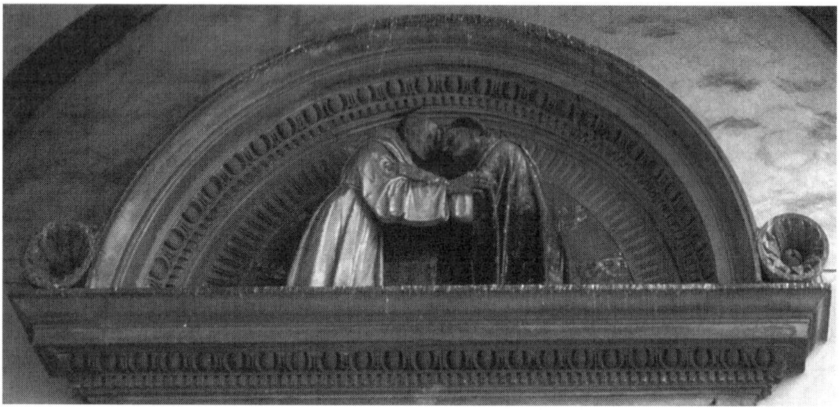

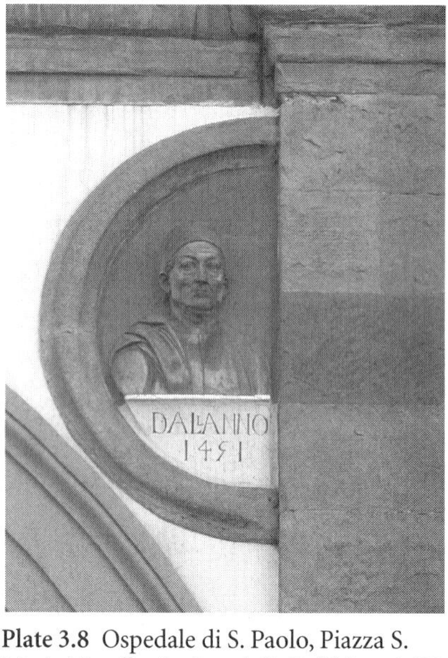

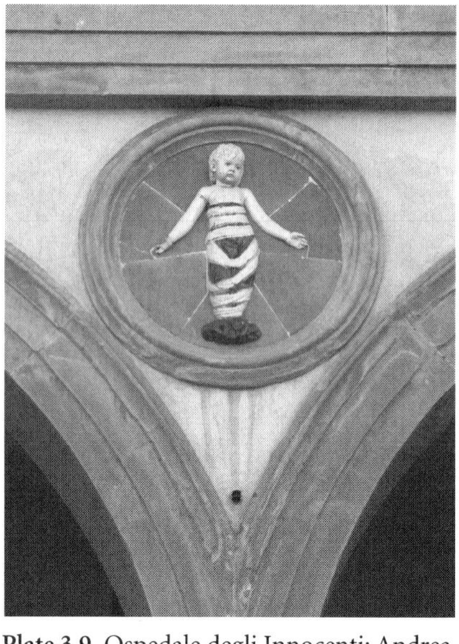

Plate 3.8 Ospedale di S. Paolo, Piazza S. Maria Novella: Andrea della Robbia, c.1498
a. Church portal lunette, *The Meeting of SS. Francis and Dominic*
b. Loggia half-roundel, *Portrait of the Hospital Director Bonino Bonini*

Plate 3.9 Ospedale degli Innocenti: Andrea della Robbia, roundel of foundling, 1487

hospital, while S. Maria Novella, the church of the Dominicans, dominated the piazza of which S. Paolo formed the southern side (Plate 3.8a). In addition to decorated tympana, a series of roundels was placed above the spandrels on the façade of S. Paolo, including Andrea della Robbia's portraits of the hospital director Bonino Bonini of c.1498 (Plate 3.8b). Benini had been largely responsible for restructuring the hospital from the early 1450s, including a new chapel in the main ward, new cloisters for both the female and male staff, and the beginnings of a new hospital church.[21]

The idea of a hospital having a loggia and associated terracotta reliefs was soon copied in Florentine subject cities. One of the best surviving examples is the hospital of the Ceppo in nearby Pistoia, which in 1501 had come under the direct control of S. Maria Nuova in Florence. Indeed, the *spedalingo* of the Florentine hospital at that time, Lionardo di Giovanni Buonafede, was to remain the director of the Ceppo until 1530. This period covered both the years when the loggia itself was built, c.1514, and when the glazed terracotta frieze of the Seven Works of Mercy was added to the façade by Giovanni di Andrea della Robbia's workshop, 1525 to 1529 (Plate 3.10).[22] What differentiated the Ceppo's façade was that many of the figures were lay rather than religious and one of the main purposes in showing them in action was to excite the piety of visitors and potential patrons to help finance the medical and spiritual functions of the hospital.

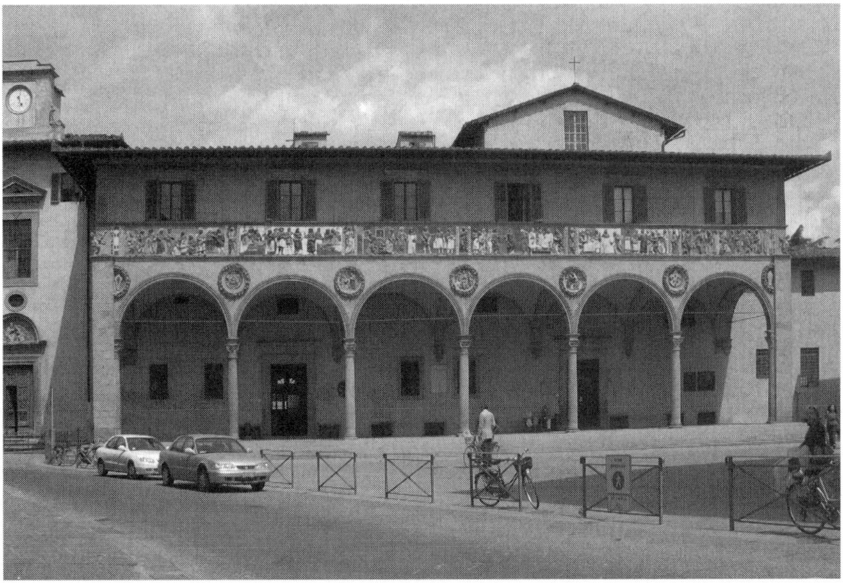

Plate 3.10 Façade of the Ospedale del Ceppo, Piazza S. Lorenzo, Pistoia, with glazed terracotta frieze by Giovanni di Andrea della Robbia's workshop, 1525–9

Recognition of the importance for the city of hospitals' charitable-medical role was reflected in public ceremonies. As seen in the Introduction, one of the best-documented was Pope Martin V's involvement in the reconsecration of S. Egidio. The wider context is described by Bartolommeo del Corazza in his contemporary *Diario*, where he discussed the events leading up to this event:

> Leaving S. Maria Novella, they went to S. Maria Maggiore, and then to S. Giovanni and to S. Liperata, and to the Canto di Balla, and turned and went to S. Maria Nuova in S. Gilio. And there the holy father dismounted, and confirmed that which had been consecrated by the cardinal of Bologna, and undertook those ceremonies that he had done at S. Maria Novella, and left there an indulgence of eight days. Then he remounted his horse and left, going by Via di S. Gilio as far as Canto alla Rondine, and turned by Borgo degli Albizzi towards Canto de' Pazzi, and then the Palazzo del Podestà and the Palazzo of the Magalotti and onto Piazza de'Signori and through Vaccareccia and through Porta S. Maria and onto Ponte Vecchio and as far as Porta a S. Piero Gattolino.[23]

This episode was part of Pope Martin V's ceremonial departure from the city, for which spectacle the commune had granted the considerable sum of 800 *scudi* to cover the expenses.[24] He had been staying at the Dominican friary of S. Maria Novella since February 1418 and this formed the point of departure for the procession, at the centre of which was the holy sacrament surrounded by a group of young boys carrying lighted candles 'with a rich and beautiful banner of gold cloth, with pendants hanging from fourteen poles, under which the holy father processed and others carrying two banners, one of the Church and the other of the pope'.[25] From S. Maria Novella, he processed to S. Egidio via three of the oldest ecclesiastical sites in the city, S. Maria Maggiore, the Baptistery and the cathedral, and then visited the two main centres of secular power, the Bargello and the Piazza della Signoria, before eventually taking the road to Rome.

The fresco offered a snapshot of one part of the ceremony, as is made clear by the series of illustrations from a breviary belonging to S. Egidio illuminated in the 1470s by Gherardo and Monte di Giovanni di Miniato (Plate 3.11).

The first illumination (Plate 3.11a) shows the pope arriving at S. Egidio riding a white horse, which had been given to him by the Parte Guelfa on entering Florence the previous year.[26] He was welcomed by the *spedalingo*, who in the following scene (Plate 3.11b) kneels before the pope. To the left of Martin V is a group of prominent citizens, also kneeling, one of whom is carrying the end of the pope's cloak, and to the right a group of kneeling clerics dressed in white. To the far right in a separate but related scene is an excited group of spectators, probably representing male members of the hospital's

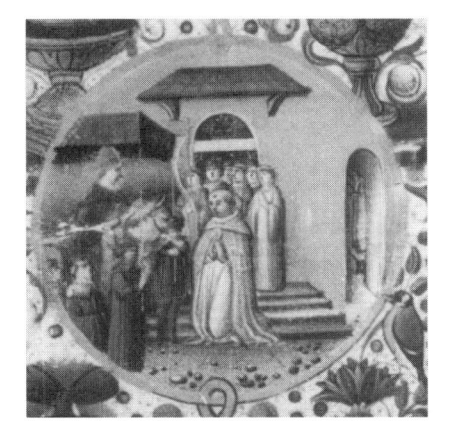

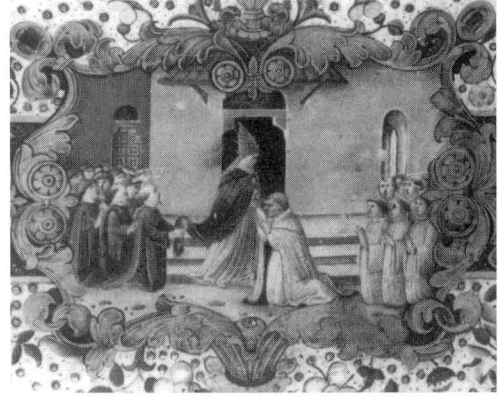

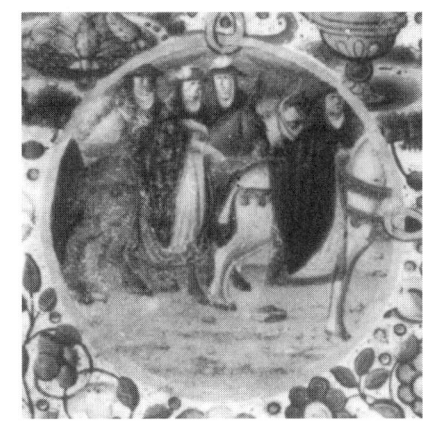

Plate 3.11 Gherardo and Monte di Giovanni di Miniato
a. *Arrival of Martin V at S. Egidio*
b. *Martin V Greeted by the Spedalingo of S. Maria Nuova*
c. *Departure of Martin V from S. Maria Nuova*
(S. Egidio, Breviary, 1474: Museo Nazionale del Bargello, MS A68, f. 161v)

staff, watching the scene from under the small projecting roof over the entrance door to the male ward. The third scene (Plate 3.11c) shows the pope taking leave of the hospital on his way to the Bargello.

This event placed S. Maria Nuova at the heart of the ceremonial life of the city, giving the hospital the same symbolic importance as other major civic institutions. Its importance for the future life of the hospital cannot be exaggerated: from this time forward S. Maria Nuova became one of the major centres of artistic patronage in Florence and, as will be seen below, the beneficiary of increased attention from the commune – some welcome and some unwelcome.

3.2 Behind the Façade: 'Capacious and Adapted and Organised to Receive any Sick or Healthy Person Who Is Wretched'

If the façade helped to define the 'beauty' of the Renaissance hospital, an important related feature was the scale and organisation of the site, as recognised in the legislators' proud statement in 1464 about the scale and adaptability of their hospitals. Following the discussion in Chapters 1 and 2 of the foundation and development of the city's major medical hospitals, the next section will examine in more detail the influence of their expanding activities on their architectural form.

Some of the most striking developments took place at the largest hospital in the city, S. Maria Nuova, at exactly the same time as the initial phases of construction of the Innocenti were under way. Although the building programmes of the whole of the S. Maria Nuova site have never been studied in detail, in the preceding chapters I have outlined some of the major elements in response to the growth in the liturgical and medical functions.[27]

The areas that have attracted most historical attention are S. Egidio, to be examined in more detail in Chapter 4, and the male ward, whose capacity more than doubled over the century from 120 to 250 beds.[28] The interest of historians in the male ward has crystallised around the debate concerning whether or not the cruciform model originated in Florence or in Lombardy. At the beginning of the century the ground plan had resembled an inverted 'L' with an eastern extension to the original hall, and then in 1409–10 work was begun on the western extension (Plate 1.9:1d) with expenses recorded for the foundations and the roof of the 'new arm of the hospital' or the 'new hospital'.[29] This was the first phase of the project, which can be seen behind the main cloister in Rustici's sketch of S. Maria Nuova in c. 1445 (Plate 1.10),[30] which was finalised in 1479, taking the form of a 'T'. As in the case of the western arm, work on the final northern section (1e) was a drawn-out affair, with evidence of some construction in about 1515, though the vast bulk of the project was not completed until the last quarter of the century.[31] This was part of a grand collaborative project between Grand Duke Francesco I and his architect Bernardo Buontalenti to modernise the appearance of the hospital to include the remodelling of the interior of S. Egidio and the construction of a loggia on the piazza.[32]

The basic structure of the women's ward was not altered in this period, though the five-year building programme begun 'on the women's side' in 1437 may have led to the enlargement of the facilities for the patients within the pre-existing space.[33] It has been seen in earlier chapters that though the women benefited from the medical and spiritual expertise of doctors and priests located in the main hospital, emphasis was laid on the separation of men and women, whether they were nurses, serving staff or the patients themselves. This led to a clear segregation of the sexes between these two *spedali*. While sacramental duties could not be performed by anybody except a male priest, the women's hospital seems otherwise to have been run almost independently, although under the overall supervision of the *spedalingo*. This partly explains why the site south of S. Egidio was so substantial. By the early sixteenth century

THE LATE RENAISSANCE: BEAUTY, SICKNESS AND THE POOR 83

women patients were looked after by a hundred female members of staff; they were made up of both live-in servants, who had committed themselves to serving the sick, and their assistants. The nurses counted among their number several whom the 1510–11 'Ordinances' described as 'skilled in surgery' with 'many remarkable cures to their credit'.[34]

The basic principle of separating male and female patients and staff into distinct wards and living areas was also a feature of hospitals such as Messer Bonifazio and S. Matteo. Their plans offer an interesting comparison with that of S. Maria Nuova; instead of evolving gradually over the course of the fourteenth and fifteenth centuries, they were purpose-built for the treatment of the sick. I shall concentrate mainly on S. Matteo since its internal history and architectural development have been much more thoroughly examined than those of Messer Bonifazio, despite the fact that the latter is usually regarded as a prototype for later hospitals.[35] Much more of S. Matteo's basic structure is still extant: the conversion of the site into the premises of the Accademia delle Belle Arti from 1784 was less dramatic than the total rebuilding of Messer Bonifazio in the later nineteenth century to become the office of the Questura.[36]

A useful guide to the layout of S. Matteo is provided by the ground plan drawn up in 1780 along with those of the other major hospitals in the city (Plate 3.12). Though building work was carried out in the later sixteenth century,

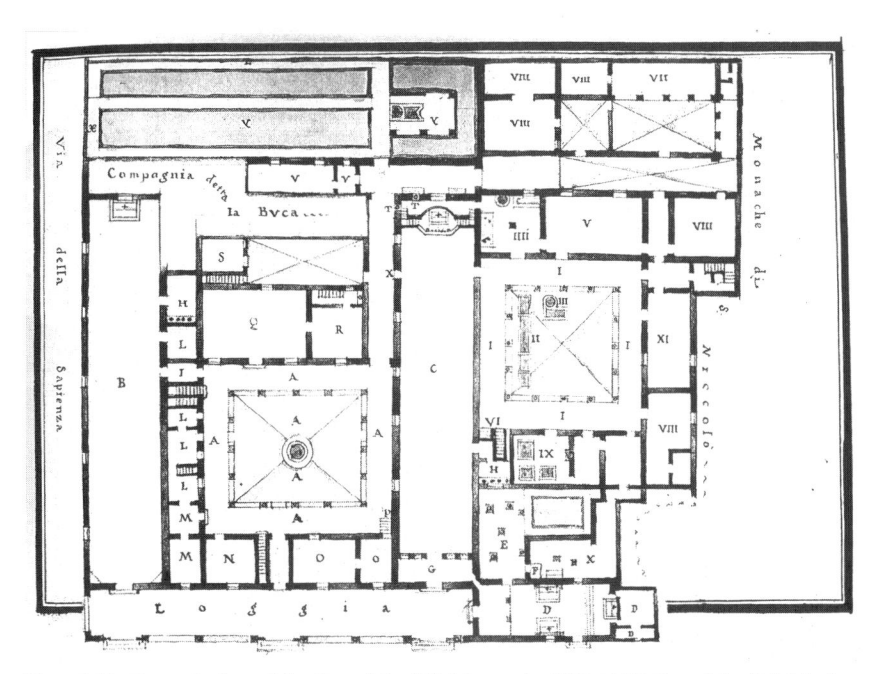

Plate 3.12 Ground plan of the Ospedale di S. Matteo in 1780 (ASF, Ospedale di S. Maria Nuova 24: Plan 5)

especially in the male cloister and church, these interventions were more a question of detail than radical change, as can be appreciated from a comparison of the basic disposition of space in 1780 and the information provided in contemporary records, including the contract between the founder, Lemmo Balducci, and the master masons, building accounts and inventories.[37]

The principal entrances to the hospital were through the loggia on what is now Via Ricasoli. In the centre was the door leading to the main cloister of the male patients (Plate 3.12: 'A'; Plate 3.14) and to the left or north was the male ward ('B'), with its entrance off the far left-hand bay of the loggia. The ward is seen clearly left of centre in Francesco Rosselli's famous 'Catena' view of Florence of 1471–80, labelled as 'SP D LELMO', the 'Spedale di Lelmo' (Plate 3.13). The measurements prescribed by Lemmo for the ward, 80 *braccia* long by 18 to 19 *braccia* wide, equivalent to 47 by 11.2 metres, correspond exactly with those on the plan of 1780.

The same measurements apply to the female ward, which lay to the south, parallel to the male ward; its main door opened off the last bay on the right of the loggia. To the south of the women's ward lay the women's cloister (I), referred to in 1401 as the 'chiostro de' lavatoi';[38] the plan shows a series of water troughs for washing linen. The hospital church, now the library of the Accademia, lay on the same axis as the loggia, at right angles to the female ward, and, according to the 1780 plan, had three entrances (D). The principal door was from the loggia, and could therefore be readily accessed by the public, while the two internal doors connected the church to the female ward and the internal hospital cemetery, which lay to the east (IX).

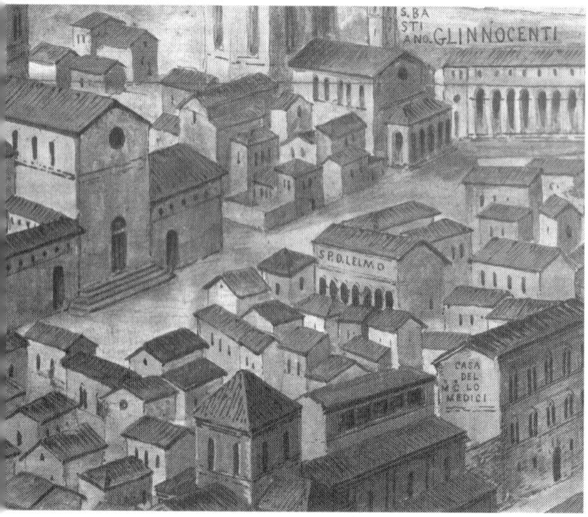

Plate 3.13 Francesco Rosselli, *Veduta di Firenze detta 'della Catena'*: detail of the Ospedale di S. Matteo, 1471–80 (Museo di Firenze Com'era)

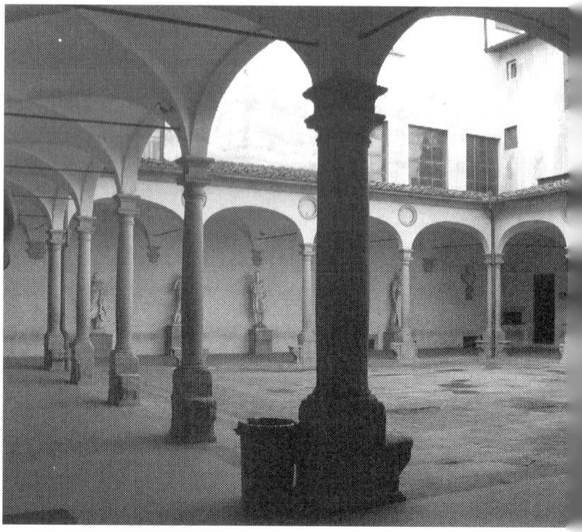

Plate 3.14 Ospedale di S. Matteo, Piazza S. Marco: male cloister

An inventory of the hospital drawn up in December 1454 by the Provveditore, one of the main officials of the Arte del Cambio, provides more information about some of the other spaces on the plan used in the fifteenth century. The tour of the site began in the men's ward and moved south towards the male cloister to a series of rooms, including the *medicheria* or surgery and the 'camera della spezieria' (Plate 3.12: 'M'). The placing of the hospital's apothecary's workshop to the front of the hospital and close to the male ward reflects its function as provider of medicines to both in- and out-patients, who would have entered from the left-hand side of the loggia. Next the *provveditore* moved to the female ward, then the male cloister and upstairs to the sleeping accommodation with eleven single rooms, including those designated for the use of two priests, Ser Giovanni and Ser Antonio da Bargha. The male refectory was the next major space visited by the *provveditore* once he had descended the stairs to the ground floor. This room, which was described as the 'large refectory of the men', can presumably be identified with 'Q' on the 1780 plan since it is the only other large space contiguous to the male cloister. Finally, he returned to the female side and the spaces identified on the 1780 plan as within the convent of the nuns, including cloister, refectory ('V') and the kitchens described in the inventory as 'above the chiostro delle donne' (IIII).

This brief survey of the layout of S. Matteo has shown the similarities and differences between this purpose-built medical hospital of the early Quattrocento and an institution like S. Maria Nuova, which had evolved over a number of centuries from more humble beginnings. Each hospital by definition shared the same basic functional spaces: wards and pharmacy, cloisters and church, kitchen and refectory, sleeping and living accommodation for staff, as well as storage areas on the first floor. But the way in which these functions were allocated across the site depended on the amount of available land. Thus, when S. Maria Nuova was founded in the late Duecento, not only did the Portinari family have the advantage of already owning property in the vicinity, but more land was being made available with the demolition of the earlier city walls. The area was further enlarged by the acquisition of the convent and church of the Frati Saccati.[39] Lemmo Balducci, on the other hand, had had to acquire a site that was already owned and partly developed by the convent of S. Niccolò, with the result that he had had to pay for the construction of both his hospital and a new complex for the nuns.[40]

The history of the different sites helps to explain why these institutions adopted different solutions to provide concrete expression of one of the basic principles that underlay their constitutions: namely, the separation of male and female patients and staff. At S. Matteo this was not, as at S. Maria Nuova, achieved by a split site with a street running between the two parts, but simply by internal divisions. In both cases, however, there were two related but separate institutions with distinct sleeping and eating quarters, although the patients would have been treated by the same doctors, barbers and apothecaries, and eaten the same food. In addition, the daily spiritual needs of patients would have been met through the celebration of Mass in separate ward chapels, though they would have shared church and cemetery.

The division between the sexes was also a shared principle of the two other larger medical hospitals, Messer Bonifazio and S. Paolo, though they adopted different solutions, probably reflecting differences in land availability. Via S. Gallo, the site of Messer Bonifazio, was much less built-up in the fifteenth century than the location of S. Paolo on the southern side of Piazza S. Maria Novella.[41] Messer Bonifazio, in common with S. Matteo, had two wards divided by a cloister, the male on the right with a portal opposite the northernmost bay of the loggia and the female to the south, as can be seen from both contemporary views and the 1780 plan of the hospital (Plate 3.15).[42] The main difference at S. Paolo was that there was apparently only one ward, which was divided internally to separate male from female patients, who also entered through different doors (Plate 3.16).[43]

It is now possible, then, to determine how some of the main architectural features of the Renaissance hospital fulfilled contemporary claims about how their *bellezza* combined with multi-functionality on an impressive scale: each possessed a loggia, although at S. Maria Nuova this was not added until the early seventeenth century. The main entrance to the hospital was normally centred halfway along the façade and led directly into one of the main cloisters. Except in the case of S. Maria Nuova until the seventeenth century, the male and female wards were built as parallel blocks on either side of the cloister (though S. Paolo's was a single and divided space), and the entrance to the hospital chapel was from one end of the loggia. The service areas such as the rooms for the administrators, kitchen staff and refectories were then all disposed around the cloisters. The living quarters of the nursing staff were normally placed above, on the first floor. At the front of the building were those spaces that needed to be most accessible to the public: first, the office of the *spedalingo*, who represented the hospital in its dealings with the public; then, the apothecary's shop, which was frequented not just by the staff, but also by those seeking medicines for treatment at home; and, finally, the church, which would have been visited by both inmates and the public.

This brings us back to the religious character of the institution: to state the obvious, the plan was based on the monastic model of cloister and infirmary hall. Each hospital also possessed a separate chapel and at the head of each of the wards was an altar at which the chaplain would celebrate Mass. The combination of the various elements of the hospital made concrete its dual function, in which the priest or spiritual doctor remained as important as the physical

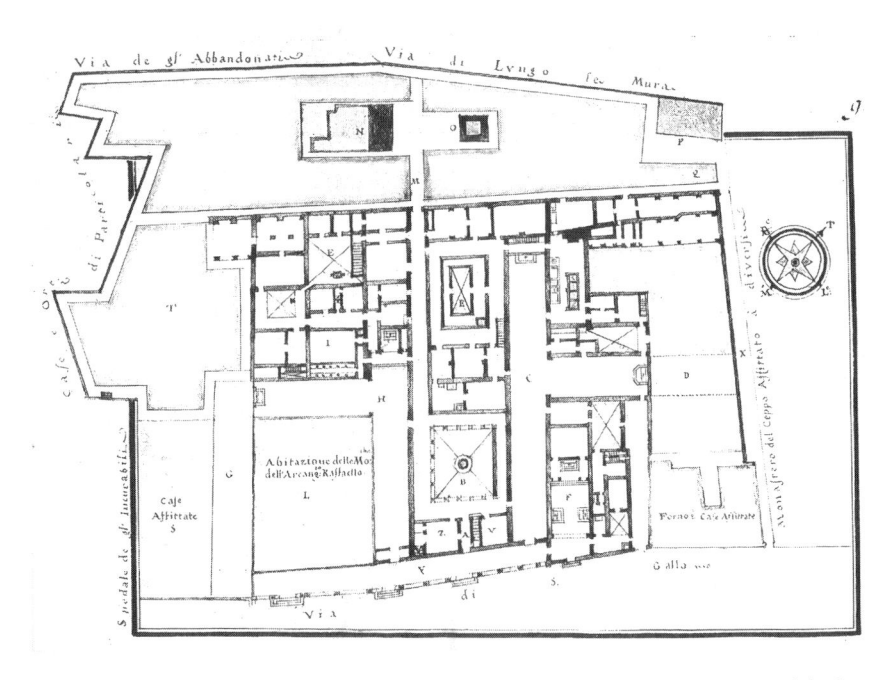

THE LATE RENAISSANCE: BEAUTY, SICKNESS AND THE POOR 87

Plate 3.15 Ground plan of the Ospedale di Messer Bonifazio in 1780 (ASF, Ospedale di S. Maria Nuova 24: Plan 9)

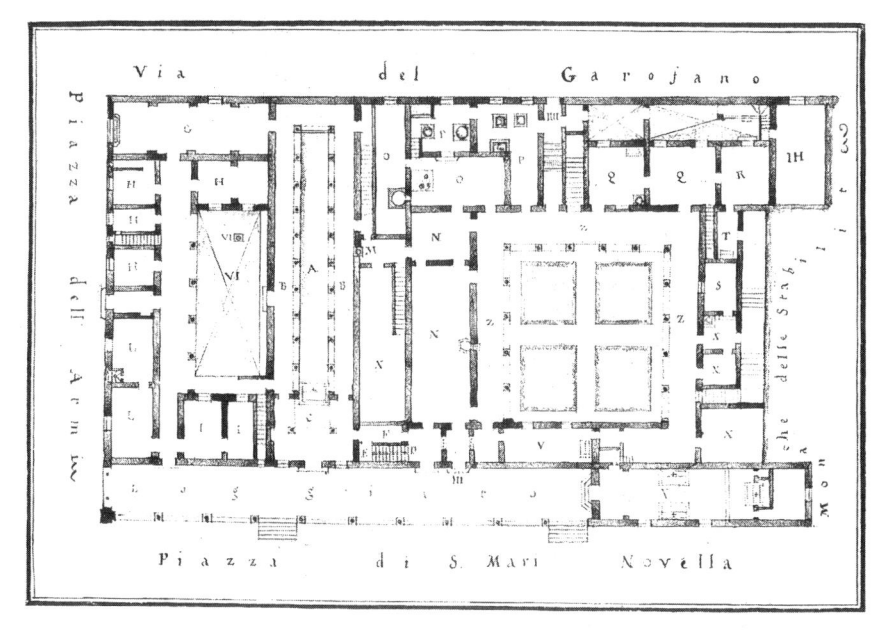

Plate 3.16 Ground plan of the Ospedale di S. Paolo in 1780 (ASF, Ospedale di S. Maria Nuova 24: Plan 7)

doctor or physician in the healing process, thus reflecting the hospital's combination of the cure of the body with the cure of the soul.

3.3 The 'System of Care'

The third main feature that contemporaries cited to justify the reputation of the Renaissance hospital was the high standard of treatment. This free service to the sick poor provided by the major medical hospitals formed part of the city's 'system of care' in the fifteenth century and included a range of charitable institutions with complementary specialisations. Indeed, when an influential figure such as Archbishop Antoninus was writing about charity in his *Summa theologica*, he distinguished between the functions of various types of hospital, emphasising the need for a network of institutions with different but complementary roles.[44]

The excellence of patient care impressed both local commentators and visitors. It was most often mentioned in relation to S. Maria Nuova, as when Matteo Villani explained why the foundation had merited a large inheritance during the Black Death. Cristoforo Landino, writing 120 years later in his *Commentary on the Divine Comedy*, waxed lyrical about S. Maria Nuova, which he called 'the first hospital among Christians':

> There are always, however difficult it may be, very white beds and always somebody who looks after the sick and provides for their needs at all times. Neither the food nor the medicines are the same for everybody, but each person is treated according to his sickness. There are always doctors, physicians and surgeons ready to give individual treatment to each person.[45]

It was, then, the combination of the diligent service of the nurses and the treatment provided by the doctors that impressed Landino. He also praised the cleanliness of the beds, suggesting frequent washing of the linen to make it 'very white', and the expert attention provided by the doctors, which included the prescription of a diet and medicine tailored to the individual patient.

A similarly laudatory description was provided by visitors, as in the case of Luther when he stayed at S. Maria Nuova in 1510–11,[46] though his comments clearly reflected his personal experience of staying in the Sapientia, a special room set aside in S. Maria Nuova for visiting clerics and laymen of good birth.[47] While the food and the cleanliness of the beds provided for the majority of patients were probably a vast improvement on their conditions at home, it is unlikely that the three hundred inmates mentioned by Landino would have received quite the same standard of service in their enormous hall-like wards as the clerics in their privileged quarters.

Clearly all these views represent the services provided by hospitals in the best possible light. Landino, like Matteo Villani before him, was stirred by patriotic fervour to represent an idealistic picture, as were the priors of the commune in their law of 1464. The same was true of Francesco Portinari, the papal proto-notary at the English court, whose dedicatory letter to King Henry VII accompanying the 'Ordinances' of 1510–11 talks of S. Maria Nuova as having added 'a welcome lustre' to Florence.[48] In his case there was also a more personal reason for wanting to praise the hospital: its foundation by his ancestor reflected glory on his family.

The reputation of hospitals in Renaissance Florence was not simply based on S. Maria Nuova, but more generally on the city's system of care. Although hospitals emerged haphazardly in the city without any apparent grand overarching design, by the fifteenth century there was an increasing awareness of the desirability of specialisation. This was certainly a reality by the time Benedetto Varchi was writing his *Storia fiorentina*. In his detailed description of the city in the late 1520s he evinces considerable pride in its hospitals, which he presents as part of a well-integrated system catering for all types of poor and sick people:

> In Florence there are two types of hospitals, some that receive male and female patients, keeping them apart, treating and looking after them until they have recovered, without charging them anything ... The other type of hospital is that which receives and gives shelter not only to travellers or to other healthy people, but also to the poor of the city, who for a night or two receive food and lodging without paying anything.[49]

Varchi makes a fundamental distinction in the typology of hospitals between those with a medical function and those with the more traditional role of providing temporary hospitality and shelter to the local poor and travellers; in a later passage he mentions another category, the foundling hospital of the Innocenti. He singles out the major medical institutions as well as the new Incurabili hospital for those suffering from the French Disease. The two features he praises in particular are that the patients are looked after until they have fully recovered and that treatment is free of charge, important characteristics that helped to persuade potential benefactors to provide funds.

If Varchi, like Antoninus before him, was impressed by the complementary roles of these institutions, ideas concerning specialisation in function were also becoming part of the language of architects, as can be seen in the treatises of Leon Battista Alberti and Antonio Filarete. Significantly, both were Florentines. Alberti also recommended that treatment of the poor should be divided into different but complementary initiatives, with the contagious separated from the non-contagious, the old from the mad. However, reflecting the debate about poor relief in Europe at this time, a harsher tone entered his voice when discussing beggars. Not only should they not be allowed to beg from door to door, he wrote, but they should not even be allowed to remain in the city for longer than three days without working, because 'no one, however disabled, is unable to do something useful for the community through his work: even the blind can be useful working for rope manufacturers'.[50]

Alberti's ideas concerning the need to separate those with different types of illness reflected contemporary ideas and practices in other parts of Italy, most strikingly in fifteenth-century Milan under first the Visconti and then the Sforza dukes.[51] This led to centralisation of resources, with small hospitals being amalgamated, and the establishment of the vast 'Ospedale Maggiore' with separate and specialised wards.[52] The foundation of the 'Ospedale Maggiore' was part of a more general movement in northern Italy, inspired in part by the Observant Franciscans, towards the centralisation of charity under a series of 'great hospitals'.[53]

That this administrative and financial reorganisation of hospital care did not take place in Florence is in part a reflection of contemporaries' self-satisfaction; in part it also derives from the fact that there was no princely power to enforce a radical rethinking of the system. This explains why the period 1450–1550 was one of retrenchment and consolidation of hospital foundations (Table 1.1). It is striking that in the century from 1450 to 1550 I have been able to discover references to only nine new hospitals in Florence, compared with twenty to twenty-five in the previous hundred-year periods.[54] The stability of these institutional arrangements is reflected in a very general way by totals provided by contemporary records: the 1427–9 Catasto listed thirty-five *spedali*, Landino mentions thirty-six in Florence in 1480 and the Decima records thirty-two in 1495.[55] These figures should probably be rounded up, for the Appendix includes at least forty-four hospitals active in Florence in c.1500. Institutional longevity is reflected in the fact that twenty-five of these forty-four hospitals survived until their suppression in the eighteenth century, first through the reforms of the House of Lorraine in the 1750s and then through the Enlightenment policies of Pietro Leopoldo in the 1780s.[56]

The lack of new foundations in this period is reflected in the pride of chroniclers and lawmakers in existing institutions. Most of the new *spedali* founded or recorded for the first time at this time were small, such as that of S. Maria degli Angioli in Via del Campuccio, established in 1489 by the Università dei Battilani (Map 1.1: 61). It had six beds dedicated to retired elderly members of their profession, the wool-carders.[57] Two other small-scale hospitals, both founded in 1508, were located near city gates and were intended to provide accommodation for travellers and pilgrims: S. Giuliano near Porta

S. Niccolò in the Oltrarno (65) and S. Rocco to the north and just inside Porta S. Gallo (66).[58] The only departure from these small foundations were the two substantial hospitals for the treatment of people sick from the main epidemic diseases: in 1479 the lazzaretto of S. Bastiano for plague victims (60) and in 1520 the Spedale della SS. Trinita for those with the French Disease (67), both of which will be dealt with in more detail below.

According to contemporaries, then, by the early sixteenth century Florence had a fairly comprehensive system of care provided by a wide range of hospitals, from the smaller for a few poor widows to the large-scale institutions for the sick and foundlings. Much of their international reputation can be attributed to admiration for S. Maria Nuova. Indeed, the very presence of this hospital is a further reason why Florence did not follow the lead of northern Italian states in reorganising and centralising its charity in the fifteenth century; it already had a 'Great Hospital'. Potential patrons channelled their charitable funds into the financing of existing hospitals rather than establishing new large-scale enterprises. Individual hospitals thereby increased their physical capacities and services to patients, two of the main characteristics of a Renaissance hospital.

The picture painted so far of the development of hospitals in fifteenth-century Florence appears to conform to the image projected by contemporaries, that, as the priors declared in 1464, 'our city above all others is copiously provided with hospitals that are beautiful and capacious'. Indeed, all this building activity took place in a period when Florence saw major construction projects involving both secular buildings, such as the Medici and Strozzi palaces, and churches, as at the cathedral and S. Marco. The *bellezza* of hospitals had thus become part of the aesthetic of the Renaissance city.

Just as it is necessary to pass behind the physical façade to understand how the Renaissance hospital functioned, so it is necessary to get behind the façade of official rhetoric and contemporary *campanilismo* – love of the bell-tower – to examine the financial implications of high levels of spending on construction and increasing running costs as the charitable system tried to cope with growing demand from the poorer levels of society. Indeed, the hundred years from the middle of the fifteenth to the middle of the sixteenth century saw a gradual but slow depreciation in the real standards of living of skilled and unskilled workers.[59] These were years of particular hardship caused by severe shortages of grain with an associated rise in the price of all basic foodstuffs. After a long period of demographic stagnation, the city of Florence now experienced a gradual growth in its population from the last quarter of the fifteenth century, though this upward movement was to suffer periods of abrupt decline, most noticeably as a result of epidemics of plague in the 1490s and, above all, in the 1520s and ending with the drawn-out siege of the city.[60]

Adverse conditions among the poor led to increasing pressure on the physical and financial capacity of the city's charitable institutions. At S. Maria Nuova, for example, there was a considerable growth in the patient population: by the early sixteenth century it admitted an average of 6,500 male and female patients each year (see below, Chapter 8). It can be no coincidence that it was in the plague year of 1479 that the penultimate extension was built to S. Maria Nuova's male ward. The number of foundlings admitted by the Innocenti also increased dramatically. When it opened in 1445 it took in sixty-two children, but by the mid-1470s this figure had increased to well over two hundred.[61] In 1506 there were 450 children in-house and 870 outside at wet-nurse and by 1540 these figures had grown to 782 and over 1,500 respectively';[62] four years later it was decided to enlarge the building's capacity in response to the growth in demand.

If government officials praised the city's hospitals as 'capacious' and 'organised to receive any healthy or sick person who is wretched', they also recognised that running these institutions was an expensive business, especially if they were being enlarged to increase capacity. Official pride was reflected not just in flowery declarations of support, but also in more practical assistance. Tax exemptions were reconfirmed from the previous century, including taxes on bequests or on contracts relating to bequests as well as gabelles on goods imported into the city.[63] Governments also granted regular contributions in kind, a common form of which was salt, at the time a valuable and much-used commodity in the preparation and conservation of food and medicines.[64]

Despite these financial and legal privileges, many hospitals continued to experience financial hardship in the fifteenth and sixteenth centuries. The neatly balanced books presented by Varchi in his discussion of S. Maria Nuova and the Innocenti are belied by other types of records for, as seen above in Chapter 2, the Catasto recorded that many hospitals were in debt by the late 1420s. This remained true twenty years later, as can be seen in a spirited letter from the Signoria to the pope when the latter attempted to tax the hospitals of the city, which argued that they had 'much larger expenses than income'.[65] The Signoria's arguments tell us much about the financial precariousness of charitable institutions in this period: here the four major medical hospitals examined above along with S. Gallo are cited in particular. The letter began by explaining that hospitals 'are all constituted and maintained by the patrimony and alms of our citizens' and that taxation would ruin them, for the Florentines 'will abstain from [giving] alms and bequests through which they are supported and of which these places have continuous need'.[66] Income from fixed assets was insufficient because of the constant demand for their services, as Varchi made clear in his discussion of S. Maria Nuova.[67]

Already by 1445 the Signoria attributed the hospitals' indebtedness to 'the large number of wretched people and male and female children who have to be cared for'.[68] This was confirmed by a petition by S. Gallo in 1449, which complained that it could no longer support the recent rise in the number of foundlings in its care.[69] The Innocenti also rapidly found itself in the same position. In 1466 a law described the hospital as in 'total poverty'; its income was insufficient to meet the expenses of looking after 201 in-house children and staff and 456 babies at wet-nurse. No permanent solution was found; by 1483 the Innocenti had an annual deficit of 3,000 lire and the director claimed that conditions were so bad that some children were actually dying of hunger.[70]

Plague was the single greatest challenge to the health and status quo of Florentine hospitals in the fifteenth century. The threat stemmed from the very real possibility that an epidemic might break out in the hospital itself, leading to the deaths of patients and staff. Epidemics also had serious economic side effects and city-states implemented increasingly strong measures to prevent the import and sale of goods from beyond the city walls at such times. Institutions such as hospitals would have suffered in the short term from a shortage of produce from their own property, just as a temporary break in communications would have interrupted the payment of rents, already a source of complaint in the 1420s.

Those factors were further exacerbated by the fact that the city had no permanent lazzaretto until the 1490s. The government therefore depended on existing hospitals to cope with crises caused by the waves of plague which returned every decade. Then, just as Florence began to put in place mechanisms to deal with plague, a new disease arrived in Europe, the Mal Francese or French Disease. Although mortality rates were not as high as with plague this fresh epidemic alarmed contemporaries owing to the drawn-out agony of those who caught it and who added a particularly unpleasant element to the crowds of disabled beggars who already littered the city's streets. It is in the context of how Florence coped with these two epidemic diseases that the relationship between hospitals and the communal authorities is best understood in this period.

3.4 Hospitals and 'the Multitude of Those Sick from Plague'

In fifteenth-century Florence hospitals bore the brunt of the human cost in the fight against plague; S. Maria Nuova was used above all to house and to treat plague victims and its nursing staff helped the sick in the city, as in 1448 when they distributed chicken soup to the poor in their houses.[71] But even in that year there was some recognition that it was not the ideal place to keep plague victims. Despite a suggestion to build a separate hospital for the infected, no plan was spelt out in detail until the reappearance of plague in 1464.[72] The priors acknowledged that in the past there would have been nowhere to place those sick from plague 'were it not for that which has been recently provided by the hospital of S. Maria Nuova of Florence'. While saying that the role of the hospital in this was 'greatly appreciated and praiseworthy', they also admitted that such activities created another problem because 'others who are sick from other illnesses become infected with the contagion of those with plague and therefore those die who should not have died'.[73]

S. Maria Nuova was not the only hospital to have suffered during the pestilence of 1464. Four years later a petition from S. Matteo recorded its financial indebtedness as a result of the epidemic, having chosen to house and treat S. Maria Nuova's patients who were sick from conditions other than plague. The *spedalingo* complained that the hospital had had to care for over a hundred sick men and women at a time, which led it to spend over 2,000 gold florins in bills to the 'apothecaries for the medicines for the sick and to the sellers of chickens and to butchers'.[74]

The problems generated for hospitals by epidemic disease finally persuaded the commune of the urgency of the need to establish a separate isolation hospital for plague victims. The subsequent decree was couched in terms of Christian charity to show the world that the city's 'door of charity was as open as in other parts of the world' to all, including those sick from plague, and was justified on the grounds that 'the greater the danger to those who look after the sick and the more these people are abandoned by everybody, the greater the merit in the eyes of God to whomever receives them and provides for their needs'.[75] The expression of such noble sentiments may have had more to do with the desire to impress other city-states with the willingness of the regime to deal with plague than with any underlying policy to receive plague victims with open arms. The Signoria would have been aware of measures taken elsewhere which left Florence behind in the battle against plague: in Venice, for example, a lazzaretto had already been opened in 1429.[76]

S. Maria Nuova was at the centre of plans for a lazzaretto in Florence. The *spedalingo* and five citizens were elected to supervise the building of a house outside the city walls to be provided with beds and all other things necessary to the functioning of a lazzaretto. The staff would consist of both spiritual and physical experts, including a priest, physician, barber, apothecary and servants, all under the personal supervision of the *spedalingo*.[77] The whole operation was financed indirectly by the hospital through its holdings in the Monte Comune, the communal debt. Normally religious institutions such as S. Maria Nuova were not allowed to sell their shares or to receive interest because they enjoyed tax-exempt status. However, in 1464 the commune provided a special dispensation so that the hospital could raise up to 3,000 gold florins on receipts from interest or sales of its credits in the state run bank, the *Monte Comune*.[78]

The close involvement of S. Maria Nuova in the administration and financing of plague provisions also had a negative side; it was ordained that while the new building was being erected, S. Maria Nuova 'must give support and receive and treat those sick from plague as it does at present'. However, this was not a long-term solution. It was declared that those sick from plague in S. Maria Nuova 'should not remain in the heart of the city', and that one or more places outside Florence should be found where they could be taken.[79] In fact, in 1464 little was done to establish a lazzaretto and so S. Maria Nuova remained at the heart of government plans to deal with threats to public health. Instead of resorting to the sale of credits in the *Monte Comune*, in 1472 and 1476 the commune provided subsidies of 500 and 1,000 gold florins to S. Maria Nuova to employ special staff (doctor, barber, servants) to look after those sick from plague, who were to be kept 'separate from the others'.[80]

When plague struck in 1477–9 it was clear that simply paying for extra medical staff was not an adequate solution. A law of April 1479 therefore declared that new subsidies were being provided 'to the new hospital which is being built on the Prato della Giustizia to treat those sick from plague'. Its finances were to be separate from those of S. Maria Nuova and were derived from fines levied by the Otto di Guardia e Balìa and other magistracies in the city; this source of income was to last for a period of three years to offset the costs.[81] The lazzaretto was to be dedicated to S. Sebastiano, the patron saint of plague victims, and the construction programme was to be administered and organised by S. Maria Nuova. When finished, it was to have two separate wards for the different sexes and a garden surrounded by a high wall to prevent the escape of diseased people and air.[82]

By mid-June 1479 extra funds were being provided by the priors to cope with the plague raging in Florence because, as they admitted, 'there would be no provision if it were not for that provided by the hospital of S. Maria Nuova'.[83] The extent of this service can be seen in a letter written at this time by the *spedalingo*, Bonini di Antonio Bonini, to Lorenzo de' Medici in which he outlined its costs, including expenses to

> supply the pharmacy with medicines we have spent 500 gold florins. Now we have to pay 100 gold florins for sugars, bought for syrups and mixtures that we have bought. And moreover we find ourselves in debt to the poultry suppliers by about 2,300 lire. As far as the expense of linen for the well and sick is concerned it is impossible to calculate; for the hospital of S. Maria della Scala spent in just this month 50 florins in clothing the dead. And the expenses increase daily.[84]

S. Maria Nuova was also looking after the sick in the city[85] by distributing bread and wine to about three hundred 'case de' morbati', which with an average of five people per household meant it was sustaining 1,500 people.[86]

S. Maria Nuova was not the only Florentine hospital to be affected by the measures taken during the epidemics in the second half of the fifteenth century. In 1464 S. Matteo had been the recipient of patients from S. Maria Nuova who were sick from 'normal' non-plague diseases at a time when the latter was still used as a lazzaretto. By June 1479 the *spedalingo* of S. Maria Nuova, Bonini, had obtained permission from the Signoria to use S. Maria della Scala as a lazzaretto. The facilities proved insufficient and in a letter written by Bonini to Lorenzo de' Medici on 5 July he recorded that they had had to be expanded on account of 'the multitude of those sick from plague'.[87] Towards the end of the month the patrons of S. Maria della Scala wrote anxiously to Lorenzo about the change of use and the expense involved, and suggested that the plague victims should be transferred to Messer Bonifazio and that their hospital should be returned to being an orphanage.[88] There is no evidence that this idea was ever put into effect. Luigi Passerini records that in the mid-nineteenth century there was still an inscription in the garden now used by nuns that read: 'In this cemetery were buried twenty thousand bodies, who died from plague in this place in the year 1479: *requiescant in pace*.'[89] Although this figure was probably exaggerated, it underlines the importance of S. Maria della Scala's role as a lazzaretto.[90]

The long and rather tortuous history of the setting up of a lazzaretto, an idea mooted a good thirty years earlier, reflects both a lack of political will, at a time of tensions among the various factions in the city,[91] and a recurrent hope that the plague would not return. It also underlines the centrality of hospitals to government measures during epidemics. This point is worth stressing both because of the implications the policy had for the hospitals themselves and because the Florentine experience contrasts with that of other major cities in northern Italy, especially Venice and Milan, which had envisaged much more substantial institutions from their inception. While the Florentine Spedale di S. Bastiano had only twenty-six beds by the 1490s, the Milanese lazzaretto had two hundred from the start.[92]

The role of S. Maria Nuova and S. Maria della Scala indicates that the lazzaretto was not yet in use: it was probably not until December 1479 that it was finished, when the priors discussed the supply of beds and linen.[93] In fact, S. Bastiano only came into its own in the 1490s, when the city was again assailed by an exceptionally serious combination of epidemic disease and severe food shortages.[94] Moreover, with the threat of plague the lazzaretto was enlarged; in November 1495 the Otto di Guardia e Balìa ordered some of the small Florentine hospitals to take one or two beds with a full complement of mattresses and linen to the new 'Spedale degli Ammorbati'.[95]

This decade of crisis must have created enormous problems for all the main elements of the city's existing sanitary structure, especially hospitals. In 1497 Florence was so inundated by the poor, in particular those from the countryside, (the *contadini*), and others from even further afield, that according to Jacopo Nardi 'all the hospitals and the other places requisitioned for plague victims were insufficient to house them'.[96] Food prices remained extremely high and contemporaries record that people actually died of hunger. There was talk in the city of an outbreak of an epidemic of 'fevers', associated with poor-quality food and unhygienic conditions.[97] The authorities now made a distinction between the local poor, including *contadini*, and everybody else and threw the latter out of the city. In mid-May 1497 the epidemic had spread to many people both in and outside the hospitals. At that time about twelve people were admitted to S. Maria Nuova every day and by the beginning of June up to twenty-four people died there each day after plague broke out among the patients.[98]

At the end of the Quattrocento hospitals still continued to play a central role during periods of dearth and disease. There was, though, a growing consensus of the necessity to separate those sick from plague from those suffering from other diseases. The establishment of the lazzaretto for plague victims should in theory have obviated the need for the direct involvement of S. Maria Nuova in the care of *appestati* (those sick from the plague) and simply left the *spedalingo* to supervise the running of S. Bastiano, but in June 1497 this neat distinction collapsed when plague broke out among S. Maria Nuova's own patients.[99] It was only during the next significant outburst of plague in Florence, during the 1520s, that proper provision was finally made for plague victims. Isolation hospitals were established for those sick with plague and the people they had had contact with; the burden of coping with plague victims was removed from hospitals and the administration of lazzarettos was assigned to the fraternity of the Misericordia under the auspices of the Ufficiali di Sanità.[100]

Plague was not the only new epidemic disease to afflict Renaissance Italy, to challenge existing sanitary structures and to demand new solutions. The most significant of these new diseases was the Mal Francese or Great Pox and its appearance as an epidemic in Italy in the mid-1490s led to the development of a new type of hospital, the Incurabili.

3.5 'The Boils of the French Disease' and the Incurabili Hospital

And in this time Florence and the *contado* were full of the boils of the French Disease, as in every city of the whole of Italy, and they lasted a long time. Though treatment succeeded in reducing the size of the boils, they continued to give much pain in all the joints and finally they returned. And no appropriate medicine was found and few died from it, but they suffered with much pain and in a disgusting way.[101]

The apothecary Luca Landucci and other contemporaries recorded that the outbreak of the Mal Francese in the mid-1490s caused widespread concern. It was the disgusting appearance or *schifezza* of the sick poor that created problems for society. In contrast to plague victims, who died rapidly, those infected with the Mal Francese remained to clutter up the streets. In Italy, as elsewhere, policies were only gradually evolved to cope with those who suffered from this new disease. Much of the initial inspiration came from individual laymen within the shadow of the Church rather than governments, although the latter supported these initiatives. Under the influence of a group of active laymen, inspired among others by the Genoese notary Ettore Vernazza and St Caterina Fieschi, a series of confraternities were established known as the Companies of Divine Love, which founded the 'Spedali degli Incurabili' to treat those sick from the Mal Francese.[102] In time a network of these hospitals was founded in many of the major Italian cities; the largest and wealthiest was S. Giacomo in Augusta in Rome, which became the mother house for all Incurabili hospitals.[103]

In Florence the Incurabili hospital of SS. Trinita was established through a combination of local and national influences.[104] According to a 1521 Bull of the archbishop, the city had for years been inundated by large numbers of poor people with incurable diseases, who were especially visible because the general hospitals for the acute sick refused them admission.[105] The Bull reflected unflattering contemporary descriptions which referred to the *mal franciosati* as travelling around on little handcarts because of the diseased condition of their limbs, and offending the visual and olfactory senses of the citizens whom they importuned for alms. A likeness of one of these beggars can be seen incised into a marble plaque in Rome outside the church of the Incurabili hospital of S. Giacomo (Plate 3.17).

In 1520 there was therefore already a groundswell of local public opinion in favour of establishing a hospital for incurables in Florence, a movement given focus by the Lenten sermon cycle of 1520 delivered in the cathedral of S. Maria del Fiore. The preacher was Don Callisto da Piacenza, an Augustinian canon regular from the Badia Fiesolana. In these sermons Don Callisto apparently (the sermons are lost) dwelt on the trials of those suffering from the Mal Francese and proposed that members of his congregation should form a society to remove these poor creatures from the streets and find a way to tend to their needs. The same day a group of 150 citizens met in the church belonging to the canons regular, S. Maria della Neve in Via S. Gallo, where under Don Callisto's guidance they founded the company of SS. Trinita, which then established a hospital of the same name to treat 'incurables'.

Although local historians have tended to present this as a spontaneous exercise by noble-minded citizens, the whole event must have been orchestrated

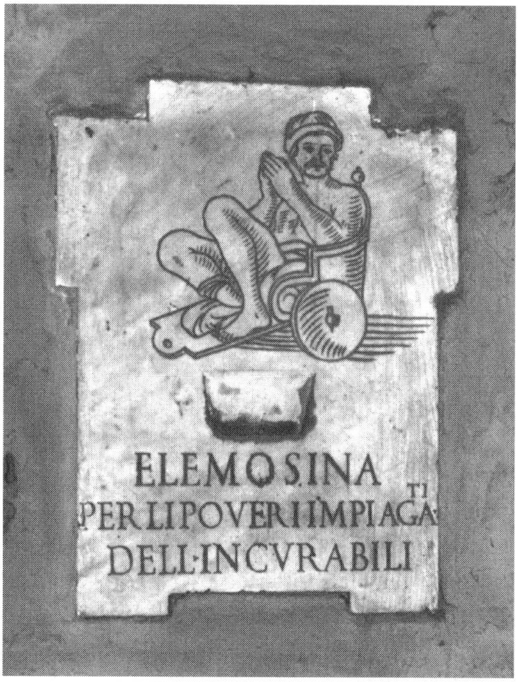

Plate 3.17 *Beggar with the French Disease Seated on a Handcart*, incised marble plaque, outside Church of S. Maria in Porta Paradisi, Hospital of S. Giacomo, Rome

from the beginning. It would not have been possible for Don Callisto to deliver one of the most prestigious sermon cycles in the cathedral without the agreement of Cardinal Giulio de' Medici, who as archbishop would have known in advance his proposed theme and message. Giulio, in turn, would have been influenced by his uncle, Pope Leo X, who was an enthusiastic supporter of the Companies of Divine Love, and would have been well aware that Don Callisto was a prominent member of the circle of Ettore Vernazza, which had recently been involved in establishing the Incurabili hospital in Naples.[106] Indeed, just as Leo encouraged the establishment of S. Giacomo in Rome, so Giulio backed the Florentine hospital. Not only was his Bull of 1521 based on Leo X's famous Bull *Salvatoris nostri* of 1515 encouraging the foundation of S. Giacomo, the hospital records also describe Giulio as the 'head, protector and founder' of the confraternity.[107]

Initially the confraternity took over two small hospitals near Porta S. Gallo, S. Caterina dei Talani and S. Rocco,[108] and began to raise funds to build new premises from leading citizens, many of whom were drawn from the influential group of Piagnoni or neo-Savonarolans.[109] Land was purchased in Via S. Gallo to the south of Messer Bonifazio; the new hospital was completed in 1534 and later extended in the 1590s by the architect Giovanni Battista Pieratti.[110] Some indication of the level of public support for this initiative is given by the fact that within the first seven months of the hospital's foundation the confraternity received nearly 2,000 gold florins in alms.[111] In April 1520 the confraternity's treasurer recorded the astonishing sum of 344 gold florins collected from the public.[112] Cardinal Giulio himself made an example by contributing 200 gold florins and the communal treasury another 330 gold florins, to be followed by an annual subvention of 43 gold florins.[113]

By 1534 the first fundraising effort had proved insufficient, however, and the senate, Senato dei Quarantotto, offered to provide the hospital with a guaranteed income from taxes on account of its reputation for 'many pious acts and great charity to the sick who are treated there'.[114] Support from Church and State continued to be forthcoming through legacies and substantial gifts from well-known individuals, such as Grand Duchess Eleonora of Tuscany and Senator Francesco Capponi, who personally underwrote Pieratti's expansion of the hospital in the 1590s.[115]

Though SS. Trinita's earliest statutes of 1521 contain little information about the types of people accepted or the treatment provided, they do indicate that it responded to public demand by dealing with the problem of the swarms of chronically sick in the streets. Four custodians were elected to 'diligently search throughout the city for those poor sick people whom they believed were oppressed by any sickness or from the Mal Francese or from another incurable disease, except for leprosy and plague'.[116] The hospital's policy was to concentrate on all incurables, including those sick from the Great Pox; when the custodians encountered 'those sick from curable diseases' they were to 'take them or cause for them to be taken to the other hospitals of the city'.[117]

Hospitals, then, played a major role in the fight against two of the major epidemics to afflict Renaissance Florence. In the widest sense this was not only part of but also contributed to a greater functional specialisation among the institutions for the treatment of the sick poor. Initially it was the larger hospitals, and especially S. Maria Nuova, that helped the city to cope with plague. But with experience the city fathers came to see that this had a negative effect on the normal patient population and created unbearable financial burdens on these institutions. This awareness, in turn, led to the emergence of the more specialised lazzaretto, which during subsequent epidemics housed plague victims, leaving S. Maria Nuova to care for those with acute diseases. Furthermore, the administrators of different types of hospital saw a clear division between the categories of people whom they did and did not admit, as at SS. Trinita, which refused admission to lepers and *appestati*. The 'incurables' were in turn declined admission by general hospitals, which normally only admitted those likely to be cured quickly.

Contemporaries recognised that specialisation and division of labour between hospitals were important aspects of health care and poor relief in the Renaissance city.[118] The idea of specialisation was taken one stage further at some of the larger institutions in other cities which housed different types of poor people separately under the same roof. For instance, S. Maria della Scala in Siena catered for both the sick and foundlings, while the vast new Ospedale Maggiore in Milan took in the acute sick and had separate provision for a whole range of conditions, including the mentally sick, *mal franciosati* and foundlings.[119] The idea of hospitals differentiating between endemic and epidemic sicknesses or acute and chronic conditions was one of the main characteristics of the new Renaissance system of care. In Florence this system encountered a severe challenge during the crises of the 1520s, but the fact that many of its main features remained intact suggests that the Renaissance hospital was more than just a pretty face and played an important role in the relief of poverty.

3.6 Crisis and Reform: 'To Keep Open the Hospital for the Benefit of the Poor of Christ'

The Crisis of the 1520s

The foundation of the Incurabili hospital in 1520 was the first of a series of measures taken to cope with epidemic disease in a decade characterised by natural and man-made disasters, including plague in 1522–4 and 1526–7, and the siege of Florence in 1529–30 with its attendant high prices and extreme shortages. In these circumstances not only were the new provisions brought in to deal with plague stretched to their limits, but so also were the charitable institutions that normally tackled poverty and sickness in the city. The 1520s were thus as crucial as the 1490s had been to the development of official policies towards the sick poor.

The 1520s saw Florence's provisions to deal with plague reach maturity. The lazzaretto of S. Bastiano was greatly enlarged and the government requisitioned a number of monasteries and other buildings as isolation centres. These complexes, together with temporary encampments of huts outside the city walls, were used to house the *sospetti*, those who had come into contact with plague victims. At the same time a full-fledged health board was established to co-ordinate the campaign during the epidemic, although there is no evidence, contrary to what is usually claimed, that it became a permanent magistracy at this stage.[120] The main work in providing food and medicines to those shut up in their houses was now no longer the responsibility of S. Maria Nuova, but was instead assigned to the greatly expanded fraternity of the Misericordia.[121]

In theory, then, during epidemics of plague the major medical hospitals should have been unaffected by rising mortality in the city. And, indeed, the basic system seems to have worked; as will be shown in Chapter 8, there was no dramatic rise of deaths among S. Maria Nuova's patients during the two major epidemics of 1522–4 and 1526–7 (Table 8.3a, b). However, the last two years of the decade show a very different picture: for many months the number of deaths was consistently higher for both male and female patients at S. Maria Nuova; male deaths represented 38 per cent of the overall total recorded for the whole period 1512–30. This coincided almost exactly with the ten-month siege of the city by the French and Imperial armies, from November 1529 to August 1530, in an attempt to restore the Medici family who had been ousted in 1527. Combined with the existing severe food shortages, a feature in many parts of Italy since 1527,[122] conditions worsened each month, exacerbated by epidemic disease.

During 1529 and 1530 all charitable institutions, and in particular the large medical hospitals, played an important part in dealing with the sick and hungry. The special Commissioners for the Poor, who were appointed in spring 1529, summarised the gravity of the situation as follows: 'Given the multiplication in the number of poor people, caused by the unexpected shortage which is increasing, it is terrible and cruel to see and hear all the people in the city who suffer and protest because they are dying of hunger.'[123] There were two main elements to the response: the first involved designating specific locations where food would be provided to the poor, the second involved housing the poor in the city's hospitals.

> And because many of these said poor people are found sick in the streets through their weakness caused by hunger [the Commissioners are authorised] to send them to the hospitals of S. Maria Nuova, Lelmo, S. Pagolo and Bonifazio of Florence ... and the said most excellent Lords order the *spedalingi* of these said hospitals ... to receive and accept [these poor sick people] in their said hospitals like the other poor sick people under pain of the anger of the Commissioners.[124]

That this policy was actually instituted is reflected in the high levels of mortality at S. Maria Nuova, especially when the price of grain reached 117s a bushel, over four times the average price in more normal times (Figure 8.4a, b).[125]

The 1520s, therefore, represented a period of crisis for the poor of Florence, with very high prices and unemployment leading to plunging standards of living as a triumvirate of natural and man-made disasters struck the city: plague, famine and war. Governments adopted a number of strategies to deal with this situation: the establishment of isolation hospitals; provision of subsidised food to victims of plague and famine; and the strict maintenance of order within the city. Existing charitable institutions also played an important part, but they, and in particular the city's major medical hospitals, paid a price for doing so.

The Medici Dukes and Reform

The attention of Duke Cosimo's predecessor, Alessandro de' Medici, had been drawn to the financial plight of the city's charitable institutions soon after his return to Florence in 1531, following a period of exile during the short-lived Republic. As well as the severe pressure on their resources caused by the large number of starving and sick people in Florence, the republic in the late 1520s had met some of the spiralling costs of the defence of the city by plundering the finances of religious and charitable institutions. The most affluent hospitals, such as S. Maria Nuova and the Innocenti, had been subjected to forced loans and heavy taxation.[126] This had put them in the unenviable position of having to liquidate their cash reserves, including returnable deposits and bequests, leaving them without the wherewithal to underwrite deposits and testamentary obligations.[127]

The wealth of hospitals also suffered as a result of the Republic's policy of razing secular and ecclesiastical property within a mile of the city walls, while more far-flung houses and farms were often destroyed by enemy action, further depriving institutions of rent and produce to feed their personnel and patients. The actual premises of some hospitals were affected where they lay close to the city walls. One of the oldest, S. Gallo, was pulled down to prevent it providing cover for the besieging army; as the 'Catena' view of Florence shows, it was quite a considerable complex outside Porta S. Gallo in c.1470 (Plate 1.3).[128] The hospital of S. Giovanni fra l'Arcora outside Porta al Prato was also demolished in the preparations for the siege, despite being run by an international order of Hospitallers, the Knights of St John of Jerusalem.

The financial state of S. Maria Nuova caused the greatest concern to contemporaries, sufficient for the subject to have been mentioned by the chronicler Benedetto Varchi, who recorded that the hospital 'was in the greatest disorder, having lost much during the war and spent much more than in normal times'.[129] On 20 October 1532 a commission of enquiry was established, to include the *spedalingo* of S. Maria Nuova, to discover the exact causes of its problems and to propose a remedy. More precise information about the reasons for its losses was recorded in a law of March 1533 in which new sources of income were granted to the hospital.[130] In addition to the 'infinite amount of damage due to the recent war', the Medicean regime blamed the financial losses on members of the republican government, who were described as 'men who had little affection for their city'.[131] In particular they were accused of having confiscated money that had been left on deposit with S. Maria Nuova; over the previous seventy years the hospital had developed a banking service that provided interest on deposits.[132]

The solutions proposed by the commission and in a series of laws over the following year involved granting privileges and providing new sources of income. The hospital was allowed to suspend payment of its debts for a period of four years. At the same time the process was speeded up for the reclamation of its own debts: 'the judges, officials and ministers of these places [should] provide quick and expeditious decisions and justice, discovering quickly the truth of the case.'[133] Then, from March 1534, the Senato dei Quarantotto provided the hospital with a series of new sources of income, including granting it a percentage of the taxes on the sale of bread and wood for the construction industry. This was in addition to annual subventions for four years of 2,000 ducats from the Monte di Pietà, the state-run pawn bank, and of 1,200 ducats from the gabelle on the sale of salt.[134] Even these substantial contributions did not resolve S. Maria Nuova's financial problems. Two years later it was described as being in 'the greatest need'. At this time it was declared that 'it must be subsidised in order to keep open the hospital for the benefit of the poor of Christ', and the hospital was given permission to suspend its debts to its creditors for a further six years.[135]

This series of privileges and financial packages was an extension of the traditional protectionist policy of Florentine governments, but on a much larger scale. However, official intervention came at a price and had long-term implications for the hospital's independence. For instance, it began a process that enabled the Medici dukes to gain greater control over the way the hospital was run, a fate shared with other hospitals in Florence, including S. Paolo, the Incurabili and the Innocenti. The commission, which had been elected in October 1532 to investigate S. Maria Nuova's finances, now became a permanent feature; each year it returned to check the hospital's accounts to make sure that its income had been spent properly.[136] Later in the century this was taken even further by Duke Ferdinand when he imposed an official to superintend the hospital's administration.[137]

Another significant strategy adopted by the Medici dukes to gain greater control over the city's major hospitals was to intervene in the election of *spedalingi*. At S. Maria Nuova this process was initiated by the Medici pope Clement VII, who in 1532 took away the right of the Portinari family to choose the *spedalingo* and nominated his own candidate, Don Angelo Morsi, abbot of the Vallombrosan monastery, leaving the Portinari with the merely formal role of presenting the candidate to the archbishop of Florence for approval. When Morsi died in 1544 Duke Cosimo quickly intervened before the new pope had time to interfere – Clement had died ten years earlier – and imposed his own nominee, a monk in the Florentine Badia, Don Isidoro da Montauto.[138] Over ten years the Medici family had therefore succeeded in reversing the basic rights of the patronal family of S. Maria Nuova which had lasted for some 250 years. However, it was important for the Medici that the Portinari should remain nominal patrons in order to combat the Church's claims to elect the *spedalingo*. Thus, in 1561, when the last male member of the Portinari family in Florence died, Duke Cosimo sought out a distant branch living in Milan and returned the patronage rights to the brothers Manetto Dionigi and Adovardo di Manetto Portinari.[139]

S. Maria Nuova was not the only hospital to fall under the influence of the creeping bureaucratisation of the Florentine state. Cosimo and his successors Alessandro and Ferdinando continued to expand their control over the more affluent Florentine hospitals.[140] The next in the line of fire was the Innocenti; in the past its patrons, the silk guild of Por S. Maria, had elected the *spedalingo* for periods of between three months and three years. Now the duke made the office a lifetime appointment and reserved to himself the right to confirm the election, thus facilitating government control.[141] These moves were not simply designed to extend Medicean power; they also reflected genuine concern over the state of these institutions. The same was true for S. Paolo, which had a chequered history in the sixteenth century as a result of conflicts between the administrators and the role of the nursing staff, especially after they assumed a more enclosed life-style following the decrees of the Council of Trent. In the late 1540s accusations of debt, falling standards of care, scarcity of patients and what Luigi Passerini described as 'a series of embarrassing scandals, over which decency requires me to draw a veil',[142] led Cosimo in 1549 to request the pope to intervene. The papal reforms, which were finally initiated in the 1570s, did not resolve all of the problems and only in 1592 did Grand Duke Ferdinand intervene decisively and turn S. Paolo into the city's first hospital for convalescents.[143]

This policy of intervention by the Medici dukes into the affairs of the major hospitals of the capital can be interpreted either as protectionism or as exploitation. Florentine historians, such as Passerini and Arnaldo D'Addario, are inclined to be positive in their portrayal of Cosimo's motives, as indeed was an American historian who declared recently that 'the Duke cared passionately about charity'.[144] There is no doubt that Florence's hospitals following the depredations of the republican regime and the siege in the late 1520s were in need of financial assistance. This was an ongoing problem and in the late 1560s, for example, Cosimo authorised substantial loans to be made by the Monte di Pietà to S. Paolo and the Innocenti (2,000 and 800 scudi respectively).[145] It seems likely that the duke was genuinely concerned about the exploitation of hospitals by unprincipled individuals. In 1557 a scam was discovered among the male nursing staff of S. Maria Nuova, some of whom had been accused of only staying long enough to learn the 'art of the apothecary or the surgeon' and then leaving without permission to practise elsewhere for profit; Cosimo ruled that such people should be exiled.[146] The various decrees concerning S. Paolo also appear to ring true, though some accusations against the staff and the care provided by the nuns do need to be questioned. For example, an investigation in the early 1570s, which reported that there were no longer many patients in the hospital, is belied by the surviving registers of those admitted for treatment between 1554 and 1603.[147] Furthermore, as the renewed statutes of 1571 remind us, 'the main aim of [those] who founded this pious place [was] to exercise effective charity towards the sick poor'.[148]

The possibility that the Medicean dukes took advantage of the financial disarray of the hospitals to gain control of their very considerable possessions should not be discounted, especially given that many of the larger charitable institutions, including the fraternities of the Misericordia and the Buonomini di S. Martino, were absorbed by the Medicean bureaucracy.[149] Furthermore, while the loans authorised by Cosimo to various hospitals may have answered their immediate needs, they also increased their dependence on him.[150] This two-edged policy can be seen in operation across a wider canvas in relation to Cosimo's general move to centralise and streamline the bureaucracy of the Tuscan state. In March 1542 he issued an edict to institute a survey of the charitable institutions in the Florentine territory and to reform those found to be inefficient and corrupt.[151] Excess funds were siphoned off and sent to the capital to finance measures to cope with the problems of two groups of society for whom existing arrangements were deemed to be inadequate.[152] The first were abandoned children over the age of three; although there was already a series of foundling homes, older orphaned children remained a problem. The second, beggars, seem to have provoked a less charitable reaction and one more typical of early modern views towards the shiftless poor, a perception no doubt provoked by the influx into Florence of the very poor during the recent period of dearth.[153]

The edict of 1542 was full of good intentions to reform existing institutions and to tackle what were regarded as some of the major social problems of the day. The administrative machinery was set in motion almost immediately by the election of a commission of five (later expanded to twelve) good men, the Buonomini del Bigallo, who were given full powers to exercise ducal authority.[154] What made this initiative particularly remarkable was that the Buonomini's power was extended over not just the city of Florence, but the whole of Medicean Tuscany.[155] Local notables were elected to survey local hospitals and charitable institutions in the state and the directors of all hospitals, except those under ecclesiastical control, were required to submit annual accounts of their income and expenditure and to send any surplus to the Buonomini in Florence.[156]

Despite the rhetoric of the 1542 decree, few hospital administrators appear to have provided the information requested until July 1543, when a new decree was issued supported by a papal bull. Over the following fourteen months reports from 104 institutions were supplied by thirty-three different territorial administrators.[157] One should not, however, exaggerate the efficiency of this system over the longer term. Just as the traditional picture of a centralised Medicean state has recently been modified to present a more nuanced view of a negotiated settlement between local and central powers, so it has also been suggested that Cosimo encouraged the Buonomini not to enforce penalties for the non-fulfilment of all aspects of the decree in order to avoid offending patricians and local interests.[158]

Once the machinery had been set in motion to raise finance the Buonomini began to implement new initiatives in the capital, made more urgent because, as the Senato dei Quarantotto noted in November 1542, 'the number of poor abandoned children has grown in the city of Florence and is increasing every day'.[159] The following month the Buonomini took over the Spedale dei Broccardi in Via S. Gallo to house abandoned boys. This hostel became an established feature of the city's charitable system, receiving support from both public and private sources. The project was seen as particularly worthy of Christian charity since the recipients were more easily controlled and the whole enterprise redounded to the good reputation of the city and its reigning family. In time the premises proved insufficient for its needs, however, particularly during the famine of the early 1590s, when the much larger convent of S. Caterina was requisitioned to meet demand.[160]

The Broccardi was intended not just to feed and house its occupants, but also to educate them and make them into moral and useful citizens. These aims were outlined in the papal Bull of July 1543, based on the Buonomini's first statutes,[161] and included the injunction that all children were to be 'instructed in the divine precepts', taught the trade to which they were most suited and then found work with an employer who would 'treat them with charity to the honour of God'.[162] Discipline was strict, with punishments for those boys who left the hostel without permission so that they 'do not have the opportunity to commit an infinite number of sins and so that they live in fear of God and love of Our Saviour Jesus Christ'.[163]

It was contemporary concern for girls and women that led to the most innovatory developments in Florentine charity in the second half of the sixteenth century: the establishment of four conservatories between 1551 and 1590. However, these foundations do not appear to have been initiatives of either the ecclesiastical hierarchy or the dukes of Tuscany. Rather, they were founded by members of the laity, although frequently guided and inspired by individual religious. Thus, both the Monastero del Ceppo (1551) and the Monastero di S. Maria e S. Niccolò (1555), which were later united, were founded by groups of patricians.[164] In 1554 a group of pious women, headed by Margherita Borromei and under the influence of the Dominican

Alessandro Capocchi, was the main force behind the Monastero delle Fanciulle Abbandonate della Pietà.[165] Towards the end of the century, in 1590, the Monastero di S. Caterina was established by three prominent men: Giovan Battista Botti, who was also closely involved in this period of dearth with initiatives for the institutionalisation of local beggars, Giulio Zanchini, who was a knight of Malta, and Girolamo Michelozzi, a knight of the crusading order of S. Stefano.[166]

The influence of the Counter-Reformation can be detected clearly in the statutes of these four hostels. Both those of S. Maria e S. Niccolò and S. Caterina declared that they had been established during periods of crisis, which necessitated many girls 'going begging through the streets', in order 'to avoid many bad things and sins'.[167] Clearly, while the preservation of female virtue may have been the underlying motive for these foundations, it should not be forgotten that periods of dearth sparked all three initiatives.[168]

The statutes of these institutions have similar aims and present a picture of a strict, almost monastic way of life; it is no accident that these institutions were known as *monasteri*. The prevailing ethos had much in common with the conventual way of life, with an emphasis on obedience and rules of silence and good behaviour, summed up in the injunction that the girls should be 'healthy in body and mind so that nobody through any blemish causes our place to be infected since it is now in such a state of cleanliness'.[169] They were employed in various ways, each working under a *maestra* or mistress, who taught them to weave or work with silk or gold thread.[170] These conservatories for girls were thus very much part of the later sixteenth-century concern for the vulnerability of both married and unmarried women, which also led to the creation of houses organised on expressly conventual lines, such as that of the Malmaritate for unhappily married women.[171]

Perhaps less motivated by Christian charity was the third initiative typical of this period: the clauses in the Buonomini's statutes that dealt with beggars.[172] Distinctions familiar from legislation in other parts of Italy and Europe were drawn based on the idea of sorting the moral sheep from the immoral goats. In the former category were those 'poor beggars over ten years of age, impotent and forced to beg in order to live', who were to be collected in the city's hospitals where they were to 'receive lodging, heat and light'. Those whom the Buonomini decided were 'able to earn their bread through working and labour' were given shelter and expected to pay for food 'from their own sweat'. Furthermore, since this was a measure designed to clear the streets of beggars, only a few licensed by the Buonomini were allowed to go on begging, and then for a maximum of three days, including impotent and sick locals and any worthy poor from outside Florence. False beggars, who simulated sickness and attempted to cheat the public into giving alms, were to be punished.[173]

These proposals to deal with beggars would have represented one of the more far-reaching programmes in early modern Italy if they had been put into practice. In the event little was done. Cosimo evidently saw them as unworkable because of the expense involved in administering and financing the scheme. Furthermore, since these measures probably represented a reaction to the effects of the 1539 dearth, when significant numbers of beggars had been attracted to the city in search of sustenance, with the amelioration of the situation there was suddenly less urgency. It was not until 1621 that Florence founded a beggars' hostel, the Ospedale dei Mendicanti, of a sort common in other Italian cities, to house beggars and provide them with work.[174] However, recent studies have shown that even these institutions did not fall into the Foucaultian categories of repression and incarceration. Instead they tended to offer temporary solutions during periods of economic downturn, when a larger proportion of the population than normal found it difficult to make ends meet, so leading to an increase in the number of people who were supported by institutions and begging.

Conclusion

The model of the Renaissance hospital that had evolved over the fourteenth and fifteenth centuries remained central to measures for coping with the poor, whether they were sick from endemic or epidemic diseases or reduced to the status of homeless beggars. All these institutions were substantial in scale, impressive in appearance and offered increasingly specialised facilities as part of the system of care developed by the Renaissance city. Many measures that historians have viewed as characteristic of early modern attitudes towards the poor actually have their roots in earlier periods. Though Cosimo's attitude towards beggars in the mid-sixteenth century has sometimes been thought of as novel, intolerance was hardly a new phenomenon and there are numerous examples of this type of policy in fourteenth and fifteenth-century legislation.[175] Similar sentiments are also to be found in Alberti's treatise on architecture written in the 1450s; the aim was to prevent the poor from 'disturbing honest citizens uselessly through begging and harassing them with their repugnant appearance'.[176]

Cosimo's reform programme of 1542 shared elements of the policies of other governments in other parts of northern Italy over the previous 150 years, when a series of states had sought to centralise their charitable resources.[177] The reason this type of initiative had not been attempted earlier in Florence may have had much to do with the dramatic changes of regime from the mid-1490s with periods of republican rule (1494–1512, 1527–30) alternating with the Medici family's dominance, and a consequent lack of political power and will to implement such drastic reforms.[178] It may also have stemmed from pride in the existing poor-relief system. New initiatives then grew out of measures to combat specific social conditions caused by epidemics or famine with the concomitant high demand on available resources. This is illustrated by the drawn-out history of the foundation of the lazzaretto in Florence. It took practically forty years to establish S. Bastiano, a project that was repeatedly shelved after epidemics had passed and only promoted again as a kneejerk reaction to the next visitation of the plague.

Another motor for change in the later sixteenth century was the Counter-Reformation which introduced a new moral component in the exercise of charity. This was exemplified by the Incurabili hospital in Florence, whose 1574 statutes now list certain moral and financial prerequisites for admission to SS. Trinita for treatment: 'those people who brought with them a certificate from their physician of having need to take the wood [Guaiacum] and a certificate from their parish priest that they are really poor and cannot afford to treat themselves.'[179] The new 'redemptive charity', as Brian Pullan has labelled it, is also seen in the campaign in the second half of the sixteenth century to institutionalise boys in the new hostel of the Broccardi and poor girls and women in conservatories. This new moral element was even more evident in the houses for *convertite*, institutions designed to reclaim prostitutes, convince them of the error of their ways and 'convert' them to a religious life in a monastic setting.[180]

Just as intolerance towards beggars was not peculiar to the sixteenth century, so the religious underpinning of charity was not new to the Counter-Reformation. Indeed, underlying the functioning of hospitals in this period is the continued importance of their religious role as part of the Church's mission to reclaim the hearts and souls of the population. Thus, to enter a hospital, hostel or conservatory for reformed prostitutes implied participation in a set of religious rituals, central to which was the celebration of Mass, underlining the complementary roles of the *medico fisico* and the *medico spirituale* in the cure of the body and of the soul.

PART II

HEALING THE SOUL

qui contra fecerit tribus dies in pane et aqua ieiunet.

De suscipiendis infirmis
et ministrandis illis. Cap. xij.

Cum ve-
ne-
runt in-
firmi i-
n' de
portari
fuerint
domui

sancti sps. tali modo fu[sa]

CHAPTER 4

'To the Almighty Physician No Infirmity Is Incurable': The Role of the Hospital church

Introduction

The church and the ward together formed the stage for the enactment of the hospital's two main functions, the cure of the soul and the cure of the body. This chapter will concentrate on the 'cure of the soul' within the context of the hospital church, which was among the most public spaces on such sites, where staff, ambulatory patients and members of the public attended Mass and celebrated annual festivals. Chapter 5 will then examine the ward as a focus of devotional activity and provider of care, leaving consideration of specifically medical treatment to Part III. Chapters 4 and 5 will be linked, fittingly, by a short section on the cloister, the intermediate space between church and ward which provided patients, visitors and staff with an area for quiet contemplation and helped to ease the spiritual pain that was thought to cause physical disease.

4.1 *Christus Medicus*

The overriding importance of the role of religion in the healing process is conceptualised in the idea of Christus Medicus and the relationship between the divine physician and the mortal physician, particularly as developed by St Augustine. Christ was portrayed as the divine physician who cured men's spiritual diseases. Disease was equated with sin and health with virtue, as Augustine makes clear in one of his sermons: 'Like a skilled physician, the Lord knew better what was going on inside the patient than the patient himself. In the case of bodily infirmities, human physicians do what the Lord also is able to do in infirmities of the souls.'[1] Augustine takes further this comparison between the human and divine physician in another sermon: 'To the Almighty Physician no infirmity is incurable … The human physician sometimes is deceived and promises health in the human body. Why is he deceived? Because he is treating

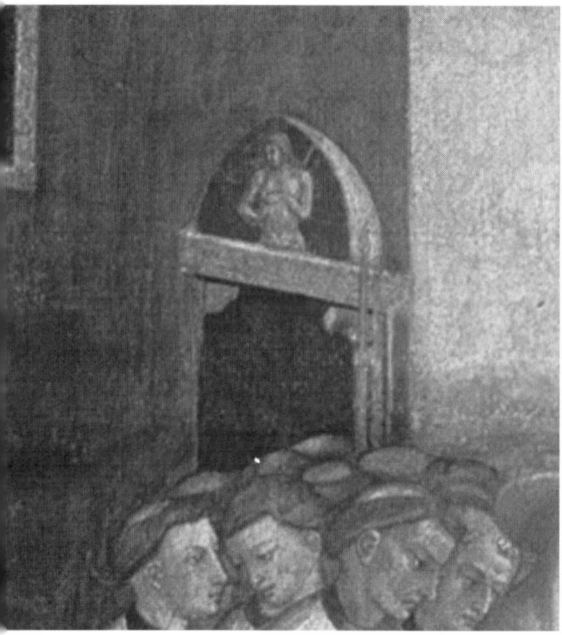

Plate 4.1 'Man of Sorrows', detail of Bicci di Lorenzo, *Martin V Confirming the Consecration of S. Egidio*, 1424–5, Salone di Martino V, Hospital of S. Maria Nuova

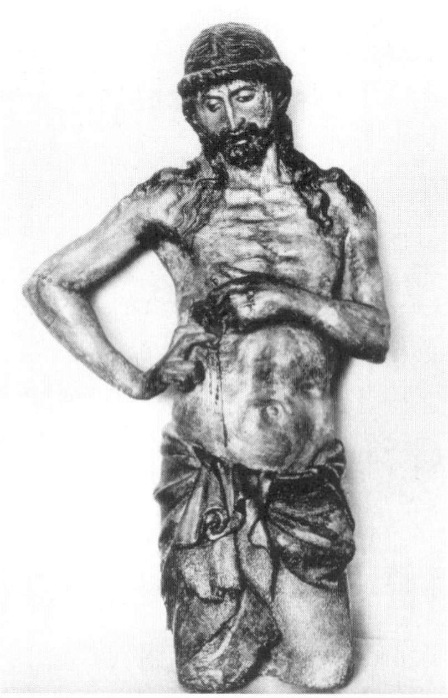

Plate 4.2 Florentine School, *Christ Showing His Wound*, c.1420–5 (Victoria and Albert Museum, London)

what he has not made. God, however, made your body, God made your soul. He knows how to restore what He has made.'[2]

Augustine's comments help to explain the ubiquity of the image of Christ in the medieval and Renaissance hospital. Emphasis was placed on representing the physical sufferings of Christ, which were associated closely with the condition of the patients and which above all pointed the way to their spiritual salvation. The importance of this image to Florence's major hospital, S. Maria Nuova, is reflected in the commissioning in c.1424 of a sculpture of the Man of Sorrows for the lunette above the door into the cemetery, as depicted in Bicci di Lorenzo's fresco discussed in the Introduction (Plate 4.1; and cf. Plate I).

For a long time this figure was identified with the painted terracotta sculpture attributed to Dello Delli in the Victoria and Albert Museum in London (Plate 4.2).[3] Although recently this attribution has been convincingly refuted, the work remains significant for us for its iconographic theme increasingly important in the second half of the fourteenth century as a fresco or panel painting, but apparently unique in Florence in this period as a sculpture.[4] Unlike the more usual image of this subject, Christ is not represented with His arms extended, but instead with His fingers inserted into His wound. The reason for this method of representation is obviously in part practical given the restricted space of the lunette. The horrifying realism of the subject also serves to underline most graphically the link between the theme of the Crucifixion and the Chiostro delle Ossa. The eyes of visitors are ineluctably drawn to the large gaping wound at the centre of the composition, thereby causing them to associate themselves with the only too visible suffering and death of Christ. Moreover, as mentioned above in Chapter 3, the position of the sculpture above the entrance door to the cemetery is paralleled by the tradition that saw the wound in Christ's side as representing a door to salvation. More generally, the theme of the Man of Sorrows also serves to reflect the pain and illness of the people who died in the hospital and were buried in the cemetery.[5] This is taken one stage further in the closed state of one of the best-known pictures associated with a late medieval hospital, Grünewald's *Eisenheim Altarpiece*, where the crucified Christ is shown covered with boils.[6]

This image of Christ was far from carrying just a negative message for visitors. Worshippers and patients would have been reminded that the suffering of both Christ and the inmates promised redemption, thus helping to justify the role of the hospital in serving the sick. Contemporary awareness of the Augustinian concept of Christus Medicus in Florence in this period is reflected in the treatise of the Dominican friar Domenico Cavalca, *Lo specchio della croce*, also known as the *Medicina del cuore*.[7] In his discussion of the first of the Works of Mercy, visiting the sick, he tells us that Christ 'came as a doctor not just to visit us, but to cure us'. Cavalca likens the corporeal sufferings of Christ to a 'bitter medicine' which He took to cure us of the 'sickness of sin ... Thus Christ acted as our midwife and took the medicine to heal us.'

If Cavalca's picture of Christ as healer points to His role as Christus Medicus, that of midwife was more familiarly associated with Mary as nursing mother and intercessor, famous for her healing powers.[8] The relationship between Mary and her Son was represented on the exterior of the hospital in a terracotta group attributed to Dello Delli of the *Coronation of the Virgin*, a theme that had played a central role in Marian imagery and been represented frequently in frescoes and altarpieces in Trecento Florence.[9] The *Coronation* is clearly represented in the lunette above the church doorway in Bicci di Lorenzo's fresco of c.1424 (Plate 4.3). Indeed, Bicci himself painted and gilded the group of figures, which stands out dramatically from the white background,[10] thus underlining the importance of Mary's role for the hospital. In contrast to the pain represented in the image of the Man of Sorrows, Christ is shown here in the joyous act of crowning Mary, representing the culmination

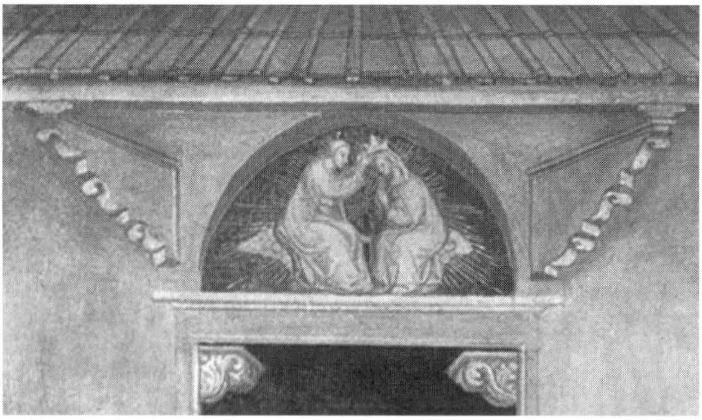

Plate 4.3 *Coronation of the Virgin*, attributed to Dello Delli, c.1424: detail of Bicci di Lorenzo, *Martin V Confirming the Consecration of S. Egidio*, Salone di Martino V, S. Maria Nuova

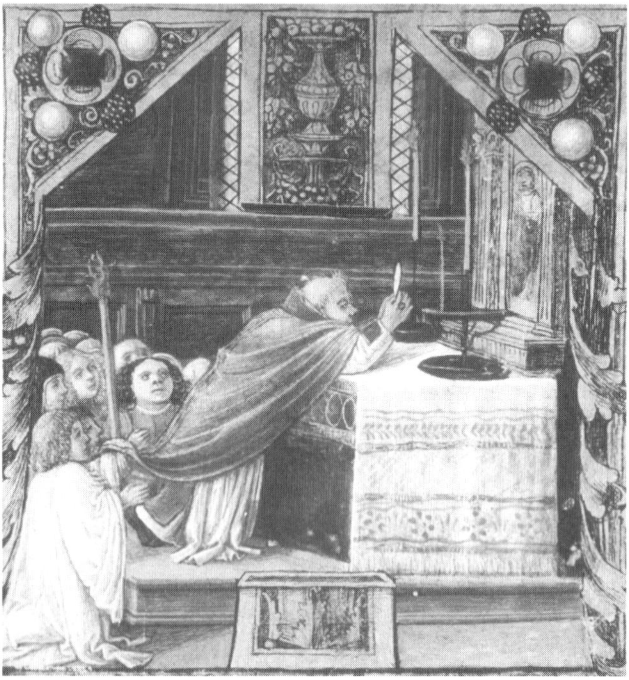

Plate 4.4 Gherardo and Monte di Giovanni di Miniato, *Celebration of Mass*, 1474 (S. Egidio, Missal, 1474: Museo Nazionale del Bargello MS 67, f. 151r)

of her bodily assumption and her triumph over death. The brilliance of the scene emphasises that it takes place in Heaven, a setting also suggested by the figures being seated on clouds, so underlining to visitors the hope of eternal felicity and drawing them into the church, where they would view the body of

Christ elevated at the central point of the Mass. It has been noted that the positioning of Christ to the viewer's left rather than right is unusual.[11] The arrangement makes sense, however, when seen in relation to the entrance to the Chiostro delle Ossa, for it makes reference to the other lunette, reminding us that this joyful scene cannot be understood without the suffering represented by the Man of Sorrows.

These terracotta figures on the façade therefore introduced the visitor to two of the main themes of the hospital through the images of two sacred figures: Christ in His role as Christus Medicus promoted both the spiritual and medical health of patients; Mary, as the new patron of the church, was a visible embodiment of spiritual purity as she was crowned by her Son, a felicity that she passes on to visitors and patients alike in her role as heavenly intercessor. These sculptures have to be thought of in relation to the Bicci di Lorenzo fresco itself, painted beside the main entrance to S. Egidio between the church door and the entrance to the main cloister.[12] This commemoration of a major event in the life of the hospital also helped to emphasise the importance of the hospital in the Renaissance city.

4.2 The Hospital Church: Devotion, Decoration and the Cure of the Soul

Hospital churches were among the most accessible parts of a hospital complex. They were usually built at the front of the site, just off the street, where a passer-by could attend Mass. Moreover, considerable sums were lavished on these spaces. It was, after all, important that the devotion of the public should be excited by the presence of splendid religious objects, helping to stimulate them to finance the running of hospitals, which were constantly in need of cash. S. Egidio became one of the most important centres for artistic patronage in mid-fifteenth-century Florence, commissioning works by some of the leading Italian Renaissance painters, including Fra Angelico, Domenico Veneziano, Piero della Francesca, Bicci di Lorenzo, Andrea del Castagno, Alessio Baldovinetti and Fra Filippo Lippi.

The patron of a hospital played a central role in the embellishment of its church and chapels. In Florence, as elsewhere, the foundation of hospitals was often associated with affluent merchants, including Folco di Ricovero Portinari at S. Maria Nuova, Lemmo Balducci at S. Matteo, Francesco di Marco Datini at the Innocenti; an exception was Bonifazio Lupi of Parma, who had been employed as a mercenary by the Florentine republic. The goal of these men in founding such institutions was partly to express Christian charity and partly to establish an institution with a commemorative function to benefit their souls in the afterlife. Other, more worldly considerations would also have been at work, in particular a desire to promote their identity in the city, as has been argued recently in relation to Giovanni Benci's patronage of the monastery of Le Murate.[13] If this was true of Benci, how much more so might it have been the case for a man like Folco d'Adoardo Portinari, who, despite his distinguished ancestry, was the representative of an impoverished branch of the family by the early fifteenth century.[14] The year 1420 was pivotal not just for the development of S. Egidio, but also for the Portinari family: in that year they extended their patronage rights from the chapel in the male ward to the choir of the church.[15] Folco thus assumed a central role in plans for the decoration of the Cappella Maggiore in the 1420s, in part probably inspired by his close association with Cosimo de' Medici, who in these years was engaged in developing his own artistic and architectural projects.[16] Folco had become manager of the Florentine branch of the Medici bank just over a month after the consecration ceremony on 16 October 1420 and remained in the post until his premature death in 1431.[17]

Much of the following section will concentrate on the religious and artistic life of S. Egidio, since it is by far the best-documented hospital church in the city, in terms of both written and iconographic evidence.[18] However, S. Egidio's development needs to be examined in relation to the development of other hospital churches in late fourteenth- to early fifteenth-century Florence. While S. Maria Nuova had taken over and extended a pre-existing church, those of the two new medical hospitals (Messer Bonifazio and S. Matteo) were built from scratch. This gave them the opportunity to build larger structures. S. Egidio was the shortest in length, even after Bicci di Lorenzo's extension of 1420 (16.5 metres); S. Matteo's was a full 6 metres longer.[19] The Innocenti's church followed within fifty years and S. Paolo was expanded and remodelled in the later fifteenth century.[20] Each shared a similar design; a long rectangular ground plan, with the main altar situated about three-quarters of the way along the length of the church, and a choir and sacristy behind.

The ground plans of all the major hospitals in the city can be reconstructed from a series of remarkable late eighteenth-century plans and in some cases from their surviving structures.[21] It is not straightforward to estimate the extent of subsequent changes to the fabric due to expansion and changes in use, but other types of documentary source can be used to flesh out the fifteenth-century reality. These include inventories and account books recording the purchase of objects for the hospital for a wide range of uses from medical, religious and administrative ones to construction projects. Liturgical manuscripts and devotional objects also help to reconstruct how churches and ward chapels were used for the cure of the souls of patrons, patients, staff and visitors.

The richness of S. Egidio's devotional life even before its enlargement and redecoration is reflected in the hospital's 1376 inventory, of which three-

and-a-half entire folios are taken up with a detailed list of the contents of church and sacristy.[22] The vast majority of items listed were associated with the liturgy celebrated in the church. The clergy attended all the prescribed hours of divine office during day and night, while all other members of staff, including *conversi* and servants, had to be present at Mass at least once a day.[23] The statutes also stipulated mandatory attendance at the hospital's main festivals of St Giles, St Luke and the Purification of the Virgin, though account books over the previous fifty years listed additional feast days, recording expenses for the purchase of food to sustain those attending vigils. In 1336, for example, chickens were bought for the vigil of S. Egidio, peaches and cherries for S. Piero in 1335, 7lb of fish for the vigil of Ognissanti and veal and beef for the festival of St Elizabeth in 1349.[24]

This regular round of liturgical observance necessitated the ownership of a substantial quantity of elaborate vestments for the clergy, as well as altar cloths and frontals, which were changed according to the calendar:

> Item a vestment of red cloth with a chasuble with a golden fringe worked with lions and a stole and a dalmatic, maniple and a tunicle with a thistle decoration made with a compass as was done in the past.
> Item an altar cloth made from purple cloth worked in gold … and with a strip above embroidered with griffins and butterflies and other decoration.[25]

S. Egidio also owned a series of service books, from missals, antiphonaries and psalters to books of offices for each day of the year and for the sick and the dead.[26] Some measure of the importance attached to this collection is suggested by the fact that the hospital commissioned leading illuminators to illustrate them, including Lorenzo Monaco in the early Quattrocento, and Gherardo and Monte di Giovanni di Miniato and Bartolommeo di Fruosino later in the century.[27]

The number, variety and high level of decoration of vestments and choral books underline the importance of S. Egidio as a hospital church in the city. This centrality is also evident in its ownership of devotional objects. Although much more is known about the larger altarpieces and frescoes commissioned in the decades following the rededication of the church in 1420, the inventory also lists smaller works with important devotional roles, such as a small portative ivory image (*tavoluzam*) of the Virgin and two angels and three crucifixes to be hung above altarpieces as well as reliquaries.[28] One made of 'gilded copper' contained the relics of St Agnes,[29] the virgin and martyr of fourth-century Rome who had a reputation for healing. According to *The Golden Legend* she had cured Constantine's daughter of leprosy and restored to life one of her tormentors, who had been killed by the devil when attempting to rape her.[30]

A possible snapshot of liturgy in action at S. Egidio is provided by one of the illuminations of the Giovanni di Miniato brothers in the missal of 1474 (Plate 4.4). Even if the view is not intended as a literal representation of the church's interior,[31] the scene of the priest kneeling in front of the altar at the culmination of Mass was nonetheless enacted in S. Egidio on a daily basis and was the central point of the liturgy, when the Host was held up to be visible to the congregation.[32] On the altar is a small panel painting representing a male saint illuminated by a taper on each side. The congregation is shown clustered around the priest's feet; their proximity reflects the constraints of the composition and the desire to represent a wide range of people including both the lay public and members of the nursing staff in a comparatively small space.

The central focus of S. Egidio was the main altar. There has been considerable confusion concerning the identity of its patrons and of the altarpiece before the arrival of Hugo van der Goes' *Adoration of the Shepherds*. Until recently it was assumed that from 1345 the main altar was under the patronage of the painters' confraternity, the Compagnia di S. Luca, which had been granted the use of the Cappella Maggiore by the Portinari family.[33] However, this was not the case and is a misunderstanding based on a confusion of the Cappella Maggiore with the main chapel of the male ward, which was known as the 'chiesa di S. Maria Nuova'. It was the ward chapel that was dedicated to St Luke and where, as the 1349 statutes of the Compagnia di S. Luca record, the captains and councillors attended Mass.[34]

Indeed, given that the church was dedicated to St Giles, it makes much more sense that the main altar should have been under his patronage than of St Luke, especially as the 1215 Lateran Council had laid down that the saint to whom the main altar was dedicated should directly reflect that of the church.[35] The identity of the subject of the altarpiece is not made clear in the 1376 inventory, but the main altar would have been the proper location for the relics of St Giles, which are listed in the inventory: 'Item, one silver tabernacle of glass with the relics of S. Egidio and other relics.' The tabernacle was a recent acquisition: two years earlier the goldsmith Francescho di Vanni had been paid 43 gold florins for its completion.[36] This was a substantial sum and reflected the importance of the ownership of Giles's relics to the hospital and to the public who attended Mass and prayed in the church.

Though the dedication to St Giles predated the establishment of S. Maria Nuova, his presence was apposite given his close association with hospitals, particularly in northern Europe.[37] Like St Martin, he had given away his cloak to a beggar, thus encouraging charity to the poor; he moreover brought about the cure of the beggar's sickness and then managed to heal his own wound. His spirituality was proven through miracles and his life as a hermit, which then took on a very practical bent when he founded and began to run an abbey, which shared with a hospital the spiritual aspiration for the salvation of souls, even if it was less open to the cure of the physical sufferings of the world. Giles is shown dressed as an abbot standing in front of S. Maria Nuova in the drawing in the Codice Rustici of c.1445 (Plate 1.10).[38]

The importance of relics in promoting the religious profile of a hospital church and encouraging the financial support of the public and secular and ecclesiastical authorities was, as mentioned in Chapter 2, well attested by S. Maria della Scala in Siena.[39] In 1359 it acquired a very important collection of relics from Constantinople, which had purportedly belonged to Constantine himself. This made the hospital church into one of the major religious centres in Siena, especially when it became the locus for the city's celebration of the feast of the Annunciation. On 25 March each year the relics were placed on display in a window on the hospital façade which was visible to the public in the piazza between the cathedral and S. Maria della Scala. It was the huge popularity of these relics that over the following century led to the building and decoration of two sacristies and the commissioning of new altarpieces and reliquaries, a programme associated most clearly with the painter Vecchietta.[40]

Even without a comparable collection of relics, S. Egidio became an increasingly important religious centre, especially after its rededication to Mary. What remains less clear at the present stage of research is the exact appearance of the interior of S. Egidio in the 1420s. Even after the enlargement of the Cappella Maggiore at the northern end, the ground plan of the original church remained unaltered. It was a simple rectangular structure with a slightly narrower, square choir, in front of which stood the main altar. No land was available for expansion so S. Egidio has essentially the same dimensions today, though its interior has a very different appearance following its remodelling beginning in the late sixteenth century (Plate 4.5).[41] For example, in 1594 the original pointed arch leading to the choir was replaced by the rounded entrance arch visible today, just as the present cupola on pendentives took the place of a quadripartite vault.[42]

A possible guide to the appearance of the interior in 1420 is provided by another illumination by the Giovanni di Miniato brothers, *Pope Martin V Blessing the Altar*,[43] though one must be cautious about accepting this image as a 'true' representation of S. Egidio since it shows a scene that had taken place some twenty years before either illuminator was born (Plate 4.6).[44] Even so, it does fit surprisingly well with Bartolommeo del Corazza's short contemporary account, which can be fleshed out using his description of the consecration of S. Maria Novella only eight days earlier since both conformed to the standard ceremony of the Roman Rite.[45] At S. Maria Novella, Cardinal Orsini 'processed into the church accompanied by friars, and went around the inside; and then he attached a lit torch to each apostle, each of which had been newly repainted

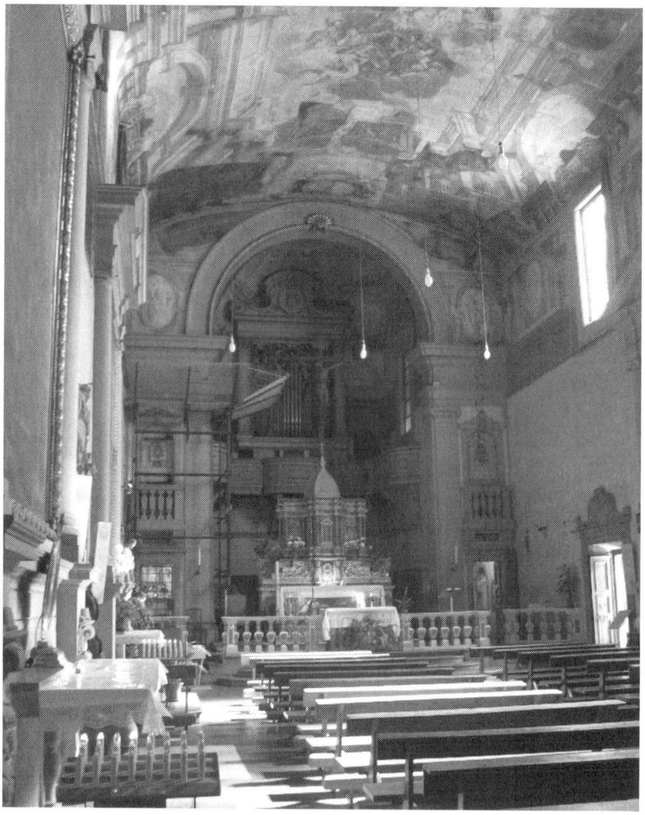

Plate 4.5 Interior of S. Egidio today

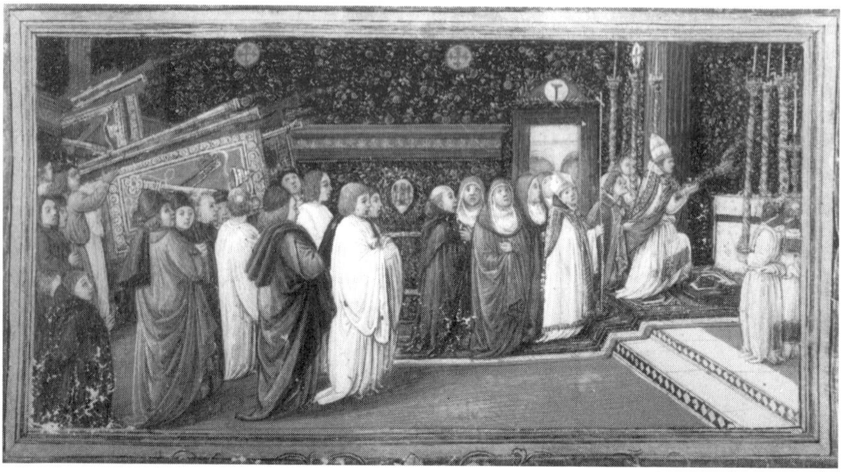

Plate 4.6 Gherardo and Monte di Giovanni di Miniato, *Pope Martin V Blessing the Altar of S. Egidio in 1420* (S. Egidio, Missal, 1474: Museo Nazionale del Bargello MS A67, f. 285r)

on every column on each side of the church.' Later on in the ceremony the cardinal returned and 'went to all of those newly painted apostles, and anointed the red cross painted in a white circle which they held in their hands'.[46] Images of the apostles would also have played a central role at S. Egidio. Indeed, Dello Delli was paid for a sculptural programme of sixteen terracotta statues of the twelve apostles and the four church fathers, which were painted and gilded by Bicci di Lorenzo's workshop in late 1424.[47]

Plate 4.6 shows the pope in the act of sanctifying the main altar, swinging a censor containing burning incense. Behind him stands the bishop holding a tall cross, and to his right is a group of clerics dressed in white carrying candlesticks, as well as a friar and *converse*, followed at a short distance by the leading members of government accompanied by the commune's trumpeters. The pope's role was described by Del Corazza briefly: 'he put the relics on the main altar, saying the solemn office ... and then celebrating the Mass ... the pope went out onto the piazza in the usual place and gave his benediction to the people: there was a very great crowd.'[48]

The image also shows some recognisable architectural elements in the church. Through the door one can see a view of a cloister – the Chiostro delle Ossa to the west of S. Egidio. Then behind the pope's hat one can see the lower part of the columns that delimited the entrance to the Cappella Maggiore, along with the white marble steps that led up to the main altar. One of the most striking elements of this scene is the complex decoration of the walls, on which was painted a series of emblems including the hospital's symbol of the crutch above the door, two consecration crosses and the Portinari coat of arms in the lower register.[49] This was not an invention of the Giovanni di Miniato brothers, as is borne out by a series of payments to the painter Meo di Bartolommeo di Fruosino on 27 September 1420 'to make a garland of laurel for the church ... and then paint the coat of arms of the patrons and to paint the vines and for gold for the vines, and for the making of the vines'.[50] What remains unclear is whether this was a temporary or permanent decorative scheme. If it was permanent and still represented the walls of the nave in 1474, the florid imagery would have provided an iconographic link with decorative elements of two subsequent commissions, the meadow that formed both the ground of Fra Angelico's predella panel of the *Marriage of the Virgin* and of Baldovinetti's fresco-cycle of the same subject in the Cappella Maggiore.[51]

The first altarpiece usually cited as having been commissioned in the fifteenth century for the main altar is by Lorenzo Monaco, a natural choice given that over the past decade he had illuminated a series of liturgical books for S. Egidio (Plate 4.7).[52] Between 1420 and 1422 Lorenzo was paid 182 gold florins for 'una tavola per l'altare di Sancto Egidio',[53] identified as his *Adoration of the Magi*, now in the Uffizi. Though a relatively small picture for a main altar

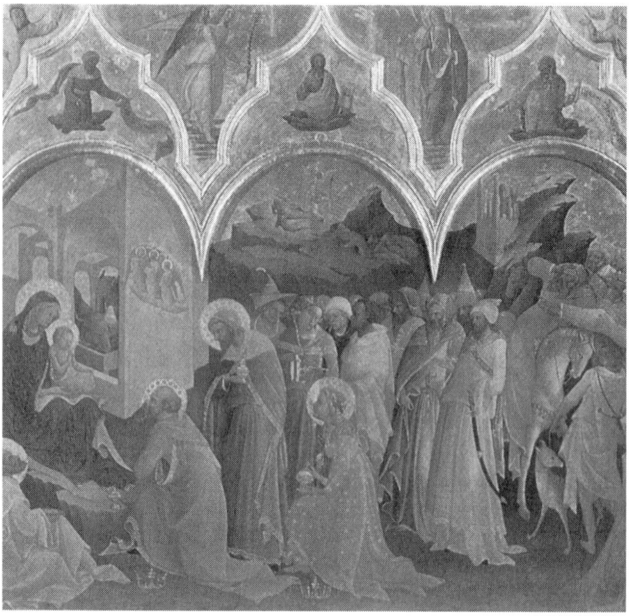

Plate 4.7 Lorenzo Monaco, *Adoration of the Magi*, 1420–2 (Galleria degli Uffizi)

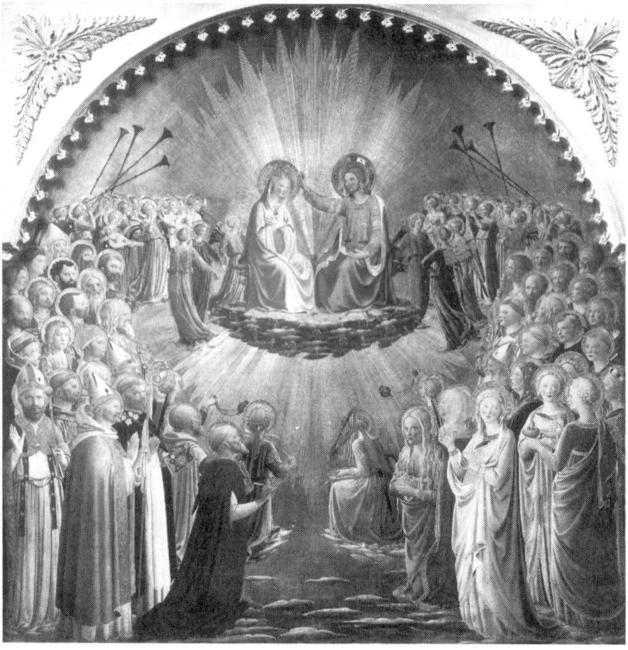

Plate 4.8 Fra Angelico, *Coronation of the Virgin*, c.1435–43 (Galleria degli Uffizi)

– it measures some 115 × 170 cm – this was more than made up for by the extraordinary richness of the clothes of the Magi and their retinue and the generous use of gold leaf in the background of the main composition and the spandrels. Despite the fact that the Virgin is off-centre to the left, she and the Christ-child are the main focus of attention. Indeed, a major theme of the composition was reflected in Bicci di Lorenzo's fresco of the *Reconsecration of S. Egidio*, which visitors would have passed on their way into the church; just as leading representatives of Church and State and the massed ranks of hospital employees paid obeisance to the pope, so the Magi paid homage to the Virgin and Child.

S. Egidio was also the location for another well-known picture from this period, Fra Angelico's stunning of altarpiece the *Coronation of the Virgin*, probably commissioned for S. Egidio between c.1435 and 1443 (Plate 4.8),[54] and now in the Uffizi, with its two predella panels, the *Marriage* and the *Dormition* of the Virgin, in the Museo di S. Marco.[55] There has, however, been considerable confusion about the placement of this picture and historians have tended to rely on Vasari's assertion 'one can see in the Tramezzo [the choir screen] of S. Maria Nuova a picture in his hand', but there is no evidence that this was its original location, if indeed there was a choir screen in the Quattrocento.[56] The other common assumption is that the altarpiece was 'painted for the nuns' choir'.[57] However, this term is anachronistic; in all contemporary documents this space was known as the Cappella Maggiore.[58] The term 'nuns' choir' derived from the later sixteenth century when, under the influence of the Counter-Reformation, lay nursing sisters took the veil. In theory, in these circumstances a more substantial Tramezzo would have been necessary so that the nuns could attend Mass without having to mix with the male members of the congregation. However, this scenario seems unlikely since they attended church on the first floor of S. Egidio behind the grille which can still be seen today (Plate 6.4b).

Whatever the exact location of Fra Angelico's painting in S. Egidio, visitors were introduced to its subject by Dello Delli's terracotta relief of the *Coronation* in the lunette above the main door. Both Dello Delli and Fra Angelico depicted Christ and Mary among the clouds of Heaven, with Mary seated on the right of her Son as she was crowned. For obvious reasons of space, what was missing from the lunette was the extraordinary host of celestial figures surrounding the main actors; in Fra Angelico's scene there are thirty-eight angels playing instruments and forty-eight holy figures in the heavenly court. The close association between the son of God and His mother was further reinforced by the church's view of Mary as the tabernacle of Christ.[59]

References to the hospital and its charitable and medical roles are made through the presence of particular saints among the members of this extraordinary celestial host, especially those shown full-length and facing out towards the viewer rather than inwards towards Christ and the Virgin. Prominence is given to Giles as the long-standing titular saint of the church of S. Maria Nuova who was also corporeally present in a reliquary on the main altar.[60] He is one of the saints nearest to the viewer and is identified by his cope, crosier and mitre, and an inscription on his hood: 'Sanct. Egidio abbas intercessor existe.' Also present was a local Tuscan saint famous for her charitable acts, St Catherine of Siena, who within living memory had tended plague victims in the 1374 epidemic and more generally the poor sick in the hospital of S. Maria della Scala, where she met with her followers in a confraternity in the crypt.[61] Other saints particularly relevant to the role of S. Egidio as a hospital church include St Lucy, who had close associations with those suffering from eye complaints as her eyes had been gouged out during her martyrdom; and St Agnes, who was corporeally present in a reliquary in the church and was also associated with curative powers in restoring sight and health. It may not be entirely coincidental that, as will be seen below in Chapter 9, treatments for eyes stand out in S. Maria Nuova's recipe collection as the most frequently cited treatment associated with the head (Table 9.4).

While iconographic evidence links Fra Angelico's *Coronation* to S. Egidio and historians have assumed that it was commissioned by the *spedalingo*, no payments have been found to Beato Angelico in the hospital's account books for these years.[62] But this is not surprising if the altarpiece was instead commissioned by the Portinari family, the patrons of the Cappella Maggiore. However, with Folco's premature death in 1431, his patronage rights passed to Pigello, the eldest of his three sons, who was then aged only ten. Given Pigello's age, it has been argued that Cosimo de' Medici became a leading influence in the choice of artists and themes for the decoration of the chapel in this period, especially since the Portinari boys are believed to have lived in the Medici household after the death of their father.[63] Furthermore, by the time S. Egidio's Cappella Maggiore came to be decorated, Pigello would have been unable to take a direct supervisory hand since he was now living in Venice and working for the Medici bank.[64] This helps to explain the choice of Fra Angelico, who was one of Cosimo's preferred painters.[65]

Cosimo's influence would also have been crucial in commissioning the new six-part fresco-cycle of the *Life of the Virgin* in the Cappella Maggiore. The programme, which was begun in 1439 and completed in 1461, has now unfortunately all but disappeared.[66] It is some indication of the hospital church's importance in the city that this work was undertaken by some of the leading painters of their generation.[67] The first phase, painted between 1439 and 1445 by Domenico Veneziano, assisted by Piero della Francesca and Bicci di Lorenzo, consisted of the *Meeting at the Golden Gate*, the *Birth of the Virgin* and the *Marriage of the Virgin*. Then, between 1451 and 1453, Andrea del Castagno painted the *Presentation in the Temple*, the *Annunciation* and the *Death of the Virgin*.[68] The cycle was completed by Alessio Baldovinetti after the death of Veneziano and Castagno, as recorded in a written agreement between the painter and the *spedalingo* on 17 April 1461.[69]

Clearly if this programme had survived it would have filled a very important gap in our knowledge of the stylistic development of fresco decoration in Renaissance Florence.[70] It was seen as a significant achievement at the time, reflected in the presence of both leading painters and the portraits of prominent Florentines in the *Marriage of the Virgin*. According to Vasari, it showed members of the Portinari family, principal among whom was Folco Portinari (probably Folco d'Adoardo rather than the founder, Folco di Ricovero),[71] together with Benadetto de' Medici, Bernardo Guardagni and the *spedalingo* of S. Maria Nuova, Messer Bernardo di Domenico della Volta. It has been convincingly suggested that if these individuals really were included in these frescoes the cycle would have represented 'a celebration of a major event in Florentine history', that is, the flight of Cosimo from Florence in 1433.[72] The figures listed by Vasari were Medici partisans who engineered Cosimo's escape from prison by bribing the jailers. The fact that S. Maria Nuova's *spedalingo* provided half the bribe of 1,000 florins presumably cemented the relationship between Cosimo and the hospital. This together with his close links with the Portinari may help to explain how Cosimo became involved in the programme for this major fresco-cycle, especially as at the time the Medici had 'no patronal rights over public chapels suitable for decoration with frescoes'.[73]

The implications of this new relationship with the Medici family for the development of S. Maria Nuova in the fifteenth century remain to be explored properly via a detailed analysis of the records of sums received and paid out by the hospital. For example, it is well known that when Veneziano was working in S. Egidio he was supplied with azure through the Medici bank in Venice where Pigello worked.[74] It is less well known that the Medici family already had connections with the hospital. In 1427, for example, S. Maria Nuova was involved in the funeral of Monna Chaterina de' Medici,[75] and in same year between 18 March and 3 July the hospital paid to the Medici bank the sum of 745 florins, at the time when Folco d'Adoardo Portinari was the head of the Florentine branch.[76] Then there were substantial financial transactions involving the hospital, the 'Monte Comune' and the Medici bank at precisely the time the decoration of the Cappella Maggiore was planned.[77]

Despite the influence of these powerful families, one should not undervalue the role of hospital directors, for they provided continuity in the relationship with artists while the interest and presence of patrons waxed and waned. For example, in 1461 it probably fell to the *spedalingo* to see through the completion of the fresco-cycle in the Cappella Maggiore since Pigello Portinari was still in Milan as the branch manager of the Medici bank and Cosimo was old and sick.

By the end of 1461, then, visitors would have seen a completely redecorated church. The next major innovation to the decorative programme was introduced by Tommaso di Folco Portinari, who, following the death of his brother Pigello in 1468, assumed his family's responsibilities as patron, despite being resident in Bruges. He probably took on this role in 1469 when he visited Florence to negotiate his new contract as manager of the local branch of the Medici bank.[78] Soon afterwards he began to send substantial sums of money to the hospital. In 1472 he gave 700 gold florins to S. Maria Nuova to establish a chaplaincy at S. Egidio and another at SS. Annunziata for the celebration of Masses every morning for his soul and those of his ancestors.[79]

About three years later Portinari commissioned the leading Flemish artist Hugo van der Goes to paint a new and substantial picture for the main altar, the *Adoration of the Shepherds*, designed to complete the cycle of the *Life of the Virgin* (Plate 4.9). It was eventually transported and put into place eight years later, in May 1483; its exceptional size meant that sixteen porters were required to carry it between the city gate of Porta S. Frediano and the hospital.[80] The decision to employ a local rather than an Italian painter may have been a matter of convenience for Portinari who was based in Bruges, but the choice of a picture on this scale also reflects his character as a 'self-confident egoist' who liked impressive gestures.[81] These years saw Tommaso Portinari becoming increasingly embroiled in the losses of the Bruges branch of the Medici bank and the sending of Van der Goes' triptych would have helped him to re-establish his presence in Florence especially as the work had a significant influence on painters working in Florence at the time.[82]

This enormous triptych with its vivid colours still has an extraordinary impact on the visitor to the Uffizi today, but it is important to examine its role within the context of S. Egidio. As can be appreciated from the view of the church as it is now (Plate 4.5), the altarpiece must have dominated the Cappella Maggiore. Its total surface area was almost 22 square metres and when fully opened it would have obscured some of the frescoes in the choir; fully extended it measured some 5.86 metres across, while the choir was only 6.45 metres wide in total.[83] However, little is known about the liturgical function of the picture or how it was displayed in S. Egidio. If this painting had been commissioned for a church in northern Europe – and after all Hugo van der Goes painted within that tradition – it would only have been opened on particular feast days, as was the case with another famous hospital commission, Grünewald's *Isenheim Altarpiece*.[84] The closed altarpiece, a severe image in monochrome grisaille, presents an extraordinary contrast to the intense and vivid colours of the *Adoration* in its open state (Plate 4.10). The exterior

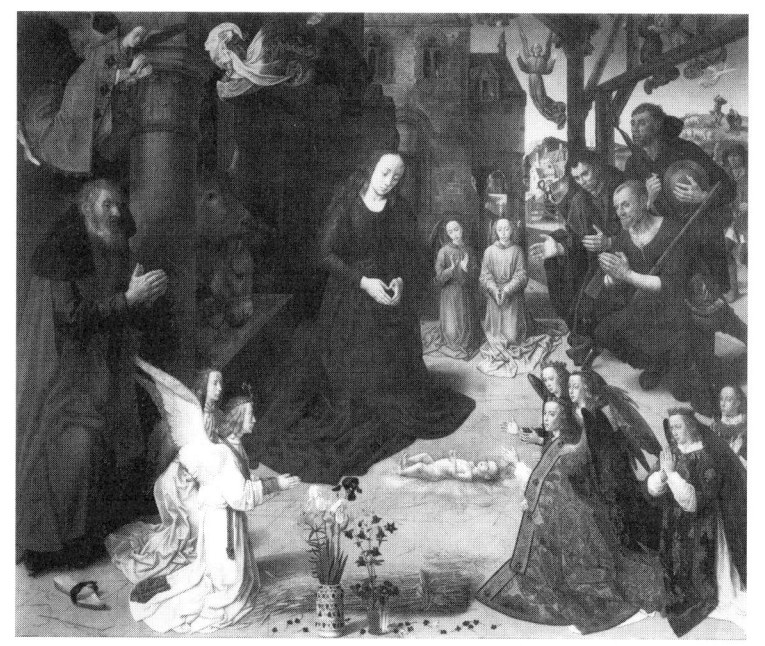

TO THE ALMIGHTY PHYSICIAN NO INFIRMITY IS INCURABLE 129

Plate 4.9 Hugo van der Goes, *Adoration of the Shepherds*, 1475–83 (Galleria degli Uffizi)

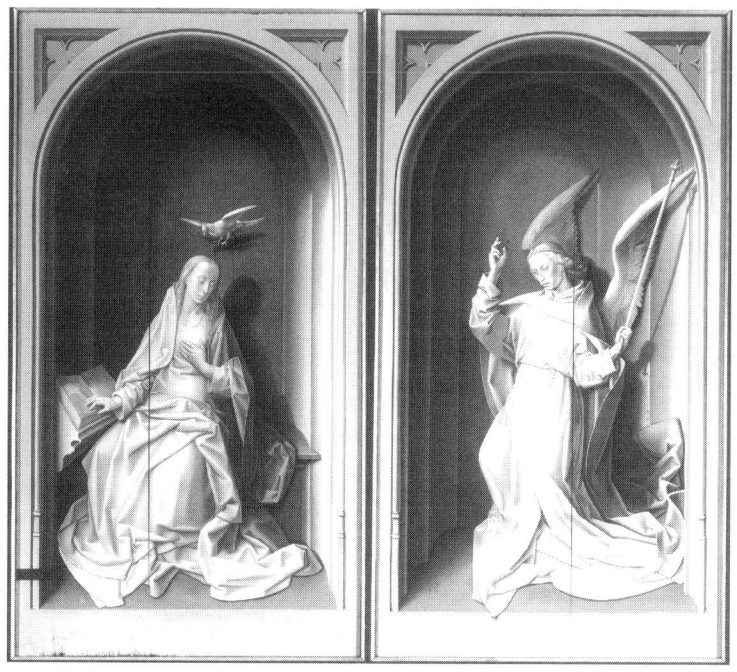

Plate 4.10 Hugo van der Goes, *Annunciation*, exterior of the *Adoration of the Shepherds*, 1475–83 (Galleria degli Uffizi)

represents the Annunciation, the moment of the incarnation of Christ when the Angel Gabriel announced Christ's birth, the scene to be revealed in all its glory once the altarpiece was opened.[85] Mary is shown modestly seated in a niche with downcast eyes. In contrast, the figure of the angel is viewed in motion as he dramatically imparts his news. It has been suggested recently that the altarpiece could have been displayed in a half-open state with the two side panels at right angles to the picture surface; in this way only the central panel of the *Adoration* would have been clearly visible.[86] However, whether the altarpiece was totally or only semi-closed, its overall size would have been much reduced, reserving its real visual impact for feast-days when it would be fully open.

An aspect of the *Adoration* that historians have only recently begun to take seriously again is the relationship between the themes of the altarpiece and the work's location in a hospital church. It has been suggested that, apart from the obvious associations between the portraits of the donors and the adorers of the Christ-child, the main subject of the picture was Mary's miraculous parturition.[87] Furthermore, it has been argued that because this was supposed to have happened without pain, she was seen as a patron saint of childbirth, providing hope to those suffering from physical ailments in the hospital. Even if the replacement of St Margaret with Mary as the patron of childbirth is not entirely convincing, the more general point is true, that the Virgin's presence provided hope to those suffering from physical ailments in the hospital. The theme of the miraculous parturition can be seen as a metaphor for salvation, most immediately for patients who were able to attend Mass in S. Egidio as well as staff, visitors and members of the patronal family.[88] As will be seen below, in Chapter 5, these themes were further developed in the decorative programme in the chapel area of the women's ward.[89]

The combined religious and medical messages of the altarpiece are further exemplified by the flowers in the immediate foreground of the picture, nearest to the congregation: the lily, iris, columbines and violets. In general terms all flowers were seen as reflecting the Christian virtues of Christ, Mary and the saints. Erwin Panofsky argued that the choice of these flowers announces the Passion of Christ, with the scarlet lily symbolising His blood.[90] The sheaf of wheat placed on the ground behind the flowers is another eucharistic reference, to the bread of the communion. Other flowers are linked to Mary: the iris is the sword that pierces the heart of the Mater Dolorosa, the seven columbine blossoms refer to the Sorrows of the Virgin, and the violets symbolise her humility.

If the flowers point to the power of spiritual medicine, the presence of the Venetian ripple glass and the Spanish albarello in the foreground point to the role of physical medicine. The glass tumbler may have referred to vessels from which patients drank, while the albarello type of ceramic jar was one of the most common containers for the simple and compound medicines stored in the on-site apothecary's workshop. Although S. Maria Nuova's albarelli would have come from nearby Montelupo, Hugo van der Goes would have been more familiar with Spanish than Italian examples.[91] The flowers themselves had important medicinal virtues. The root of the iris, shown in the albarello, was used to cauterise wounds, while both the carnations and columbines in the ripple glass were seen as having particularly efficacious roles in healing: the latter was applied to wounds and administered internally for stomach pains.[92] A further reference to the connection between hospitals and the care of the sick is contained in the presence of St Anthony Abbot among the saints adoring the Christ-child in the left wing of the altarpiece. His presence is explained in the first instance by his being the eponymous patron of Tommaso Portinari's son, Antonio.[93] But there was also a well-known association between the saint and those suffering from St Anthony's Fire or ergotism. The fact that these patients were treated at another Florentine hospital, S. Antonio, rather than at S. Maria Nuova may help to explain the lack of any specific reference to this illness here, in contrast to the horrifying realism of diseased bodies in the *Temptation of St Anthony* scene in the *Eisenheim Altarpiece*.[94]

Another thematic connection between the iconography of the picture and the function of the hospital is the emphasis on the adoration of the shepherds, which is given unusual prominence in the composition. This represented a shift from the subject of Lorenzo Monaco's *Adoration of the Magi*, which had probably formed the previous centre of the high altar. While Monaco had emphasised the richness and affluence of the kings, Van der Goes instead underlined the humbleness of the shepherds. One should not push this point too far – such an approach was typical of Flemish art and we know nothing about Portinari's instructions to Van der Goes – but it does nonetheless link to a tradition in Italian art of representing the poor in hospitals as part of their programme of advertising their good works.[95] The best-known examples are the patients in the frescoes in the Pellegrinaio or pilgrims' ward at the hospital of S. Maria della Scala in Siena (Plate 5.6),[96] but closer at hand was the fresco-cycle in the Cappella Maggiore of S. Egidio. Vasari stresses the beauty of the scene in the Presentation to the Temple 'where Our Lady is shown mounting the steps of the temple; above which were depicted many poor people'. This aspect of the fresco was dismissed by Gaetano Milanesi, the editor of Vasari's *Vite*, as a 'very trivial idea which is totally inappropriate to the theme of the picture' – ironic given that the presence of the poor is central to the purpose of the hospital.[97] If the sick poor were depicted in a sanitised painted version in S. Egidio, in the hospital's main wards they would have been found in all their gore amid the stench of sickness.

My discussion of the church has concentrated on underlining the connections between S. Egidio and S. Maria Nuova. This has been done by linking the spiritual and medical roles of the hospital with certain iconographic themes associated with individuals or objects represented in the altarpieces, sculptures and fresco-cycle in the church. In this way I have sought to move beyond the piecemeal approach that usually typifies studies of the redecoration of S. Egidio. Although the fresco-cycle has disappeared and the major altarpieces have been dispersed, it is important to consider them as an integrated whole in order to understand properly the liturgical function of the church and its role within the medico-spiritual mission of the hospital. I have also underlined the impact on S. Egidio of its rededication in 1420 to the Virgin Mary and how this served as an incentive for commissioning the new decorative programme, beginning with Dello Delli and Fra Angelico's representations of the *Coronation of the Virgin* to the fresco-cycle and extending to the *Adorations* by Lorenzo Monaco and Hugo van der Goes. These altarpieces were part of a thematically integrated programme, for S. Egidio's main altar was framed by the frescoes in the choir of episodes in the *Life of the Virgin*. Furthermore, the immediate context for the main altarpiece, which was the first thing a visitor to S. Egidio would see, would have been the flanking walls on either side facing the nave. According to Vasari, these were painted by Baldovinetti and were much praised, especially for the 'bellissima' figure of St Giles, underlining his continued importance as patron of the hospital.[98]

I have also emphasised the role of the church of S. Egidio as the focus for the daily celebration of the canonical hours – except for prime, which took place in the wards – and the hospital's three main festivals of St Giles, St Luke and the Purification of the Virgin.[99] Indeed, over the course of the fourteenth and fifteenth centuries their celebration became more elaborate, especially after the reconsecration of S. Egidio. The ceremony in September 1420 formed a turning point in the life of the hospital church. Pope Martin V took the first step to guarantee its new, more public persona when he granted five years of indulgence and five *quarantane* (forty days of indulgence) to anybody who visited S. Egidio on the day of its reconsecration.[100] The Florentine commune followed the papal lead, suspending the hospital's debts for a period of eight days from 8 September.[101] It also became involved in making public the hospital's feast-days, as a payment in 1428 reveals: 'To the town-criers of the commune on 3 September to announce the feast [*sagra*] of S. Egidio, that is on ninth of this month, £2.'[102]

The festival of S. Egidio continued to be a central event in the hospital's calendar and its celebration became increasingly splendid over the century. For example, on 7 September 1493 a lump sum of £7.18.0 was paid 'for masses and for vespers for the festival of San Gilio, and for the *sagra*', and the following year on 2 September £8.4.4 was paid to 'nine priests, the preacher and eleven clerics and for 103 S. Gili and for two loads of laurel, all for our festival of S. Gilio'.[103] Here a clear distinction was made between vespers on the eve of 9 September and the *sagra* or festival of St Giles, when Mass was celebrated, a sermon was delivered and twenty members of the clergy were present. Indeed, the significance for the city of not just the feast day of St Giles, but of other festivals at S. Egidio is reflected by the importance of the preachers, including Antoninus, who delivered the Lenten sermon cycle in the church when he was archbishop of Florence.[104]

The increasing splendour of feast-days at S. Egidio was part of a more general trend towards greater elaboration of festivals in Florence at the level of the commune, the Church and the many religious fraternities in the city.[105] This is a subject that remains to be properly investigated through an examination of the surviving collection of S. Egidio's liturgical manuscripts.[106] Indeed, the importance of the church's missals, breviaries and antiphonaries is underlined by the fact that they were of an equal standard with the much-better-known collection of the contiguous convent of S. Maria degli Angeli.[107] The high level of artistry of the miniatures can be seen in one of the largest and most prominent scenes for one the hospital's missals, the *Annunciation*, painted by Gherardo and Monte di Giovanni di Miniato in 1474 (Plate 4.11). Mary and the Angel Gabriel are positioned on either side of an open window through which can be seen a valley with a beautifully painted view of a village clustered around a church. The fineness of this and the miniatures contained in a breviary commissioned by the hospital at this time (Bargello MS A68) underlines the importance placed on these liturgical books and the availability of finance to underwrite such projects. The care lavished on the miniature emphasises the centrality of the Virgin Mary in the liturgy of S. Egidio. Not only did this reflect her importance in the liturgy of the Church as a whole and in the devotion of the laity to her cult; it also reflected her humanity as the mother of Christ, who weaned and protected Him as an infant and child, a role that was especially relevant in an institution that provided both physical and spiritual healing to the poor made weak and defenceless through infirmity.

The commissioning of liturgical and devotional objects, often as part of building programmes, obviously implies the expenditure of considerable sums of money. As has been seen, the financing for some projects derived from the hospital's own coffers, while for others it was the patron who paid. In the case of S. Maria Nuova the Portinari had been the dominant influence since its foundation. However, as in so many wealthy and prestigious institutions in Renaissance Florence, it is not surprising to discover the hand of the Medici at work, especially from the 1430s, when leading members of the Portinari family were either under age or living away from Florence. Once begun, Medici

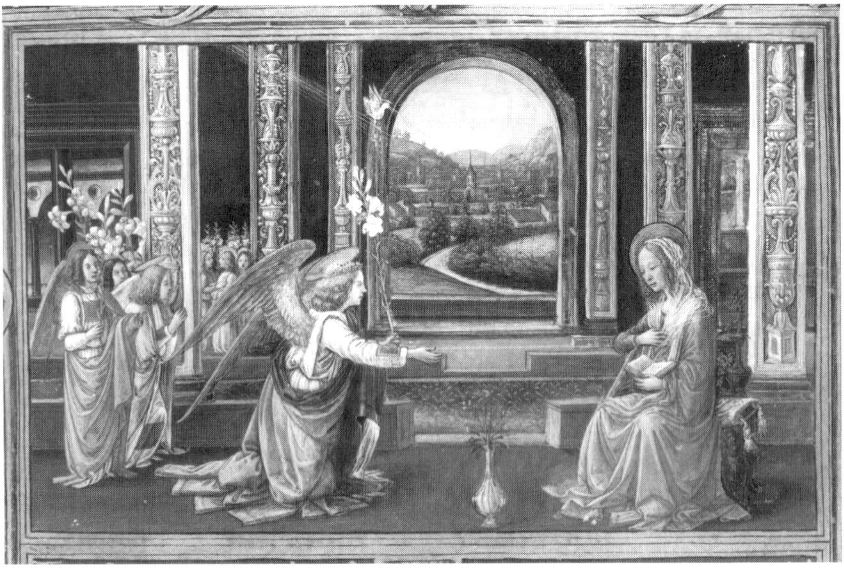

Plate 4.11 Gherardo and Monte di Giovanni di Miniato, *Annunciation of the Virgin* (S. Egidio, Missal, 1474: Museo Nazionale del Bargello MS 67, f. 5r)

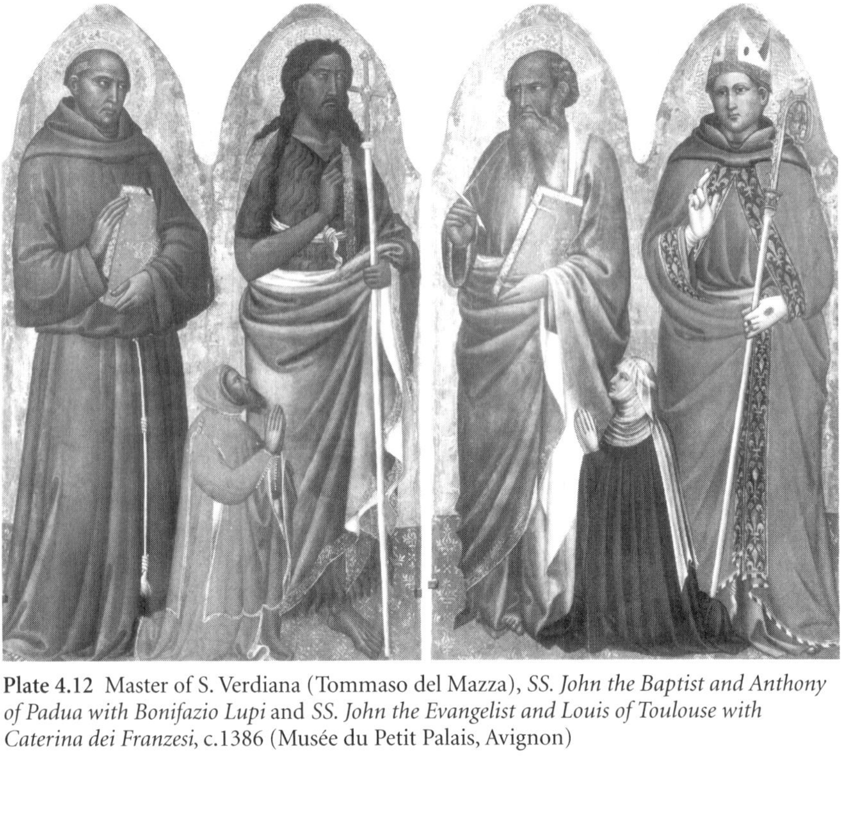

Plate 4.12 Master of S. Verdiana (Tommaso del Mazza), *SS. John the Baptist and Anthony of Padua with Bonifazio Lupi* and *SS. John the Evangelist and Louis of Toulouse with Caterina dei Franzesi*, c.1386 (Musée du Petit Palais, Avignon)

involvement in S. Maria Nuova continued, for they, like other Florentines, obviously felt great pride in this institution, as reflected in Giovanni de' Medici's comment about the hospital in his letter to Francesco Sforza in June 1456: 'it is a great and excellent thing.' Indeed, when *spedalingo* Bonino di Antonio Bonini wrote a begging letter to Lorenzo de' Medici in 1479, he invoked a long tradition of Medici financial support: 'always relying on the long established customs of your family who, from the time of the blessed memory of your great-grandfather Giovanni, were always a supporter of this hospital and hospital director, and everybody since has continued to provide the same support.'[108]

The sustenance of S. Maria Nuova by these leading families was part of a general feature of Renaissance society which led to the patronage of a wide range of charitable and religious foundations. Hospitals, along with other secular and ecclesiastical buildings, also came to form part of the Renaissance aesthetic, which promoted civic and individual pride. Public appreciation of their social role in looking after the bodies of the sick poor was matched by appreciation of their religious role in making available to their patients the spiritual medicine provided by Christus Medicus. In addition, the hospitals themselves provided an important individualised religious service for their patrons by holding commemorative Masses for their souls.

4.3 'For the Salvation of his Soul and of his Successors': Hospital Churches and Commemoration

A general development in the religious practices in the city shared by S. Egidio and other hospital churches in the fifteenth century was the multiplication of commemorative Masses on behalf of their benefactors and patrons. Hospitals became ever more involved in the administration of estates and benefited financially from bequests, arranging for the commissioning of devotional objects and funerary chapels both in their own and in other churches in the city.[109]

S. Egidio, for example, became increasingly associated with the Portinari following the extension of the family's patronal rights from the ward chapel to the hospital church in 1420. This division of spiritual responsibilities between church and wards underlines the centrality of the role of S. Egidio in the spiritual life of the hospital and as an important chantry chapel. In the act of foundation of 1286 Folco di Ricovero Portinari repeats that he had created the hospital 'in memory of his soul and those of his relatives' and part of his endowment paid for these commemorative Masses.[110] When Portinari died in 1289, he was buried, as he had requested, 'in the chapel of my hospital of S. Maria Nuova', also known as the 'Chiesa di S. Maria Nuova', that is, at the northern end of the men's ward. It was only in 1313 with the departure of the Frati Saccati, who had previously lived on the site, that S. Egidio became the main hospital church and that one can date the growth of its importance in the liturgical life of the institution over the original 'chiesa di S. Maria Nuova';[111] by 1374 seven of the eight daily canonical hours were celebrated there and only one in the hospital ward.[112]

In the Trecento Folco di Ricovero's descendants continued to be buried in the ward chapels, but in the Quattrocento the hospital church assumed greater prominence in their afterlife, culminating in the representation of Tommaso and his wife in Hugo van der Goes' *Adoration of the Shepherds.* Thus when Folco d' Adoardo died in 1490 he was buried in S. Egidio, despite the fact that Tommaso had had him jailed for fraud for six months in 1487–8 when he worked for him in the Medici bank in Bruges.[113] Tommaso's attachment to the hospital is reflected in the fact that he chose to die there in 1501.[114]

Bonifazio Lupi and Lemmo Balducci did not elect to die in their respective foundations, but the hospitals nonetheless performed important commemorative roles. In his petition to the Florentine government Bonifazio had stated that he wished to establish a hospital, 'In memory of his soul and those of his heirs', next to which was to be built 'a chapel where divine office can be celebrated'.[115] This was the church of St John the Baptist, where the first Mass took place on 6 February 1386, as confirmed by a Bull of Urban VI, who granted an indulgence to any visitor to the church on the Baptist's feast-day.[116] The hospital church later recorded its annual obligation to Messer Bonifazio Lupi: 'We have to hold in the church or indeed in the chapel of our hospital a solemn office with twelve priests who say Mass, supplying the choir with tapers and honourable candles each year on 21 January for the soul of Messer Bonifazio Lupi da Parma.'[117] Large numbers of candles were consumed. In January 1477, 34lb of wax was burned, including 'tapers and candles to hang [in the church] and to give to the priests to hold'.[118] In addition to this annual commemorative service, Mass was celebrated daily in the church or chapel ward as well as regular festivals, as recorded by a payment in 1475 to the organist Giovanni di Sandro detto Monachetto from Prato. He was contracted to play the organ 'every Sunday, the feasts ordered by the Church, Christmas and Easter or other festivals that should be celebrated in church'.[119]

The demand by the patron for commemoration led to the commissioning of a series of altarpieces for the hospital church, at least one of which can be identified clearly with the patron since the two lateral panels contain portraits of Bonifazio and his second wife, Caterina.[120] This large altarpiece of the *Virgin and Child*, now in the Musée du Petit Palais, Avignon, is by the Master of S. Verdiana, recently identified with Tommaso del Mazza (Plate 4.12).[121] Another was one of Niccolò di Pietro Gerini's late works, the *Crucifixion with*

SS. Paul, Mary Magdalene, Luke, Bartholomew, Catherine of Alexandria and Peter Martyr (c.1400), today in the Accademia Gallery in Florence.[122] Given the presence of the donors and its substantial size (in its open state it measures 67.7 × 50cm), Tommaso del Mazza's altarpiece was probably intended for the high altar and was most likely in place for the celebration of the first Mass in December 1386.[123] In the side panels Bonifazio is accompanied by SS. John the Baptist and Anthony of Padua, a reference to the original dedication of his hospital and to his city of origin, while Caterina was flanked by SS. John the Evangelist and Louis of Toulouse, the latter a reference to the French connections of her family, the Franzesi. Given that Bonifazio did not die until 1389, it is quite possible that he discussed his general requirements with the *spedalingo*, who then commissioned Del Mazza and oversaw the execution of the altarpiece. This was a common model, as suggested by the well-known case in the early sixteenth century when the *spedalingo* of S. Maria Nuova commissioned Rosso Fiorentino to paint the *Virgin and Child Enthroned* (Galleria degli Uffizi) in fulfilment of the wishes of Francesca Ripoi, an affluent patient who had died in the hospital.[124]

The *spedalingo* is also likely to have played a central role in commissioning the second substantial picture associated with the hospital at this time, Niccolò di Pietro Gerini's *Crucifixion* triptych. Though Bonifazio Lupi himself was no longer alive, his widow, Caterina, who did not die until 1405, had been made an executor of his will and, together with the merchants' guild of the Calimala, maintained a supervisory role of the building and decoration of the hospital.[125] As in the case of Del Mazza's altarpiece, there is a clear association between saints depicted in Gerini's polyptych and the patrons. The main theme of the altarpiece, the crucifixion of Christ, carried a complementary message to Del Mazza's *Virgin and Child*, just as did the two terracotta lunettes on the exterior of S. Maria Nuova. Indeed, the scene of the Passion was one for which Gerini was well known, for he had completed fresco-cycles on this theme for a number of important Franciscan friaries in the 1390s.[126] One of the main characteristics shared by all these cycles and by the central panel of this painting is the emotional charge he brought to the scene. In the central panel the mourning women are shown turning away in sorrow from the crucified Christ, while St Francis is represented in a familiar pose, kneeling at the foot of the Cross, which he grasps firmly while he looks upwards towards the feet of his Saviour. The presence of Francis reflects in a general way the influence of the Observant movement with its renewed emphasis on the themes of the sufferings of Christ, and in a specific way Messer Bonifazio Lupi and his wife Caterina's membership of the Franciscan Third Order. One of the most interesting aspects of the composition is, moreover, the relationship between the figures in the central and side panels. It has been suggested that the enormous size of the saints in the wings of the painting relative to those in the central scene reflects the Crucifixion's iconic function.[127] The six saints represented the important association between the hospital and its founders, the inclusion of Catherine of Alexandria accorded honour to Bonifazio Lupi's wife, and the presence of the physician saint Luke underlined the obvious connection with the hospital's role in healing.

The same mixture of medical and spiritual healing characterised the decorative programme for the hospital church of S. Matteo, where a series of surviving inventories provides a good idea of the contents of its interior in the fifteenth century.[128] Once again, the main purpose behind the acquisition and commissioning of the altarpieces was the observance of the church's liturgy and the commemoration of the souls of patron and benefactors, as reflected in the contract with a new chaplain in 1441: 'Frate Bartolomeo di Giovanni from Zürich from Low Germany ... is obliged in the future to say ... Mass every day in the hospital or anywhere he wants and then to assist the other priests in the singing of the Great Mass and other offices according to the wishes of the hospital director and especially vespers and matins in the church'.[129]

Priests also participated at the funeral of the inmates and staff, as in the case of Monna Salvestra, who was buried on 7 November 1461:

> And on the said day, for 19lb 2oz of candles to give to thirty-eight priests and friars and clerics who came from various places and from S. Marco and light the church around the choir and on the altars and other surrounding areas.
>
> And on the ninth, thirteen Masses were said and a beautiful office for her soul and £6.15s was given to the priests and clerks for the vigil and the Masses, so that between wax and payment to the priests and clerics the total [spent] was £17.6s.[130]

This description tells us not only about the splendour of the occasion, with a large quantity of candles to light the hospital church and substantial numbers of priests and friars to sing Mass, but also something about the layout of the space. As at S. Egidio, there was a choir and separate altars in the body of the church.

The most detailed entry in the early fifteenth-century inventory of the hospital's contents was a description of the main altarpiece, the *S. Matteo* by Andrea di Cione or 'Orcagna' and Jacopo di Cione (Plate 4.13a):

> A most beautiful and old altarpiece with the figure of S. Matteo, which belonged to the Cambio guild [of bankers], and we know that when the said guild had the altarpiece made it cost 120 florins or thereabouts. And the said

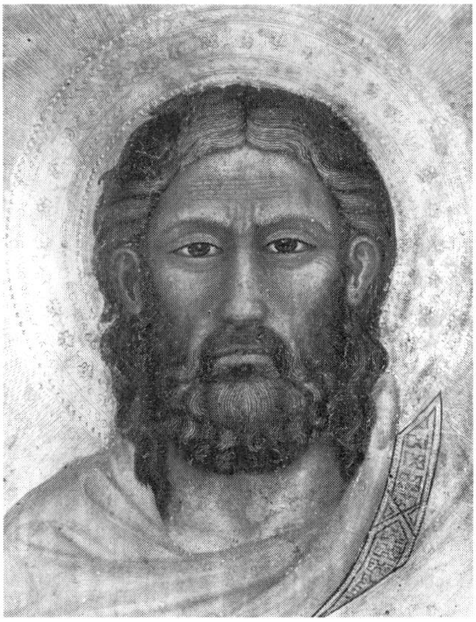

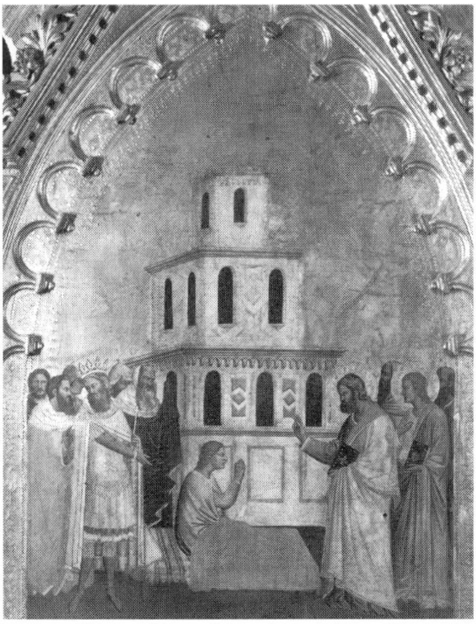

Plate 4.13 Andrea di Cione, 'Orcagna', and Jacopo di Cione, *S. Matteo* 1368 (Galleria degli Uffizi) a. Detail of head; b. S. Matteo in his counting-house

altarpiece was in Orsanmichele on the pilaster belonging to the said guild, and when the captains of Orsanmichele ordered that all the altarpieces of all guilds should be removed from the pilasters, this altarpiece was taken away and was carried to the guild's [residence]. And then the guild gave the said altarpiece to these hospitals.[131]

The 'hospitals' – the plural refers to both the male and female wards – had been fortunate when the captains of Orsanmichele decided in 1402 that the guild altarpieces displayed in the interior of the confraternity's oratory should be replaced by frescoes.[132] This saved a considerable outlay and meant they acquired a picture depicting their main patron from one of the leading workshops in the mid-Trecento. The occasion may also have provided the Cambio guild with a useful way to recycle a picture that had become redundant at Orsanmichele. Indeed, the description of a well-known picture commissioned a mere thirty-five years earlier as 'old' ('anticha') may suggest that the style was already regarded as old-fashioned.[133]

Orcagna's achievement can still be appreciated today, although the context and lighting of the Uffizi are a far cry from the work's original setting on the main altar of the hospital church where it would have glowed in the mellow light of candles and oil lamps. This magnificent altarpiece was constructed in three sections, with the large standing figure of St Matthew taking pride of place in the central panel, flanked in the side panels by four small scenes from his life. What impresses above all is the power of the saint, emphasised by the extensive use of gold leaf in the background and by the emphatically hieratic tone of the composition.[134] The central panel was largely by Jacopo di Cione and most of the four smaller side panels were probably by Orcagna, as suggested by the harmonious and strongly architectonic nature of the composition. The subject of the third panel, the miraculous resurrection of a boy, was particularly appropriate to its new setting, though the scene most relevant to the Cambio had been the *Calling of S. Matteo* which showed the saint in his counting-house (Plate 4.13b), reflecting and justifying the activities of the guild itself, represented in the gold coins on a red background in the four tondi in the cusps of the side panels.

This discussion has stressed the need to examine the function of these hospital churches in relation to the lives of the hospitals more generally and the role of their devotional objects in the treatment of the bodies and souls of patients and staff. Equally I have emphasised the importance of these churches as centres for the patronage of well-known Renaissance architects, painters and sculptors at a time when the main hospitals of the city were founded or expanded. Hospitals acquired pieces by the popular workshops of Niccolò di Pietro Gerini and Lorenzo di Bicci and by artists such as Lorenzo Monaco, who combined panel painting with manuscript illumination, and later by other leading members of their generation such as Castagno, Veneziano and Hugo van der Goes. Those who commissioned these works of art shared the same range of aspirations and needs as those who patronised the parish, conventual and monastic churches throughout Florence, from commemoration and self-aggrandisement to the promotion of the ideal of *bellezza*. It has also been seen that hospitals attracted patronage from a range of sources, from individual businessmen to craft and professional guilds. Indeed, hospitals reflected a wider move in Renaissance society from corporate to individual patronage, especially with the growing influence of the Medici family in all aspects of the life of the city.

If the hospital church was the main public religious space within the hospital complex, the other centre of devotion was the ward chapel, which will be examined below, in Chapter 5, after a short transitional section on cloisters.

4.4 *Tranquillity and Transition: The Hospital Cloister*

Cloisters mediated between the sacred and the secular, between those spaces devoted to the spiritual and those devoted to the medical, as at S. Maria Nuova where the Chiostro delle Medicherie – where the surgery was based – separated the church from the men's ward (Plate 4.15).[135] As in the monastic context, they provided a tranquil space for contemplation and the reading of devotional

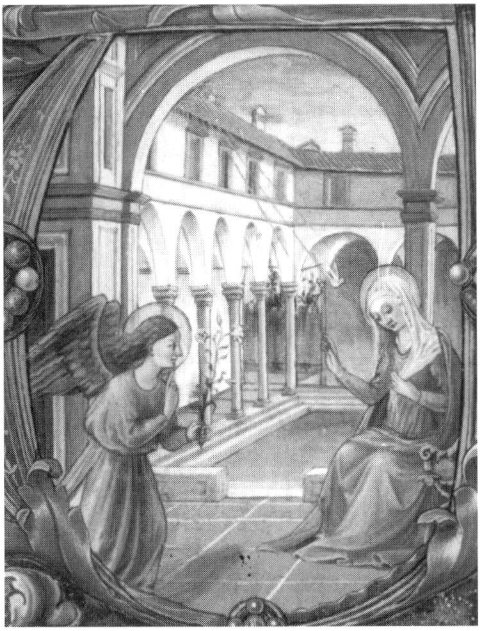

Plate 4.14 Gherardo and Monte di Giovanni di Miniato, *Annunciation of the Virgin Mary*, showing view of hospital cloister (S. Egidio, Missal, 1474: Museo Nazionale del Bargello MS 67, f. 220r)

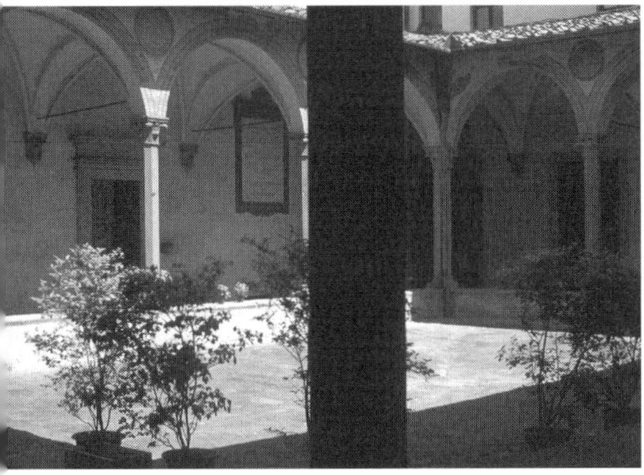

Plate 4.15 S. Maria Nuova: Chiostro delle Medicherie

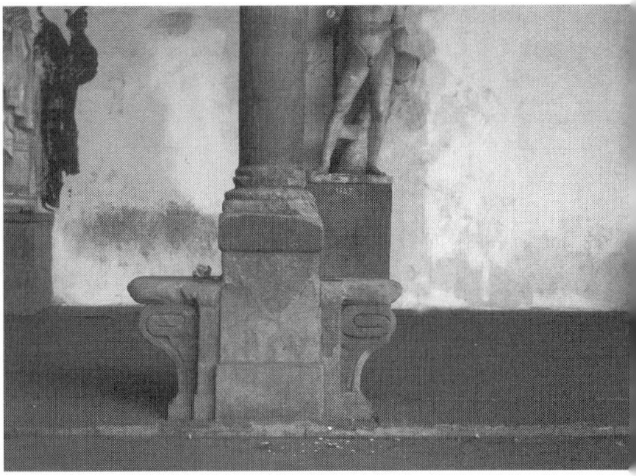

Plate 4.16 S. Matteo, Piazza S. Marco: male cloister, ledge at base of plinth

texts, as reflected in Gherardo and Monte di Giovanni di Miniato's *Annunciation* for S. Maria Nuova's missal, where the Virgin Mary is shown seated in the cloister of the hospital (Plate 4.14). At a more prosaic level cloisters also provided shelter. As Filarete notes in his description of the Ospedale Maggiore in Milan: 'on leaving the hospital [i.e., ward] one can go to all those parts under cover.'[136]

Cloisters in hospitals, as in monasteries, fulfilled a wide range of functions. Given their location, they also performed a therapeutic role; the tranquillity of the cloister would have helped all patients to recover the proper balance of the 'accidents of the soul', one of the six non-naturals that governed health.[137] If cloisters performed a similar role for men and women, their relative positions on the site nonetheless led to some differences; since the female living quarters were usually placed further away from the public face of the hospital than the male. The male cloister often constituted one of the main entrances into a hospital, as can still be seen at both S. Maria Nuova and S. Matteo. After walking through the loggia and along a short passageway, visitors would have found themselves in a light and harmonious space where they could orientate themselves and pass on to other areas or meet patients and personnel. This was usually facilitated by the design of the internal colonnade, for each column was mounted on a low wall that provided a space on which to sit and talk or wait for treatment, as can be seen in the illumination of the Annunciation scene in Plate 4.14. In contrast S. Matteo's colonnade extends down to the ground and each column is supported by a low plinth into which small projecting ledges were built to provide single seats (Plate 4.16). One disadvantage of the male cloister's more public role was that it was less secure. For this reason there was a separate locked room off the cloister which was used as an archive: 'A little room where the books are kept.' The holdings in this storeroom were not only numerous, since they included many of the hospital's administrative records, but also of value because they included a 'register in which is kept Lelmo's testament covered with wood and leather, almost grey, with a number of big nails' on each of the outer covers.[138]

In contrast, female cloisters were located further away from the public face of the hospital, as in monastic communities where the more private areas were positioned in the 'deeper' spaces to limit public access.[139] This reflected the strict sexual segregation of a community, as laid down in the rules governing hospitals. S. Maria Nuova's female cloister survives today as a splendid airy space with a double colonnade and a low wall supporting the columns (Plate 4.17); exactly when the upper gallery was added remains to be discovered, as does the extent of its original decoration.[140] At both S. Maria Nuova and S. Matteo these courtyards were distanced from the street by a number of rooms, and because they were more secure they were used as storage spaces.[141] The 1454 inventory of S. Matteo records that the women's cloister contained forty-two locked chests and coffers, where they kept the female servants' clothes, shirts and kerchiefs as well as bedclothes and clothes for the patients.[142]

Studies of monastic cloisters in fourteenth-and fifteenth-century Tuscany have shown that many of their walls and vaulted ceilings were frescoed. Furthermore, the period in which the cloisters of the new medical hospitals were built or remodelled coincided with the period characterised as a 'boom' in Florentine cloister decoration (c.1420–50), seeing the creation of works

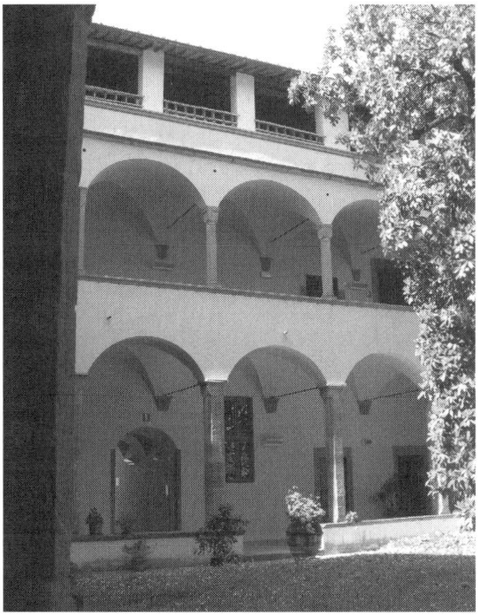

Plate 4.17 S. Maria Nuova: female cloister

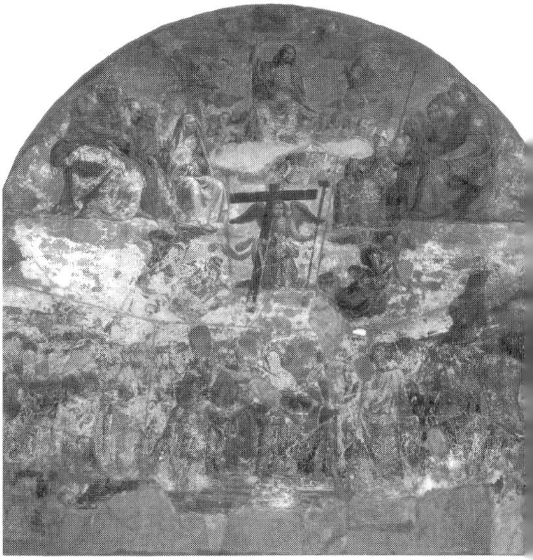

Plate 4.18 Fra Bartolommeo and Mariotto Albertinelli, *The Last Judgement*, 1499–1500 (Museo di S. Marco, Florence)

ranging from Masaccio's *Sagra* and Fra Filippo Lippi's *Scenes of Early Carmelites* in S. Maria del Carmine to Paolo Uccello's *Creation Scenes* in the Chiostro Verde at S. Maria Novella.[143] Even so, little evidence survives about hospitals commissioning large-scale frescoes in their cloisters and, although little has been written about the subject, it seems unlikely that such cycles would have remained unknown. Instead, when Florentine hospitals did employ artists to paint large-scale frescoes they tended to be for the church, ward chapels or façade, all of which had a similar function as a form of 'self-advertisement and self-representation' to attract public attention and patronage.[144]

Smaller rather than large-scale commissions were more typical of hospital cloisters, in common with the more restrained programmes of the cloisters of Observant convents, as at S. Marco.[145] Devotional images in the cloister, as in other parts of the hospital, emphasised the religious character of the institution and the importance of spiritual medicine in healing. Thus in 1454 S. Matteo's male cloister included a 'little altarpiece of Our Lady in a little tabernacle' and a 'little crucifix in a little tabernacle with two doors',[146] so guaranteeing the presence of both Mary and Christ, who between them represented the promise of divine intervention and redemption.

Most cloister decoration was in lunettes above doorways, emphasising the cloister's importance as a transitional space, as with entrances from loggias into hospital churches and courtyards. The architectural feature of the tympanum provided a readymade frame for the painting, sculpture or terracotta image and a natural focus for the eye of the visitor. This is evident in a contract with the painter Stefano d'Antonio di Vanni for a painted overdoor for one of the entrances into S. Maria Nuova's male cloister. Vanni, who had begun as a member of Bicci di Lorenzo's workshop, had recently been employed by the hospital of S. Matteo on a fresco-cycle in one of its dormitories.[147] The contract of May 1470 sets out in detail the hospital's requirements:

> Maestro Stefano d'Antonio di Vanni painter to paint a lunette over the door in the middle which goes into the cloister of our hospital ... he must paint Our Lady who has in her lap the dead body of Our Lord, as it is done in the Pietà. And at the head of Our Lord should be St John the Baptist and at His feet St Mary Magdalene. The background must be of fine gold and the surrounding cornice and also the moulding of the doorpost in fine gold, and thus fine gold must be put in every other place and he must work with good colours, and for blue he must use fine ultramarine and paint foliage above the cornice with the appearance of marble and in the doorpost he must put foliage like that of the door which goes into the women's hospital, and all the materials, gold and colours, should be paid for by him. And he should have for payment of this work 72 *lire piccioli*. And this work should be finished before the end of July 1470.[148]

The amount of detail provided here follows the practices of the time and reflects a creative dialogue between patron and artist. In this case, the contract demonstrates the desire of the *spedalingo* to make sure that the fresco would include the appropriate subject matter and also certain decorative motifs such as the painting of 'foliage', which was to be 'like that of the door which goes into the women's hospital'. The hospital also specified the use of two particularly expensive ingredients, 'fine gold' for the background and surrounding cornice and doorpost, and ultramarine blue, presumably for Mary's dress. The fresco would have provided a splendidly luminous spectacle for anybody passing through the door into the cloister. It would again have reminded the viewer of the road that led from physical suffering to spiritual redemption, a path that would have been eased by the intervention of three intercessionary saints: the two Marys and John the Evangelist.

The painting of over-doors was as common a practice in many parts of hospitals as in monastic complexes, and subjects were chosen to underline the religious role of the institution and of the area beyond the door.[149] S. Matteo paid 30 gold florins in 1412 to Mariotto di Nardo 'to paint two lunettes in the said hospital; [in the] one above the door of the church of S. Matteo he painted

S. Matthew and [in] the lunette above the door of the women's ward he painted the figure of the glorious Virgin Madonna and S. Maria [Maddalena?]'.[150] The S. Matteo fresco would have led one into the church and reflected the principal subject of the Orcagna altarpiece on the main altar, as did Lorenzo Monaco's *St Nicholas* in the lunette above the door of the men's ward, a reminder that these saints were joint patrons of the hospital. Then a *Pietà*, painted by Lorenzo Monaco between 1415 and 1420 'in the first door on the left-hand side as one enters the men's ward', underlined that the suffering of Christ and of the sick was not in vain because it led one closer to God.[151]

All these decorative programmes have to be seen within the wider context of the liturgical life of the hospital, for, as has been well said in relation to S. Marco, the 'painting of frescoes over doors refers to the importance of axes, and routes of liturgical processions'.[152] If at S. Marco the liturgy of space has been well discussed, this remains a virtually unexplored area in Florentine hospitals. However, one has only to remember the importance of festivals in the religious life of hospitals to understand the liturgical significance of spaces such as cloisters since members of the clergy and the staff would have processed from one area to another. Hospital statutes tend to skate over the details of their liturgical life, but these can be inferred by reading between the lines. Take the case of a funeral of a male patient at S. Maria Nuova. After a period of lying in front of the altar in the ward, his body was carried in procession through the cloister to the church where Mass was sung and then through to the cemetery in the Chiostro delle Ossa.[153]

Indeed, the only large-scale fresco for a Florentine hospital cloister to survive from this period was in the Chiostro delle Ossa, *The Last Judgement* by Fra Bartolommeo and Mariotto Albertinelli, 1499–1500, a theme appropriate to its role as the hospital's cemetery (Plate 4.18).[154] Though commissioned by the Dini family for their family tomb, the cemetery was intended principally for the burial of those who had died in the hospital. If the frescoes and tombs linked the living with the dead, the cloister's main inhabitants were the bodies and skeletons of the sick poor; there is no evidence that there was a separate ossuary. Ferdinando Del Migliore, writing in the late seventeenth century, recounts that the hospital's burial registers recorded 360,000 burials in the Chiostro delle Ossa between the time of the hospital's foundation and 1657, when it was closed to make way for the construction of the new female ward.[155] Both Del Migliore and Giuseppe Richa's descriptions of the cemetery were deliberately conceived to show how the sight of skeletons encouraged visitors to dwell on the thought of death:

> all the walls were covered with piled-up bones and well accompanied by whole skeletons which were fitted into niches in such a way that nowhere

else could one see such a plentiful display after the manner of that created by Leo X at the church of S. Salvadore known popularly as 'de ossibus'. The custom was for many Florentines to take their children to see these bones and to say to them: 'Children, remember that this is our end and that our flesh is weak!'[156]

Conclusion

The hospital cloister, then, fulfilled a series of functions, which had much in common with those within the conventual context. These were modified in so far as the hospital was a more public institution, especially in relation to those areas intended for male rather than female patients and staff. The fact that the cloister like the church was an essential feature of these architectural complexes underlines the ecclesiastical origins of hospital design. This was, though, an unusual period for hospital architects. Not only were a number of substantial new hospitals for the sick and for foundlings built or begun within a forty-year period, it was also a time that was typified by important construction projects within the city as a whole. The fact that the loggia became an essential feature of the Renaissance hospital façade suggests that innovation was possible and even desirable. The extent to which this innovatory spirit might have been carried further forward in the ward, the area of the hospital that most differentiated its activities from the monastic model, will be seen in the next chapter.

CHAPTER 5

'Splendid Houses of Treatment Built at Vast Expense': Wards and the Care of the Body and Soul

Introduction

A visitor to Florence in the mid-fifteenth century walking past one of the large new hospitals or foundling homes would have been struck immediately by their elegant loggias, but from the street there was little to indicate the extent of the substantial complex behind these façades. A native Florentine, on the other hand, would have been much more likely to have been aware of and even to have visited the main elements of the sites: their churches and cloisters, examined in the previous chapter, and their very substantial wards. It was the ward that brought together some of the main characteristics of the Renaissance hospital: 'beautiful and sufficient and suitable to receive any sick or well person who is wretched.'[1]

If the ward made concrete the beauty and utility of the Renaissance hospital, it is also the area where two of the main themes of this book intersect, the complementary roles of religion and medicine. This combined function is well summarised in a visually striking mid-seventeenth-century view of the interior of the Corsia Sistina, the main ward of Rome's largest hospital, S. Spirito in Sassia (Plate 5.1). It is the sheer volume of space, still impressive today, that would have struck contemporaries in the late fifteenth century. The same would have been true of S. Maria Nuova's vast cruciform ward when it was completed a hundred years later.

The Corsia Sistina, like Florentine hospital wards of the period, combined the cure of the body with the cure of the soul. Individual beds lined the walls of the ward, each enclosed by curtains to maintain heat and privacy. This image probably shows it more crowded than normal; the four extra rows of temporary beds would have been added as a response to the demands of a Jubilee year or an epidemic. The view is taken from the crossing, in itself highly symbolic, and shows an impressive neo-classical altar where the daily celebration of Mass would have been visible by patients in all wings of the ward. The

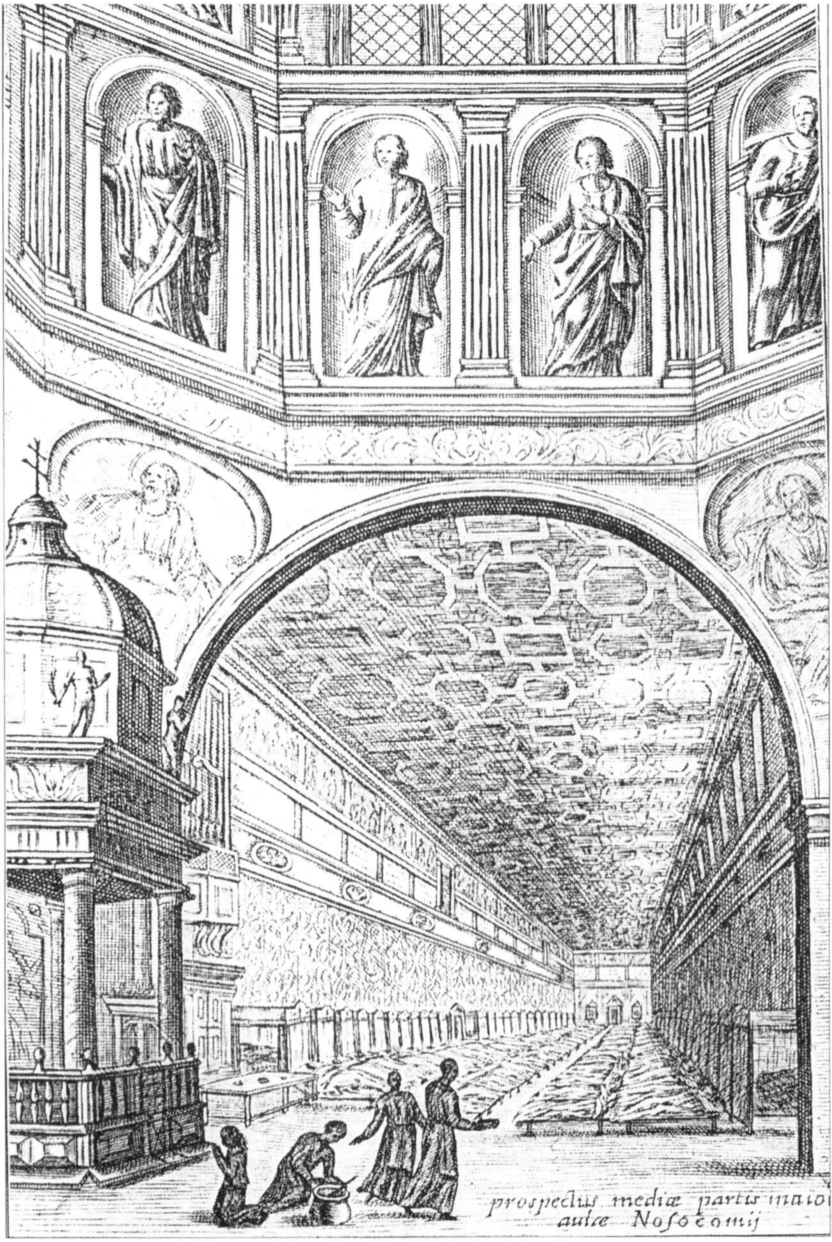

Plate 5.1 *The Corsia Sistina, Hospital of S. Spirito, Rome: View from the Crossing*, from P. Saulnier, *De capite sacri ordinis* (Rome, 1649)

'SPLENDID HOUSES OF TREATMENT BUILT AT VAST EXPENSE'   149

organ just behind the altar indicates that Mass would have had a musical accompaniment, while the group of nursing staff in the foreground includes one kneeling in prayer.[2] Hospital chapels and wards, like their churches, were also visited on feast-days by potential patrons, who would have been encouraged to follow the example of Pope Sixtus IV and leave money for their expansion and decoration.[3]

This chapter will explore the dual themes of the physical and spiritual care provided in the wards of hospitals in Renaissance Florence by examining their evolving structures, their use of space and the role of their material culture from altarpieces to beds.

5.1 Wards Seen from the Outside

Local pride in the appearance of hospitals ensured their prominent representation in contemporary views and maps alongside other important sites. Often the façades stand out more clearly than the wards, which are represented schematically. Pietro del Massaio's 1472 view of Florence (Plate 1.1) provides a clear representation of Messer Bonifazio, showing three parallel buildings, the church and two wards, separated by a cloister. On the façade of each building above the loggia there is an oculus beneath the gable of the pitched roofs.[4] Francesco Rosselli's 'Catena' map of c.1471–80 (Plate 3.13) shows the loggia of S. Matteo prominently (marked as 'SP D LEMMO'); the male ward runs along Via della Sapienza, with the female ward parallel.[5] In Massaio's view of S. Maria Nuova (Plate 1.1), S. Egidio is clearly visible with the roof and façade of the parallel men's ward, but the whole complex for women south of the piazza is completely hidden by the mass of the cathedral. In his view of S. Paolo, prominence is given to the main ward, which stands above the surrounding buildings and is covered by a pitched roof.[6]

These early views of the larger Florentine hospitals provide a third dimension to our picture of the hospital ward, by definition lacking from plans. Even if representation of detail should not be interpreted too literally, contemporaries were clearly struck by the height of wards. Though the front elevations of the new hospitals tend to be obscured by their loggias, the façade of S. Maria Nuova's male ward remained clearly visible parallel to S. Egidio (Plates I and 1.10). The façades of both church and ward come to a point under their pitched roofs, but are differentiated by their fenestration. Above the main entrance to S. Egidio there is an oculus and above the ward an elongated mullioned window to illuminate the long, tall space beyond. The front elevation of the ward was further distinguished by a relief image above the window of a crutch, the symbol of the hospital, which appeared in other parts of the site and on the uniforms of the staff.

Plate 5.2 S. Maria Nuova: entrance to female ward today, Piazza S. Maria Nuova (now the Archivio Notarile)

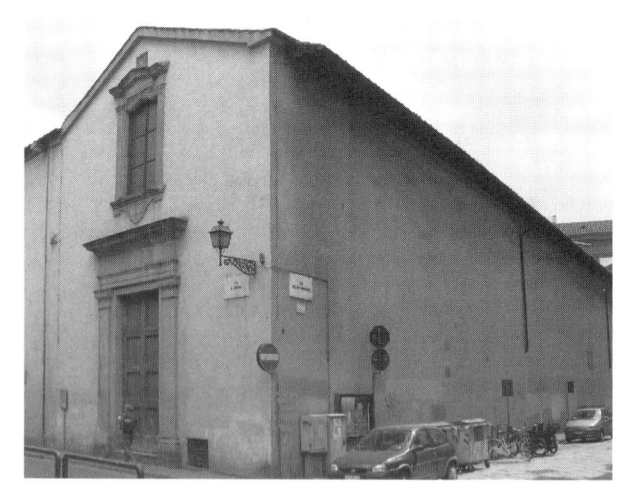

Plate 5.3 Stefano Bonsignori, *Plan of City of Florence*: detail of S. Maria Nuova, 1584 (Museo di Firenze Com'era)

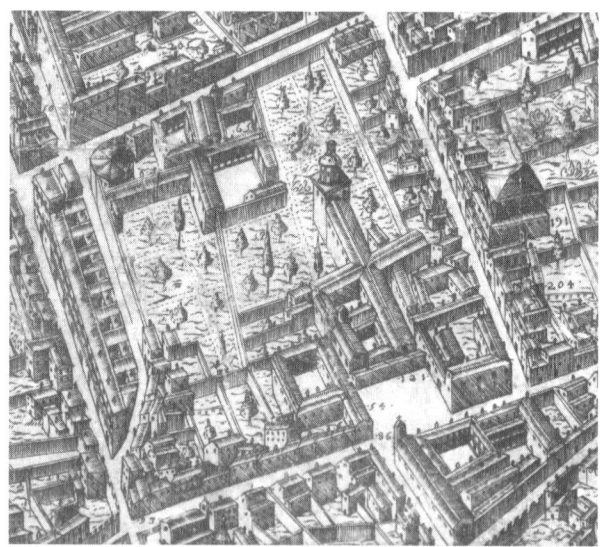

The entrance to the women's complex on the southern side of Piazza S. Maria Nuova was considerably more modest, as befitted a space that was less accessible to the public, lacking its male counterpart's elongated window and steeply pitched roof. The overall appearence today is not dissimilar to that of Bonsignori's plan of 1584, though the bell-tower, which surmounted the northern end of the ward, has disappeared (compare Plates 5.2 and 5.3). However, a number of changes had already been undertaken before Bonsignori's view, most noticeably in 1577 when the ward altar was demolished, a door cut into the northern wall and a new luminous window added.[7]

5.2 Ward Interiors: 'Beautiful and Sufficient and Suitable to Receive any Sick or Well Person Who Is Wretched'

If the façade of the Innocenti has long been seen as typical of the Renaissance hospital, another characteristic element is S. Maria Nuova's enormous cruciform ward. Indeed, given the long-standing debate between Tuscan and Lombard historians over the origins of the cruciform ward, it is worth summarising the evidence for its evolution.[8]

S. Maria Nuova's Cruciform Ward: A Paradigm?

Until the early fifteenth century the ground plan of S. Maria Nuova's male ward resembled an inverted 'L' (see above, Chapter 3). The first phase of the new western extension was begun in 1409–10, though it was not finished to form a 'T' until 1479 (Plate 1.9: 1d). This building programme was undertaken under the active directorship of *spedalingo* Bonini in response to demand for more space, especially during epidemics.[9]

The planning and completion of the northern arm of the male ward (Plate 1.9: 1e) have given rise to a long-standing debate over whether Tuscan or Lombard hospitals provided the model for the cruciform ward plan. Local Florentine historians have invested a great deal of energy and emotion in attempting to prove that this design originated at S. Maria Nuova. According to a charming legend, recorded by Giuseppe Richa in his *Notizie istoriche delle chiese di Firenze* (1759) and repeated by subsequent historians, in 1312 a comet in the shape of a shining gold cross appeared for three nights in the sky over the hospital. This was apparently taken by the *spedalingo*, Lorenzo di Jacopo da Bibbiena (1308–32), as a sign that the ward should be created on a cruciform plan, an idea then allegedly inherited by *spedalingo* Orlando Pierozzi da San Casciano (1332–48) under whose aegis the eastern section was built.[10]

The legend hardly stands up to scrutiny. No explanation is provided for the lack of progress for this grand design across so many years; if it had really been a priority, S. Maria Nuova's endowment during the Black Death would surely have provided sufficient funds for the construction of the two final wings of the cruciform shape. A more probable explanation is that the ground plan of a 'cross' envisaged by those who ran S. Maria Nuova for most of the fifteenth century was not cruciform at all but a 'T'. Thus, when S. Maria Nuova employed Antonio da Urbino and Bettino da Imola in 1413 to paint 'the roof of part of the cross', the reference was to a 'T' shape rather than to an incipient cruciform.[11] This was the shape of the Greek letter 'Tau', made famous within the context of hospitals dedicated to St Anthony of Padua, which, along with S. Maria Nuova, adopted the emblem of the *gruccia* or crutch.

Discussion of the influence of Tuscan hospitals on northern Italy is based primarily on the correspondence of Francesco Sforza, duke of Milan, in the 1450s when he was considering the foundation of the Ospededale Maggiore of the Lombard capital. In early April 1456, having laid the foundation stone, Sforza wrote to his ambassadors in Siena and Florence for information about S. Maria della Scala and S. Maria Nuova. The surviving report on the Siennese hospital, drawn up by the rector himself, dealt principally with its administration, finances and personnel.[12] Also included, however, was a brief description of its architectural layout. From this account and more recent reconstructions of S. Maria della Scala, it is evident that by the mid-fifteenth century the hospital had two long parallel wards, 'Pellegrinai', which contained 130 beds for the male sick and pilgrims. Between these wards was a corridor and, although the rector described this link as 'per crucem', the ground-plan is a long way from the famous Lombard cruciform design with its intersecting arms.[13]

In Florence Cosimo de' Medici, having heard of Sforza's plans for a new hospital, offered the services of an unidentified Florentine engineer.[14] But it was Cosimo's second son, Giovanni, who from June 1456 acted as the intermediary in Francesco Sforza's search for inspiration since the previous year he had been at the Milanese court.

The Florentine Antonio Averlino, best known as Filarete, is the architect most closely identified with the Milanese Great Hospital, as an important part of his *Trattato di Architettura* is devoted to his design for the hospital. On 4 June 1456 Sforza wrote a letter to Giovanni de' Medici, now in Florence, in which he 'presented' both Filarete and Maestro Giovanni di Sant'Ambrogio who were coming 'in order to see in its entirety all of that hospital of your city and examine it and to obtain the design ... and discover if your hospital can be improved on in any way, so that we can have the best possible design'.[15] Though Sforza may have favoured Filarete, Giovanni de' Medici obviously wanted him to leave his options open. In his letter to Sforza later in the month, he says that he has been 'shown everything here of S. Maria Nuova which is a great and excellent thing ... and because there are numerous masters here who are most worthy I have ordered them to produce a number of different models and I will send them to Your Lordship'.[16]

Clearly S. Maria Nuova provided inspiration, but it was seen by Florentines themselves as a model that could be improved upon; hence the idea of sending a number of designs to Sforza. Indeed, when Giovanni wrote again in August he mentioned that he had asked his *capomaestro*, Bernardo Rossellino, to design a model which he was sending to Milan 'and it is taken partly from ours here [i.e., S. Maria Nuova], but it is much more beautiful because this one was built in a number of stages and if we had to construct it today it would be more beautiful and with more order than it is today'.[17]

Sforza appears to have agreed and, indeed, there were more obvious models to follow nearer home. The mid-fifteenth century was, as noted above in Chapter 3, a period when the hospital 'systems' of many northern Italian cities were reorganised and centralised. This also provided the opportunity to create a new architectural model for the Renaissance hospital. The prototype appears to have been that of S. Matteo in Pavia, which was begun in 1449 and completed seven years later. The main ward was shaped like a Greek cross with arms of equal length, inserted within a courtyard and surmounted by a double loggia. Though the papal bull of 1449 that gave permission for the erection of the hospital mentioned that it was like the Florentine and Siennese hospitals, this was obviously a reference to the length of the wards rather than their ground plans.[18] Other substantial hospitals were also begun in this period, including those at Mantua (1451), Brescia (1447), Cremona (1451) and Bergamo (1457).[19] Though Mantua had a cruciform plan, the others were closer to extant Tuscan models: Brescia had long wards like S. Maria della Scala in Siena and those at Cremona were similar to S. Maria Nuova's partly built 'T' plan.

Simply looking at the chronology of the completion of these hospitals in Lombardy suggests their obvious importance as an influence on Sforza and his architectural advisors when considering their options for the design of the Ospedale Maggiore. Though Sforza had sent his advisors to examine Tuscan hospital architecture, the design of the cruciform wards of northern Italy may have proved more influential for the eventual development of S. Maria Nuova's large cross-shaped ward rather than the other way around, especially as the Florentine 'model' was not realised for another century.

Over the years there has been much confusion over when the final arm of S. Maria Nuova's male ward was completed, but recently it has been shown convincingly that this did not take place until the late sixteenth century, under the supervision of the architect Bernardo Buontalenti.[20] It is possible, as in the case of the western wing, that it was already begun in the early sixteenth century, as suggested by the fact that the confraternity of artists, the Compagnia di S. Luca, had been forced at some time before 1515 to move from its meeting place at the chapel at the head of the male ward. As the 1563 statutes of the Accademia del Disegno record: 'The Portinari then built the ward [*spedale*] of the said S. Maria Nuova and attached to the said chapel the cross of the said ward for the sick.'

The importance of the construction of the fourth arm in the life of S. Maria Nuova is reflected in a contemporary description of the foundation ceremony on the feast of the Annunciation, 1575:

> Today, on the 25th of the said month [March] 1575, Friday, the day of the Annunciation of the Santissima Vergine, the Most Reverend Don Vito

Buonaccolti, monk of Monte Oliveto, *spedalingo* of this hospital, laid the first stone. In [the said stone] was carved the holy name of Jesus around which was written 'Santa Maria Nova, anno saluto 1575 addì XXV di marzo' and in two holes that were made in the stone were put two lead vases in which were put the following relics: and first a number of *Agnus Dei* blessed by the most holy Pope Pius V, a golden ducat with the image of the Madonna and an eagle, around which was written 'Federigo a great friend', three 'grossi' of the Madonna on which was written 'Virgo protege Pisa'. The said *spedalingo* first said the Mass of the Holy Spirit in our church, and then led the procession with all the male and female members of our family, along Via della Pergola. They then entered through the door in the wall behind the garden made for the Compagnia de' Bianchi, which meets next to our hospital with a crucifix which was much venerated, and the *spedalingo* having taken [with him] the wood of the holy crucifix, a relic of our house, sang the *Te Deum* and other appropriate hymns and orations.[22]

The involvement of the whole *famiglia* in this ceremony is reminiscent of the other great event in the life of S. Maria Nuova, Martin V's confirmation of the consecration of the enlarged church of S. Egidio.

Further ceremonies that took place at subsequent stages in the development of the ward were also attended by representatives of the grand-ducal court. On 16 May 1575 a marble plaque engraved with the names of the *spedalingo* and Bernardo Buontalenti was placed at the north-western corner of the new ward, together with a lead container with six old gold and silver coins, two gold rings, and six medals with images of the grand duke, the projected design of the ward and the Virgin Mary. To underline the importance of the occasion two representatives of the grand duke were present: his court architect, Buontalenti, and Ser Pierantonio de' Bardi, the general of Francesco I's cavalry.

By the time the final arm of the male ward with its chapel had been completed in 1581 its capacity had grown considerably, as can be appreciated from Bonsignori's map of the city in 1584 (Plate 5.3). The longest section was from north to south; another 33 metres had been added to the first section of 39 metres, making a total of about 72 metres. The transverse arms were shorter, but even so their combined length was a not inconsiderable 43 metres. Unfortunately virtually nothing survives of the original structure so it is difficult to reconstruct the appearance of what was by far the largest male ward in the city. Obviously the aim of the extension was partly religious and partly medical, providing a much more theatrical and flamboyant centre for the devotional activities in the ward. However, capacity had also been increased. In the late fifteenth century the male ward had had room for 120 beds; this would have been increased by about another forty if each bed was allowed roughly the

'SPLENDID HOUSES OF TREATMENT BUILT AT VAST EXPENSE' 155

same amount of space. Assuming dual occupancy, this would have meant a potential capacity of up to 320 sick patients.[23]

Open Wards: Form and Function

All other wards in Florence's hospitals in this period conformed to the traditional open-ward design. A typical example was the women's ward at S. Maria Nuova, which, in common with the whole female complex, has been virtually ignored by historians.

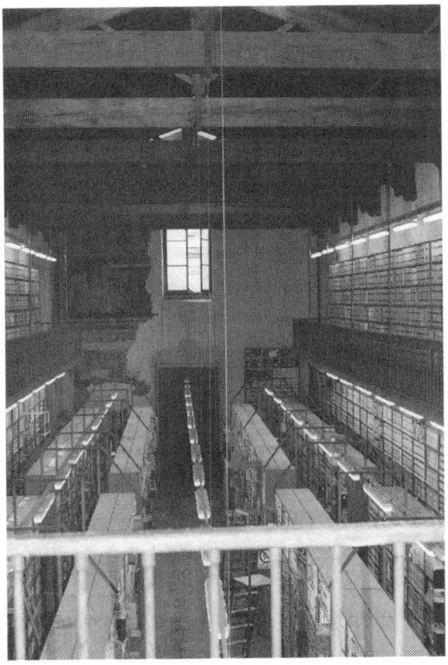

Plate 5.4 S. Maria Nuova: interior of the female ward today (Archivio Notarile, Florence)

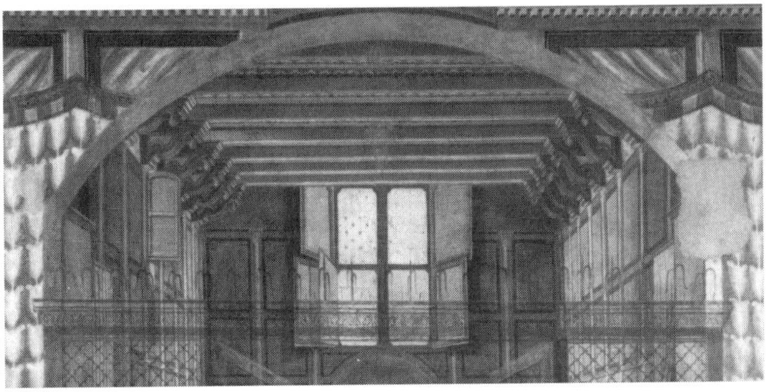

Plate 5.5 Domenico di Bartolo, 'Sala di San Piero', detail of *Care of the Sick*, 1440–4, Pellegrinaio ward, Hospital of S. Maria della Scala, Siena

In fact this ward is one of the most complete sections of the hospital to have survived, as one can see from Plate 5.4. Although the function of this area has changed from housing patients to housing the files of the Archivio Notarile, this new role has not led to radical restructuring of the interior. The sick poor shared the same need as the manuscripts of a growing archive for an ever-increasing amount of space. Today the walls are no longer lined with beds but tall bookshelves, accessed by means of a balcony. Evidently the hospital administrators had not considered building a new floor as a practical response to the growing demand for bed space. Hence the proposals in the sixteenth century to construct another female ward parallel to the existing one on the other side of Via delle Pappe, though this project was eventually abandoned in the seventeenth century in favour of the new cruciform structure north of the piazza.[24]

The choice of the original women's ward as the site for the city's Archivio Notarile and its continued use to this day offers some indication of the building's capacity. It follows the traditional plan of an open ward, with the northern-most section reserved for the chapel where Mass was celebrated daily. It stretched south from Piazza S. Maria Nuova to the parallel street, Via dell'Oriolo, and was some 56 metres in length, 17 metres longer than any of the individual sections of the male ward.[25] Despite this length, conditions must have been very crowded by 1500. While the hundred beds in the male ward were spread out over a total area of 115 metres, in the female ward seventy beds were squashed into about half that space. The problem would have been magnified by the fact that each bed probably contained two patients and three by 1595, as Henry Piers recorded when he visited Florence.[26] Twenty-three years later, when Grand Duke Cosimo II visited the hospital, the situation had grown worse for four or even six women were now forced to share the same bed.[27] This practice may already have been in place a hundred years earlier; cross-infection would certainly help to explain S. Maria Nuova's higher female mortality.[28]

The open-ward plan can also be seen today in S. Matteo's women's ward, which is now the Sala delle Toscane of the Galleria dell' Accademia. Three major structural changes have been made to take account of its new function to display plaster casts and sculptures. The first was the removal of the altar and altar rails at the northern end; the second was the bricking-up of the high windows near the roof and the opening of new, larger ones to produce more light; the third, again to produce greater illumination, was the demolition of the *verone* or balcony at the top of the stairs giving access to the floor above.[29] While there is some continuity in use – it is still employed to provide a service to the public – a major difference is the secularisation of the space and the abandonment of the ward as a centre of spiritual and medical healing.

The dimensions of the wards at S. Matteo, Messer Bonifazio and S. Paolo were fairly similar, at just over 50 by 10 metres.[30] The ward size at S. Matteo remained unaltered from the time Lemmo Balducci stipulated the measurements in his 1385 contract to the drawing of the hospital plan in 1780.[31] Though it was over 2 metres shorter than S. Maria Nuova's women's ward, it was also wider, giving a total area of 1,600 square metres compared with 1,020.[32] Even so, since the length of a ward determines the number of beds, the loss of almost 3 metres meant fewer patients.[33]

These figures add a new dimension to our understanding of the way in which spaces within wards actually worked and the implications this had for patient care and survival rates in different hospitals (see below, Chapter 8). They also point to the need to examine further the extent to which these spaces were developed in response to demographic pressure. At the Innocenti, for example, though much of the building had been completed by 1445, when the first abandoned baby was accepted, the site continued to be enlarged in response to the growing number of abandoned children and live-in staff.[34] Though it was less grandiose in scale than S. Maria Nuova and the Innocenti, this period also saw the remodelling of S. Paolo under Michelozzo,[35] and at Messer Bonifazio, though not expanded in the fifteenth century, funds were raised by the *spedalingo* in 1565 to extend both the male and female wards in response to demand.[36]

This rapid survey of the plans and dimensions of the wards of the main medical hospitals in Renaissance Florence suggests their close dependence on the ground plan of monastic infirmaries. The model of the open ward remained a powerful influence and what has often been seen as a revolution in hospital architecture, the cruciform plan, was merely an outgrowth of existing ideas. Indeed, throughout Europe the open ward or hall remained the prevalent type of design from the Middle Ages until the eighteenth century. This can be seen, for example, from a reconstruction of the monastic infirmary at Cluny, dating originally from about 1135, which was built on an enormous scale. When completed, it measured some 65 metres long, 34 metres wide and 27 metres high with accommodation for between eighty and a hundred patients. Other examples of these substantial open wards still survive today in northern Europe, and include the infirmary of the abbey of Ourscamp in northern France of 1210 (49 metres long) and the hospital of Nôtre Dame des Fontenilles at Tonnerre of 1293 (88 by 19 metres).[37]

Height and the Circulation of Air

Another striking characteristic of open wards was their internal height, a phenomenon that has more often been noted than explained. The simplest and most straightforward explanation is the strength of tradition; namely, that since the hospital ward was an outgrowth of the monastic infirmary, which in turn depended on the church model, designers of wards simply relied on what they knew best from the ecclesiastical context.

The reliance on existing models can be seen at S. Matteo where Lemmo Balducci self-consciously copied features such as the loggia in front of the recently completed Spedale di Messer Bonifazio. He looked as well to S. Maria Nuova for inspiration for the roof: 'Then the said masters were contracted to make the roof of the said hospital, above the above-mentioned walls, and they must make twelve supporting beams for the said roof to that size and height and dimensions of wood and according to the model of the hospital of S. Maria Nuova.'[38] Balducci went on to stipulate the measurements of the wards, including the height of about 11 metres: 'up to the height of 18 to 19 braccia, as the said Lemmo wants.'[39] Just as visitors in the fifteenth century would have been struck by the ward's height – it was exactly double that of the cloister they had just left[40] – so are visitors today to the two surviving women's wards, at S. Matteo and S. Maria Nuova, since their basic structure has not been altered since the fifteenth century.

The preference for height can be explained by the central role of air in contemporary theories about the nature and transmission of disease. It was believed that disease could actually be created in the air through the escape of noxious fumes into the atmosphere from the 'putrefaction of things and matter',[41] whether evil smells from low-lying boggy areas or rotting flesh. Giuseppe Richa suggested that an important consideration when Lemmo Balducci chose a site for his hospital of S. Matteo was that the place should be 'wide and with good air'.[42] The best-known application of this theory is in contemporary discussions of the plague, which was seen as a 'vapore velonoso': hence the decision to site lazzarettos outside city walls.[43]

Even if the Renaissance nose was not as olfactorily precise as that of Jean-Noël Hallé in late eighteenth-century France; the hospital smells that he described cannot have been very different from those of the wards in fifteenth-century Florence:

> There is a stench that is similar to the one exuded by clothes, and there is a mouldy smell that is less noticeable but nevertheless more unpleasant because of the general revulsion it arouses. A third, which might be called the odour of decomposition, may be described as a mixture of the acidic, the sickly and the fetid; it provokes nausea rather than offending the nose. This mixture accompanies decomposition, and is the most repellent among all the odours to be encountered in a hospital.[44]

One finds similar comments in relation to Tuscan hospitals in Giovanni Targioni Tozzetti's *Notizie degli Aggrandamenti delle scienze fisiche in Toscana* (1780), where he wrote: 'The buildings of these hospitals are truly beautiful and commodious, but are not healthy for the patients, lacking ventilation and the easy expulsion of air, so necessary in hospitals ... Thus very often the pestilential sickness called *febbre di spedali* originates and multiplies in the hospitals themselves; sores easily become corrupted and many diseases get worse.'[45] Preoccupation with smells and the transmission of disease was hardly confined to the seventeenth and eighteenth centuries. Marsilio Ficino, for example, writing in 1478 about how individuals might preserve themselves from catching plague, advised them to 'Keep away from trapped air which is enclosed and humid; and remember that air, which does not move often and is not renewed and where sun with dry wind does not purge the air sufficiently, becomes corrupt and full of poisonous putrefaction like water which remains still.'[46]

Sick patients were believed to have an innate ability to create disease within themselves. The basis of this process was again putrefaction caused by malignant humours within the body and the sick thus spread disease by exhaling corrupt air. Hospital wards were therefore designed to ensure the circulation of air and to encourage it to rise from the level of the beds towards the roof. This would have been achieved in part by the design of open-plan buildings with a simple roof 'a cavaletti', that is, a pitched roof of beams with an external covering of tiles allowing smells and infected air to escape. Aeration of these spaces was also necessary for the upward movement of fumes from stoves used to heat the wards during colder seasons. Filarete in his design for the Ospedale Maggiore in Milan provided four fireplaces, one in each arm of the cruciform ward, supplemented by braziers down the central aisles.[47] But there was also an awareness of the need to avoid materials that would have generated smoke; the fireplace in S. Maria Nuova's infirmary used to heat water in a copper cauldron was 'stoked not with smoking wood, but with a great heap of charcoal'.[48]

Windows were another way to promote circulation of air, as Tommaso del Garbo advised anybody who visited those with plague: 'Notaries, confessors, relations and doctors who visit those sick from plague on entering their houses should open the windows so that the air is renewed.'[49] Extant evidence about the placement, type and size of windows in wards and whether or not they could be opened is scarce and difficult to interpret, especially as the fenestration of surviving hospital buildings has frequently been changed over the centuries. Those windows depicted most clearly in contemporary views were in the front elevation, though it seems likely that these were glazed and fixed shut, being designed as a source of light rather than to encourage the circulation of air. Examples include the tall mullioned window of S. Maria Nuova's male ward, as shown in Bicci di Lorenzo's fresco (Plate I), and the oculi under the pitched roof of the façade of the hospitals of Messer Bonifazio and S. Paolo, as represented in the 'Catena' map and the Ptolomy views (cf. Plate 1.1). These windows were probably made of glass.[50] During the final phases of construction in August 1420, Francesco di Giovanni and Bernardo di Francesco, described as 'making windows of glass', were paid for 'a glass oculus for the church' and 'a glass window of the said church on the cemetery side'.[51]

Windows on the side elevation of hospitals could potentially have promoted cross-draughts in wards and thus removed the infected air of disease. These are represented rather schematically in contemporary views of the city, with the wards of S. Maria Nuova, Messer Bonifazio and S. Paolo all having a series of rectangular round-topped windows, as did the Corsia Sistina at S. Spirito in Rome (Plate 5.4). Despite the fact that the size, construction and materials of windows are central to an understanding of the illumination of wards and the circulation of air, little has been written on the subject. Other types of buildings in the period tended to employ solutions that were cheaper than glass and to use materials, such as linen or cloth soaked in oil, that would have been translucent.[52] While earlier medieval hospitals in northern Europe, such as leper-houses, initially used stretched polished skins, by the later Middle Ages the windows of the larger institutions for the poor sick in both England and France were glazed with clear glass.[53]

A picture of the materials used in the ward windows can be reconstructed through the evidence in account books. In January 1420, for example, S. Maria Nuova paid 5s to buy 'studs for the cloth-covered windows', whereas five years earlier Niccholò di Piero, described as a 'master of glass windows', had been paid the not inconsiderable sum of £65.15s for 'a glass window next to the chapel of the male ward' and 'a glass window opposite the crucifix in the hospital'. Though these glazed windows reflected their positions of prestige within the ward, they may also have been part of a campaign to replace all windows with glass.[54]

Scattered evidence suggests that at least some ward windows could be opened. When S. Maria Nuova's women's ward was being constructed in 1327, the hospital paid £29.8s 'for rope for the windows of the new hospital' and £10.10s 'in pulleys for the women of the said hospital'.[55] The rope and pulleys were used to open the windows which, as has been seen, were sited high under the roof. Shutters were also opened in the same way, as seen in both Masaccio's fresco the *Tribute Money* in the Brancacci Chapel and in the view of S. Maria della Scala's infirmary in Domenico di Bartolo's fresco in the Pellegrinaio (Plate 5.5). Later known as the Sala di San Piero, the infirmary is represented in the fresco as being well lit by a large glazed window with four panes and hinged wooden shutters at the end of the ward. On the left side there is another smaller window with a shutter.[56]

The explanation for the height of wards, like so much in hospital design, is therefore partly religious and partly medical. Like the nave of a church, a ward was long and relatively narrow and provided a dramatic vista of the altar to facilitate patients' participation in the celebration of Mass. The considerable height would have enabled the smells and fumes generated by disease and insanitary conditions to move up towards the roof, away from patients and staff alike. Continuing concern about these issues, in particular the relatively small dimensions of these openings, led architects in subsequent centuries to enlarge the windows. Ferdinando Del Migliore records that when the architect Giovan Battista Pieratti was employed in 1650 by *spedalingo* Ricasoli to redesign parts of the northern complex of S. Maria Nuova, he 'enlarged the windows [of the men's ward] in order to make it easier to air these spaces and get rid of any bad air that was produced by the exhalation of so many sick people'.[57] Later still, when the female ward of S. Matteo was being converted for the use of the Accademia delle Belle Arti, the architect noted the small size of the windows near the roof, deliberately bricked them up and opened new, larger ones to produce more light.[58]

So far I have concentrated on the design and structure of hospital wards, but avoided discussion, except in general terms, of the function of these spaces. If it is self-evident from a twenty-first-century perspective that wards were primarily intended for the medical treatment of the sick, this was far from the case in the Renaissance, when the priest was seen as playing as important a role as the physician in healing patients.

5.3 The Care of the Sick and the Material Culture of Health

Domenico di Bartolo provides a comprehensive guide to both the spiritual and medical roles of the ward in his well-known fresco the *Care of the Sick* at S. Maria della Scala (Plate 5.6).[59] Looking from right to left, we see first the removal of the corpse of a patient who has died in the hospital. His body, covered by a blanket bearing the hospital's insignia of a ladder, is being carried on a bier by two men dressed in white coats. They are about to pass a very sick man, who is attended by a well-fed Augustinian friar, listening to his confession and administering the last rites. Further on, a seated man with a severe gash in his right leg is attended by a surgeon and a crowd of the hospital's brethren. Finally we see a wasted-looking patient on a litter, above whom stand a consultant physician and an assistant discussing his case.

While useful as a general introduction, this image conflates a whole series of events in the life of a hospital patient from entry to exit, alive or dead. In order to reveal best how wards functioned as centres of care – the role of physicians and surgeons will be dealt with in detail below, in Chapter 7 – I shall follow a patient through his or her time in hospital, largely in relation to the material culture associated with this experience.

The descriptions of the arrival and reception of patients in written records such as statutes often portray the sick poor as 'almost like Christ in their

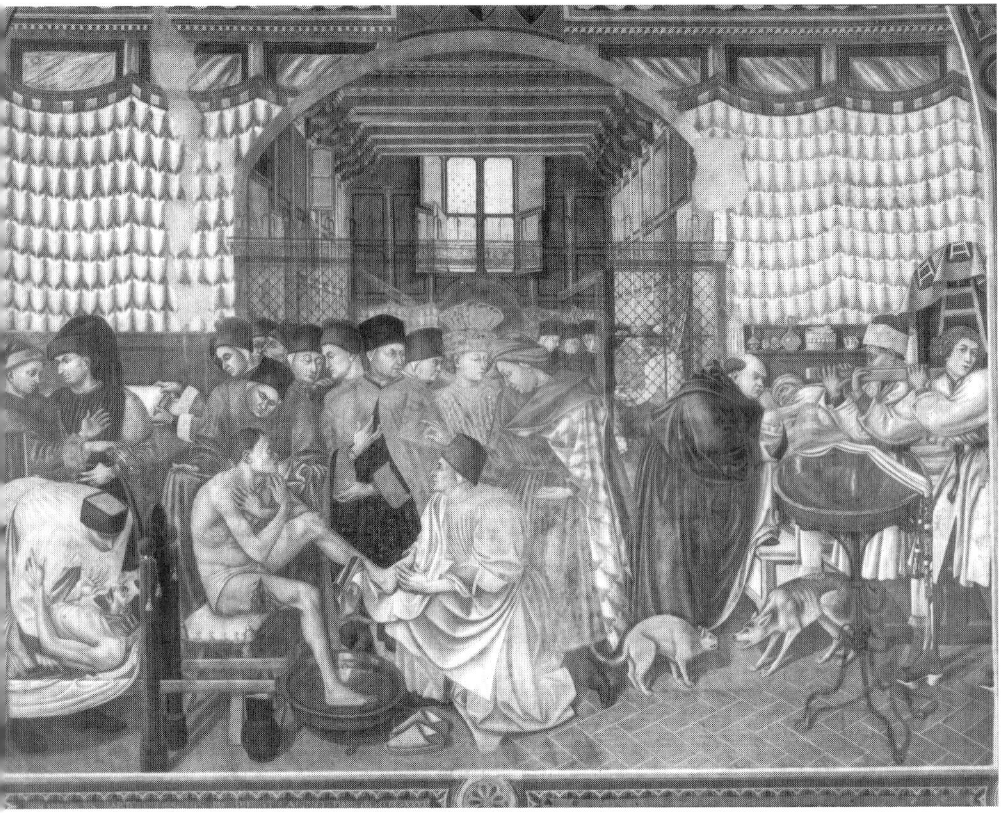

Plate 5.6 Domenico di Bartolo, *Care of the Sick*, 1440–4, Pellegrinaio ward, Hospital of S. Maria della Scala, Siena

persons'.⁶⁰ The association between Christ and the poor refers to the idea of Christ the Pilgrim; in the context of the hospital the patient is seen as sharing Christ's sufferings as a stage towards salvation. The hospital is therefore presented as the institutional embodiment of two of the Seven Works of Mercy: housing travellers and pilgrims, and tending to the sick.⁶¹

Once the patient had passed through the main doors of the hospital he or she was met by members of staff who began the admission procedure to the ward. This process was described in general terms in the 1374 statutes of S. Maria Nuova in relation to the duties of hospital staff, who were to receive the sick 'diligently and charitably, tend to and comfort, and refresh, nourish and clean [them], and administer to all their needs, and treat them [*medichino*] with all their strength and charity'.⁶² Emphasis was placed on diligent care of the sick, who were to be comforted, fed, cleaned and given medical treatment.

A more detailed description concerning the reception of the sick is contained in S. Maria Nuova's 'Ordinances' of 1510–11:⁶³

How the sick are received

In the middle of the infirmary there is a little bed covered with a cloth on which the sick are laid when they first arrive. As soon as they are admitted the infirmarer comes to them to determine the nature of their illnesses. He assigns the feverish and those with skin lesions or wounds to empty beds ... and he sends one of the head nurses to wash the sick person's feet and another sub-infirmarer to get [their clothes].

This description runs together a number of stages in the admission process, which can be reconstructed through various types of evidence. On arrival they were usually taken to the chaplain to confess their sins and subsequently to 'greet the Body of Christ', as shown in one of the illuminated scenes of S. Spirito's *Liber regulae* of about 1350 (Plate 5.7).[64] Patients were then passed on to the hospital servants, who washed their feet, a service that was both hygienic and symbolic, recalling Christ's practice at the Last Supper. It can be seen at the centre of Domenico di Bartolo's *Care of the Sick* (Plate 5.6). The right foot of a wounded male patient is shown immersed in a water-filled copper bowl supported by short legs, while his left foot is being dried by one of the male nurses on a large black-bordered towel. Slippers have been placed alongside

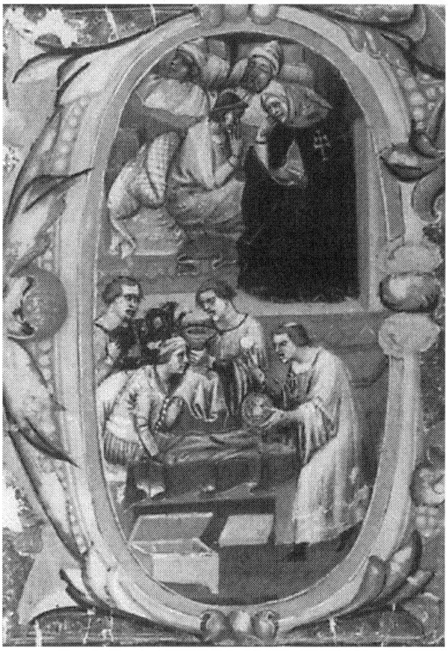

Plate 5.7 Circle of the Master of the S. Giorgio Codex, *Chaplains Confess Patients*, Hospital of S. Spirito, Rome, *Liber regulae Sancti Spiritus*, c.1350 (ASR, Ospedale di S. Spirito 3193, f. 49r)

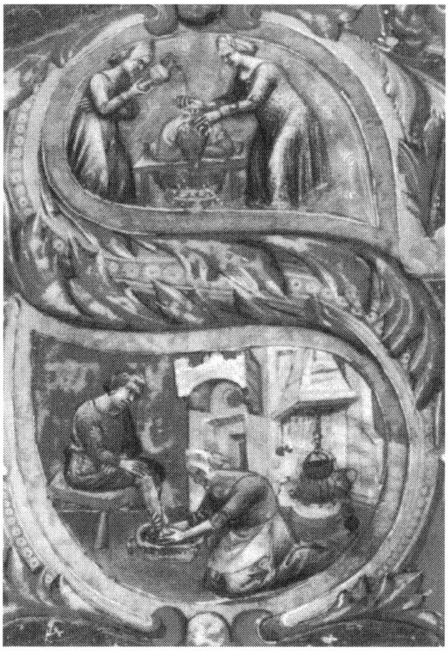

Plate 5.8 Circle of the Master of the S. Giorgio Codex, *Nurses Delouse Patients and Wash their Feet*, Hospital of S. Spirito, Rome, *Liber regulae Sancti Spiritus*, c.1350 (ASR, Ospedale di S. Spirito 3193, f. 128v)

the bowl for the patient's feet once they have been washed and dried. Further to the right is another copper bowl, mounted on a tripod with an embroidered towel. Bowls were also recorded in inventories, as at S. Matteo, which owned 'two iron bowls for cleaning the sick', two copper ones 'to wash hands' and a caste-iron warming pan for the beds.[65]

Once patients had been undressed, their clothes were taken away to be stored, a practice made clear in S. Maria Nuova's instructions to the sub-infirmarer:

> Once the sick person has been assigned to a bed, he comes, collects all the clothes taken off by the patient and wraps them up. He notes his name, father's name, place of origin, family name and the amount of money he is carrying, if any, and he writes all this on a label attached to the bundle, which he places in a storeroom called the Pergola ... This depository is lined with chests or cupboards identified by the letters of the alphabet and the bundle is placed in the cupboard corresponding to the patient's initial. Thus, when a patient recovers and wishes to leave, it is easy to find his effects once he tells his name.[66]

A new set of hospital clothes was then issued to the new inmate, as detailed by S. Maria Nuova's statutes: the sub-infirmarer was to fetch 'slippers, a leather robe, a shift, a cap, and two pillows for him. In the winter we ... use caps made of wool; in summer the clothes and caps are made of linen, and we use tunics without sleeves.'[67] Providing clean clothes had both a practical and a symbolic function. Changing into clean clothes carried an obvious hygienic benefit since, as explained by S. Maria Nuova's early sixteenth-century 'Ordinances': 'Because many of the poor arrive teeming with lice, we separate out their clothes and store them in the same way but in a different place.'[68] The delousing of patients by the nursing staff is shown vividly in another illumination to S. Spirito's *Liber regulae* (Plate 5.8).

New clothes also symbolised leaving behind everyday life and entering a new environment dedicated to the cure of the body and the spirit. Indeed, the garments provided by the hospital also reflected the semi-monastic environment of the institution, as can be seen in Pontormo's fresco in the Sala delle Toscane, which shows little difference between the garb of the nurses and that of the women patients, both of which were based on a nun's habit and covered body and head (Plate 6.6). The material itself was plain, usually grey, and made from *panno romagnolo*, a coarse undyed woollen cloth.[69]

As the discussion of the processing of patients has shown, once they entered the hospital they became numbers in a complex system. Not only were their own clothes numbered, so were the patients themselves. Throughout their stay

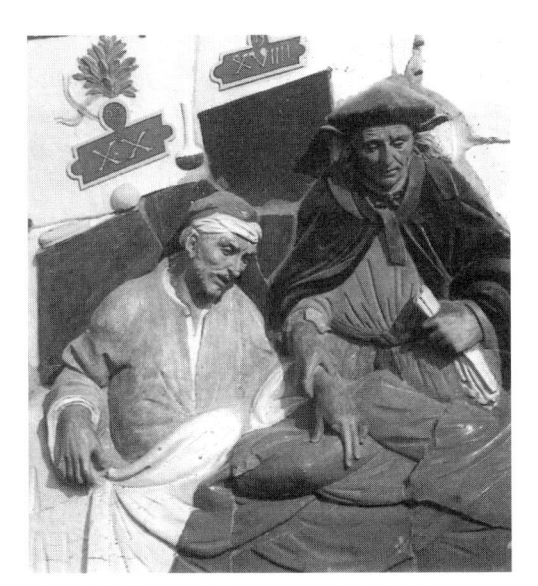

Plate 5.9 Giovanni di Andrea della Robbia's workshop, *Care of the Sick*, 1525–9, Ospedale del Ceppo, Pistoia (detail showing bed numbers)

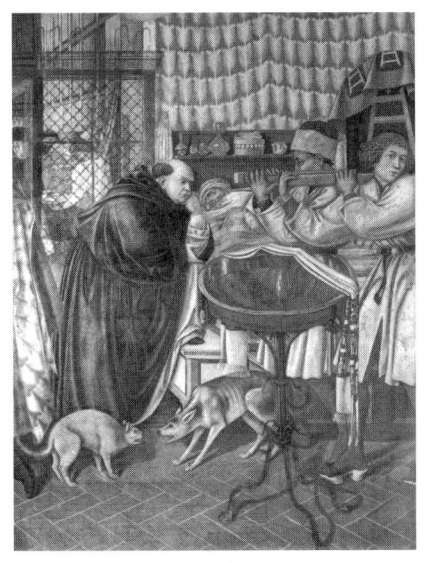

Plate 5.10 Domenico di Bartolo, 'Confession of a Dying Patient', detail from *Care of the Sick*, 1440–4, Pellegrinaio ward, Hospital of S. Maria della Scala, Siena

patients carried these personal numbers, which were recorded at entry and exit, and thus became absorbed rapidly in the daily routine of the ward. The system of numeration can be seen in use in the Ceppo in Pistoia. The terracotta frieze of the ward scene shows that each bed was numbered above the headboard for rapidity of identification (Plate 5.9). It is worth examining the structure and appearance of beds to add to our understanding of patients' day-to-day experience of their immediate environment.

The simplest kind of bed was the litter, visible on the left-hand side of Domenico di Bartolo's *Care of the Sick* (Plate 5.6), which was used to place a patient on when he or she arrived at hospital for admission. This practice is recorded too at S. Maria Nuova in the clause in the early sixteenth-century 'Ordinances' on the reception of the sick: 'In the middle of the infirmary there is a little bed covered with a cloth on which the sick are laid when they first arrive.' Larger numbers of litters could then be brought in during emergencies, as in the case of the four rows of temporary beds in the seventeenth-century view of the Corsia Sistina (Plate 5.1).

The most common type of bed in the hospital, as in the home in Quattrocento Italy, was the *lettiera*.[70] This consisted of a series of planks joined together by a frame, distinguished from the most basic litter form of bed by its headboard to which a shelf or cornice was attached, as in the scene showing the dying man on the right-hand side of Domenico di Bartolo's *Care of the Sick*

(Plate 5.10). Behind the bed was a shelf on which there were a number of receptacles for medicaments; the two flasks may have contained water or wine, while pomegranate was used for the treatment of stomach pain – the fruit was also a symbol of the Passion, a reminder of the spiritual function of the hospital through which the dying patient might attain salvation. In the domestic setting beds often had benches or chests around them, again as shown in Domenico di Bartolo's fresco, where the friar is shown resting one of his feet. A variation on this theme is contained in Filarete's description of his plans for the Ospedale Maggiore in Milan:[71]

> The beds were fine and good. The bedsteads were 2½ braccia wide and 3½ braccia long [1.5 × 2.1 metres]. At the head of each bed was a cupboard, or a little window. When it was opened, the door made a little table where the sick could eat … At the foot of each bedstead there was a small chest where things could be kept in case of need.

Contemporary images of wards often show that beds could be enclosed by curtains to maintain privacy and heat (Plate 5.1). Heat was also provided by blankets and covers. The 1454 inventory of S. Matteo's men's ward listed all the necessary accoutrements for their thirty 'beds for the sick with different symbols',[72] including 29 straw mattresses, 30 bolsters, 29 smaller pillows and 18 pillowcases, some described as 'in good condition', sheets, 30 blankets and a series of covers – 8 white, 22 red, 6 striped and others with a long pile.[73] These different colours probably reflected the tastes of individual patrons who had provided the covers and distinguished beds reserved for people with specific conditions or linked to benefactors. The women's beds were similarly equipped, except that each of the twenty-four beds had two mattresses in addition to the straw *sachoni*, they were given softer ones containing wool flock or feathers (*materasse*).[74] Many covers were red, as in the case of the miraculous bed at the Ceppo discussed below, while others were white or in a yellow-and-red herringbone design.[75]

Another common feature was the painting of images on headrests or footboards, a practice also found in the domestic context.[76] At S. Maria Nuova Nicholò *dipintore* was paid 2 lire in October 1375 'to paint a bed with S. Piero Martire and coat of arms', in January 1377 Filippo di Guido received 8 lire 'for eight beds which he painted for us in the ward of the men and women', and in March 1379 2 lire were paid to Jacopo di Corso *dipintore* 'to paint two beds belonging to Tedaldo Tedaldi'.[77] The largest amount of evidence comes from S. Matteo, particularly during the first decade of the fifteenth century, when the administration sought outside sponsorship to furnish the hospital. Thus 20 *soldi* were paid in April 1409 to Piero di Michelino, 'painter in the workshop of

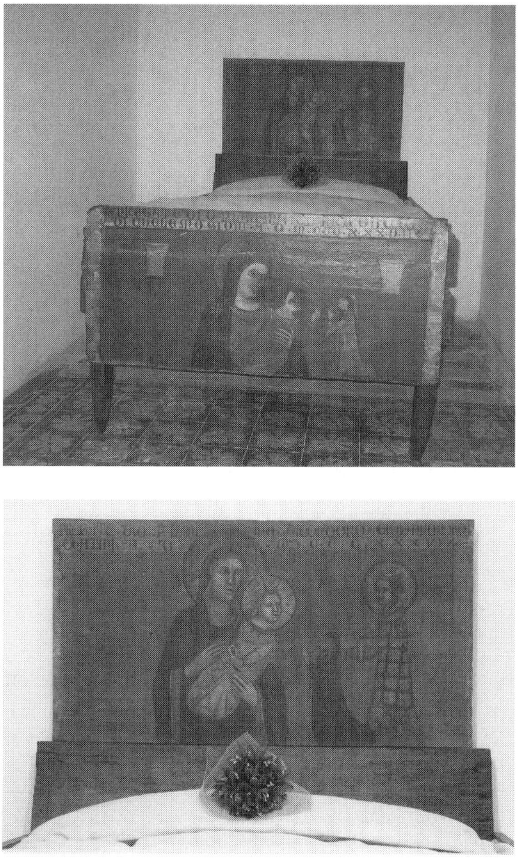

'SPLENDID HOUSES OF TREATMENT BUILT AT VAST EXPENSE'   167

Plate 5.11 Hospital bed from the Ospedale del Ceppo, now in the church of S. Maria del Letto, Pistoia, 1336–7
a. View of whole bed; b. Detail of painted headboard

Ambruogio di Baldese', 'for a bed that he is painting in the men's ward with the coat of arms of Andrea di Chomo, the money-changer', while an inventory lists 'a bed with the sign of Remigi Malifici, who was the scribe of the said wards'.[78]

The painting of beds thus both commemorated an individual and linked him with a particular saintly intercessor. The only Tuscan fourteenth-century hospital bed I know to have survived is from the hospital of the Ceppo in Pistoia and shows the Virgin and Child (Plate 5.11). It has survived because of its association with the miraculous cure of a young girl in hospital after the appearance of the Virgin at her bedside. The head and footboards also contain images of the kneeling figures of the patron, who was identified by the coat of arms painted at the foot of the bed. In other cases where headboards were not painted, small devotional images were hung above the beds, as with S. Maria Nuova's tabernacle of Our Lady above the 'litter where the sick are sat when they come to hospital' repainted by Davide di Tommaso Ghirlandaio in 1490.[79]

These various contemporary views of hospital interiors provide us with a guide to the main activities in a ward and a general idea of the roles of the personnel. They also provide a clear visual representation of objects listed in hospital inventories. Moreover, many of these scenes, whether the Siennese frescoes, the Pistoiese terracotta frieze or illuminations from the *Liber regulae* of S. Spirito in Rome, demonstrate the interdependence of the physical and spiritual care of patients. In the next section I shall turn to examine in greater detail how the ward functioned as a religious space.

5.4 *Wards and the Cure of the Soul: 'When He Is Dead they Clothe him in Linen, and Place him on a Bier in the Middle of the Ward Where the Chapel Is'*

Anybody entering a ward of one of the large hospitals in Renaissance Florence would have been struck immediately by the long vista stretching down the tall hall past rows of beds towards the chapel, which formed the focus of the patients' devotional life. The chapel itself would have been dominated by an altarpiece and probably framed by a fresco-cycle. Something of the drama of all this was captured in a sketch by an epileptic, Giovanni Ortolani, when he was a patient at S. Maria Nuova in 1849 (Plate 5.12). The drawing shows the interior of the male ward as seen from the crossing looking towards the impressive chapel built by Bernardo Buontalenti at its northern end in 1575.[80] The design was simple and bold and consisted of a large triumphal arch of *pietra serena* mounted on substantial Doric columns, the top halves of which are still visible today (Plate 5.13). The arch was surmounted by a cupola and the spandrels decorated with the four evangelists by Alessandro Allori.[81] The windows in the cupola, which can be seen from the exterior in Buonsignori's 1584 view of the hospital, provided a light source to illuminate the altar immediately below. The centrality of the altar was further enhanced by the tabernacle designed by Giambologna to stand over the sacred area. The altar was completed on 1 May 1591 and consecrated by Bishop Giovanni Battista Milanesi, but transferred in the late nineteenth century to the church of S. Stefano al Ponte following the destruction of the male ward (Plate 5.14). The altar is a relatively simple example of an architectural ensemble, much less ambitious in conception and execution than Giambologna's well-known Altar of Liberty for the church of S. Martino in Lucca twelve years earlier: two columns of grey and white marble are mounted on the marble altar and support a broken entablature, leaving a frame for an altarpiece.[82]

This theatrical design must have presented an imposing sight to patients on arrival. Indeed, the altar would have continued to impress when viewed from the perspective of any one of the beds that can be seen lining the walls in

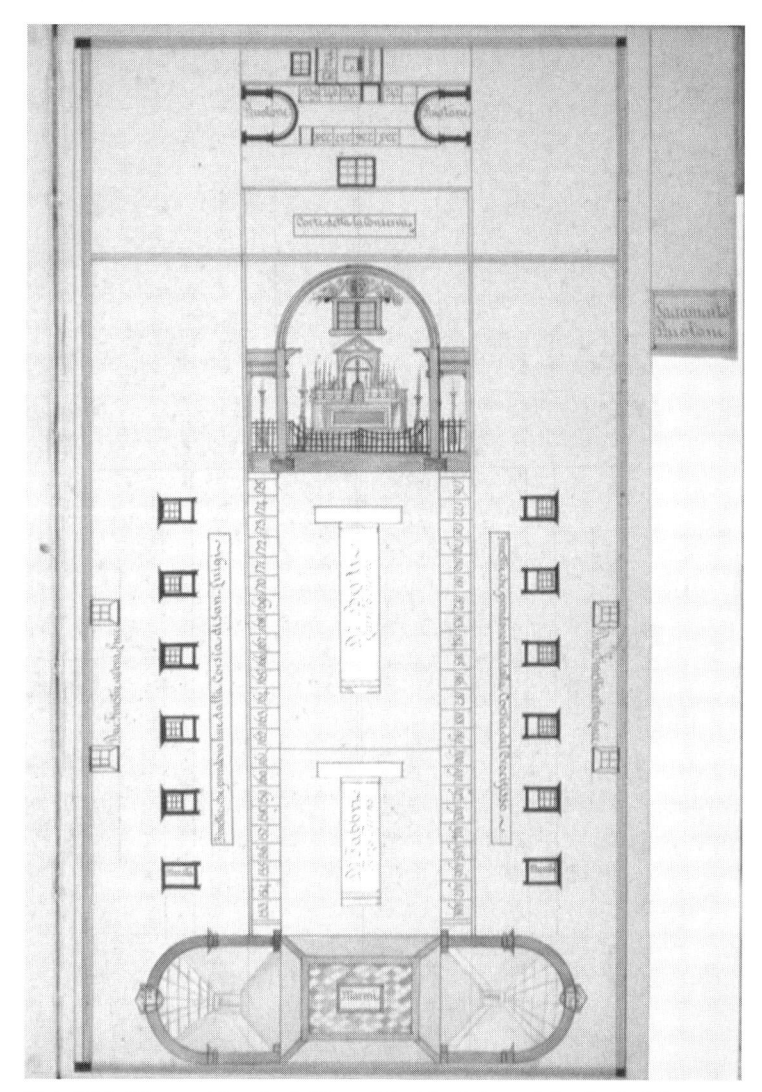

Plate 5.12 Giovanni Ortolani, *View of the North Arm of the Corsia del Sacramento* showing Buontalenti's chapel, male ward, S. Maria Nuova, 1849 (ASF, Ospedale di S. Maria Nuova 717, c. 32)

Ortolani's sketch, especially during the drama of the liturgy of Mass. This scenographic view would also have been designed for visitors, who might have included relatives of patients or wealthier individuals who nursed out of a sense of Christian charity, or visiting gentlemen whose itineraries included hospitals among the main monuments of the city.[83]

The centrality of the chapel in ward life led all major hospitals to commission well-known artists to paint their altarpieces and to design their chapels

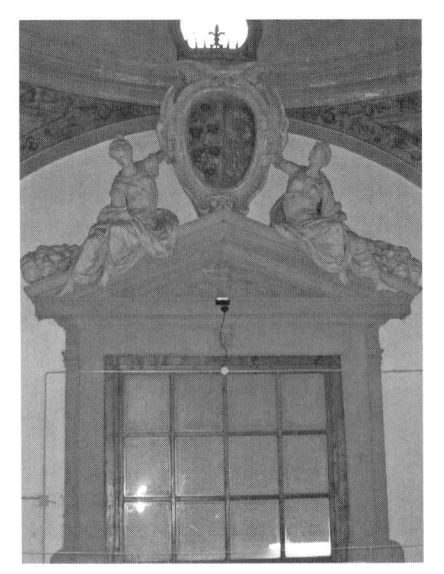

Plate 5.13 Arch of Buontalenti's chapel, male ward, 1575, S. Maria Nuova

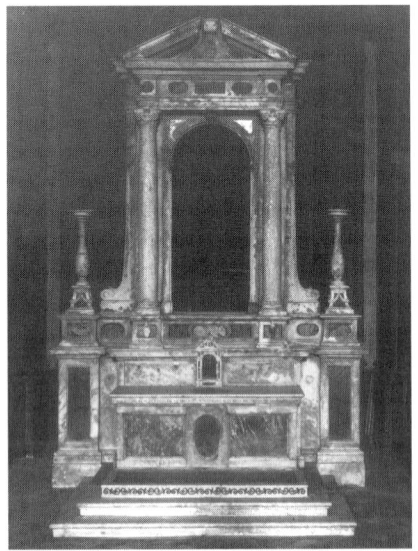

Plate 5.14 Giambologna, altar for male ward, S. Maria Nuova, 1591 (now in S. Stefano al Ponte)

and tabernacles. Individuals, families and corporations all helped to commission artistic programmes, for instance, the Portinari, Balducci and Lupi, and the guilds of the Cambio at S. Matteo, the Notai at S. Paolo and the Seta at the Innocenti. Confraternities also met in ward chapels; one of the best-documented was the painters' company of S. Luca, which had been founded in 1339 in S. Maria Nuova's male ward (and not in S. Egidio as many generations of historians have believed).

Patrons, whether individual or corporate, shared similar motivations for artistic commissions, the foremost among them being the promotion of their own spiritual health in this life and the next. The celebration of Mass in ward chapels catered for a series of consumers, including staff and individual and corporate patrons, but above all the patients, whose physical treatment was bound up intimately with their spiritual health. It is knowledge of their presence that helps us to interpret the altarpieces, frescoes and sculptures commissioned for wards.

Ortolani's view of S. Maria Nuova's men's ward presents an atmosphere of Baroque drama, but a more restrained idea emerges from the women's ward, which still contains fragments of the original early fifteenth-century fresco-cycle in the chapel area (Plate 5.15).[84] The workshop responsible was that of Niccolò di Pietro Gerini, a well-known and popular artist, who was employed by a wide range of ecclesiastical institutions to paint frescoes, including

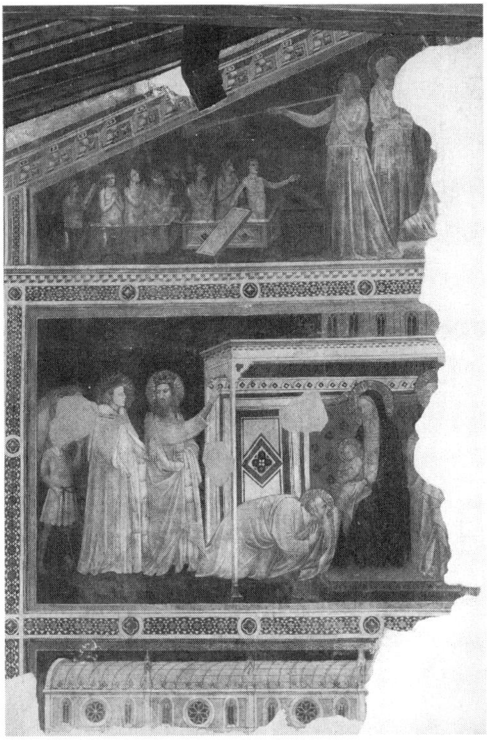

Plate 5.15 Niccolò di Pietro Gerini: *The Last Judgement* and *The Adoration of the Magi*, fragments of fresco-cycle, 1414, female ward, S. Maria Nuova (Archivio Notarile), Florence

Passion cycles for Franciscan friaries, in their chapter-houses in Pisa and Prato and the sacristy of S. Croce in Florence.[85] Lay religious corporations were also among Gerini's clientele, including confraternities, such as the Florentine company of Gesù Pellegrino, who commissioned the *Christ with Saints* now in the Galleria dell'Accademia,[86] and other hospitals like Messer Bonifazio, which had employed him to produce a large triptych of the *Crucifixion* in the hospital church.

Gerini's commission from S. Maria Nuova can be traced to a series of payments in 1414 totalling over 77 gold florins:

To Niccholò di Piero painter on the said day [23.xi.1414] for the paintings listed below, done for the women's side:
First for the Madonna of the Snow with surrounding decoration 8 flor.
and for the Natività di Cristo with decoration 10 flor.
and for S. Lucia and S. Agnese and S. Cecilia 9 flor. and
of the pediment above the tomb 2 flor.
and S. Lisabetta 2 flor.
and the Twelve Apostles 9 flor.

and for the front above the altar and window 10 flor.
and for all the arch with two prophets and decoration 6 flor.
and in addition the 4 [figures] under the arch: S. Giorgio, S. Margherita, S. Barbera and S. Giovanni Batista 7 flor.
and also for the Pietà on the front of the well of the women's hospital 2 flor.
and for the painting above the door of the women's hospital 12 flor.[87]

The documents relate principally to the decoration of the women's chapel at the northern end of the ward. Though the basic space remains today as it was in the early fifteenth century (Plate 5.4), the altar has been demolished and in 1577 a door was cut into the northern wall and a new luminous window added. Furthermore, under this programme of reconstruction the walls were repainted by Alessandro Allori, probably with faux-architectural features, covering over Gerini's original fresco decoration.[88] Thus, though the information provided in these payments to Gerini enables one to identify various elements of the ward chapel, it is not always immediately obvious either how they fitted together or in some cases what their relationship was to the extant frescoes in the Archivio Notarile.

The altar would have been in the centre of the wall, framed by frescoes and illuminated by a glazed window.[89] The theme of the cycle, the Life of Christ, explains the payment for the *Nativity*, the surviving frescoes of the *Adoration of the Magi* and *The Last Supper* which are still to be seen to the left of the present window (Plate 5.15), as well as a *Pietà*, which has been detached and stored by the Soprintendenza.[90] Other scenes may have been painted on the contiguous walls and to the right of the new window; the payments to Gerini probably represent the final stages of a decorative programme that had been ongoing from at least the previous autumn.[91] There may also have been a parallel cycle of the Life of the Virgin in the ward, for the entrance hall to the Archivio Notarile still contains detached panels of the Visitation and the Annunciation.

Other clues to the appearance of the altar bay of the women's ward are contained in the payments to Gerini in 1414. He was paid to decorate the 'elevation [*faccia*] above the altar and window' and the arch, which contained two prophets and underneath four more figures: St George, St Margaret, St Barbara and St John the Baptist. Other saints in the chapel area included Elizabeth, Lucy, Agnes and Cecilia. The presence of many of these figures is explicable by their association with healing and the poor: the Sicilian saint Lucy had distributed her goods to the poor and, as mentioned above, was associated with eye complaints; Elizabeth of Hungary was famous for founding and working in her hospital in Marburg; and Barbara was the patron of those in danger from sudden death.[92] Elizabeth was clearly of central importance to

'SPLENDID HOUSES OF TREATMENT BUILT AT VAST EXPENSE' 173

S. Maria Nuova's female ward since forty years earlier the *Storia di S. Lisabetta* had been painted there by another artist, Tuccio *dipintore*.[93]

These frescoes, covering the north and also probably the northern side walls, must have been a remarkable sight for patients as they lay in their beds. Even given the fragmentary nature of the two sections that remain, the message is clear: in the lower register Mary is the central actor in the *Adoration of the Magi*. The image of the mother of Christ was one with which the female patients would have associated themselves, especially as many of them would have shared Mary's experience of giving birth. The Virgin was also present as advocate and gentle intercessor and this too would have underlined the message that their present sickness was only a stage, for health lay at the end of their sufferings: improved physical health – for most patients left cured – and the possibility of spiritual health, as they were reminded by looking at the top register of the *Last Judgement*, given that suffering purified the soul. Not long after this programme had been completed, the hospital turned its attention to S. Egidio and did not resume its redecoration of the wards until the mid-fifteenth century after work had been completed in the church.

There are no traces of a fresco-cycle in the women's ward of S. Matteo (the Sale delle Toscane of the Galleria dell' Accademia), but an extant altarpiece can be identified from this period.[94] This is a large panel painting by Mariotto di Cristofano in the Accademia executed between 1445 and 1447 (Plate 5.16),[95] listed in S. Matteo's 1454 inventory of the women's ward as a 'large altar with an altarpiece painted on each side with a crucifix above'.[96] The contract with Mariotto on 6 December 1445 laid down the subject matter:

> Today Gerolamo, prior of the hospital of S. Matteo [di Lemmo] from Montecatini, and Ser Simone, chaplain of the said place, and Monna Nanna, the head of the female ward of the said hospital, contract the painter Mariotto di Cristofano to paint an altarpiece for the altar of the women's ward and that the said Mariotto should contract a carpenter and the said Mariotto should paint the said altarpiece and do it as well as he can and knows. And the said altarpiece should be painted in front and behind: in front Our Lady with these saints, that is [blank], and behind the resurrection of Our Lord Jesus Christ.[97]

The subject of the mystical marriage of St Catherine of Alexandria was determined by those responsible for commissioning the painting – *spedalingo*, chaplain and head of the female staff.[98] The choice of the saints for the front of the panel was particularly appropriate for a female ward, as they were almost exclusively women and indeed it could be argued that the *Mystical Marriage of St Catherine* would also have had particular appeal (Plate 5.16a). As the

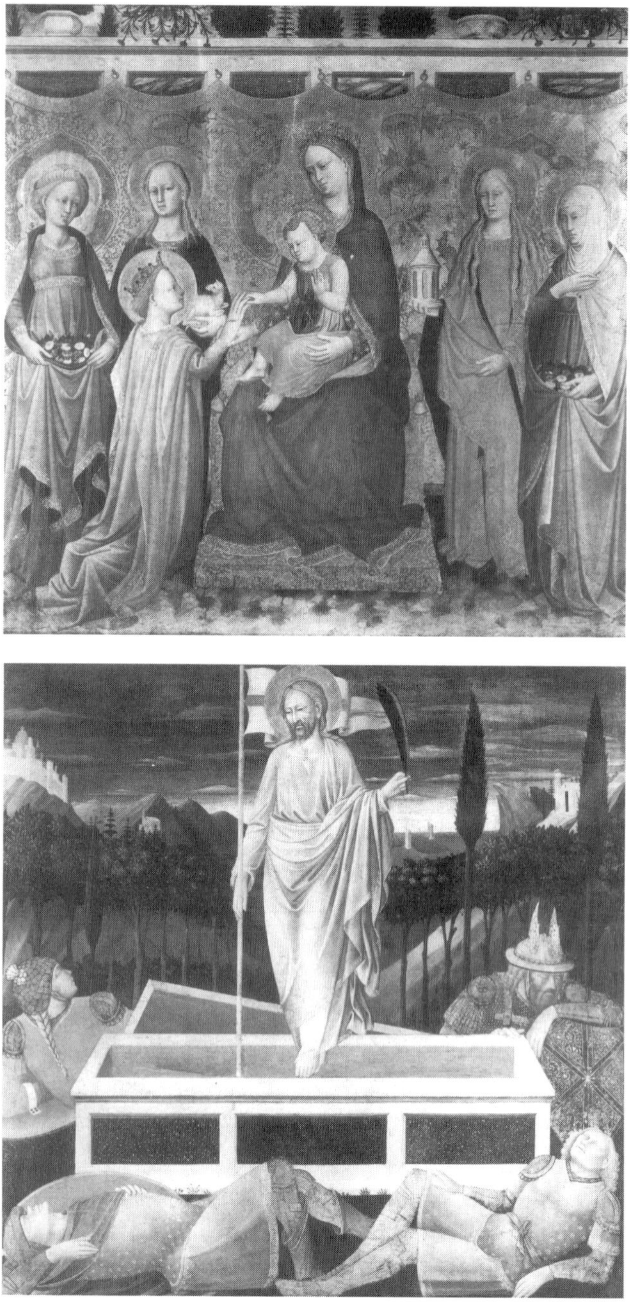

Plate 5.16 Mariotto di Cristofano, 1445–7 (Galleria dell' Accademia, Florence)
a. *Mystical Marriage of St Catherine of Alexandria with Saints*;
b. *Resurrection of Christ*

contract stipulated, the Virgin and Child were at the centre of the devotion of both the spectator and the adoring figure of St Catherine of Alexandria, who is represented as kneeling before the Christ-child for her mystical marriage. On either side of the Virgin are St Agnes and Mary Magdalene, flanked by SS. Dorothy and Elizabeth and shown offering flowers to the Virgin and Child. In this way salvation, as represented by Christ, was combined with examples of female purity to aid the recovery of the female patients in the ward. Both Catherine and Agnes had dedicated their lives to the service of Christ, their heavenly husband. Many of these saints associated with healing were also represented in S. Maria Nuova's women's ward, including Elizabeth of Hungary and Agnes, who restored the sight and health of the Roman youth who had been struck down by the ire of God when he attempted to violate the saint's bodily purity. There was also a strong contemporary association between Mary Magdalene and conversion to a holy life in the service of the sick, one of the best-known examples of which was Beata Margherita of Cortona, who is believed to have founded that city's Spedale della Misericordia.[99] The presence of the ointment jar was a reminder of the role of both Mary Magdalene and the nursing staff in the ward. The jar in the picture contained the healing salve with which Mary anointed the feet of the living Christ and which also served for the preparation of the body after death; similar jars in the hospital would have contained unguents to treat the sick.

The painting of both sides of the altarpiece suggests that they were to be viewed from the front and back and that the scenes were intended to be read as complementary. A very different image appeared on the reverse of the picture, which would have been seen as one entered the ward from the eastern end (Plate 5.16b). If the subject of the altarpiece most visible to those who frequented the ward was one of hope showing the Christ-child and the mystical marriage of St Catherine, the reverse showed the Resurrection and the salvation of mankind through the suffering of Christ. This darker, more brooding image of the emergence of Christ from the tomb represented both literally and metaphorically the birth of hope for a new age with the sun rising behind the familiar Tuscan scene of cypress trees and hills.

Mariotto's altarpiece stood at the end of the women's ward, raised on an altar and facing down the hall so that the patients could see the image during the celebration of Mass. Even at night it would have remained visible from the further end of the ward; its extravagant gold-leaf background would have glowed in the warm light of candles and lamps on the altar.[100] Some context for the altarpiece is provided by inventories. We know, for example, that in 1454 the altar was surrounded and separated from the rest of the ward by a rail. This was to delineate the sacred space and to avoid moral and physical pollution of the Host, thought especially necessary owing to the potential presence of menstruating women.[101] On either side of the altarpiece were two wooden candlesticks with iron candleholders to provide light during Mass.[102] By 1591 the inventory records that S. Matteo had acquired a 'head of St Antoninus' – presumably a sculpture rather than the original, which was owned by the Buonomini di S. Martino.[103] In addition, there was a large crucifix, probably made of wood and suspended above the altar, similar to that owned by the Spedale di S. Fina in San Gimignano.[104] Finally, S. Matteo's ward chapel contained two lecterns, to be placed on either side of the altar to hold its liturgical books.[105]

As far as is known, the cost of both Gerini's frescoes and Mariotto's altarpiece was underwritten by the hospitals themselves. At other times it was patrons who paid, as when the painters' company of S. Luca commissioned a certain Andreuzzo *dipintore* for the main altarpiece in the chapel of the male ward of S. Maria Nuova,[106] described by Vasari as 'an altarpiece of St Luke, who was shown painting a picture of Our Lady; and in the predella he showed on one side the men of the confraternity and on the other the women, all kneeling.'[107] The picture of Luke painting the Madonna referred to both the main activity of the members of the painters' guild and to the saint's role as physician. The painters' company in fact held a number of meetings at this chapel, including their festivals of Luke and Mary Magdalene, when Mass was followed by the membership's procession through the hospital.[108] On the first Sunday of each month it also gathered there to celebrate 'masses and divine offices in honour of God and of S. Luca and of all the celestial court' and to accept new members. The example of the company of S. Luca shows how the ward chapel, while being principally designed to provide spiritual medicine to patients, served other constituencies, including the staff and corporate and individual patrons.[109]

Ordinarily Mass was celebrated daily by a priest in all wards at prime or vespers. Members of the household were required to be present, including the *spedalingo*, who 'should encourage the negligent to attend services, warning them and punishing them if they do not'.[110] Festivals were also celebrated there when patients and staff alike listened to sermons delivered from a small pulpit, as in the scene by the Giovanni di Miniato brothers showing a preacher talking to an attentive crowd of hospital *commesse* (Plate 5.17).

Given the central significance of medicine for the soul in the treatment of patients, the main role of the ward chapel was to act as the centre point for the administration of sacraments. The four main ways in which patients participated in devotional activities were listed on a board displayed in the ward: 'In the first section we write the names of those patients making confession; in the second we record those about to receive the Eucharist; in the third those commending their souls to God; and in the fourth those receiving extreme

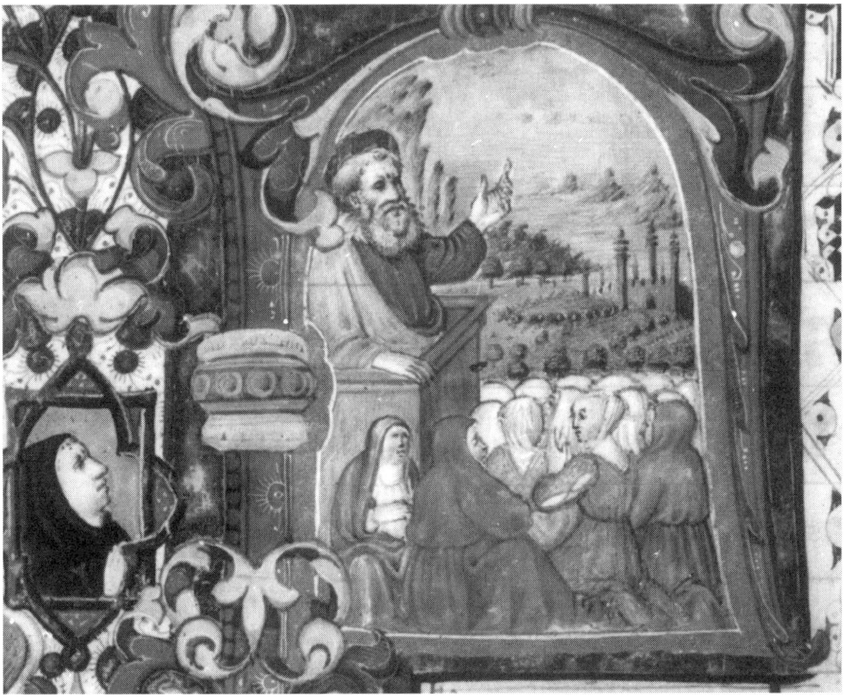

Plate 5.17 Gherardo and Monte di Giovanni di Miniato, *Friar Preaching to S. Maria Nuova's Commesse* (S. Egidio, Missal, 1477: Museo Nazionale del Bargello MS 68, f. 17r)

unction.'[111] S. Matteo's inventory recorded that the hospital owned two seats on which friars sat to hear the confession of patients. The friars, probably from either the nearby churches of S. Marco or SS. Annunziata, would have sat beside the patients' beds to hear their confessions, as in Bartolo di Domenico's representation of the fat Augustinian friar in the Pellegrinaio ward at S. Maria della Scala in Siena (Plate 5.10). Furthermore, given the international character of their clientele, S. Maria Nuova employed priests who spoke English, Spanish, French and German so that foreigners could make confessions in their native tongues.[112]

The second section of the board listed those to receive the Eucharist, which required the presence of a tabernacle next to the altar to house the Host. In the mid-Quattrocento S. Maria Nuova commissioned two superb new marble tabernacles from leading artists of the time. The first, for the men's ward, was undertaken by Luca della Robbia between 1441 and 1442 and in 1477 Andrea Verrocchio was commissioned to produce two small bronze images to fill the openings in the tabernacle. The first of these was a circular disc, now in the Bargello, with a three-dimensional dove placed inside the angel's wreath; and the second was a small bronze plaque covering the doorway into the tabernacle. The subject of the relief on the plaque was the 'Body and the Blood of Christ'. Christ is shown standing with His left arm wrapped around the crucifix, while His right is extended above a chalice into which His blood streams, a graphic reminder of His suffering and a reflection of the daily miracle that takes place at the high point of Mass.[113]

In 1450 Bernardo Rossellino was commissioned to produce a tabernacle for the women's ward and Lorenzo Ghiberti the small door or *sportello* to cover the space where the Host was stored (Plate 5.18).[114] Reading from the top, patients would have been able to see the full iconography of the Christian message: in the triangular pediment at the top was God the Father raising His right hand in benediction and holding a globe in His left. The central section of the tabernacle was framed by two Corinthian pilasters and two adoring angels. It was here that the patients' promise of salvation lay through Christ's sacrifice: the Holy Spirit symbolised by the sculpted dove and above all the Host housed inside the tabernacle. Angels are shown crowding out from doors on either side of the *sportello* guarded by Ghiberti's figure of God enthroned in majesty, directing the eye to the Host within.[115] The bold inscription, 'Oleum Infirmorum', was added after 1565, when the tabernacle was used to store the

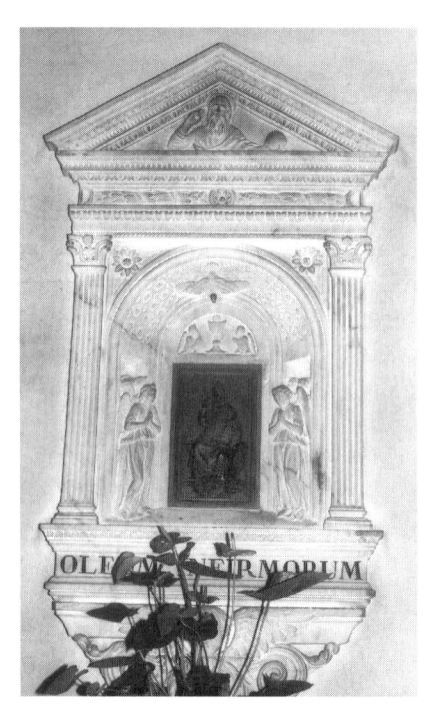

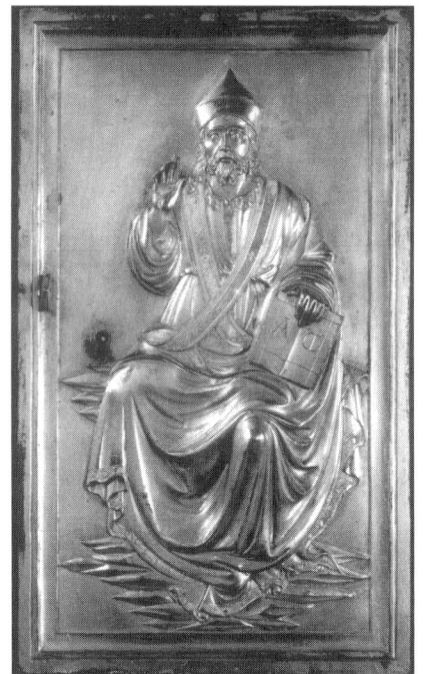

Plate 5.18 a. Bernardo Rossellino and Lorenzo Ghiberti, tabernacle from the women's ward, Hospital of S. Maria Nuova, 1450 (now in S. Egidio)
b. Lorenzo Ghiberti, *Sportello*, 1450 (detail)

blessed oil to anoint the sick and dying.[116] Finally, in the lowest register was the symbol of the hospital, the crutch, framed by a circular wreath.

The last section of the board set up in the ward listed those receiving extreme unction. The way in which the space of S. Maria Nuova's wards was used in this drama surrounding the death of a patient was described in S. Maria Nuova's early sixteenth-century 'Ordinances':[117]

> When a patient is close to death, we place before him an image of Christ on the cross, and a nurse watches over him, never leaving him and reading the Creed, the Lord's Passion and other holy texts. When he is dead, the head nurse comes with his assistants; they take the dead man from the bed, clothe him in linen, and place him on a bier in the middle of the hospital, where the chapel is, with a consecrated candle at his head and a lamp at his feet. At the appointed time a bell rings, and the priests come with a cross. Two lay brothers light two torches, and the others take the body and bear it into the church, where the funeral service is sung. After these rites they go to the cemetery; and the corpse is buried by a servant appointed for the task.

This passage demonstrates how the space of the ward was used in the liturgy of death for male and female patients. There was a series of actors who performed in the drama of a patient's last moments. The first was the priest, who would already have confessed the dying person. Then, while the nurse patiently read devotional texts aloud, the image of Christ was placed before him to represent the road to salvation and to underline the message of the value of physical suffering in the service of spiritual health.

Once the patient had died, his body was treated with the respect due to the dead: he was dressed in a clean white linen shift to represent his new state of purity now that he had passed to the next stage in his soul's journey. Then followed a period of public exposure in the middle of the ward in front of the chapel, as represented in an illustration in the *Liber regulae* of S. Spirito in Rome (Plate 5.19).

The dead patient thus laid out in front of the altar at the centre of the ward's devotional activity would have reminded the sick of the transitoriness of life. The body was then carried through the cloister, which linked the spiritual life of the ward to the hospital church, where the funeral service was held under the eyes of the patron saint of the hospital, the Virgin Mary, represented in the fresco-cycle of her Life and Van der Goes' *Adoration of the Shepherds*. Finally, the patient was buried in the cemetery of the Chiostro delle Ossa, a process also graphically represented in S. Spirito's *Liber regulae* (Plate 5.20).

After death, the ward chapel took on another important role, the commemoration of the souls of patients and patrons. In this way the ward played an

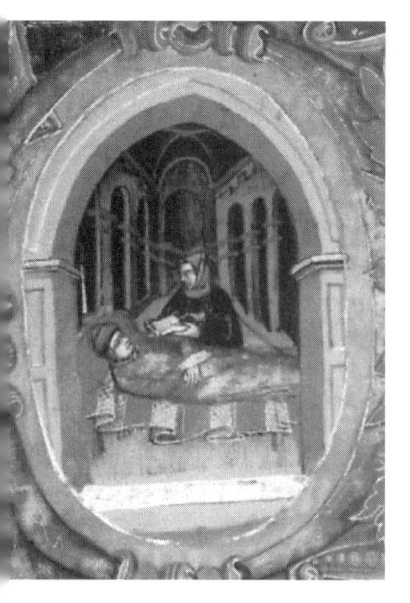

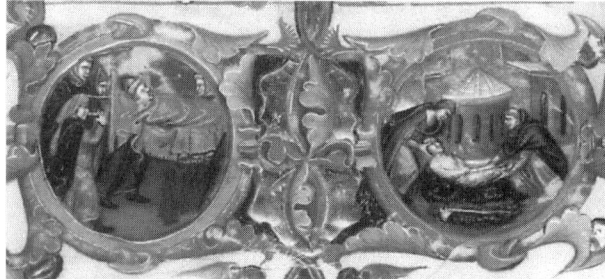

Plate 5.20 (*above*) Circle of the Master of the S. Giorgio Codex, *Death and Burial of a Patient*, Hospital of S. Spirito, Rome, *Liber regulae Sancti Spiritus*, c.1350 (ASR, Ospedale di S. Spirito 3193, f. 162v)

Plate 5.19 (*left*) Circle of the Master of the S. Giorgio Codex, *Corpse of a Patient in Front of Ward Chapel*, Hospital of S. Spirito, Rome, *Liber regulae Sancti Spiritus*, c.1350 (ASR, Ospedale di S. Spirito 3193, f. 162v)

important chantry function and the patients along with the priest participated in remembering the souls of the founders of the hospital to whom they owed their health. Indeed, S. Maria Nuova was unusual among Florentine hospitals since the founder, Folco di Ricovero Portinari, his son Manetto and grandson Accerito were all buried in the chapel of the male ward since this had been the first hospital church.[118] Folco's tomb, according to S. Maria Nuova's eighteenth-century historian, was 'next to the left-hand wall in a raised tomb under a stone arch in which the Portinari arms and letters are cut into the stone in front of the said tomb'.[119] It can be seen today in S. Egidio along with marble slabs commemorating other members of the family, having been transferred there in the late nineteenth century when the ward was destroyed (Plate 5.21). This tomb type, known as an *avello*, is a simple but imposing structure of *pietra serena* consisting of an arch surrounding a flat rectangular tomb; on the front of this example are carved three panels including the Portinari coat of arms.[120]

In the early 1450s Andrea del Castagno was commissioned to paint an important new *Annunciation* for the women's ward.[121] Ferdinando Del Migliore and Giuseppe Richa recorded that the altarpiece contained life-size portraits of two members of the Portinari family, the founder Folco di Ricovero and Castagno's contemporary Falganaccio, so it must have been of considerable dimensions and provided a constant reminder to the patients to pray for their benefactors.[122]

The presence of the altarpiece and tombs in the ward chapel underlines its important commemorative role for the souls of the Portinari family. But the

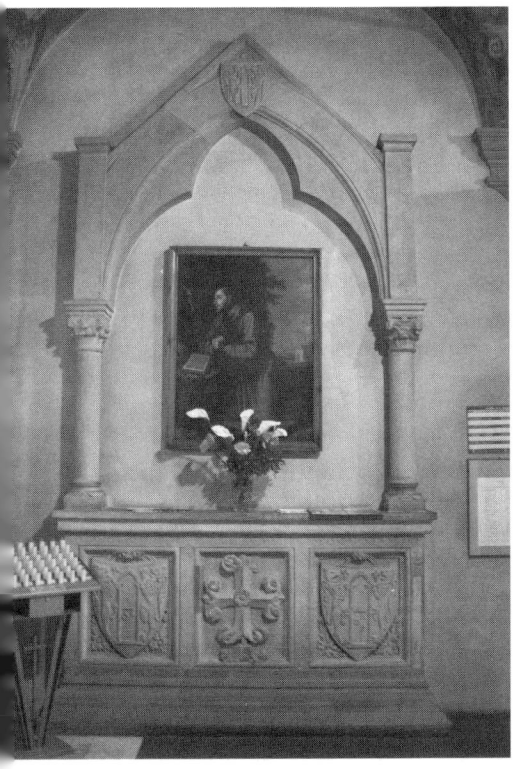

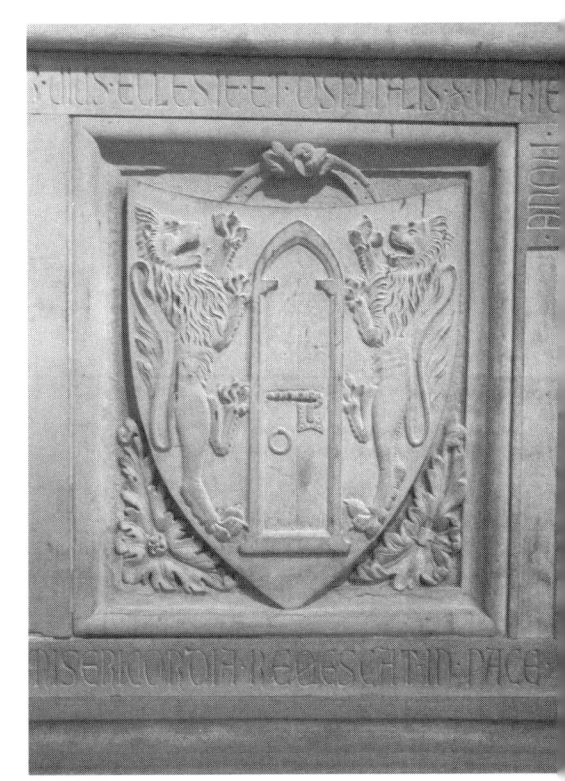

Plate 5.21 a. Tomb of Folco di Ricovero Portinari, 1289 (S. Egidio)
b. Detail of the Portinari coat of arms, 1289 (S. Egidio)

latter did not have exclusive rights over commemorative masses. For example, in 1464 one of the hospital's priests, Ser Apollonio di Francesco d'Assisi, left S. Maria Nuova a farm the proceeds of which were to pay for two of the hospital chaplains to say a series of masses for his soul in the chapel of the women's ward, including the Mass of the Dead every Monday and a special celebration of the festival of the Visitation of the Virgin, as well as a commemorative meal at which his family members were to be present.[123] Testators also bequeathed money to pay for the day-to-day devotional activities in a ward, as in the case of the widow Monna Margherita, daughter of Bartolo Bonini, who in 1415 left 50 gold florins to the hospital of S. Matteo to pay for a lamp that was to 'remain alight day and night in front of the figure of the Trinity in the women's hospital'.[124] Later in the century Ser Jacopo di Bonaiuto left the considerable sum of 900 gold ducats to S. Matteo, a part of which was paid to the 'Donne dello Spedale di Lemmo' for the celebration of twenty-four masses, twelve of which were to be on the feast of St Barbara. Indeed, such was Ser Jacopo's attachment to this saint that he bequeathed another 270 gold florins for the foundation of a chapel in the hospital dedicated to her.[125]

Just as corporate patrons were involved in devotional activities in hospital churches, so they could be part of the commemorative role of the hospital ward, as in the case of the painters' company of S. Luca, whose monthly service was held 'for the health of the souls of the deceased men and persons of the said company and of those of the hospital who had been buried there'.[126] In this way it fulfilled one of the most important functions of a confraternity, to remember the souls of past members, a role that it extended to include the spiritual health of the deceased patients and staff.[127] On 22 July, the feast-day of Mary Magdalene, it also held a *rinovale* or commemorative Mass in the chapel in front of the confraternity's altarpiece of St Luke. The twenty-four men present, who each paid 2s for the candles burned, had to 'remain devoutly in silence and pray to God for all faithful Christians who had died and especially for [the souls of] those of this company in Purgatory'.[128]

The example of the commemorative role of the company of S. Luca adds to the list of those who participated in the devotional activities of the chapel in addition to the group for whom the ward was principally intended, the sick patients. This underlines what has been suggested above, that wards – especially those for men – were spaces open to others in addition to those who lived and worked in the hospital. On special events the ward became a centre for public ceremonies, as in May 1369 when the chapel of S. Maria Nuova's male chapel was reconsecrated by the bishop of Florence following the completion of a rebuilding programme.[129] A substantial number of people would also have been present on each subsequent occasion when a new section of the ward was completed. The growing permeability of the male ward of S. Maria Nuova reflected the increasingly elaborate ceremonies that took place in these spaces, as has been seen from the foundation of the new chapel designed by Buontalenti on 25 March 1575 when, in addition to the *spedalingo*, Don Vito Buonaccolti, and his staff, representatives of the Tuscan grand duke, were present (see 5.2 above).

The extent to which the male ward became an almost public liturgical stage is reflected in the ceremony surrounding the funeral of Don Vito, who died with almost theatrical precision exactly one month later:[130]

> On 25 of April 1577 at about 15.00 hours the above-mentioned *spedalingo* of S. Maria Nuova passed to a better life and he was buried on Friday evening at about 22.00 hours....
>
> The body ... was placed [on Thursday evening] in the crossing of the male ward dressed in the robes of an abbot with mitre, pastorals and gloves; early in the morning, that was, Friday 26 April, he was visited by all the

monks, and then the priests of the house, having previously celebrated vespers, now celebrated matins and the lauds of the dead, and then he was carried through the exit opposite to the pharmacy until [the moment when] he was carried through Florence, that is along Via di S. Egidio, protector of this hospital, to the Canto alla Rondine, from the Stinche prison, from the Badia, from the Canto de' Bischeri, along the Opera di S. Maria del Fiore, from S. Michele Visdomini, through the Via di Cresci, and lastly to the church of the said hospital ... around which were about 200 lit candles ... and because he was a member of the Congregazione del Pellegrino the office of the dead was sung according to their order, together with the chaplain of S. Lorenzo and the priests of the said parish and [the priests] of our house ... and he was placed in the tomb of the *spedalinghi*, praying our Lord God that through His mercy he will be placed among the glory of the blessed. Amen.

Thus, just as in life during the foundation ceremony for the new wing of the male ward, so after death Don Vito remained at the centre of the drama. His body, having been displayed overnight in the centre of the male ward and visited by monks, priests and other members of the hospital family, then became the focus of public attention as it was processed through the streets of the city before being returned for the funeral service in S. Egidio and eventual burial. The importance placed on this whole event was reflected in the number of people who took part in the procession, with representatives from thirteen different churches, including all the major mendicant orders. There were also fifty-five male members of staff, including priests, doctors and lawyers. The whole affair was expensive, costing over 120 gold florins.[131]

By the late sixteenth century, then, the men's ward of S. Maria Nuova had become a dramatic centrepiece in public ceremonies involving leading members of Church and State. A comparison between these ceremonies of the 1570s and that of the rededication of S. Egidio in 1420 suggests that public attention had turned from the outside to the inside of the hospital. This development can be seen as a response to the requirements of the Counter-Reformation and the Tuscan grand duke for greater display of the pious and charitable works of both Church and State.

This series of ceremonies helped to promote the public image of S. Maria Nuova and above all its male ward as a paradigm of architectural design in the same way that the consecration of S. Egidio by Martin V had promoted the fame of the hospital church. Furthermore, while S. Maria Nuova had previously taken pride of place in the Florentine republic's public-health strategy, in the following century it came increasingly to form the centrepiece of the campaign to promote the image of grand-ducal beneficence.

These very public ceremonies should not be allowed to overshadow our perception of the everyday activities of the city's main medical hospitals. The ward of any major Florentine hospital can be seen as a stage on which was enacted a series of medical, social and religious services.

Conclusion

In this chapter I have discussed a large number of subjects that need further examination, particularly the architecture of Florentine hospitals and the identity and role of the devotional objects commissioned by or donated to these institutions. In this and the previous chapter I have emphasised those aesthetic aspects that contemporaries thought particularly remarkable about Tuscan hospitals: their scale, design and *bellezza*. The next chapter will concentrate on another aspect of their reputation, the care provided by the nursing staff, which in turn provides a wider context for the theme of Part III, their medical role. By examining these topics in this order I have sought to avoid the trap of adopting an overly anachronistic view. While the medical developments afoot in Florentine hospitals were remarkable in this period, their religious role was no less important. Hospitals' dedication to the sick poor was always justified in terms of Christian charity and all members of staff, including the *spedalingo*, the *conversi* and servants, were admonished to take diligent care of the sick 'for the health of their souls'. Religious imagery was also central to descriptions of the 'poor sick', who were envisaged as 'almost like Christ in their persons'. This was no pious throwaway line, but central to the very purpose of the hospital and the role of the staff. Each patient was to be looked after as though he or she were the Son of God. This reflected the image of Christ the Pilgrim, popularised in Florence through the religious confraternities dedicated to the cult.[132]

As has been seen, just as the function of a hospital reflected its dual religious and medical role, so its form did too. This was an unrivalled period in Florentine history for the building and decoration of hospitals and provided the opportunity for innovation at a time that saw many important architectural developments. Indeed the main elements of their design grew out of and adapted existing models. The loggias that fronted Florentine hospitals have been seen as novel, especially that of the Innocenti, but they also depended on a long tradition of secular and ecclesiastical architecture. Furthermore, the scale of some of the largest wards was remarkable, with the ground plan of the majority based on the monastic infirmary and with the advantage that it could be easily extended in modular form as a Greek cross through the development of a cruciform plan, enabling all patients to participate in the celebration of Mass in the ward chapel. On the other hand, the long rectangular form also enabled the administrators to fit in a considerable number of patients along the walls and in an emergency they could add separate rows of beds along the central aisle. The model was also suitable for the medical and nursing staff, who could thus more easily keep an eye on their charges.

The physical care of patients, which has formed one of the themes of this chapter through the examination of the material culture of health, is also an important theme of the next chapter, which looks in more detail at the benefits provided both for and by the nursing staff.

CHAPTER 6

SERVING THE POOR: THE NURSING COMMUNITY

> Our servants are completely dedicated to the care of the sick.... Let these few words suffice concerning their patience, dedication and hard work. Everyone knows how dirty, smelly and disagreeable the sick are; one must accept their importunities with patience.
>
> S. Maria Nuova, 'Ordinances', 1510–11, p. 183

Introduction

The dedication of the nursing staff was one of the main characteristics of the Renaissance hospital identified by contemporaries. The reality of looking after large numbers of sick people was not usually put in such stark terms as it was by the authors of S. Maria Nuova's 'Ordinances'. However, the latter shared the same aim as the majority of commentators who presented a more sanitised view of the role of the staff: to emphasise their dedication and piety. Laudatory comments about hospital nurses in Florence tended to concentrate on S. Maria Nuova, as in Matteo Villani's remark that it 'is always full of sick men and women, who are served and treated with much diligence and an abundance of good things to eat, and the sick are looked after by men and women of a saintly life'.[1] One hundred and fifty years later Luther in his *Table Talk* also underlined the commendable role of the 'attendants' and the 'noble women in veils' who were 'extremely diligent' when they served him at S. Maria Nuova.[2] Although one has to take all these comments with a pinch of salt – Villani because of his commitment to praising the role of the hospital during the Black Death and Luther because his observations reflected his experience as a priest staying in the Sapientia – it would be churlish to deny their very real enthusiasm and pride in the duties performed by the nursing staff.

Curiously, given this admiration, little attention has been paid to the nurses or serving staff of Florentine hospitals or even those of other major Italian cities.³ The aim of this chapter is to re-establish their central role in the care and treatment of the poor sick and at the same time to explain the appeal of this job dealing with 'dirty, smelly and disagreeable' patients.

6.1 Entering the New Life

I shall begin with the fairly typical case of Monna Ginevra, who was admitted to S. Matteo as a *commessa* in 1520:

> I record how Monna Ginevra the daughter of Sandro d'Antonio del Pescaia deceased, at present a servant of Monna Gostanza, widow of Bononcino Baroncini, has given to us a deposit of 17 gold florins and 1 lire ... she is to be looked after always in all her infirmities and employed here as a *commessa*, as though she was one of ours of the house. And when the said Monna Ginevra reaches the age of sixty years and she can no longer work (today she is about thirty-three years old), the said hospital should receive her in-house and give her board, lodging and clothing.⁴

Monna Ginevra shared a similar type of contract with other *commesse* or *commessi*, through which individuals committed themselves to an institution, provided either goods or services, or the two combined, and in return received varying degrees of material support for the rest of their lives. In this way the hospital gained property and voluntary personnel to serve the sick, while the individual gained material and spiritual security.

As mentioned in the Introduction, this type of arrangement was part of a venerable tradition within the monastic context, though these 'corrodians' or *conversi* as they were known were not residents and were not actively involved in the running of the monastery.⁵ It was with the appearance of substantial new hospitals in the growing cities of medieval Europe that an extended form of contract emerged to enable the individual to exercise a more overtly charitable and pious role in an institution where he or she lodged. They were known by a bewildering variety of names as diverse as oblates, corrodians, *converse*, *commessi*, *devoti* and *frati*,⁶ and their contracts had much in common, even if the details varied according to the needs of the individual and the hospital.

In Florence, for example, S. Maria Nuova had by 1374 a range of resident staff called 'conversi, oblati, familiari, servigiali perpetui'.⁷ Their status was similar to members of the Third Orders, many of whom themselves ran hospitals.⁸ S. Paolo was run by a group of Franciscan Tertiaries, but in its earlier history at least differed from the other medical hospitals in that members – including women – were free to live at home.⁹ This rather ambiguous status attracted the attention of both the secular and ecclesiastical authorities and eventually led to the emergence of a properly defined resident community. But the lack of clarity in earlier times often led to conflicts between patrons and staff over rights of appointment and control of the growing property portfolio.[10] A popular solution that was adopted by many hospitals in Florence was the appointment of guilds as patrons and governors of hospitals.[11]

Other groups like the friars of S. Gallo lived according to the Rule of St Augustine,[12] as did the Hospitaller Orders, such as the Knights of St John of Jerusalem, who ran the Florentine hospital of S. Giovanni tra le Arcore, or the Antonites of the Spedale di S. Antonio.[13] The friars or Frati of S. Maria della Scala in Siena, shown dressed in black and white in Domenico di Bartolo's fresco the *Care of the Sick* (Plate 5.6), were Tertiaries who as laymen had the option of living at home.[14]

The variation in terminology between different hospitals, compounded by the elasticity in the use of titles even within the same institution, makes it difficult to calculate the number of people within different categories.[15] Roles also changed over time, as Carole Rawcliffe has noted for England: 'by the 14th century a two-tier system had developed in some English hospitals: the routine task of caring for the sick was assigned to female servants/corrodians and professed sisters undertook less demanding work.'[16] Furthermore, not all hospitals depended entirely on voluntary labour to nurse the sick. At S. Paolo, for example, Frate Giovanni di Vanni was employed as an *infermiere* between 1338 and 1370, while the case of Lorenzo d'Antonio da Verona, who 'came to stay in the hospital to serve the sick for 2 lire a month' on 15 September 1442, shows that it was also possible for a non-Tertiary to be both paid and a resident.[17]

The staff of medieval and Renaissance hospitals were, then, characterised by the variety and flexibility of their titles and roles, with some resident, some employed, and many often sharing similar contractual arrangements.[18] It is here that one has to lose any twenty-first-century preconceptions derived from a modern, secular hospital. The surviving contracts between *commessi* and hospitals in medieval Italy suggest the distinctions between patient, nurse and resident were far from clear-cut, as reflected in the case of Bartholomeo di Bastiano di Michele, admitted as a servant to the hospital of S. Matteo on 19 August 1517:

> Because the said Bartholomeo is not very well we have agreed with him that he should look after the sick in as far as he knows and feels able, with this proviso that he does not have to stay on duty for the sick at night, because, as has been said, he is not very well ... we know that he has come here to live and die and to save his soul by being kind to the sick and well ... and he has

a great wish to get better completely so that he can work all day and be on duty for the sick also at night.[19]

Evidently Bartholomeo was not in good health and had come to S. Matteo both for physical and spiritual security. His acceptance, sweetened by his donation of 40 gold florins to 'the poor in our hospital', was celebrated through an admission ceremony that marked the transition of the individual from non-institutional life to one dedicated to serving the poor.

The investiture ceremony was simple and based on the induction of the *spedalingo* himself,[20] as reflected in two brief descriptions from S. Gallo and S. Maria Nuova. At S. Gallo applicants presented themselves at the altar of the hospital chapel where they were welcomed by the *spedalingo*. He 'wrapped the *commesso/a* in the altar cloth' and, taking the supplicant by the hands, he received in the name of God the oblation of the goods and person, following which the supplicant swore obedience to the commands of the superior and to serve devoutly the clientele of the hospital: abandoned children, the sick and pilgrims.[21]

According to a small fourteenth-century codex entitled 'The Way of Dressing the Girls Who Have Newly Arrived to Serve in Perpetuity the Sick Women of the Hospital Here of S. Maria Nuova',[22] the ceremony took place in the hospital church of S. Egidio in the presence of the *spedalingo* and other members of staff. It began with the 'girl novices' kneeling in front of the hospital director, who asked them what they desired, to which they replied with humility: 'We ask God's mercy and that of His most holy mother [the] Virgin Mary and [of] your honest and good company.' The priests responded by singing the psalm *Miserere mei Deus* followed by a series of orations and responses, and the novices then exchanged their normal clothes for their new habits. During this process hymns were sung and finally there came 'the blessing, which the director of the said hospital gives finally to the newly dressed girls'.[23]

The putting on of the new habit and its blessing symbolise the entry of the novices into the hospital community and their dedication to their new life.[24] One of the most striking features of contemporary views of hospital interiors from all over Europe in this period was the presence of the figures of the nursing staff in their recognisable habits, which distinguished them from other hospital staff.[25] Emphasis was placed on simplicity of material, design and colour. S. Maria Nuova's household were required to 'wear a simple habit of coarse and inexpensive grey cloth marked with the seal of the hospital, a crutch cut from red or green cloth; the rector should bear this symbol on the left side, the others on the right' (Plate 6.1).[26] The habit of *commessi* is clearly represented in Bicci di Lorenzo's fresco the *Confirmation of the Reconsecration*

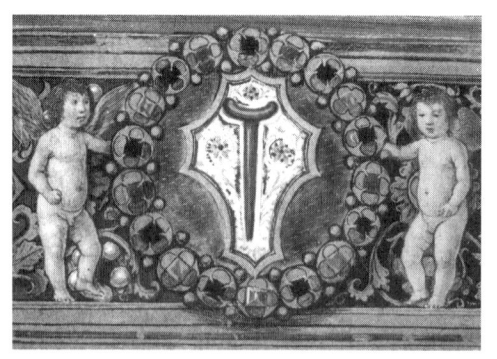

Plate 6.1 Gherardo and Monte di Giovanni di Miniato, *A Crutch,* symbol of the Hospital of S. Maria Nuova, *with Two Putti* (S. Egidio, Breviary, 1477: Museo Nazionale del Bargello MS A68, f. 116v)

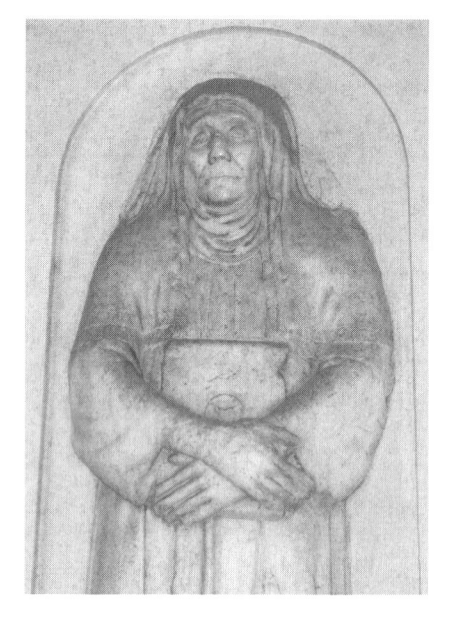

Plate 6.2 Tomb slab of Monna Tessa, Hospital of S. Maria Nuova

of S. Egidio (Plate I). They are shown watching the central moment of the ceremony outside the church when the *spedalingo* knelt before Pope Martin V and kissed the papal ring. The grey-clad hospital personnel are ranged behind the *spedalingo*, some standing and the others kneeling. They are identified clearly as *commessi* both by their grey habits and their wide range of hairstyles, distinct from the friars' tonsured heads.

Though the *converse* were not shown in Bicci di Lorenzo's fresco, other contemporary images confirm the simplicity of the female habit.[27] They are represented a number of times in the scenes of hospital life in S. Egidio's missal of the mid-1470s. In the scene showing Martin V inside S. Egidio four *commesse* stand behind the bishop by the door leading into the Chiostro delle Ossa and watch as the pope censes the altar (Plate 4.6). Each is dressed simply like a nun with a dark grey hood and habit falling from her shoulders to her feet and covering a simple white tunic. The one at the front looking out may represent the *prioressa*, the head of the women's section of the hospital. Her habit can be seen in more detail on Monna Tessa's white marble tomb slab, and shows her head covered with two layers (Plate 6.2). The outer covering – dark grey in the illumination – is part of a short cloak that covers her shoulders and is fringed and embroidered at the bottom. The white underlayer is bunched around her neck and forms part of the habit which falls to the ground. To symbolise her position as head of the women's section, Monna Tessa is shown holding a parchment-covered manuscript embossed or illuminated with S. Maria Nuova's emblem of the crutch, probably containing the rules of the women's hospital. Other *commesse* wore a similar but slightly less elaborate habit, suggesting that Monna Tessa's may have represented the clothes worn by the leading female members of the hospital, particularly for formal religious ceremonies.[28] The working clothes of the average *commessa* can be seen in a series of images in the same manuscript. One by Mariano del Buono shows St Elizabeth of Hungary visiting a patient in bed accompanied by two nurses, who wear a dark habit over a white tunic with a white apron and wimple (Plate 6.3).[29]

Though these habits had much in common, the founders of some hospitals prescribed designs of their own. Bonifazio Lupi's will specified that the garments should be characterised by simplicity: a grey cloak 'of little value' without any pleats, open in front and closed by two or three buttons of the same material, worn over a grey tunic down to the ground; the head was covered by a hood of the same colour. In this way, then, the cognoscenti could have distinguished the *commesse* of Messer Bonifazio from those of S. Maria Nuova, especially as the hospital's insignia was emblazoned on each of their habits. The *commesse* of S. Maria Nuova had the familiar symbol of a crutch on their left shoulder, while those of Messer Bonifazio had a white Agnus Dei and a cross against a background of a yellow cloud, reflecting the original dedication of the hospital to St John the Baptist.[30]

Applicants had to fulfil certain requirements in order to be accepted into this 'new life'. They had to guarantee they were prepared to dedicate themselves

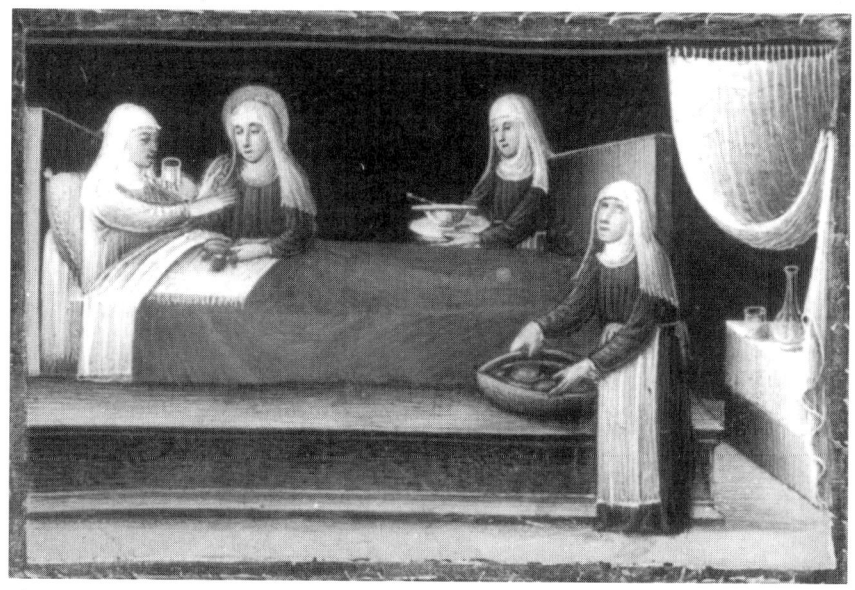

Plate 6.3 Mariano del Buono, *St Elizabeth Visits a Patient in Bed* (S. Egidio, Breviary, 1477: Museo Nazionale del Bargello MS A68, c. 148)

entirely to service in the hospital without outside distractions and that they would be morally upstanding members of the community. From the time of its first surviving statutes (1330) S. Maria Nuova declared that 'No married person, male or female, and no member of a religious order may be accepted into our household or wear its habit', though exemptions could be obtained.[31] The same rules applied to the staff of Messer Bonifazio,[32] but the S. Maria Nuova model was not universal. Both S. Matteo and the Innocenti entered into agreements with married couples. In 1445 when the foundling hospital opened its doors, two of the most illustrious members of the community, Lapo di Piero Pacini and his wife Dianora, both became *commessi*.[33] While S. Paolo began with staff members from the Franciscan Third Order who were allowed to be married and live at home, the expansion of the hospital led to the growth of resident staff, among whom was a group of female Tertiaries whose premises were gradually expanded over the fifteenth century.[34] However, the latter refused to accept control by their male colleagues and in 1516 became a community of nuns with their own rule, obtaining their independence from the *pinzocheri* and answering directly to the archbishop of Florence.[35]

6.2 'For the Health and Tranquillity of his Soul'

Once they had been accepted into the hospital community, the basic spiritual requirements for each *commesso* or *commessa* at S. Maria Nuova were much more rigorous than those likely to have been demanded of a lay man or woman living at home, but much less rigorous than for a monk or nun. Hospitals in Florence, as in late medieval England, allowed a degree of freedom from religious observance to those engaged in charitable work, but still imposed strict discipline.[36] Thus, members of the hospital community had to fulfil the basic yearly requirements of the Church, as laid down by the 1215 Lateran Council: annual confession and communion. Men could go to any priest in the city, but female staff had to confess in the hospital either in the church or ward chapel, reflecting concern that they might fall into bad company if they left the site.[37] However, they were not restricted in their choice of confessor. They could request a specific priest to come to the hospital to hear them, an important concession in this small and relatively enclosed world since it gave individuals freedom to confess to a priest whom they did not meet on a daily basis.

There were also daily obligations, for every member of the *famiglia* had to attend Mass once a day in one of the ward chapels,[38] while the priests were required to be present at 'all the hours of Divine Office, day and night, in the hospital church'.[39] There were also important occasions in the hospital's liturgical year when the *commessi* and *commesse* would have been found together

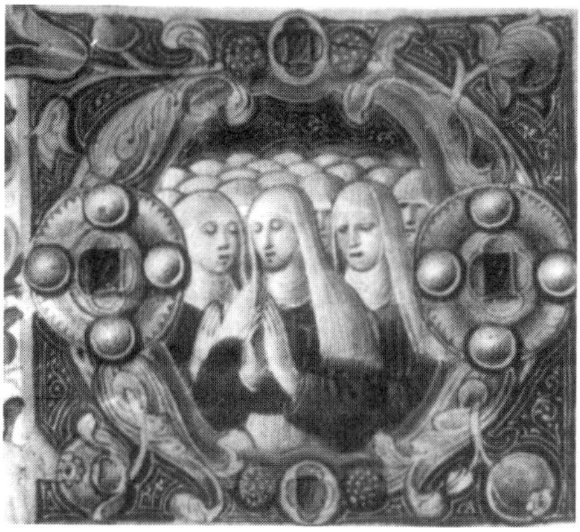

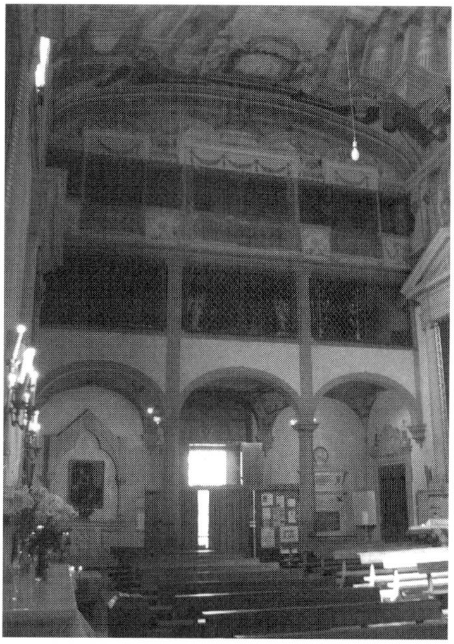

Plate 6.4a. Gherardo and Monte di Giovanni di Miniato, *Commesse Praying* (S. Egidio, Breviary, 1477: Museo Nazionale del Bargello MS A68, f. 137r)
b. Nuns' grille, S. Egidio

in S. Egidio, though, as in churches run by secular or regular clergy, they would have sat separately. Plate 6.4a gives some idea of the appearance of the massed congregation of *commesse* on one of these occasions. A sea of white-hooded women are shown with humble downcast eyes and hands joined in prayer, a scene that would not have been unrealistic if the majority of the one hundred *commesse* had been packed into S. Egidio for a special occasion.

It was only with the Counter-Reformation and its greater emphasis on rules for enclosed female communities that special galleries were built for the *converse* on the first floor of S. Egidio where they would have crowded behind a grille from which they could see but not be seen (Plate 6.4b). In this period, too, a tunnel was built under the piazza in order to link the women's ward with the church, thus obviating the risk of female members being waylaid by men and getting wet in the winter (see Plate 6.8).

Even before the Counter-Reformation's reform of lay female religious groups,[40] strict rules were enforced for the segregation of male and female staff in the living areas. This was especially necessary given that these were mixed- rather than single-sex institutions. It was seen as essential to keep the sexes apart in order to avoid potential disruption and to preserve the chastity of the women and to avoid the 'miasma of sin'.[41] Hence S. Maria Nuova's injunction concerning the women's quarters: 'They do not allow men to enter unless they are visiting patients, and one of them [the older male servants] accompanies male visitors at all times until they have left the hospital.'[42]

Exceptions were made for the clergy: 'The sacristan of our church and an elderly priest of blameless life and irreproachable habits hear the women's confessions and administer to them the sacraments both day and night.' Even these people of 'irreproachable habits' had to be accompanied by two older male servants, who remained in the vestibule when the priests were admitted into the women's ward.[43] The women's quarters and hospital were closed at dusk, at which time the key was taken by one of the lay brothers and thereafter:

> If a patient needs the sacraments, they call for a priest by ringing a bell. If a sick woman is brought to the hospital during the night for a legitimate reason, the hospital is opened to receive her. They ring the bell once if a patient wants the sacraments, twice if she wants communion, and three times if she needs extreme unction.[44]

The *spedalingo* also visited the female section once a month to admonish them 'to follow a good and honest life ... [and to] investigate whether there had been any scandal among them'. If any were found, a series of stepped punishments followed, equally applicable to the male staff. The aim was to humiliate the miscreant, as in the case of punishments meted out to the members of religious confraternities.

> On the first offence he must sit on the floor in the middle of the refectory and eat bread and water for three meals, while the others look on and eat at table. On the second intentional offence, he must eat seven times in this way. On the third offence, he must be deprived of every office, benefice, service, function and honour of the hospital, without respect to age or status, according to the judgement of the hospital director.[45]

If the miscreant proved truly recalcitrant, he or she was expelled from the community. It is some measure of the increase in power of the *spedalingo* over the fourteenth century that, while in 1330 he could not expel anybody without prior reference to two respected members of the community and the patronal family, by 1374 he could. If the expelled person wished to return and the *spedalingo* agreed, he still had to obtain the consent of 'four of the lay brothers, the servants and the governors and patrons of the hospital'.[46] Though the *spedalingo* was the embodiment of authority, he himself was subject to the statutes,[47] for example, if he wished to go outside the hospital he 'must be accompanied by one of the oldest and most senior members of the household, and he must not spend the night outside it without legitimate reason, and then only with a companion'.[48]

Discipline, then, characterised this community whose exercise of charity both helped the sick poor and its members' own spiritual development through the daily practice of one of the Seven Works of Mercy. As with confraternities, one of the great advantages of being part of the 'family' of a hospital community was the guarantee of a proper funeral and free burial in the hospital church or cemetery.[49] For example, when Monna Salvestra, widow of Antonio di Vanni Mannucci and daughter of Piero Pupi, died on 7 February 1461 as a *commessa* of S. Matteo:

> she was dressed as a widow and placed in a bier in the middle of the hospital ward, that is near the surgery towards the door. She was placed in an open bier surrounded with many benches, and the women of the house wearing their cloaks and also her female relatives sat on the benches and at the head and foot of the bier [where] two large candlesticks were placed with candles weighing 6 lb each. And she was buried in the tomb next to the door which opens onto Via del Chocomero.[50]

This description of a funeral service is more detailed than most, reflecting Monna Salvestra's high social standing, underlined by the use of her surname and the presence of her relatives and the whole community. As with funerals of patients, Monna Salvestra's took place in front of the chapel in the women's ward. Her body was dressed to reflect her status as a widow, though others such as Monna Antonia, the widow of Giovanni da San Miniato, who died in November 1508, requested to be dressed 'in grey with the belt as worn by a nun of the Third Order of S. Francesco'.[51] The practice of leaving the corpse visible to the participants meant they could each take their own personal farewell and at the same time be reminded that death was inevitable and of the need to live their lives with greater charity.

While at S. Matteo, then, members of the nursing staff could be buried in the hospital church, at S. Maria Nuova this privilege was reserved for members of the patronal family or *spedalingo*.[52] *Commesse* also chose to be buried elsewhere: Monna Filippa, the daughter of 'Lucchese deceased from Lucca', who had lived in S. Paolo, elected the church of the Camaldolese monks.[53]

The most splendid funeral ceremonies for members of staff were reserved for the hospital directors, as in the case of Messer Fenzio di Bertoldo on 24 August 1506:

> *The death of Messer Fenzio, who was our* spedalingo
> Today, 24 August 1506, in the evening two hours after twilight Messer Fenzio di Bertoldo Ciccioni from S. Miniato al Tedesco, who was our *spedalingo*, passed from this life. Friars from S. Marco were present and our male

servants and our women of the house, that is Monna Tomasa prioress of our hospital with her other companions and others from the house, who all recalled that he had had a good life and had provided a good example so that God should receive him in peace.

Then when he was dead we opened his chest and examined his purse; present were Fra Giovan Domenicho, the prior of the convent of S. Marco and Ser Simone di Filipo da Montelupo our chaplain, and Messer Tomaso Spini the scribe in our hospital...

Then the next day, that was Monday the 25th of the said month of August, the office was held in honour of the said Messer Fenzio, to which were invited all the priests of S. Maria del Fiore and the friars of S. Marcho, a good number of whom came, and also our lord consuls came with all the members of the [Cambio] guild to honour the above-mentioned [Messer Fenzio]. Given that a certain Girolamo de' Cicioni, a relative of the above-mentioned Messer Fenzio, was in Florence, our lord consuls invited him and together with him they came for this tribute and as everybody assembled and sat in the loggia, Marsino ... a Servite friar, entered the pulpit and preached. And, moreover, all the *spedalinghi* came with their chaplains and servants and each one brought four candlesticks and then they all processed on Piazza S. Marco and along Via Largha and returned by S. Nicholò. And all entered into S. Matteo and then buried him in the tomb of the *spedalinghi* with a large number of candles around the whole church and many candlesticks large and small and all the priests had a taper and his body was put into a coffin and then placed into the said tomb and everything which will be spent appears in this book at page 20 and we [had] the wax from [the company of] Angelo Rafaello.[54]

In common with other contemporary descriptions, the account presents the funeral as having three different stages,[55] beginning with Messer Fenzio's last moments. The deathbed scene was a public event, with friars from S. Marco present along with the male and female staff of the hospital, including the prioress of the women's ward, Monna Tomasa. The description reflects the influence of the handbooks for dying well, which advocated that the moribund person should provide an example to those present, who could then recall the good life of the deceased which would ensure he or she would be received by God in peace.[56]

The events of the following day were even more public, when the office of the dead was celebrated followed by the interment. In addition to the friars of S. Marco, the cathedral canons were present and the consuls and members of the Cambio guild, a relative of Messer Fenzio, the other *spedalinghi* of the city and their chaplains and servants. The size of this gathering in part explains

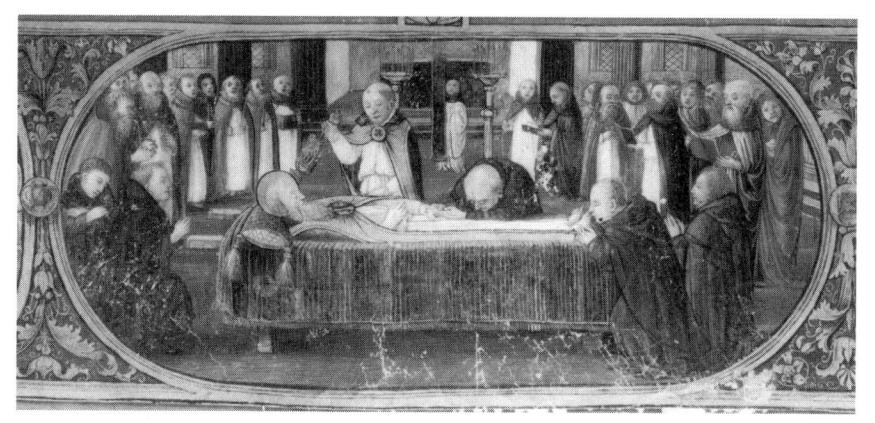

Plate 6.5 Gherardo and Monte di Giovanni di Miniato, *The Funeral of S. Egidio* (S. Egidio, Breviary, 1477: Museo Nazionale del Bargello MS A68, f. 28v)

why the first part of the ceremony took place outside the hospital, though the proceedings described also follow contemporary practices of display at funerals reflecting the importance of the person commemorated. At least some of these people took shelter from the heat in the loggia while they listened to the funeral oration by the Servite friar Fra Marsino; others would have stood in the street and piazza immediately outside the hospital. After the sermon this large group of clergy and laity then processed from the piazza down to the cathedral and back via the neighbouring convent of S. Niccolò. On returning, they 'all entered S. Matteo' for the interment. Like the loggia, the church would have been crowded and the scene may have shared some of the features of the funeral of S. Egidio illustrated in S. Maria Nuova's breviary of 1477 (Plate 6.5). In the foreground the corpse lies in his richly worked robes on a bier, while a priest censes his body and colleagues and relatives pray for his soul and others take leave of him and kiss his feet and hands. In the background more priests were singing the office of the dead and the scene, as at S. Matteo, is illuminated by candles.

Such an elaborate ceremony was reserved for patrons and hospital directors; the majority of men and women who worked in a hospital could not have expected anything so splendid. Messer Fenzio's ceremony was also much more public than an average hospital funeral, which would only rarely have been attended by members of the Cambio guild and the staff of other hospitals.

6.3 *'Patience, Dedication and Hard Work'*

A general guide to the role of the nursing staff at S. Maria Nuova is provided by the 1510–11 'Ordinances': 'They shelter and tend the sick poor who come

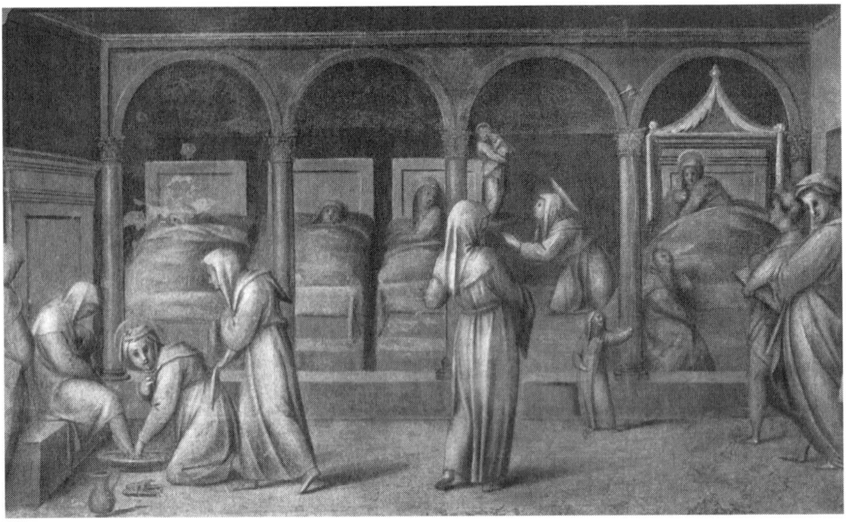

Plate 6.6 Jacopo Pontormo, *Scenes in a Ward*, 1513–14 (Galleria dell' Accademia, Florence)

to the hospital as they would Christ Himself. They must receive them with their own hands, care for them, console them and warm, feed and wash them with compassion. They must tend to their needs and treat them with all care and charity.'[57] These activities required the presence of a large staff with a series of complementary functions, especially in a hospital like S. Maria Nuova which treated about six thousand patients annually. An infirmarer was in charge of each ward (called variously *prioressa* or *la maggiore* in the case of the women's section),[58] who was assisted by four deputies or head nurses, each of whom had seven assistants under their command. The women's section had in total 'a hundred women [who] live in the women's part of the hospital, perpetual servants and assistants, humbly dressed like the men',[59] who included not just nurses but those involved in cooking, cleaning and doing laundry for the whole hospital. The whole operation at S. Maria Nuova was on a much larger scale than at any other hospital in Florence; a hundred years earlier the hospitals of Messer Bonifazio and S. Matteo had staffs of 26 and 36 respectively to look after about 62 and 108 patients.[60]

Detailed discussion of the treatments provided for the sick will be left to Part III, but it is worth outlining in general terms here the responsibilities of the nursing staff in the ward before we look at the way the hospital worked behind the scenes. The chapter devoted to 'how the sick are received' in the 'Ordinances' outlines the complementary roles of the infirmarer, the head nurse and the sub-infirmarer:

As soon as they [the sick] are admitted the infirmarer comes to them to determine the nature of their illnesses. He [or she] assigns the feverish and those with skin lesions or wounds to empty beds and sends one of the head nurses to wash the sick person's feet and another to the sub-infirmarer to get slippers, a leather robe, a shift, a cap and two pillows for the patient.[61]

The infirmarer had the greatest responsibility in identifying the ailments of the patients and therefore in deciding on their initial treatment before the arrival of the physician or surgeon. This role reflected his or her knowledge and experience, though the 'Ordinances' also state that the nurses included 'several skilled in surgery, for experience is the mistress of all things'.[62] Frustratingly, this statement about women's medical roles is not developed further here, though, as will be seen in the next chapters, some recipes in the hospital's *Ricettario* were attributed to women who worked in the ward. Studies of hospitals elsewhere in Europe have also documented other medical activities carried out by women. In France in this period institutions appointed 'sage-femmes' ('wise women') in addition to the male medical staff, though any medical function they performed would probably have stemmed from their role as midwives – this would have been less true of Italian hospitals, which tended to exclude pregnant women.[63] *Commesse* would also have worked in the garden, cultivating herbs used to treat patients, a practice recorded in smaller hospitals in late medieval England.[64]

The more menial role of the sub-infirmarers in fetching and carrying patients' clothes is expounded in another chapter of the 'Ordinances' which outlines their general duties:

Our nurses take turns in the hospital as described above, running to and fro among the sick as they call. To some they bring hot water, to others an infusion of barley water, to others a julep or sweet drink. They must hold some up, carry others, restrain others, and to others bring bedpans. Some of the sick cry out, others shiver, others are delirious. But the nurses bear it all and serve with piety and patience.[65]

The grim reality of dealing with large numbers of sick people in quite cramped conditions, particularly in the women's ward, is not usually made so obvious, but here the disagreeable aspects are stressed to emphasise the dedication and piety of the nurses. This is in stark contrast to that depicted by Pontormo in his fresco of c.1513–14 (Plate 6.6),[66] which shows the women's ward of the hospital of S. Matteo, now the Sala delle Toscane of the Galleria dell'Accademia. However, even a superficial comparison between the fresco and the actual space suggests that it was by no means intended as an accurate 'realistic' representation.[67] Rather, it is a curiously idealised picture, possibly commissioned by a patient as a votive panel in thanks for her recovery. The main goal appears to have been to trace a curative narrative about a female saint.[68] Even so, it did reflect accurately the *commesse*'s habits and patients' clothes. The fresco is divided into three scenes: the far right-hand side represents the saint's own illness; she is shown in her bed, which is separated from the others and surmounted by a canopy. The middle scene shows her activities as a healer as she prays to the Virgin and Child. Finally, she is seen washing the feet of a newly arrived patient in a scene that may reflect a not-uncommon ceremony in hospitals on Maundy Thursday when affluent women symbolically came to show their Christian charity by washing the feet of the poor.[69] More generally, charitable ladies visited hospitals to tend to the poor, a practice celebrated by an anonymous poet when recounting the virtues of Lucrezia Tornabuoni in fifteenth-century Florence.[70]

Pontormo's fresco underlines the close relationship between the physical and spiritual roles of the nursing staff in dealing with patients. In the following sections I shall turn to other aspects of the lives of the nurses outside the ward.

6.4 *Living and Working for the Community*

In earlier chapters I discussed how the plans of Florentine hospitals developed in response to the growth in their medical and spiritual functions. This led me to an exploration of the role of their more public spaces, the church and ward. However, as can be seen when examining the layout of their sites, there was also a series of areas where the staff lived and worked away from the public gaze.

Eating and Sleeping

The placement and functioning of hospital refectories reflect how the male and female communities lived together. The positioning of refectories at S. Maria Nuova, S. Matteo and S. Paolo had much in common. Those for men were placed along the rear edge of their cloister, close to the ward and the main administrative offices (Plates 1.9: 7, 3.12: Q, and 3.16: G). In contrast, women's refectories were set in 'deeper' space: S. Matteo's, for example, was behind the female cloister, which itself was separated from the front of the hospital by service rooms and the cemetery (Plate 3.12: V).[71] If the male eating space was closer to the public face, it was also more open to outsiders; male visitors were invited to join the staff at meal-times and even to eat at the table of the *spedalingo*.[72]

The statutes of S. Maria Nuova provide most information about regulations governing behaviour at staff meal-times and probably tell us a good deal about the practices of other Florentine hospitals. As in monasteries, meals were taken communally, with the sexes divided, and emphasis was placed on the religious character of the occasion.[73] All present were enjoined to 'eat charitably the same food prepared at the same time', except when somebody was unwell, in which case he or she was given a specially prescribed diet. The refectory was laid out to reflect the status of the staff. There were five tables, with the top table reserved for the *spedalingo* and the clergy, an equivalent hierarchy of seating reflected in the female refectory with the head infirmarer, or prioressa, taking the place of the rector. At the next two tables on the right and left were the perpetual servants and those responsible for the hospital's food and clothing; everybody else sat at the remaining tables. There were, furthermore, strict rules governing the occasion. Once the food arrived from the kitchens it was taken to a small room behind the refectory and handed through a window to each diner, who took his or her place at the sound of a bell. Then 'Grace is sung and everyone sits down while a cleric mounts to a lectern and reads'. At the end of the meal the *spedalingo* 'gives a signal and those present rise and go to the church and give thanks'. Despite the refectory occupying a substantial space, the size of the staff necessitated two sittings twice a day, at midday and in the evening.

The religious nature of the occasion was emphasised by the reading of a spiritual text and by the presence of important visual stimuli to devotion. For example, in the 1440s Andrea del Castagno was living at S. Maria Nuova and working on the cycle of the *Life of the Virgin* in S. Egidio. During this period he also painted a fresco of *The Last Supper* in the male refectory, though it did not survive the massive rebuilding programmes in the late nineteenth century.[74] The presence of devotional objects was also recorded in inventories.[75] The women's refectory at S. Matteo contained 'a wooden cross' decorated with 'a garland of silk flowers' and 'a book of the Holy Fathers bought by the women, covered with a towel' and 'a beautiful missal covered with a red cloth, [which] is new'.[76]

The way each refectory worked reflected the different levels of permeability of the spaces. The women's section was more separate and physically withdrawn, whereas the male remained more open to the outside. Less accessible to the public, even for men, were the rooms on the first floor. The staff dormitory was usually above the refectories, a logical location given that each required a considerable space to house a substantial number of people (Plate 6.7: F and I).[77] S. Maria Nuova's 1376 inventory identified twelve other bedrooms associated with named individuals, some of whom would have been the priests employed by the hospital. These rooms were simply furnished with a bed and covers and often contained a small devotional object, such as an image of the Virgin, which was illuminated by a candle.[78] As in the refectory, emphasis was

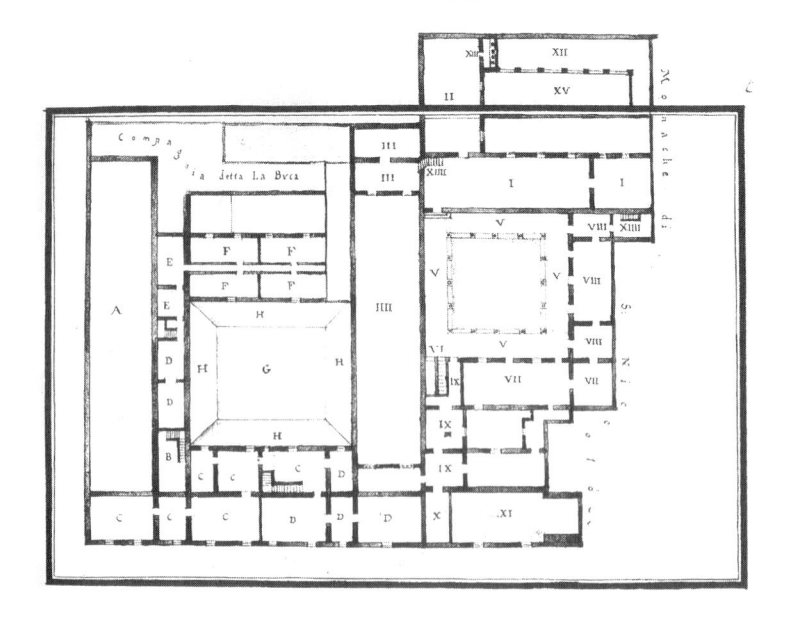

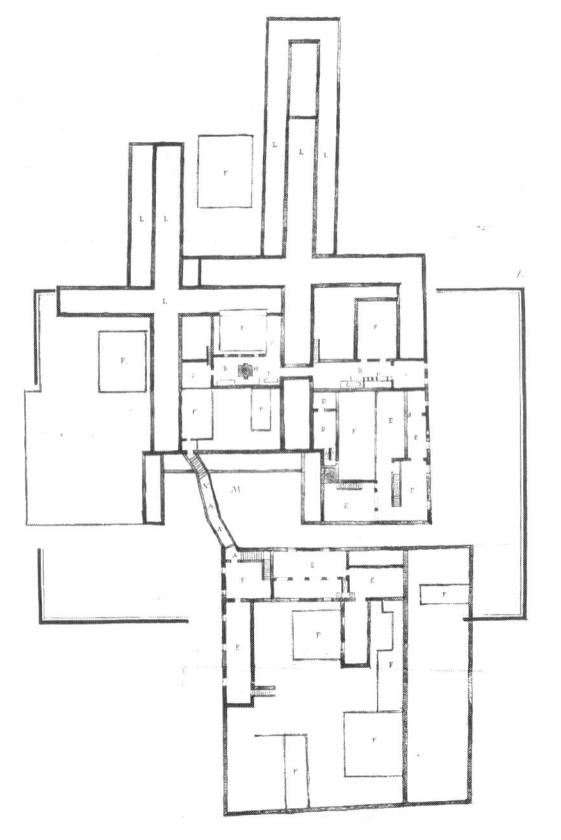

Plate 6.7 Plan of first floor of S. Matteo, c.1780 (ASF, Ospedale di S. Maria Nuova 24: Plan 6)

Plate 6.8 Plan of the cellars, Hospital of S. Maria Nuova, c.1780 (ASF, Ospedale di S. Maria Nuova 24: Plan 1)

placed on simplicity. The inventory of both the male and female dormitories at S. Matteo suggests that these rooms had the minimum to ensure the comfort of the staff. Each had twelve *lettiere*, beds made from wooden frames, with a mixture of straw and feather mattresses, sheets, feather pillows and a series of covers, some in bright red. In addition, each bed had a shelf, bench and a lockable chest for the occupant's possessions.[79] Then, underlining their religious vocation, the women's dormitory contained an 'altarpiece of Our Lady at the head of the said dormitory'.[80]

Consideration of refectories and dormitories provides a reminder of the need to widen any discussion of the role of the staff beyond simply looking after the sick if we want to understand how the hospital really functioned. The performance of these extra duties was, moreover, associated with a large number of areas within hospital complexes that tend to receive less attention because they were less public.

It would be an exaggeration to suggest that the duties of hospital staff were more than mundane. Though many tasks were shared by men and women, there was certainly some gender-based specialisation. Thus, those tasks associated with the preparation and cooking of food and cleaning and laundry were assigned to female staff,[81] which explains why by the early sixteenth century S. Maria Nuova had come to require some hundred female *commesse* and assistants.

Preparing the Food

At S. Maria Nuova a large number of women were involved in the preparation of food, changing duties every week according to a rota to provide variety.[82] There were two distinct, though related, operations involved in feeding the community: the first concerned the staff, the second the patients. Often women prepared and cooked the food in the kitchens, which were always in close proximity to their residential areas (S. Paolo: Plate 3.16: O; S. Maria Nuova: Figure 1.1: 13; S. Matteo: Plate 3.12: IIII).[83] Meanwhile another ten women would be busy preparing the dough for the bread, which was baked in a house next to the hospital and delivered by the baker's employees.[84]

Once cooked, the food was delivered to the two staff refectories. For the women at S. Maria Nuova this was simple because the refectory was contiguous with the kitchen, but food intended for male staff was collected by two men, the steward and under-steward, and carried across the piazza. Following the Counter-Reformation, when pressure was exerted on the *commesse* to lead a more sheltered life, the cooks carried the prepared food through the end of the female ward behind the chapel and placed it into a revolving hatch, in a manner akin to the way abandoned babies were left in the turning box at the Innocenti.[85]

The food for the sick was also prepared by the women in the kitchen and at S. Maria Nuova once again had to be taken across the piazza for the male patients, while at the majority of hospitals it would simply have been passed straight from kitchen to ward. The early sixteenth-century 'Ordinances' of S. Maria Nuova provide a detailed description of the various tasks involved in feeding the patients. The scale of these operations must have been considerable given that there were the occupants of 240 beds to feed – which meant at least double the number of patients.[86] The whole process was very time-consuming and was divided into two stages, the first of which was the distribution of the chicken soup for which S. Maria Nuova was so famous:[87]

> Before meals we offer to the seriously ill a soup made from puréed chicken. At the sound of a bell, a servant brings a pot full of this liquid from the women's quarters and places it on a bench in the middle of the hospital ... the infirmarer comes and ladles out the soup into cups with a serving spoon and the servants stand by. The nurses have a brass basin that holds a napkin and two cups. One contains water flavoured with lemon, damson or another such fruit. The nurse uses the other cup to carry soup to the beds. The sick person drinks it, washes his mouth with the water, wipes it with the napkin, and the nurse leaves him.

Once the seriously ill had been attended to in this way, the staff moved on to the second stage, which was to feed the rest of the patient population:[88]

> At dinnertime a servant takes the loaves of bread and cuts them into many pieces. Other attendants bring two napkins to each patient. The sick person spreads one napkin on a board rather like a table, which is kept at the head of his bed, and he uses the other to keep himself clean. The attendants bring water to each patient to wash his hands, cold in summer and hot in winter, and towels to dry them.
>
> Meanwhile the infirmarer orders a bell to be rung once, and then, after an interval, again. Between these two signals, trays are brought to a place called the Distributorium, where there are all sorts of wooden dishes and other utensils. There a table is spread ... they make up trays of food for each sick person, which are handed out by the servants and others in attendance. These carry the food to each patient as the infirmarer calls out his name and bed number... In winter they bring each patient glowing coals in an earthen vessel so that he may warm his hands to eat. While the sick are eating, three servants go round the ward serving excellent wine. Each person receives an appropriate amount of the particular wine – white, red, smooth, sweet or dry – suited to his illness and his appetite. All this is done in silence... At the

end of the meal ... the sub-infirmarer and the head nurse on duty smooth the beds and order dirty sheets to be changed. During this process those who are able to get out of bed; if they cannot we straighten their beds as well as we can.

Some of these stages in the feeding of patients are depicted in Plate 6.3, an illumination from S. Maria Nuova's breviary of 1477. A female patient, probably a sick *commessa*, is shown sitting up in bed, about to drink from a glass, possibly containing the hospital's 'excellent wine', which has just been handed to her by St Elizabeth. The other two nurses bring two dishes, the first a bowl with a ladle, possibly containing chicken soup, while the second carries a tray on which there are two plates of food.

Of course, these literary and pictorial depictions of peaceful well-ordered meals in a hospital ward were idealised. It is highly unlikely that silence was maintained throughout, especially given the presence of patients delirious with fever and of others who had recently undergone surgery without anaesthetic. Indeed, since the statutes freely admitted that 'everyone knows how dirty, smelly and disagreeable the sick are', it seems likely there would have been a correspondingly high level of noise at meal-times. That aside, however the passage quoted above does provide one with a good idea of the procedures associated with the feeding of the sick and of the number of people involved, repeated on a smaller scale at all the major hospitals for the sick in the city.

Another way of examining the implications for the resources necessary to feed such a large community is to attempt to reconstruct the appearance and contents of a hospital kitchen through evidence left in inventories, as in the case of S. Matteo's of 1454.[89] Although, to judge by the 1780 plan, the kitchen was not very spacious (14 × 13 *braccia* or 8.2 by 7.6 metres), it contained 245 different objects. The first thing one would have noticed on entering would have been 'a large dining table in the middle of the kitchen with three trestles'. Along the walls were a cupboard and a number of chests, some of which were evidently in a poor or 'sad' condition. One chest was for the bread and others were for lasagne, salt meat and eggs, evidently regarded as essential to a kitchen and hence stored in significant quantities. More fragile containers were also kept in chests, including oil jars and glass receptacles, such as tumblers and 'guascade', glass bottles with a narrow foot and neck, and eating bowls for staff and patients. There was also a wide range of metal objects, some of which were for serving food, and included copper bowls (seven), pans (eleven) and jugs (nine); and a large number of tin receptacles for patients and staff: twenty-seven small plates, twenty-seven eating bowls and forty-seven smaller bowls. Finally, there was a wide variety of iron implements for cooking, including tripods, spits and ladles.

S. Maria Nuova, whose culinary operation was considerably larger than S. Matteo's, also used contiguous spaces either on the same floor as the kitchen or in the basement. The 1376 inventory of the hospital lists, for example, the following objects kept in the 'room for oil':[90]

Item 555 earthenware jars for oil.
Item 1 large pottery vase for oil.
Item 2 flagons for oil.
Item 1 small cask for vinegar [*aceto salmarum trium*].
Item 2 chests full of flour.
Item 2 chests for keeping bread.
Item 1 chest for wheat and 1 for bran.
Item 1 lead basin.
Item 3 bread bins with 3 chests to keep flour in.
Item 6 tubs for flour.

The 1510–11 'Ordinances' also mention other rooms associated with the production of food and drink, such as the slaughterhouse where 'each month we slaughter 1,200 rams, 700 lambs, 500 young goats, 400 calves and 100 pigs'.[91] There was also a wine cellar, where the steward 'stores wines of every kind separately: sweet, smooth, dry, white and red – 5,000 or 6,000 casks a year'.[92]

In addition to storage areas on the ground floor, some hospitals also used passages and cellars in their basements, as can be seen in the 1780 plans of S. Maria Nuova, S. Matteo and the Innocenti. The plan of S. Maria Nuova's basement shows a vast network of areas, many of which still survive (Plate 6.8). Some were identified specifically as cellars and it was here that the so-called 'Leonardo's Vat' was to be found. The plan of the Innocenti suggests that the area under the foundling hospital was used even more extensive: 'Under this hospital in the cellars there are three refectories, a kitchen, rooms for the casks and wood, and the water that goes via the pump to the kitchens', and 'under the loggia there are the holes for grain.'[93]

Gardens and Growing Food

The garden was another important area associated with food production. As Benedetto Varchi mentions in his survey of Florentine hospitals, they 'all have very long walls surrounding their gardens',[94] an observation confirmed by Bonsignori's plan of the streets of Florence which shows large unbuilt areas behind each of the city's major hospitals (Plate 5.3). At S. Maria Nuova, despite the intrusion of the northern-most arm of the male ward and the recent construction of Buontalenti's chapel, there was a considerable area of land under cultivation in 1584. The garden surrounded the northern leg of the male ward on three sides and indeed stretched north to Via degli Alfani; on the west it shared a boundary wall with the garden of its neighbour, the convent of S. Maria degli Angeli, and to the east another boundary wall ran along the back of the gardens of a row of houses on Via della Pergola which belonged to S. Maria Nuova. By 1780, after two hundred years of construction, the garden had been diminished considerably in size and was reduced to a small area just south of Via degli Alfani (Plate 2.6: IV).

Bonsignori and the 1780 plan also show an area under cultivation to the south of the piazza, labelled in the late eighteenth century as the 'Nuns' Garden' (Plate 2.6: IX). It may have been here that the *commesse* kept poultry. By the early sixteenth century eight women were involved in tending to the chickens, hens, geese and ducks, which numbered about a thousand. Indeed, poultry constituted an important part of the hospital diet for both the sick and healthy. Already by the early 1370s the hospital was spending about 1,000 lire a year on fowl – 'flying meat with two feet' – 14 per cent of its total food bill.[95] The 'Ordinances' record that by the early sixteenth century the hospital had an annual consumption of twenty thousand chickens and eggs.[96] Other hospitals in Florence also had areas for keeping poultry, as can be seen from purchases made by the Innocenti in the 1450s, which included 'five pairs of pullets for producing chicks'.[97] The rest of the gardens would have been used to grow fruit and vegetables to help supply the kitchen's needs, and herbs for both culinary and medicinal purposes.

In addition to cultivation by servants and nursing staff, the grounds were also tended by part- or full-time gardeners; by 1510 S. Maria Nuova had three full-time gardeners on its payroll.[98] These humble employees, like the *contadini* who worked their farms, were very rarely represented in the iconography of hospitals' activities, which usually concentrated on the important medical and nursing personnel. One exception was the gardener or peasant who appeared in the very centre of the Della Robbia terracotta frieze on the façade of the Ceppo in Pistoia (Plate 3.10). He is shown humbly holding his hat in the background behind the hospital director. His clothes distinguish him from the other figures dressed in black and white; he wears a white shirt, brown jacket, blue doublet, white stockings and green hat.

The newer hospitals to the north of S. Maria Nuova also had their own gardens, the sizes of which depended on the land available at the time of foundation. In many cases the Bonsignori map of 1584 and the 1780 plans show a surprisingly close fit between the areas under cultivation in the late sixteenth and the late eighteenth centuries. For example, S. Matteo had a rectangular garden behind the hospital with a well at its eastern end (Plate 3.12: Y). This area was parallel to, and about the same length as but somewhat wider than the loggia; in the late eighteenth century it measured some 124 *braccia* long and

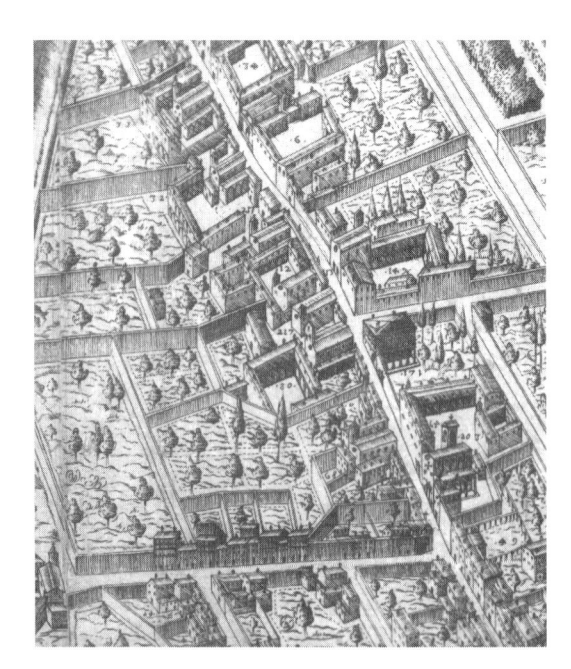

Plate 6.9 Stefano Bonsignori, *Plan of City of Florence*, 1584: detail of Via S. Gallo (Museo Firenze Com'era)

Plate 6.10 Upper terrace of women's hospital, S. Maria Nuova

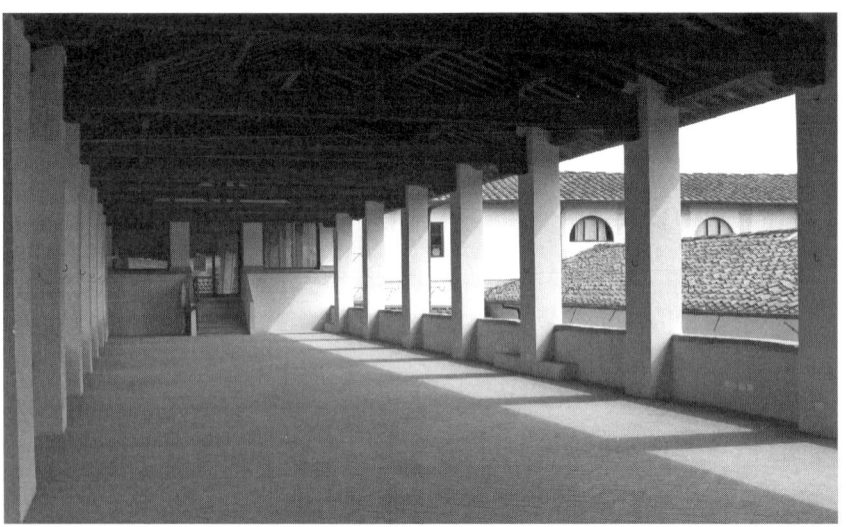

62 wide, or 73 by 36 metres. Immediately to the east, on the far side of Piazza SS. Annunziata, was the Innocenti, which had an even more substantial area under cultivation. This was made possible because, as the 'Catena' map of Florence shows, in 1471-80 there were no buildings between the hospital and Borgo Pinti other than those belonging to the institution itself (Plate 3.13). The 'Orto' of the Innocenti consisted not only of the large rectangular space

behind the hospital, but also of various other areas under cultivation possibly by the foundlings themselves (V: 'Orti per le Nocentine').[99]

While the space around S. Matteo was restricted by pre-existing buildings,[100] hospitals in Via S. Gallo benefited because the surrounding areas were less built-up. Bonsignori's map of the city in 1584 shows both Messer Bonifazio and the Incurabili hospital fronting onto Via S. Gallo and large gardens behind (Plate 6.9). Messer Bonifazio's market-garden, measuring some 49 *staiore* (Plate 3.15: M), also contained a house for the gardener and a press for making oil from olives supplied from the groves on its estates.

Laundries and Keeping Clean

Laundry was another activity essential to the running of hospitals. Not only were large numbers of sheets and pillowcases, blankets and bedcovers soiled regularly by the 5,500–6,000 patients admitted each year, but there was also the dirty bed linen belonging to members of staff.[101] S. Maria Nuova's 1510–11 'Ordinances', for example, recorded just how many women were involved on a day-to-day basis: 'Fifteen do the laundry, scalding, cleaning, washing, drying and folding it each day. The rector of the hospital appoints one woman to keep the linen clothes, another the woollens, and another the bed linens, the napkins and the cloths.'[102] The washing and care of clothes and bed linen and covers was undertaken by women in the washrooms normally situated next to the female ward (Plate 1.9: 14). At S. Matteo these were also close to the facilities in the cloister with its main water supply from the well and series of troughs for washing and soaking linen. Indeed, the 1454 inventory lists the following stored in the women's cloister: 150 pairs of sheets, 50 pillows and cushions, 200 napkins, 189 bedshirts for men and women, some new and some old, and 150 used aprons for women. Two further large *cassoni* or linen chests contained a substantial store of linen used for liturgical purposes in the church and wards (Plate 3.12).[103]

Each of these areas associated with washing or storing linen was also situated close to the stairs leading up to the first floor and to the terraces where the women dried the wet linen (S. Matteo: Plate 6.7: IV and XII; S. Maria Nuova: Plate 6.10). At S. Paolo too the washrooms were situated at the rear of the female cloister, above which were the 'stanze per la biancheria' (Plate 3.16: P). These spaces still survive in some of the hospitals in Florence and, as can be seen at S. Maria Nuova, the covered terraces were ideal for drying linen (Plate 6.10). They were of considerable size and, since they were situated on the highest point of the female complex, they were both out of the way of the main activities of the hospital and likely to have been the breeziest. The Innocenti also had large terraces, many of which survive and would have been used in cloth production, an activity in which some of the girl foundlings were involved.[104]

Keeping the hospital community fed and clothed, and cleaning the wards, dormitories and refectories were colossal tasks for a hospital on the scale of S. Maria Nuova, although the activities of the city's other major medical and foundling hospitals in these respects should not be underestimated either. It was vital therefore that these institutions should continue to attract a steady stream of staff by offering regular and secure employment. Though not highly paid, working in or for a hospital was an attractive proposition, especially for single women, whether widowed or never married, in an economy like that of Renaissance Florence which offered much short-term or seasonal work but few guarantees during individual or general crises. It was through offering security of employment that hospitals managed to maintain a supply of personnel, especially through flexible contracts that benefited both the individual and institution.

6.5 Identity: 'Men and Women of a Saintly Life'?

S. Matteo provides some of the most detailed and complete records of such contracts.[105] In the 1490s, for example, the hospital had arrangements with fifty-two individuals,[106] 63 per cent of whom were women. The predominance of females can be explained in general terms by their marital status and in a more specific sense by the nature of the contracts. It is striking that only seven of the thirty-three women represented here were married; fifteen were described as widowed and eleven more had evidently never been married, since they were simply identified in the records by their Christian name followed by that of their father.[107] It is instructive to compare these figures with those for the general female population over the age of twelve in fifteenth-century Florence. While 21 per cent of the *commesse* of S. Matteo were married, 46 per cent were widowed, and 33 per cent were unmarried, the proportions in the city as a whole were 53, 25 and 19 respectively. Thus, those women who were alone either because their husbands had predeceased them or because they had never been married was as high as 79 per cent at S. Matteo compared with 44 per cent in the population at large.[108]

These crude figures suggest that this type of contractual arrangement with a hospital was a form of survival strategy for single women who, as both economically and legally more defenceless than men, found it a convenient way to provide for their own support. But it would be a mistake to concentrate exclusively on women, for this type of contract was also attractive to single men (58 per cent of the nineteen males).[109]

S. Matteo's contracts reveal that this type of arrangement was socially selective since the majority of hospitals provided a financial sweetener when suitable applicants joined the community. Some indication of the social backgrounds of about half of these people is provided by the data on their occupations or those of relatives, though, the sample being so small, the conclusions drawn can be no more than impressionistic. Most of the men or the male relatives of *commesse* (twenty) were artisans or small mastercraftsmen. A handful were employed in, for example, the textile industry as weavers, dyers or tailors (six),[110] or in the construction industry (three) or as barbers, who may have worked for the hospital itself (two). Those who had been servants were mostly women, with a few exceptions, such as the messenger of the Florentine government. Some received recommendations from members of the patronal family (seven), though an employer did not have to be a Portinari to make arrangements with the hospital to look after their servants, as has been seen with the example cited at the beginning of the chapter, Monna Ginevra, the servant of Monna Gostanza Baroncini, who was admitted to S. Matteo in 1520.

There was also a scattering of *commesse* from better-known families such as the Frescobaldi and Sassetti. The hospital, not unnaturally, was proud of its connections with these families, especially as these individuals brought with them larger endowments. Even when records of *commesse* were less complete in the 1430s, the hospital scribe made a point of recording their names when they came from patrician families; those named included widows from the Salvi, Antinori and Spinelli families, two of whose husbands had been silk merchants, as well as the daughter of Manetto di Neri de' Medici.[111]

The contents of their rooms also reflect their financial status. Some had very few possessions, either because they were very poor or had left them with their family, while others appear to have brought everything with them. Monna Caterina, who died in the hospital of Messer Bonifazio on 2 September 1470, left forty-one different objects.[112] Most of these were made of cloth and were either the contents of her wardrobe – various cloaks, gowns and a 'widow's mantle like that of a nun which is in sad condition' – or her bed – two pillows, eight sheets, one in a 'sad' condition, and a warming pan. The inventory of a male *commesso* of S. Matteo who died some forty years later, a German called Giovanni di Ghuglielmo *tedescho*, was also dominated by clothes and included gowns, cloaks, eight doublets – only two of which were in good condition – together with caps and hats, shirts and socks, although what really attracted the scribe's attention were two silver buckles, one of which had 'a metal tip with fifteen riveted silver bars mounted on a faded satin ribbon'.[113] A similarly detailed description of the more valuable possessions found in the room of one of S. Maria Nuova's *commessi*, Giovanni Anguilla, is contained in the inventory made of his room after he died in March 1528. This includes: 'A pair of knives with ivory handles and with silver blades and a fork because the said Giovanni said in confession that he had lost it and a pair of small scissors; two cornelian stones mounted in gold with a value of three ducats and the other of one-and-a-half ducats.'[114]

This type of contract was evidently attractive to people from a wide range of backgrounds and was common to many hospitals in this period. In order to assess how representative the S. Matteo sample is, I shall compare S. Maria Nuova's 'Book of *commessi* and perpetual servants' for 1541–6 when 183 different people received regular payments.[115] These registers are broader in their scope for, while many people entered into the same type of contractual arrangements as at S. Matteo, others received payments under the terms of bequests administered by the hospital.

The more inclusive nature of these registers helps to explain some of the differences when compared with S. Matteo; a slightly higher percentage were men (43 per cent compared to 37 per cent), and though the proportion of women who were ever married was much closer to that of the city as a whole (S. Maria Nuova: 77 per cent; city: 78 per cent; S. Matteo: 67 per cent), there were more widows (34 per cent compared to 25 per cent). Even so, most women were married, as in the case of 'Monna Antonia, daughter of Luca di Malabura deceased and wife at present of Batista di Bernardino di Biagio, cloth weaver of the parish of S. Maria d'Ognissanti'. If Monna Antonia worked for S. Maria Nuova it would suggest that, as at S. Matteo, it was possible for employees to live at home, despite the proviso in the hospital's statutes that 'no married person, male or female … may be accepted into the household' or be allowed to own property.[116]

The register also supplies information about the social or occupational background of 69 per cent of the men or male relatives of *commesse*; of these 46 per cent were identified by occupation and another 23 per cent by surname. The latter figure is particularly significant because it suggests that over one in five came from relatively well-established families. Even if not all of these families were among the most affluent in the city, there were nonetheless representatives from some of the leading lineages, including the Albizzi, Antinori, Capponi, Davanzati, Ridolfi, Rucellai, Strozzi and, as one might expect, members of the patronal Portinari family.

Despite the presence of impressive family names, the majority of the people represented in this register were from humbler backgrounds, and lived in and worked for the hospital. In addition to the 46 per cent of people identified by occupation, the 31 per cent without an identifying label or patronymic after their Christian name would have been from a lower rather than a higher social or economic group. Table 6.1 shows that the vast majority were artisans, though with an important administrative and professional element (15 per cent). Six, for example, were medical men who probably either had been or still were associated with the hospital in that capacity, such as the 'plague doctor'

Francesco di Lando d'Antonio 'called Cechone' and the barber Antonio di Domenicho di Lorenzo, or suppliers, like the apothecary Bartolomeo di Biagio, who worked at the workshop at the 'Chapana', and whose wife Monna Nana was listed as a *commessa*. There was a wide variety of textile workers (13 per cent), reflecting the importance of the cloth industry in Florence. In comparison with the recipients of alms from charitable confraternities or even with the patients of the hospital itself, there were fewer day labourers. Rather, there was a larger proportion of small independent masters with their own workshops, such as dyers and weavers, as well as a couple of *lanaioli* or wool merchants.[117] This was also true of those in the third occupational category in Table 6.1, which included goldsmiths, blacksmiths, cobblers and slipper-makers. One part of the economy over-represented here, and among the poorest in the city, was servants and others employed in the service sector (14 per cent),[118] reflecting the arrangement at S. Matteo where employers paid a lump sum to a hospital to provide their old servants with a living in retirement; for example, S. Maria Nuova's *commessa* 'Sandra daughter of Pagholo di Menichuccio da Cerreto Guidi deceased … who had been the servant of Monna Maria di Portinari'.[119] Others had worked for S. Maria Nuova itself but were now retired, as in the case of Climenti di Michele Sassetti 'our gardener' or Antonio di Piero Machini, labourer on the property owned by the hospital at Badia a Ripoli.

Table 6.1 Hospital of S. Maria Nuova: occupations of *commessi* and male relatives of *commesse*, 1541–6

1. Administration and professional		
Notary (Ser)	3	
Master (Maestro)	1	
Customs' officer	1	
Merchant	1	
Medical:		
barber	3	
plague doctor	1	
bone doctor	1	
apothecary	1	
	12	(15%)
2. Textiles		
Silk dyer	1	
Cloth dyer	2	
Messenger of the wool guild	1	
Washer of clothes	1	
Weaver	2	
Untangler of wool (*Scioglitore di lana*)	1	
Wool beater	2	

Table 6.1 continued

Wool merchant (*lanaiolo*)	2	
Carder	1	
second-hand clothes' dealer	2	
haberdasher	1	
	16	(20%)
3. Leather, metal, wood and stone workers		
Knife-maker	1	
Cobbler (including slipper-maker)	7	
Smith	1	
Goldsmith	1	
Blacksmith	1	
Wood carver	1	
Saddle-maker	1	
Binder	1	
	14	(17%)
4. Food and drink		
Baker	2	
Miller	1	
Chicken-seller	1	
	4	(5%)
5. Service		
Servant (female)	7	
Piper	2	
Shop-keeper	1	
Carrier	1	
	11	(14%)
6. Labourers		
Gardener	3	
Labourer	2	
	5	(6%)
6. Religious		
Friar	4	
Nun	7	
Monk	2	
Tertiary (at the Orbatello)	1	
Priest	5	
	19	(23%)
Total of trades	81	(100%)

(81 represents 46 % of total *commessi* of 177)
Source: SMN 5792

The single largest category of *commessi* and *commesse* was the religious, including members of both regular and conventual orders as well as four secular priests. The priests and friars were probably either employed or had been employed by the hospital, as in the case of Ser Tommaso di Sano da

Montelupo 'at present chaplain', while two of the friars came from the nearby churches of SS. Annunziata and S. Marco. The nuns even included three from the enclosed Order of the Murate, who received payment in kind.

Such variety underlines the attractiveness of entering into agreement with a hospital for an individual or couple. This would have been particularly true when they came from outside Florence, for, as in the case of patients themselves, hospitals supported those without a network of family and friends to support them during times of crisis. Unfortunately, the provenance of relatively few individuals who worked for Florentine hospitals was recorded, which may indicate that most were actually from the city.[120] In the case of S. Maria Nuova's seventy-two *commessi* and *commesse* whose geographical origins have been identified, eighteen were from the city, fifty-one from the *contado* and three from northern Italy. The final pages of this chapter will examine in greater detail the form of these contracts, especially those of S. Matteo in the late fifteenth and early sixteenth centuries.

The main characteristic of this type of contract that made it so attractive was its flexibility; it was almost infinitely adaptable to individual circumstances. The basis of the arrangement was simple: an individual approached the hospital with a sum of money, a house or piece of land that would remain the property of the institution after their death. In return the hospital provided a carefully determined amount of food, drink and firewood to be delivered to the individual's lodging, which was either his or her own property or belonged to the hospital. Alternatively an individual was lodged in a room within the hospital itself.

The way this arrangement worked in practice can be seen in the contract drawn up in 1487 with Monna Lisa, the widow of Domenico *dipintore*.[121] Monna Lisa gave 60 gold florins to the hospital, in return for which S. Matteo delivered each year to her house 12 bushels of wheat; twelve barrels of wine; one barrel of olive oil; 40lb of salt meat; and half a pile of wood (*catasta*) with four loads (*some*) of twigs for kindling. Monna Lisa also made provision for her daughter after her death. She agreed to give to S. Matteo her house and 25 gold florins, in return for which her daughter was to receive board and lodging within the hospital itself. In this way Monna Lisa was provided with all the basic necessities and guaranteed that her daughter would have the same should Monna Lisa die before her child had married.

Given that the majority of people who entered into this arrangement with S. Matteo were female, I shall begin with their contracts to throw further light on their motivation in becoming *commesse*. In general terms I have suggested that this arrangement provided extra financial security for widows, who represented almost half of S. Matteo's *commesse*. Little detail is given in the records about their age or physical condition, but some at least may have been in poor health; in some cases their first contact with the hospital was as a patient. For example, on 12 April 1442 Monna Druda, 'widow of Benedetto known as Marzo' from the Valdichiana in the Casentino, 'who is at present sick in our hospital on the women's side', gave 50 gold florins to S. Matteo on the understanding that she would remain there as a resident *commessa*.[122] Evidently she was suffering from a chronic condition because three months later she was still described as 'sick in our said hospital'. On 3 July she donated further sums of 80 and 41 gold florins, a substantial total for a *contadina*. In return the hospital director recovered three sums from people to whom she had lent money 'some time ago': the weaver Antonio di Berto, Tommaso di Zanobi di Ser Benozzo and his mother, and the shoemaker Tommaso di Francesco from Peretola. The records provide no information about whether Monna Druda had habitually lent money or why these four people should have benefited from her generosity, except for the shoemaker who had received the 40 florins for 'his needs'.

Another widow with a chronic condition was also called Monna Lisa; she 'had lost the sight of her eyes'.[123] She asked to be admitted because she wanted to 'live in a pious place and [lead an] honest life in order to save her soul' and, indeed, 'live and finish her life in the said hospital of S. Matteo'. Her petition was accepted and she was lodged in the women's ward 'like the other *commesse*'. Clearly she was accepted because of her blindness and widowhood, although her admission was also seen in both social and monetary terms. She was the widow of Domenicho di Giovanni, but it was the connections of her deceased father, the fisherman Ghirighoro known as 'Zuchaio', to which she drew attention in the agreement. He had been the nephew of Tommaso del Fante Pini, mace-bearer for 'Our Magnificent Lords', the Signoria of the city. Evidently she felt that an association with the Florentine government, however tenuous, would persuade S. Matteo to grant her petition more readily. The hospital's acceptance of Monna Lisa was not based entirely on Christian charity; her family, showing genuine concern for her fate after she had been widowed, made provision for her by paying the hospital in kind. They diverted to her the grain, oil, wine and wood that the Vallombrosan monastery of S. Salvi delivered annually to the family under a similar arrangement.

The search for a secure enviroment in which to live was also a consideration for single men. In 1519 Bartholomeo di Bastiano di Michele from the parish of S. Pier Gattolini gave 40 gold florins to the 'poor of our hospital' and petitioned to enter the service of S. Matteo, where he wished 'to live and to die and to save his soul and to be loving to the sick and well'.[124] He was given reduced duties because he was unwell; he was therefore only obliged to 'look after the sick in as far as he knows and is capable' and was excused from working at night. However, he also said that 'he had a great desire to be cured completely in order to work both day and night'. These sentiments have a ring of truth because, as the *spedalingo* records, these words were taken down by him since 'the said Bartholomeo does not know how to write and wishes and is content that I write for him'.

The desire of these petitioners to become *commesse* or *commessi* and to 'finish their life' in the hospital may indicate that in addition to being sick they were elderly. On 24 December 1506 Corso di Stefano di Corso da Lucolena di Valdarno di Sopra, who was suffering from quartian fever, petitioned for admission as a *commesso* 'for the health and tranquillity of his soul'. The hospital's acceptance of his gift of only 10 gold florins suggests that it did not expect him to survive long; he declared he was 'about seventy-eight years old'.[125]

Another elderly man, an eighty-year-old member of a Florentine patrician family, Bartolommeo di Tommaso Sassetti, gave the hospital 50 gold florins in July 1492 on the understanding that he could come to stay in S. Matteo for the rest of his life.[126] His contract, based on that of 'chaplains and the other *commessi*', provided him with a room for his own use, with a sink, a *necessario* or latrine, a fireplace with a regular supply of wood, and a bed with covers and sheets which were cleaned regularly. In common with the rest of the staff, he had the right to eat in the refectory, though he could also eat in his room; if he chose to supply his own food it could be cooked in the hospital kitchen. His contract was also flexible and made provision for him to leave the hospital temporarily either at times of plague or to visit his children, though the hospital was careful to stipulate that it did not have to provide him with anything during his absence. Finally, if he fell ill 'he should be looked after with love because this was the main reason he committed himself to the hospital, though should he require another doctor [instead of the one supplied by the hospital] then he must pay him from his own funds'. The decision of the eighty-year-old Bartolommeo to live in the hospital and not with his children reflected his belief that he would receive better care there than at home when he fell ill.

Age was also a factor in the choice of admitting nursing staff, and the preference was for mature rather than younger applicants. As has been pointed out in relation to English hospitals in this period, older staff were thought useful in preventing discipline from being undermined through the 'miasma of sin'.[127] In May 1521, a patient, Monna Piera, described as 'rather sick' and about forty years old, offered S. Matteo 50 florins to allow her to live and work there. However, after some discussion her application was turned down partly on the grounds that 'she was still too young' and partly because it did not have need of her services at the moment, especially as she was already doing a good job for the hospital as a cashier at its property in Fibbiana. This was not an outright rejection; after seven years she was allowed to come and live in the hospital, by which time presumably she was regarded as sufficiently mature. Obviously both the hospital and Monna Piera felt that she had a right to reside in S. Matteo; it was referred to as her 'tornata', the same term used for a widow's right to return to her own family after the death of her husband.[128]

The question of the age at which the nursing staff were employed was obviously of some importance to Tuscan hospitals. For example, Odile Redon has shown that those admitted to S. Maria della Scala in Siena were all over forty, and many over sixty. This accords well with the ages of many of the people who ran the smaller hospitals in Florence and its *contado*; both *spedalinghi* and their wives tended to be in late rather than early middle age.[129] Elsewhere, too, there were strict rules governing the age of nurses. The Grey Sisters of the Third Order of St Francis, for example, at the Hôtel-Dieu of Wisbecq in France, had to be over thirty.[130] At St Giles's Hospital in Norwich they were to be over fifty, and at the Savoy in London, based on the example of S. Maria Nuova in Florence, they had to be over thirty-six and either virgins or respectable widows.[131]

There was, though, clearly a delicate balance to be struck between employing nurses who were sufficiently mature to work in a hospital and those who were too old to look after patients. The example of Monna Piera, the *cassiera* at Fibbiana, suggests that forty-seven was regarded as a suitable age to retire and become a *commessa*, coinciding roughly with the belief that old age began at forty-five.[132] Some idea of how long hospitals might expect their nurses to continue working is provided by the example of Monna Ginevra, the servant of Monna Gostanza di Baroncino Baroncini: 'And when the said Monna Ginevra reaches the age of sixty years and can no longer work – today she is about thirty-three – the said hospital should receive her in-house and give her board, lodging and clothing.'[133] This can be interpreted in two ways: that at sixty a woman was expected to have become incapable of work through old age or simply that she had a right to retire at that age.

S. Matteo also showed concern for those at the other end of the spectrum, the very young. This was an equally vulnerable period in the life-cycle, especially when a parent was very poor or had a physical disability. In July 1471 a blind man called Barone di Giuliano from Lamporecchio, in the Pistoiese countryside, had out of desperation brought his six-year-old son Michele to S. Matteo:

> The said Michele had been sick from a serious illness and because the father is poor and blind and travels around begging he did not know what to do with his son, whom he now gives to our hospital to stay perpetually in the said hospital to serve the sick and to do as he is ordered by me [the *spedalingo*] and by my successors and this is what is said to the boy so that he will obey the wishes of Barone his father.[134]

Although unusual, this case shows that the hospital was willing to relax its rules and to look after a child without any financial inducements. Despite the scantiness of the information, it is clear that Michele's father was at the end of his tether. He had presumably nursed the child – there is no mention of a mother – during a severe illness, possibly in the previous spring or winter, and realised that the life of a beggar was not suitable for a sickly child. Hence his recourse to a charitably minded hospital, especially since foundling homes such as the Innocenti concentrated on infants. There is furthermore no suggestion that the child was merely abandoned, given that it is recorded that he was bound to obey the wishes of his father. Why his father chose S. Matteo rather than a local Pistoiese hospital such as the Ceppo can only be surmised; Barone may have left Lamporecchio some time before to beg in Florence and that is perhaps where Michele had fallen sick.

Hospitals like S. Matteo also at times helped orphans, as in the case of Maria, daughter of Martino di Giovanni Antonio Martini deceased, who came to 'stay in the hospital' in April 1496. As part of the agreement her mother's brother, a second-hand clothes' dealer called Giovanni di Benedetto, who had presumably taken care of Maria on her father's death, gave the *spedalingo* the sum of 50 gold florins on the understanding that Maria would be 'well treated'. In the event the hospital did not have to look after her for long; she died only eight years later.[135]

Recommendations were also received through confraternities. In 1488 another young girl, Ginevra d'Andrea Portinari, was accepted by the hospital at the request of the procurators of the charitable confraternity of the Buonomini di S. Martino, who deposited a dowry of 19 gold florins for her eventual marriage.[136] That the girl had a surname reflects the fact that by this date the Buonomini concentrated on helping people of good family who had fallen on hard times.[137] It is intriguing that S. Matteo was approached rather than S. Maria Nuova, where the Portinari family owned the patronal rights. The choice probably reflects S. Matteo's more open society; the rules governing the life of a *commesso* or *commessa* at S. Maria Nuova were particularly strict and left the individual with much less flexibility in negotiating terms with the hospital. In the event Ginevra announced that 'she did not want a husband, but preferred to serve the poor of this hospital', so S. Matteo was allowed to keep the 19 gold florins, much as a convent would keep a dowry when a girl became a member of its community.

These examples point to the slippage between categories of people accepted by a hospital, especially between staff and patients. They show, moreover, that people often chose to have a formal association with a hospital because it guaranteed some financial security. The arrangement was also attractive to those who were not obviously sick or elderly and who entered into a contract with S. Matteo based on providing a sum of money in return for a steady income in kind and then served the hospital's patients.

There was therefore much variation in contracts, which could be tailored according to individual needs. For instance, instead of paying a lump sum to be a paying guest, as Bartolommeo di Tommaso Sassetti had done, another method was to pay an annual rent. In 1490 the widow Monna Antonia agreed to give 24 gold florins each year so that she could 'stay here in our hospital' and in return S. Matteo agreed to 'look after her in health and sickness and we must lodge her in the body of our ward and give her sufficient for her sustenance'.[138] It was also possible to have a separate room, as in the case of Gianotto, or Giovannetto, di Lionardo, 'who is at present [25 August 1433] trumpeter of the Magnificent Lords of Florence'.[139] In his petition to the consuls of the Cambio guild, the patrons of S. Matteo, he asked to be given a 'room furnished with a bed for his lifetime'. He also asked that his liberty of movement should not be infringed in any way and that he should not have to wear the habit. In return he would provide 60 gold florins; on his death all his goods were to come to the hospital in order to help it look after the Poor of Christ'. Finally, he requested that the agreement should be recorded in 'an authentic book of the house in honour of the changing wheel of fortune'. Priests negotiated similar contracts. In 1439, for example, Lapo di Jacopo Franceschi gave 300 gold florins invested in the Monte Comune and in return he obtained a room in S. Matteo, the right to eat with the clergy but with the minimum number of obligations: 'he is not obliged to do anything or officiate at Mass or say Mass more than he wishes.'[140]

S. Matteo also offered this type of arrangement to couples (twelve of fifty-nine contracts in the 1490s). Many decided to remain living in their own houses, receiving an annual payment of wheat, wine, oil and fixed quantities of wood in return for donating a sum of money or property. Others decided to live together in the hospital and either worked exclusively for the hospital or in conjunction with another job outside.[141] On 28 October 1516 the builder Maestro Santi di Pasquino Pieri and his wife, Monna Maddalena, came to live at S. Matteo.[142] They began by giving 25 gold florins, agreeing to dress and shoe themselves, and brought with them a bed with linen and wool covers and other goods. In return they received a room with a further promise that should they ever be in need the hospital would provide them with clothes. Although they agreed to work for the hospital, Santi was also free to follow his trade as a builder in the city. A final clause of the agreement established that the contract could be terminated either if they did not like their room or if the hospital was unhappy with their service, but 'we do not think that this will happen because we hope and desire that they will be faithful and loving of the people and of the place'.

Conclusion

This discussion of the *conversi* and *converse* at S. Matteo has underlined the adaptability of their contracts, which provided for lay men and women who sought to develop their charitable impulse in looking after the poor sick and to provide financial security for old age. The hospital benefited because it had the dual advantage of increasing its patrimony and attracting staff at the same time. Such contracts could be adapted more broadly to cover any relationship that involved the exchange of services and goods. *Commesse* entered for life rather than on the basis of short-term employment.

These kinds of contractual relationships were characteristic of hospitals throughout late medieval Europe, whether in Barcelona, Paris or York.[143] Despite variations in terminology between institutions and regions, from *donati*, *commessi* and *conversi* to corrodians and brothers and sisters, these arrangements had much in common. They all stemmed from the same model of *conversi* or *oblati* associated with monasteries, institutions that, like hospitals, were a characteristic feature of Western Europe. In some ways monasteries can be seen as loose models for hospitals, both in terms of organisation or architectural plan and in providing a secure social and spiritual environment for inmates. However, this analogy should not be pushed too far because the hospital environment was far more permeable to the outside world, and the *converso* or *conversa*, though often living according to a religious rule, retained lay status. Indeed, it is the very flexibility of these contracts that helps to account for their popularity. If these arrangements helped provide individuals with security in an uncertain world, they also guaranteed them spiritual solace through participation in a common charitable enterprise. It is this charitable mission, as will be seen in Part III, that explains why medical staff might accept little or no salary, as in the case of the doctor Maestro Bandino di Maestro Giovanni Banducci who was contracted to the Innocenti in 1445 solely 'for the love of God and the salvation of his own soul'.[144]

PART III

HEALING THE BODY

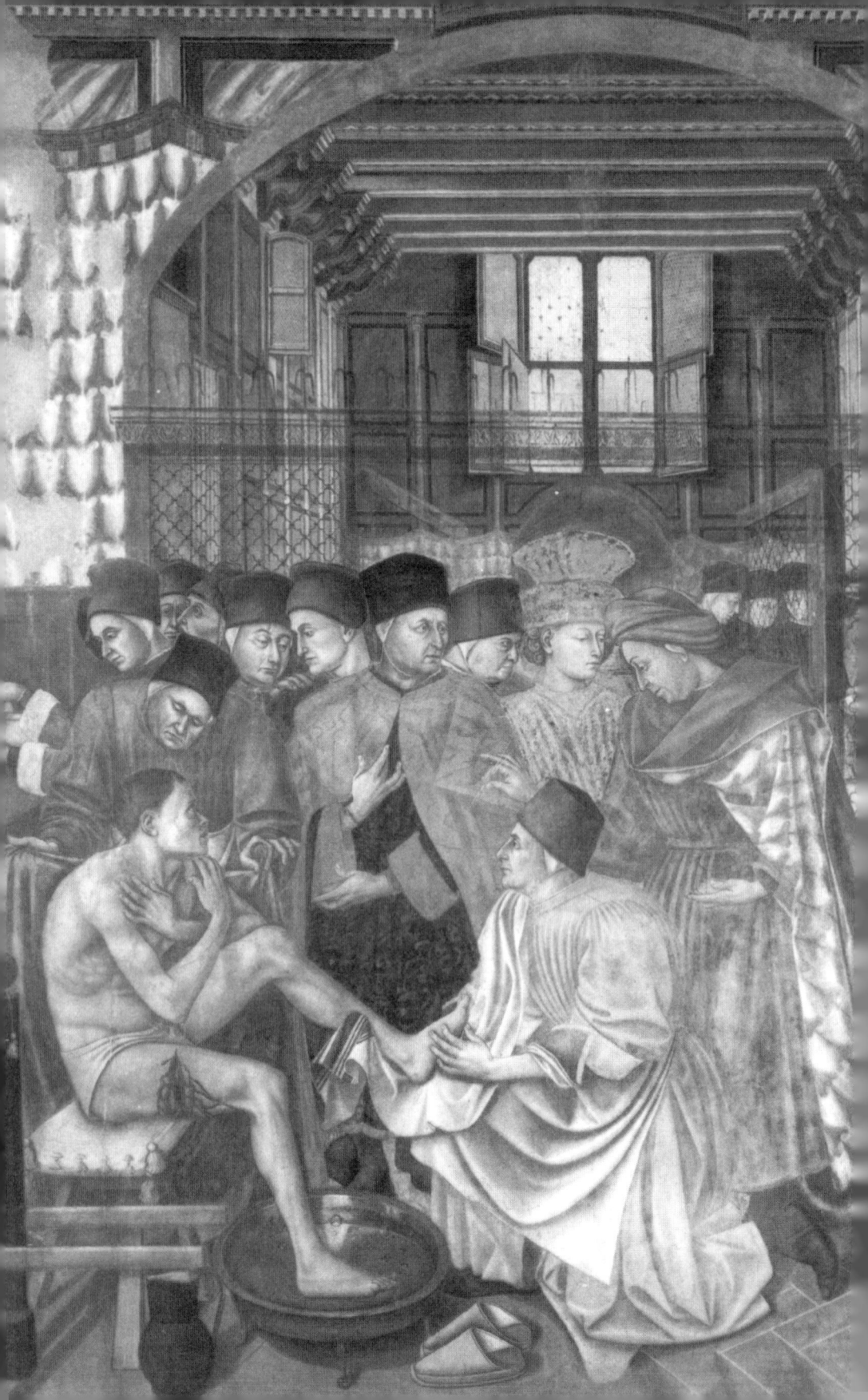

CHAPTER 7

Treating the Poor:
Doctors and their Duties

In the hospital two things can be seen and practised [upon], namely diseases and their symptoms.

G. Da Monte, *Consultationum*[1]

Introduction

The statement quoted above from the bedside discourses of Gianbattista Da Monte was taken down by his students at the hospital of S. Francesco in Padua. While this view was hardly new, what has made it particularly influential in the historiographical tradition is its association with the medical curriculum of the University of Padua where Da Monte was elected as the first professor of practical medicine in 1539.[2] His appointment has been portrayed by historians as having important implications for the way medicine was taught and practised in Padua, reflecting the new programme of the medical humanism preached by Niccolò Leoniceno, Da Monte's intellectual father.

It is important, though, to avoid falling into the trap of attributing too innovative a role to Da Monte as one of the 'great men' of medical history. His contemporaries suggested that his advocacy of bedside teaching was based on well-established practice, even if he did much to emphasise its central importance to the curriculum.[3] Gabriele de Zerbi in his *Advice to Medical Men* (*De cautelis medicorum*) of 1495 suggests that a good doctor was one who as a young man had obtained plenty of experience through having observed in hospitals a variety of patients, diseases and skilful practitioners at work.[4] The hospital itself played a central role in the development of Renaissance medicine, a role that is often ignored by historians of medicine, who concentrate instead on the development of learning within the university world, the evolution of the medical profession or the careers of individual physicians.

The skilfulness of medical practitioners was regarded by contemporaries as one of the hallmarks of the Renaissance hospital. It was within the hospital that many of the practices that have been identified as characteristic of Renaissance medicine were brought together. First, as Da Monte noted, the hospital was the best place in which to observe the widest range of symptoms and diseases under the same roof. In this way it provided a unique context in which doctors might develop their experience and implement practices learned from classical and Arabic medical authorities, whose writings were being retranslated and theories refined according to the techniques developed by the medical humanists. This process involved not just the intervention of the physician and surgeon, but also the apothecary's systematic development of the simple and compound medicines of classical writers, such as those found in the *Materia medica* of Dioscorides. The great advantage of the pharmacy of a major Renaissance hospital was that it could be developed on a far bigger scale than in any other institutional context, given the constant demands of patients for treatment and the wherewithal to pay for substantial supplies of medicines.

If Renaissance hospitals provided a crucial 'laboratory' in which doctors could develop their medical experience, they also played a useful role in the development of their careers. The evolution of the profession was another important feature of late medieval and Renaissance medicine, with the formation and growth of medical corporations. Indeed, there were close links between hospitals and medical guilds and colleges, and in Florence close associations with other major guilds appointed as patrons to safeguard the fortunes of these affluent institutions. Links were also fostered with medical faculties, not just through individuals who practised in hospitals and taught in the University or Studio of Florence and later Pisa, but also through the requirement of colleges of physicians that young doctors should pass a period practising in the major hospital of S. Maria Nuova to gain experience, as Da Monte mentioned, of a wide range of symptoms and diseases.

This chapter will examine in greater detail the relationship between hospitals and doctors both from the point of view of the hospital, which thereby obtained the services of leading practitioners, and the doctors themselves, whose employment by these major charitable institutions provided them with wide experience and access to political and professional patronage networks in the city. The reputation of the Renaissance hospital for medical excellence was based on this mutually beneficial relationship.

7.1 From Physicians to Eye Doctors to Women 'Skilled in Surgery'

Medical practitioners are assigned pride of place in the few surviving contemporary representations of Renaissance hospital wards. The panel of the *Care of the Sick* is given particular prominence by Giovanni di Andrea della Robbia's workshop in the frieze *The Seven Works of Mercy* for the façade of the Ospedale

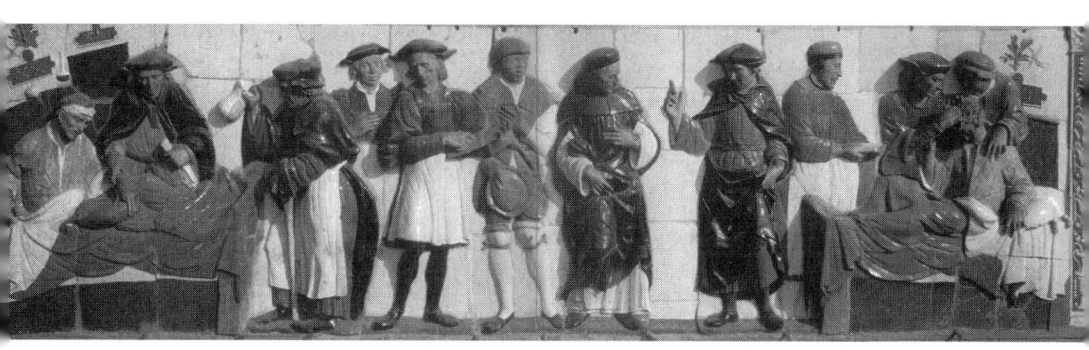

Plate 7.1 Giovanni di Andrea della Robbia's workshop, *Care of the Sick*, 1525–8, façade, Ospedale del Ceppo, Pistoia

del Ceppo in Pistoia (Plate 7.1). This scene shows the practice of both internal and external medicine by portraying the visits of two medical experts. The physician on the left concentrates seriously as he listens to the pulse of an elderly patient whose gaunt features and open mouth suggest he is in some pain, while his assistant inspects a Jordan flask containing the patient's urine, the other major form of diagnosis. On the other side of the panel a surgeon examines the head of a patient in bed. In contrast to the old man being examined by the physician, this man is young and was probably wounded in a street brawl. Head fractures were among the most common conditions treated (see below, Chapter 9).

Contemporary representations of wards tended to emphasise the role of physicians and surgeons, but in fact hospitals employed a wide range of medical practitioners, including male and female empirics who specialised in particular conditions. It is important, however, to avoid imposing a rigid distinction between these various types of practitioner. Both private patients and institutional clients viewed the medical marketplace as being made up of a range of practitioners with complementary skills. Even highly renowned ones such as Lanfranc of Milan recommended that certain complex operations should be left to specialists; characterising surgical intervention for bladder stones as a 'fearful operation', he suggested that it should be left to an experienced empiric.[5] Empirics achieved institutional recognition in their profession and were enrolled in the guild of the Arte dei Medici e Speziali in Florence.[6] Indeed, the breadth of contemporary definitions of 'doctor' can be measured in relation to the variety of people admissible to the guild according to its statutes of 1349: 'all those who practise physic [internal medicine] or surgery, setting bones, and treating mouths, whether they use writing or not, are understood to be doctors.'[7]

Recognition of the complementary roles of these various practitioners helps to explain why hospital records sometimes fail to distinguish between one type of doctor and another. Indeed, practitioners were sometimes identified in tax records not as a physician or surgeon but as a 'hospital doctor'.[8] The few surviving contracts do specify the types of activity expected from a particular practitioner, but frequently the only reference to his presence in a hospital in the Trecento is in the form of a payment to 'nostro medico' or to the 'medico di casa'. It can also be difficult to distinguish the role of a surgeon from that of a barber; both played a medical role and could qualify for matriculation in the Arte simply by their experience. Even though hospital records usually describe the duties of both as 'to cut the hair of the staff and patients' and 'to let blood', the surgeon performed more specialised operations and was usually more socially elevated than the barber.

Table 7.1 Medical practitioners at the main medical hospitals in Florence, 1320–1500

	14th c. N	14th c. %	15th c. N	15th c. %
Physicians	2	8	27	31
'Doctors'	4	16	19	22
Surgeons	9	38	23	27
Barbers	9	38	17	20
Total	24	100	86	100

Table 7.1 includes the vast majority of medical practitioners working in Florence's four major medical hospitals between 1320 and 1500[9] and shows that their numbers increased across that period. This reflects the growth in employment opportunities with the expansion of the two older institutions, S. Paolo and S. Maria Nuova, and the foundation of S. Matteo and Messer Bonifazio. The period also saw an increase in institutional demand for medical staff from foundling homes with the expansion of S. Gallo and S. Maria della Scala and the creation of the Innocenti.[10]

In addition to the growth in the overall number of hospital doctors, the Quattrocento saw an increase in those with more qualifications, reflecting the ongoing medicalisation of hospitals. Before the Black Death S. Maria Nuova principally employed specialised practitioners, including Ser Cione, 'a wound doctor', and two eye experts.[11] When S. Paolo began to employ medical staff in the 1340s it opted to have a surgeon.[12] Then after the Black Death both hospitals employed the same physician, Maestro Fruosino di Cino della Fioraia, a well-known individual in Florence, who was not only associated with the university but was also a member of the prestigious Parte Guelfa, one of the collegiate groups that advised the communal government.[13] The hospital of S. Gallo also passed from employing one surgeon in 1353 to having two physicians in 1387.[14]

This process continued in the Quattrocento, when physicians came to represent almost a third of all medical employees (31 per cent), though this proportion may actually have been higher and included some listed in the records as 'medico' or 'nostro medico' (Table 7.1). For example, Maestro Giorgio da Capri, characterised by Benedetto Dei in 1470 as 'Master Giorgio the Greek, eater of caviar',[15] was employed by Messer Bonifazio and S. Maria Nuova in 1475 and 1486 as 'medicho dello spedale', whereas his contract with S. Matteo in 1469 had specified that his duty was to 'treat as a physician our patients … with every diligence'.[16] Practitioners could also appear in hospital records with a dual function, like Maestro Domenico di Maestro Giovanni, who was employed by S. Maria Nuova as 'nostro medicho d'ossa e di fisica'. He derived his experience as a bone doctor from his father, Maestro Ciuccio da Orvieto, and his claim to physician status from a medical degree. His usefulness to the hospital is suggested by the fact that it employed him for almost thirty years.[17]

Flexibility in the use of terminology is equally evident with barbers and surgeons. For example, Maestro Giovanni Battista was described in a salary payment by the hospital of S. Matteo in 1468 as a 'medicho della barba'. This suggests a barber who had also trained as a surgeon, though to muddy the waters he was also employed by Messer Bonifazio 'as a surgeon and when needed as a physician'.[18] The Innocenti employed Maestro Piero di Puccio in 1449 as both a barber and a doctor; by 1482 he was described as 'a former doctor'. When he was replaced in the following year, it was with the surgeon Maestro Vezzano di Giovanni Benvenuti.[19]

Records of the employment of in-house medical staff as reflected in Table 7.1 fail to give a complete picture of all contacts between hospitals and practitioners. Before hospitals established their own pharmacies, as at S. Maria Nuova in the first half of the Trecento, doctors were also involved in ordering medicines from apothecary workshops with which they were associated.[20] Other doctors sold them copies of medical works, such as Maestro Agnolo *medico*, who in 1383 supplied 'a book called *Serapione*', a well-known pharmacological work from the fourth century, or Maestro Giovanni, who sold 'a book of medicine for the master of the house called *Silogisme*'.[21]

This association between apothecaries and doctors working for hospitals reflects the close formal and informal contacts between these two professions, especially as both were included in the same guild.[22] Doctors formed partnerships with apothecaries to import drugs or invest in their shops as well as seeing patients at their pharmacy or *spezieria*. There were also close family ties. Maestro Simone di Cinozzo di Giovanni Cini, for example, was a prominent physician who was the son of an apothecary. He worked for S. Matteo in the mid-fifteenth century and was involved intimately with the government of the guild, was a member of the College of Physicians and taught at the Florentine Studio.[23] These close associations can only have benefited hospitals, especially before they had established permanent pharmacies on their premises.

The growth in the relative number of physicians employed by hospitals is part of a wider phenomenon in the city of Florence. There was a dramatic increase in the proportion of physicians among medical practitioners recorded in the city's tax records between the mid-fourteenth and mid-fifteenth century from 35 to 64 per cent.[24] One explanation for this lies in the growing exclusivity of the Florentine medical profession as the guild tightened up its admission procedures in order to combat the perceived threat from immigrants and empirics, who were seen as flooding the marketplace during the decades following the Black Death.[25] If guild and tax records suggest progressive marginalisation of medical practitioners other than physicians,[26] one should nonetheless not underestimate the continued demand for surgeons and empirics. The number of surgeons and barbers employed by the four major medical hospitals remained substantial (forty-six) and this number may have been higher if, as seems likely, some of those categorised as 'doctors' were in fact surgeons.

7.2 'To Recognise the Variety of the Sick and to Know the Qualities of Urine': The Physician's Task

> Maestro Donato d'Aghostino Bartolini, doctor of physic and of surgery, came to an agreement on this day, 9 April 1445, with Girolamo d'Antonio, our *spedalingo*, to come to our hospital as a doctor to treat any need that arises in any person who falls ill, whether a member of the staff or in the wards [*spedali*], equally on the side of the men as on the side of the women.[27]

The duties of a hospital physician like Maestro Donato d'Agostino Bartolini were laid out in general terms in his contract of employment, though usually little detail was provided about his precise duties other than to say that he 'practises medicine here in the hospital'.[28] This was also true of contracts with other institutions such as foundling hospitals or monasteries.[29] S. Matteo stipulated that Maestro Donato should treat both men and women who fell ill, whether patients or staff, and was to be available as and when he was required.

Hospital statutes occasionally provide more details about the duties of physicians. The rule of the hospital of Altopascio, granted by Pope Gregory IX in 1239, is one of the earliest surviving hospital statutes in Tuscany. It contains a surprising amount of information about medical treatment, probably because Altopascio was run by the Order of the Hospitallers of St John. The hospital had four 'expert doctors', who were required to recognise the 'variety of the sick' and to know 'the qualities of urine'. In other words, they were expected to possess a sound theoretical grounding in the principles of physic, to make an initial diagnosis through visual evidence and to undertake an inspection of a patient's urine to determine the quality of his or her malady. This was seen as an ongoing process; doctors had to examine the patients 'attentively and often', particularly through uroscopy.[30]

S. Maria Nuova's 'Ordinances' were unusually informative about the role of their medical staff in the early sixteenth century.[31] Unlike other Florentine hospitals, which normally had only one physician, S. Maria Nuova employed nine, including six senior doctors and three house doctors. The 'Ordinances' declared grandly that the former were always 'the best in the city' and their role was discussed in reverential terms. They came to the hospital each morning at a set time and were greeted with a flurry of activity. When the head nurse on duty espied one of the consultants he rang a bell, which was a sign to the apothecary's assistant, who 'runs to meet the doctor, bringing a white linen garment with which he covers his clothes'. The senior doctor then began his daily ward round accompanied by the infirmarer and one of the house doctors. As they went 'from bed to bed', the junior doctor and apothecary explained to him 'the nature of each patient's illness and its symptoms, his state of mind, and what has been done for him up to that point'. The senior doctor 'then carefully prescribes treatment, which the pharmacist's assistant writes down in a book'. The senior doctors were the experts who passed definitive judgement on these cases as part of their busy practice. The provision of a white linen garment, as today, both symbolised their prestige and more prosaically protected their normal clothes from becoming besmirched. On their departure 'water is poured for them so that they may wash their hands'. The clothing and the cleansing rituals can be seen as having important symbolic and practical functions, reflecting first their entry and then exit from the healing space and emphasising their importance compared with the subservient roles of those who attended them on their rounds.

The prestige of physicians was also emphasised in contemporary views of hospital interiors. Instead of the white coats apparently worn in reality, physicians are shown in robes that represent their professional standing and distinguish them from the serving staff, as in Domenico di Bartolo's frescoes at S. Maria della Scala. The physician can be seen on the left-hand side of the *Care of the Sick* dressed in a red cloak and hat. He is represented holding a urine flask, as prescribed in the Altopascio statutes, explaining to the man on his right his diagnosis of the very sick man on the litter at their feet (Plate 7.2).

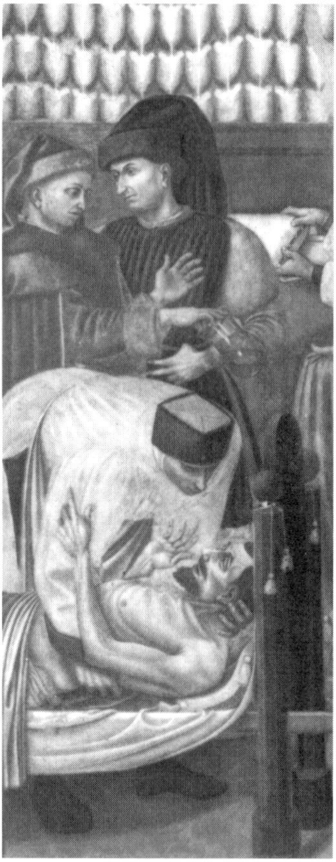

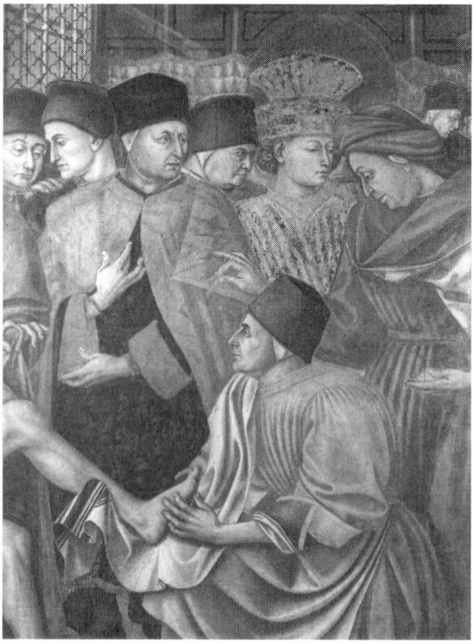

Plate 7.2 Domenico di Bartolo, 'The Physician', detail of *Care of the Sick*, 1440–4, Pellegrinaio ward, Hospital of S. Maria della Scala, Siena

Plate 7.3 Domenico di Bartolo, 'Surgeon with Pincers', detail of *Care of the Sick*, 1440–4, Pellegrinaio ward, Hospital of S. Maria della Scala, Siena

Senior physicians, whether in these images or as described in hospital statutes, were represented as visiting dignitaries who dispensed advice. In S. Maria Nuova's 'Ordinances' they were contrasted with the three younger doctors (*adstantes*) who lived in so that they were 'always in the hospital looking after the sick' to make sure that the treatments prescribed by their senior colleagues were being implemented. Moreover, their constant presence meant they were able to 'attend immediately to people who are brought in wounded or otherwise ill'; with the infirmarer they were required to 'direct the treatment of the sick, dividing up the beds and patients'.[32]

Junior doctors therefore relied on their senior colleagues' knowledge of the more theoretical side of physic and the apothecary's expertise in the preparation of medicines. As the 1510–11 'Ordinances' of S. Maria Nuova underline, working in the hospital also gave junior doctors experience in a wider range of diseases than was likely to be encountered in private practice: 'They are young men and, in the course of seeing a wide variety of illnesses and using many different remedies, they become increasingly skilled and expert, since, as they say, experience is the teacher of all things.'[33] They received no salary, but were paid in kind: 'board and a large and pleasant room worthy of their position.'[34] Indeed, by the mid-sixteenth century the College of Physicians sometimes prescribed a period of clinical practice at S. Maria Nuova before granting a licence to practise physic, as in the case of 'Maestro Lorenzo di Michele Poggini, physician in Florence'. He had obtained a doctorate at Pisa about four years previously, but was told he 'must for six months apply himself to treat patients at S. Maria Nuova and he cannot treat anybody outside the hospital, but must frequent other practising doctors to see their prescriptions and treatments'.[35]

The majority of senior physicians were paid, though the amount they received was small compared with the rates they could expect from private patients. In the early fifteenth century S. Maria Nuova paid an average of 2 gold florins a month to physicians such as Maestro Ambruogio di Giovanni and Maestro Antonio di Gianotto da Castelfranco.[36] Neither of these men was rich; indeed, Maestro Antonio described himself in his tax return of 1427 as 'dying of hunger'.[37] However, salary was not linked to prestige; in the same period Messer Bonifazio paid even less, 6 gold florins a year, to Maestro Cristofano di Giorgio Bradaglini, who played an unusually prominent part in the political life of both the doctors' guild and the commune.[38] To put these sums in perspective it should be remembered that a skilled mason or smith would have earned a maximum of 50 gold florins a year and a better-paid foreman about 72 gold florins.[39] In each case the sums paid by these hospitals would have represented only a small proportion of a doctor's salary, bearing in mind that a well-paid physician would have been expected to earn much more than a construction worker. Though 60 gold florins per visit for a particularly affluent private patient was exceptional, the annual income of Maestro Iacopo di Coluccino da Lucca in 1385 amounted to 185 gold florins, of which his salary as hospital doctor would have constituted only a fraction.[40]

A number of other factors have to be taken into account to understand the level of salaries paid by hospitals to their senior physicians. The first is that being a hospital physician represented only one source of income in a busy practice and senior doctors only came for short visits. A physician's clientele would have included a wide range of private patients and institutions, from the commune to monasteries and convents as well as hospitals. Indeed, contracts with institutions were highly sought after since they partly guaranteed a practitioner's annual income, which was subject to the vagaries and instability of the marketplace.[41] For example, Maestro Cristofano di Giorgio Brandolini is recorded as working for both Messer Bonifazio and S. Gallo in 1405 and Messer Bonifazio and S. Paolo in 1425.[42] An even better-known hospital doctor was Antonio di Ser Pagholo Benivieni, who between 1475 and the end of the century practised first at Messer Bonifazio, and then at S. Matteo and S. Maria Nuova.[43] Others worked for S. Maria Nuova and the foundling hospital of the Innocenti, which employed medical staff to care for their abandoned babies and children, who were clearly at risk given the high incidence of mortality among the very young.[44] Yet other doctors had more connections with religious houses, working for hospitals occasionally rather than regularly. An example of the range of institutional contracts of a Florentine practitioner can be seen in the case of the *ricordanza* or diary of Maestro Baccio di Lodovico Alberighi in the years 1516–30. He was employed as a surgeon by S. Maria Nuova in 1528 'to take blood and [do] other tasks on the women's side' and at the same time by S. Gallo. He also worked for no fewer than six male and female religious houses, including SS. Annunziata, S. Maria degli Angioli, S. Miniato, S. Benedetto outside Porta a Pinti and S. Orsola.[45]

Fees to hospital doctors often included payment in kind. Those who were resident, such as Maestro Bernardo di Maestro Nichol da Migliazi at Messer Bonifazio, might be provided with 'a bedroom furnished with everything that was necessary and living expenses for his mouth with the others of the house and [eating] at the table of the prior'.[46] The privilege of dining at the prior's table reflects the status of the physician within a hospital. Other types of non-financial benefits included those provided by the Innocenti from the 1450s, a capon on All Saints' Day and a kid (*chavretto*) at Easter, and twelve bushels of barley each year.[47] The Innocenti was exceptional in not making any monetary payments to its physicians. The first two it employed, 'the venerable and famous doctors of medicine Maestro Mariotto di Niccolo and Maestro di Francesco di Domenico', were 'hired and confirmed as doctors of the said hospital, for the love of God and the salvation of their souls, without any salary'.[48]

Working for a hospital was thus also an expression of Christian charity. When in 1477 the bishop of Pistoia wrote to Lorenzo de' Medici to recommend his candidate to become the new physician of the Ceppo he underlined the purity of his motives for the post, 'for the *onore* and for the *utilità*' of the hospital.[49] Furthermore, as the intervention of Lorenzo suggests, hospital appointments played a part in the wider patronage networks and helped practitioners to establish contacts and gain influence in the city and guild. But the religious context helps one to understand why doctors would have worked for hospitals at such reduced rates; the position gave them prestige in both professional and spiritual terms, for through charitably treating the bodies of the sick poor they were able to help heal their own souls. In a broader sense, the role of the doctor was seen as complementary to the role of Christus Medicus, the ultimate healer of body and soul.

7.3 To Shave, Let Blood, Cut and Medicate: Surgeons and their Surgeries

Contemporary images of hospital interiors also show surgeons at work in the ward. In the Della Robbia terracotta frieze at the Ceppo in Pistoia, one is shown dressed in a grey tunic and hat undertaking the examination of a patient's head wound (Plate 7.1). The surgeon's garb here appears simple compared with the more impressive cloak of the physician, underlining their

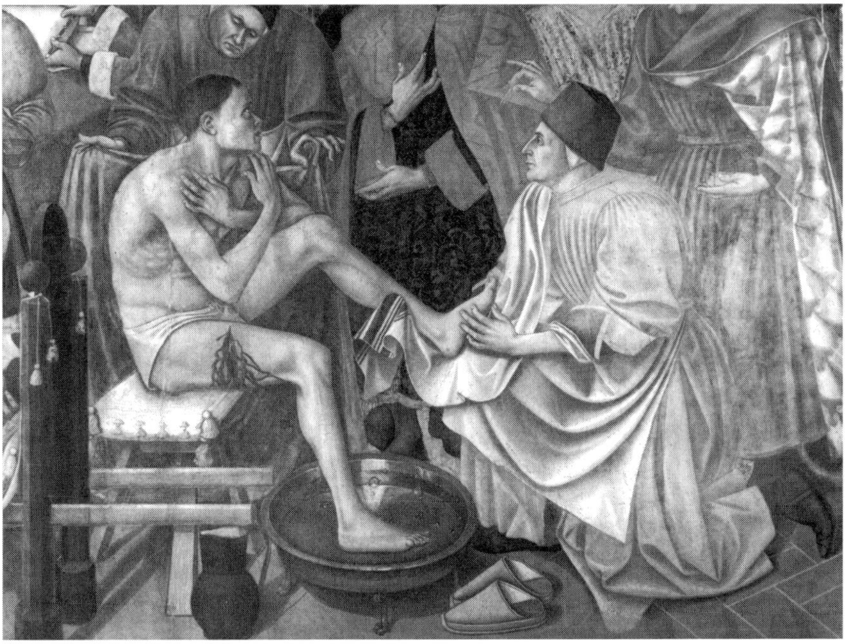

Plate 7.4 Domenico di Bartolo, 'Wounded Male Patient', detail of *Care of the Sick*, 1440–4, Pellegrinaio ward, Hospital of S. Maria della Scala, Siena

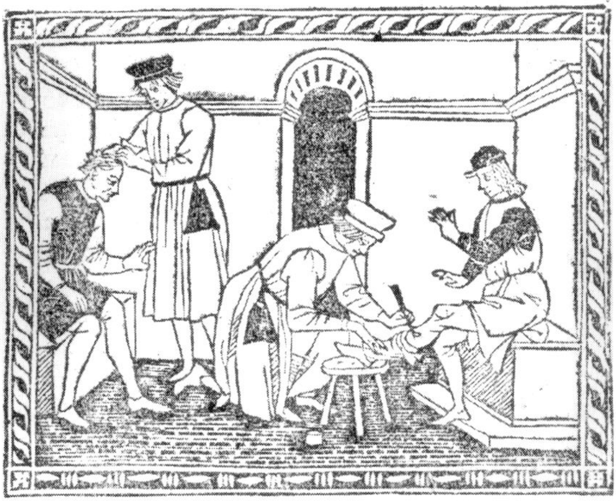

Plate 7.5 'The Medicheria', frontispiece, Peter of Spain, *Thesaurus pauperum* (Florence, 1497) (Wellcome Institute Library, London)

relative status in the hospital. At Siena, in contrast, Domenico di Bartolo represents the principal surgeon of S. Maria della Scala at the very centre of the *Care of the Sick*, tending to the young man with a deep leg wound (Plate 7.3). His placement in the picture together with his more splendid costume suggests higher status than at the Ceppo; he wears a red turban on his head and his red cloak is cast back over his shoulder to reveal a grey-blue lining with the same decorative pattern as the hangings behind him.

The functions of surgeons depicted in these scenes are reflected in general terms in S. Maria Nuova's 'Ordinances', which boast that 'we employ a surgeon to treat them [patients], the best in Florence ... The surgeon must spend two hours in the morning and two in the evening attending the sick.'[50] Furthermore, given the scale of the hospital's operation, the surgeon was 'assisted by three lay brothers, who have learned surgery through long experience'. Domenico di Bartolo shows the surgeon surrounded by a crowd of male nursing staff (Plates 7.3 and 7.4).

As seen above in Chapter 6, S. Maria Nuova's *commesse* also played a medical role. There were 'several skilled in surgery', as the compilers of the 'Ordinances' remarked in a slightly amazed tone: 'These [women] have many remarkable cures to their credit and are even more trusted than the men.'[51] The practice of using the skills of resident female staff in surgical procedures may have been far more widespread than is usually suggested by the literature on Renaissance hospitals. Normative records did not normally describe the activities of staff in detail, particularly those lower down the professional scale. Any medical procedures undertaken by nursing staff would have been part of their normal activities and done on an ad hoc basis by individuals with the relevant interest and experience. These women described as 'skilled in surgery' may have gained their experience either through being the daughters of medical practitioners or through helping male surgeons to treat women patients.

Two of the hospital's female practitioners, Monna Caterina and Monna Francesca, were identified by name in S. Maria Nuova's early sixteenth-century *Ricettario*, a collection of all the recipes purportedly 'tried and tested' in the hospital.[52] Each woman was described as a 'medica di casa' and the recipes they prescribed suggest they were treating conditions needing surgical procedures or external medicine. Both provided a recipe for a green unguent for *capi rotti* – literally 'broken heads' – described by the compiler in words that recall the comments of the author of the 'Ordinances' as the recipe which worked miraculously – 'la ricietta di mirabile operatione'.[53] Another recipe of more general application was Maestra Caterina's 'Fine black unguent made by Maestra Caterina doctor of the house and it is good for pains and wounds and for cuts and fractured heads that are wounded or any other sickness and it is applied with great success.'[54]

Male surgeons received a salary and were employed on a variety of contracts, as can be seen at Messer Bonifazio in the first fifteen years of its existence. In the year 1404–5, in addition to two physicians the hospital employed Maestro Niccolò, a bone doctor from Parma, who was paid 3 gold florins a year 'to visit and treat the sick with his craft when the need arises'. Also there was Pagolo di Pagolo from Piazza di S. Giovanni who was employed on an annual salary of 4 gold florins to shave the staff and patients every fifteen days.[55] Then three years later a *medico cerusico* or surgeon, Guerriero di Michelotto from Pescia, was employed to replace one of the earlier medical practitioners. He was to come to the hospital twice a day, for an hour in the morning and another in the evening, to tend to the sick at 18 gold florins a year.[56]

Hospitals thus employed a number of practitioners at different salary levels, from 3 florins for the bone doctor, double for physicians and six times as much for the surgeon. This distribution reflected both the expertise and the level of activity of each practitioner, with Guerriero di Michelotto's twice-daily visits more onerous than the more occasional visits of Maestro Niccolò from Parma and the two physicians. This basic pattern continued throughout the century at Messer Bonifazio, with the average annual fee paid to barber-surgeons remaining at approximately 24 lire for shaving and letting blood on a regular but not daily basis. However, amounts paid to more full-time practitioners increased over the fifteenth century. For example, in 1468 S. Matteo paid 40 gold florins a year to Maestro Fruosino d'Andrea to come to the hospital each morning for an hour or more to treat in- and out-patients and to shave and let the blood of patients and staff.[57] Another type of contract was arranged with Maestro Giovanni di Francesco Machi, who began working for S. Matteo in 1471 at 20 gold florins a year.[58] He fulfilled two roles, as both *medico cerusico* and apothecary. He had to promise 'to serve at any time, equally at times of pestilence which God pleases [to visit on us] as at any other time'.[59] When his salary was reduced to 40 lire (7.3 florins) he was more than compensated by additional payments in kind of twenty-four bushels of wheat, twelve barrels of wine and a house to rent – presumably at a subsidised rate – 'behind our hospital ... so that he can conveniently serve our patients'. He certainly needed to have a convenient place since he was required to be available day and night.

Hospital doctors therefore enjoyed a wide variety of employment contracts depending on their qualifications, the amount of time which they spent in treating the sick and their own religious and charitable motivations. In general, less well-qualified surgeons were paid more than physicians; the latter spent much less time in the hospital and were prepared to work for reduced fees. Such was the case with the distinguished doctor Maestro Donato d'Agostino Bartolini, who was contracted in 1445 to work as both a doctor of physic and as a surgeon for S. Matteo for only 6 gold florins and 24 bushels of wheat (worth just under 3 gold florins each year).[60] Payment to practitioners in a mixture of cash and kind was not uncommon and suggests that both hospitals and practitioners were prepared to negotiate flexible contracts.

More detail about the duties expected of a hospital surgeon can be found in S. Matteo's contract with Maestro Fruosino d'Andrea of July 1468:

> I record that today, this day of 20 July 1468, Messer Lucha di . . . our *spedalingo*, agreed with Maestro Fruosino d'Andrea barber that the said Maestro Fruosino must come, or send his assistants, to shave and look after all the members of staff of the hospital, the healthy as well as the sick, well and diligently, once every fifteen days in the winter and every ten days in the summer.
>
> And in addition to this the said Maestro Fruosino must come personally each morning, or his assistant, for an hour or however long is needed to remain in our *medicheria* to medicate and to treat well and diligently all our male and female patients whom we have in our hospital as well as the staff, and furthermore to deal with all the medical needs of all those who come from outside.
>
> And furthermore the said Fruosino is obliged to let blood and to draw teeth and to be available as needed for all our male and female patients and the *famiglia* of the house.[61]

Maestro Fruosino's first regular job was 'to shave and look after' all patients and staff, which would have included washing their hair, as mentioned in S. Matteo's contract of 1442 with the company of barber-surgeons of Giovanni di Martino, whose workshop was down the road at the Column of S. Zanobi on Piazza S. Giovanni.[62] These tasks reflected those of the traditional barber-surgeon, reminding us that, despite their pretensions to status and membership of the medical guild, surgeons shared their origins and often functions with the more lowly barbers. Hair was cut more frequently in the summer – defined more exactly in another contract as from Easter to All Saints' Day[63] – as it grows more rapidly in warm weather and it was believed that frequent washing in cold weather might lead to infection. This was the reason given a hundred years later by the Incurabili hospital to justify only providing Guaiacum Wood treatment for the Great Pox during the summer months; going out into the cold after being in a warm environment led to the risk of ill health.[64]

Such menial tasks were probably undertaken by Fruosino's assistant, while he concentrated on preventative medicine and the treatment of specific complaints. He would have let blood on a regular seasonal basis as a form of preventative medicine in order to rid the body of excess humours, which were regarded as dangerous if allowed to collect and corrupt in the body. He would also have recommended purgation using laxatives, enemas and cauterisation or cupping.

As far as surgical procedures were concerned, only his role as a dentist was mentioned – described elsewhere as drawing 'denti tristi' (literally, 'sad teeth')[65] – though undoubtedly, as in S. Matteo's contract with Maestro Nicholo di Gianghano di Nicholo in 1511, he would have been employed for the 'healing of all wounds and sores that come to be treated in this hospital'.[66] Some conditions were also treated by specialists, as in the case of the eye doctor Maestro Filippo who in the 1350s had removed cataracts for the hospital,[67] while in the Quattrocento other surgical specialists included the bone doctors Maestro Giovanni di Maestro Ciuccio da Orvieto (1406 and 1415)[68] and Maestro Domenico di Giovanni dell'Ossa (1435),[69] and in 1456 Antonio 'medico da Norcia', whose geographical origins suggest he was a specialist in hernias and possibly urogenital infections.[70] Recipes for the latter alone formed 11 per cent of all those listed in S. Maria Nuova's *Ricettario* of 1515, suggesting a common complaint (Table 9.3).

The location where treatment was provided by hospital surgeons depended on the severity of the patient's condition. If the iconographic evidence is to be believed, the ward played an important role. Domenico di Bartolo shows S. Maria della Scala's surgeon at centre stage carrying pincers in his right hand to be used in the treatment of a young man with a deep wound to his right-hand thigh from which blood is flowing copiously (Plates 7.3 and 7.4). On the right-hand side of Della Robbia's workshop's frieze at the Ceppo in Pistoia, a surgeon inspects the head wound of a young man in bed (Plate 7.1). Recipes for these parts of the body formed a significant percentage of those in S. Maria Nuova's *Ricettario*: 28 per cent of the overall total of 840 were to treat the head and another 12 per cent were to treat cuts, bruises, fractures and ulcers of the limbs (Tables 9.3 and 9.5).

Surgical patients who could walk were taken to the *medicheria* and surgeons such as Maestro Fruosino were contracted to be available there every day to treat residents and out-patients alike; his contract stipulated he had to be available 'to all those who come from outside, to treat them according to their needs'.[71] An idea of its appearance can be gained from an image printed as the frontispiece of a copy of Peter of Spain's *Thesaurus pauperum*, which was published in Florence in 1497 and owned by S. Maria Nuova (Plate 7.5). The representation of the interior of the *medicheria* is schematic. It shows a small room with an arched opening at the rear and patients sitting on two benches along the walls. On the left a surgeon inspects a man's head and cleans a wound, a process that is evidently causing pain because the patient raises his left hand towards the surgeon. The patient on the right appears to be in even greater pain; he raises two hands in supplication, while the surgeon probes a gash in his left leg. The image thus reflects both the brief written descriptions of surgeons' duties and other iconographic representations of doctors treating external wounds. It is significant that it should come from the *Thesaurus pauperum*, which was one of the most widely circulated works of remedies for the treatment of over fifty common complaints and diseases and would have been a standard work for hospital surgeons and their assistants.

Inventories provide more evidence of the contents and appearance of a hospital *medicheria*. The simplest was apparently that at S. Matteo, where the inventory listed a litter for patients, a bench where the doctors sat, a wardrobe that held unguents, a brass pan for heating unguents, a number of brass or iron tongs, and 'a chest without bottom to receive the alms', presumably from grateful out-patients.[72] S. Maria Nuova's inventory of 1588 revealed a much larger space full of objects.[73] The first thing seen on entering the room would have been a brass-topped counter and around the walls five large cupboards which held a wide range of instruments used by the surgeon. Four boxes were kept on the counter and contained instruments for regular use. Two smaller boxes were used to carry instruments into the wards to treat bed-ridden patients. Also visible on or near the counter was a range of items used on a daily basis, including basins for washing, cauldrons and pans for heating unguents, and oils and metal tools for cauterisation.

The cupboards contained a wide range of surgical instruments, mostly made of metal and divided according to use. There were winches for setting broken legs, 6 saws (though described as in poor condition) for amputation, 26 bone-scrapers or raspers for removing infection, 5 small instruments for opening abscesses, 3 small instruments for prodding or digging into open wounds, 24 'irons' for the extraction of bullets, as well as knives and files for slitting open wounds and filing down broken bones. Other instruments were used to treat sexual or gastro-intestinal dysfunctions, including two 'serpents' or worm pipes, two syringes, an iron for cutting the penis, presumably for the cancerous effects of the Great Pox or French Disease, and a 'key' for treating anal fistula.

The combination of evidence from contracts, contemporary images and inventories has underlined the wide variety of surgical procedures undertaken by the large medical hospitals of Florence, a story that could undoubtedly be repeated for many of the major hospitals in other Italian city–states. These procedures followed the recommendations of established practitioners and textbooks, such as the book on surgery by William of Saliceto (1210–80/85), which was owned by S. Maria Nuova in the late fifteenth century.[74] All in all, such evidence goes some way to justifying the claims of contemporaries that the Renaissance hospital did indeed provide a significant medical service to its patients, based on the most 'modern' surgical techniques.[75]

Hospitals, then, were seen as useful places for the medical profession to gain experience of a wide range of conditions, to increase their prestige through association with the largest medical centres in the city and to obtain a regular income. Remuneration was moreover seen in terms of the honour and reputation that would accrue to the professional man who, through offering his services to the poor, demonstrated that he was selfless and public-spirited. Given the importance of these factors, what type of practitioners were chosen by hospitals? Did they, as S. Maria Nuova's 'Ordinances' claimed, actually correspond to the 'best in the city'? In the following sections I shall move from the role of hospital doctors within the institutional context to their wider role in Florence. A reconstruction of their socio-economic backgrounds, involvement in guild and communal politics and in the life of the Studio will also help to further our understanding of how hospitals themselves formed part of the personal, political and professional networks of the Renaissance city.

7.4 Hospital Doctors: 'Always the Best in the City'?

The period that saw the evolution of the main characteristics of the Renaissance hospital also saw what has been described as the gradual 'political déclassement' of medical practitioners.[76] Plague, it is argued, had created a vacuum that was filled progressively by non-native Florentines, who because they were not full citizens were excluded from political life. Medical practitioners thus became increasingly marginalised within the power structure of the Arte dei Medici e Speziali as other guild members, principally apothecaries, came to dominate.[77]

Table 7.2 Geographical origins of doctors in the guild (1409–44) and of hospital doctors in the Quattrocento (where known)

	Guild		Hospitals	
	N	%	N	%
Florence	18	20	14	35
Territory	27	30	17	43
'Foreigners'*	46	50	9	23
Total	91	100	40	100

* From outside the Florentine state
Source for guild: Park, *Doctors*, p. 77: Table 2.3

In order to see how far hospital doctors fitted into this general picture I shall begin by reconstructing their geographical origins. Though little substantive evidence survives from the Trecento, for the following century it is possible to trace the provenance of 57 per cent of the seventy practitioners documented as working for Florentine hospitals. One obvious difference when compared with all those matriculated in the Arte dei Medici e Speziali in this period is that the proportion of 'foreigners' was lower (23 compared to 50 per cent: see Table 7.2). Contracts with hospitals tended to go predominantly to residents of Florence (35 per cent) or of the Florentine state (43 per cent). The latter were mostly from four of the largest towns that had recently fallen under Florentine rule making it easier to work in the capital: Volterra, Prato, Pisa and Arezzo.[78] This underlines the attraction of Florence as a commercial and banking centre where rich private patients and affluent monastic foundations and hospitals provided more secure employment. Within the medical profession as a whole, this attraction extended to those from outside the Florentine state, including Novara, Padua, Parma and Venice.[79]

Table 7.3 Geographical origins of hospital physicians, doctors and surgeons in the Quattrocento (where known)

	Physician		Doctor		Surgeon		Total	
	N	%	N	%	N	%	N	%
Florence	10	48	2	28	2	16	14	35
Territory	9	43	3	43	5	42	17	43
'Foreigners'*	2	9	2	28	5	42	9	22
Total	21	100	7	100	12	100	40	100

* Outside Florentine state

Breaking down the geographical origins according to type of practitioner, Table 7.3 shows that the majority of physicians who worked as hospital doctors were from Florence (ten of fourteen), whereas surgeons were split equally between the Florentine territory and further afield. Some were from northern Italy; Maestro Niccolò of Parma was employed by Messer Bonifazio in 1404–5 as a 'bone doctor', possibly through connections with the founder's family who lived in Parma.[80] In contrast to Maestro Niccolò's more empirical approach, the rather grand-sounding *cerusico* from Padua, Maestro Girolamo di Messer Niccolò, a surgeon colleague of Ficino's father at S. Maria Nuova in the mid-1470s, may very well have received training at the celebrated medical faculty of his native city.[81]

This analysis points to some interesting differences between hospital doctors and all medical practitioners working in Florence. Most significantly, substantially more hospital doctors came from the city and its territory, 78 per cent compared to 50 per cent of all guild matriculants, forming an exception to the general move towards employment of 'foreigners'. The fact that the vast majority of practitioners from Florence were physicians lends support to contemporary claims that the city's hospitals really did attract well-known doctors, though it should be remembered that these men represented an elite whose careers were better documented than those of the majority of hospital doctors. This difference is reflected in the returns of six hospital doctors registered in the Catasto of 1427, one of the most detailed fiscal records in Renaissance Europe. These six physicians and four surgeons were employed by the four major medical hospitals in Florence in the 1420s.[82] They represented a wide economic range, with net wealth ranging from 8,736 florins to 400 florins. Their average net wealth was 2,956 florins, 500 florins more than the average of all doctors' households in the city. This placed them high up the occupational hierarchy of Florence, below bankers and wool merchants but above lawyers, apothecaries and stationers.[83] Two examples of affluent physicians will suffice. Maestro Lionardo di Maestro Agnolo di Ser Tignoso da Bibbiena, who worked for S. Maria Nuova in 1415 and had a net wealth of 5,741 florins, emigrated from Bibbiena, probably at a time when the commune offered tax exemptions to medical practitioners to work in Florence.[84] Maestro Domenicho di Piero Toscanelli, who was employed by S. Maria Nuova some forty years later and was worth 8,736 florins net,[85] was the brother of the medical humanist Paolo Toscanelli and held a number of the main offices in the Arte dei Medici e Speziali.

To concentrate on the wealthier, better-documented practitioners skews the evidence, however. Hospital doctors shared the general discrepancy in wealth between physicians and surgeons in the city, for hospital physicians were over twice as wealthy as their surgeon colleagues (3,534 as against 1,661 florins). Indeed, the figure for the average wealth of the four surgeons is misleading because one very affluent individual, Maestro Giovanni di Ser Bartolo di Maestro Giovanni Fratellani da Radda, had a net wealth of 4,819 florins.[86] The others had an assessment of 400–758 florins and were probably more representative of surgeons and empirics employed by S. Maria Nuova in the second half of the Trecento, who included hernia and bone doctors, a dentist who worked as a herbalist and a cobbler who removed cataracts. For example, in 1351–2 Maestro Francescho di Nolo was listed between the 65th and 70th percentile in the city's wealth table and his successor, Luca di Ceco, was actually excused the Prestanza indirect tax because he was a *miserabile* and too poor to pay tax.[87] These less affluent surgeons were more representative of the average medical practitioner in the city; according to the Catasto of 1427, nearly half of all doctors in Florence had a pre-tax assessment of 600 florins or less.

This analysis of the provenance and financial standing of hospital doctors has shown that not only S. Maria Nuova but all the major medical hospitals attracted well-known practitioners. Their records suggest that a higher percentage of their doctors came from Florence and its territory than was true of the profession as a whole, reflecting the growing proportion of physicians among hospital medical staff. Hospital records also reflect the general bifurcation of the profession, for the vast majority of surgeons were less affluent and from further afield. I shall now return to examine this more elite group and their participation in the wider world of the city through membership of the guild, commune and Studio.

7.5 Professional Networks

About one in five of all hospital doctors (twenty-two of 110) has been traced as serving the guild or commune in the period 1320–1500. However, in common with general developments in the medical profession in Florence, the vast majority ceased to be involved in both political arenas after the third decade of the Quattrocento. Furthermore, while surgeons participated in the guild leadership in the late Trecento, their power was rapidly overturned by physicians as they came to be excluded from effective influence in the Arte.

We can look at the example of two hospital surgeons who had an active political life, but with different degrees of success. The first is Maestro Giovanni di Giusto da Castel S. Niccolò, who was associated with S. Maria Nuova in 1384.[88] He came from a relatively modest background – his father was a crossbowman – and his Prestanza tax returns between 1379 and 1413 demonstrate that he remained of relatively modest means. Unlike some of his more affluent and powerful contemporaries, he was three times elected guild consul, but this did not lead to communal office.[89] In contrast, the surgeon Maestro Giovanni del Maestro Ambrogio Solosmei, also associated with S. Maria Nuova, was many times guild consul and was even twice elected a prior of the city. Part of his success may be attributed to his background since he came from one of the new families that had established themselves in Florence after the great plague and that had become one of the main medical dynasties in the city.[90]

Maestro Cristofano di Giorgio Brandaglini, who died in 1425, was a hospital physician who became successful in all walks of life. In the early Quattrocento he was associated with the hospitals of Messer Bonifazio, S. Paolo and S. Gallo.[91] He was the son of a second-hand clothes' dealer and joined the silk guild before starting to pursue a medical career. However, once embarked on the latter, he was elected consul of the Arte dei Medici e Speziali twenty-two times between 1382 and 1425. He also rose to political prominence, becoming a prior of the city four times and was elected to the coveted post of Standard-Bearer of Justice.[92] Indeed, he has been described as a member of the 'inner core' of the regime in the early Quattrocento,[93] receiving commissions from the commune, including the direction of the refurbishment of the baths of Bagno a Morbo near Volterra.[94]

The careers of those hospital doctors involved in guild and communal politics in the late fourteenth to the early fifteenth centuries conform to the general pattern for city practitioners, since the majority came from outside Florence and made their way up the political ladder through the guild structure to the commune. Yet this type of advancement was denied to many and, even when they were personally wealthy, their political role remained limited. Another pattern was that many of their sons failed to build on their achievements and therefore did not succeed in establishing medical dynasties, in marked contrast with their lawyer contemporaries. Instead their social mobility was often characterised by a sideways movement, as in the case of Simone di Cinozzo, who worked at S. Matteo in the 1450s. His father was an apothecary, but his son became a *linaiolo* or cloth merchant and the first member of the family to serve in the Signoria, but wearing a linen rather than a medical hat.[95] One exception to this rule was the Toscanelli family, who did establish a medical dynasty. As such, wealth was passed down from generation to generation, as were links with clients and major hospitals. The first member who came to prominence was the affluent S. Maria Nuova physician Maestro Domenico di Piero. His origins are obscure; we know neither the occupation of his father nor how he acquired his wealth. His son Maestro Piero del Maestro Domenico di Niccolò was also a physician who at least had financial dealings with S. Maria Nuova, while his grandson Maestro Lodovicho was described in 1486 as 'nostro medicho nello spedale'.[96]

Employment by a major medical hospital not only provided income but also promoted one's reputation among patricians looking for family doctors. The best-known example is Marsilio Ficino's father, Diotifeci d'Agnolo da Figline, who worked for S. Maria Nuova and was Cosimo de' Medici's doctor, and was described by his son as 'outstanding among his contemporaries'.[97] Cosimo's son Piero then employed as his house doctor Maestro Mariotto di Niccholò di Gerino Gerini da Castiglione Aretino, who treated Giovanni Rucellai's daughter-in-law and worked for S. Maria Nuova and the Innocenti.[98]

Even if few medical men made a successful political career in the guild or commune after the third decade of the Quattrocento, there were two important arenas in which they were able to develop their own powerbase, the College of Physicians and the Studio.[99] Membership of the College, a branch of the guild established in 1396, was restricted to doctors with a university doctorate, which excluded the majority of practitioners below the level of physician who had qualified for membership of the guild through taking its own examination.[100] Little is known about the College in this period, but membership evidently lent prestige. The leading physician Cristofano di Giorgio Brandaglini, who worked for three hospitals, was a member until his death in 1425, as were others who belonged to the 'solid middle class', including S. Maria Nuova's physician Maestro Domenicho di Maestro Ciuccio da Orvieto and Maestro Bandino di Maestro Banducci da Prato, who also worked for S. Paolo and the Innocenti.[101]

Public recognition was also achieved through association with the Florentine Studio, well known for medicine, theology and the arts.[102] As with the College, there was considerable rivalry between the Studio and the guild, since members of the latter resented the exclusion of native Florentines both from the university's rectorship and all the major chairs. Even so, there was a close association between members of the College and the Studio, underlining the continued importance of the former as an alternative powerbase to the guild, especially when the Studio was closed during plague epidemics and after it moved to Pisa in 1473.[103]

Hospital doctors first came to be associated with the Studio by taking a degree, like Maestro Tomaso di Baccio d'Arezzo, who obtained his in 1402 and was employed by S. Matteo within eleven years of his graduation. More unusual was Ficino's father, Dietifeci d'Agnolo, who obtained his doctorate late in life after he had already been working for S. Maria Nuova for a couple of years.[104] A physician could also be involved in another's doctoral examination by presenting a candidate or simply by being present, as was Maestro Ugholino di Piero da Pisa at the examination of Ficino's father.[105] In both cases their presence refected that they were members of a privileged circle.

The most public and prestigious form of association with the Studio was employment as a reader or professor. All hospital doctors who taught at the Studio were physicians – with one exception, the surgeon Maestro Bartholomeo di Nicholò Babachari da Lucha. He taught surgery at the Florentine Studio between 1415 and 1419, a few years after being employed at S. Matteo.[106] Subsequently physicians took over the teaching of surgery at the Studio; S. Matteo's Maestro Bartholomeo di Chambio was trained in both physic and surgery.[107] Another well-known university teacher, Maestro Donato d'Aghostino Bartolini, received his doctorate in the autumn of 1431 and went to work for S. Matteo after teaching logic, philosophy and medicine for fourteen years.[108] Maestro Simone di Cinozzo di Giovanni Cinozzi followed a similar career path, although he may have combined working for S. Matteo and the Studio since he taught medicine intermittently between 1432 and 1446.[109] He was also a busy committee man, serving ten times as a consul of the Arte dei Medici e Speziali and for fifteen years as a member of the College after leaving the Studio.[110]

The teaching of medicine provided another potential link between hospitals and the Studio. There is a well-established historiographical tradition for the presence of a medical school at S. Maria Nuova in the later Middle Ages, even dating back to the institution's foundation.[111] However, no convincing evidence has ever been cited for a fully fledged 'school', though bedside teaching did take place, as is suggested by the chapter in S. Maria Nuova's 'Ordinances' on junior doctors: 'in the course of seeing a wide variety of illnesses and using many different remedies, they become increasingly skilled and expert, since, as they say, experience is the teacher of all things.'[112] This recalls Da Monte's suggestion that 'In the hospital two things can be seen and practised [upon], namely diseases and their symptoms'. The writers of both these texts placed emphasis on learning about therapy through the administration of simple and compound medicines and therefore the manipulation of the six non-naturals.

It is one thing to assume that hospitals provided junior doctors with experience of diseases and treatments and quite another to infer the presence of 'medical schools'. While there is no evidence in this period of any formal association between Florentine hospitals and the medical faculty,[113] the presence of university's readers in medicine on their staff suggests informal links. After all, at the most general level the statutes of universities teaching medicine assumed that part of a student's training was to accompany senior doctors on their visits and in this way to learn from experience.[114] Even after 1472, when the Studio moved to Pisa, medical students from Florence may have remained in their native city and 'practised for six months with one or more physicians', as was prescribed, for example, by the 1409 statute of the College of Arts and Medicine at Pavia.[115] As we saw above, the Florentine College of Physicians from the mid-sixteenth century delayed granting licences to young physicians until they had gained more experience by working for a period at S. Maria Nuova.

The other myth that has grown up around S. Maria Nuova in the Renaissance concerns the teaching of anatomy and the establishment of a school of anatomy, neither of which took place until much later than is asserted by many of the general works on the hospital. Anatomy remained a grey area given the Church's prohibition of the practice. Corpses used for the regular human dissections prescribed by both the College of Physicians and the Studio derived from only one legitimate source: men and women who had been condemned to death.[116] Even so, it was obviously possible to gain access to bodies of people who had died in S. Maria Nuova in the early sixteenth century, as was recorded by Leonardo da Vinci in a well-known anecdote:[117]

> And this old man a few hours before said to me that he was more than 100 years' old and he had not felt anything lacking in his body, other than

weakness, and thus seated on his bed in the hospital of Santa Maria Nuova of Florence without any movement or any sign of a symptom passed from this life. And I anatomised him to discover the cause of such a sweet death, which came about less because of the lack of blood that had fed the heart and the other inferior members which I found very arid, weakened and dry, which I described in great detail at the anatomy, but because it was deprived of fat and of humours which blocked the parts.

This passage alone provides ample evidence of Leonardo's knowledge of Galenic humoral medicine and his fascination with the workings of the human body and the reasons for this 'dolce morte'. While the anecdote suggests by its very casualness that dissection of patients at S. Maria Nuova did take place, it is stretching the evidence too far to suggest that it must have been common practice. The contemporary doctor Antonio Benivieni records in his *De abditis* a series of dissections of patients carried out for the same reason as that given by Leonardo: namely, 'to discover the hidden causes of death'. However, it is striking that Benivieni only mentions dissections of private patients and none at S. Maria Nuova, despite his employment there as house doctor.[118]

It is only after the mid-sixteenth century that links between Italian hospitals and the study of anatomy can be pinned down more definitively. Girolamo Cardano in the 1545 edition of his *On the Bad Practice of Recent Physicians* emphasised the need for doctors regularly to dissect patients who died in hospital, probably a reference to the practice at the Ospedale Maggiore in Milan. As Nancy Siraisi has pointed out, what was new was Cardano's stress on only dissecting specific organs rather than the whole body to determine the effects of a specific disease, paralleling Gianbattista da Monte's observation about hospital patients in Pavia.[119] There is no evidence that dissections were being organised for doctors at S. Maria Nuova in this period. Only in July 1563 did there appear an institutional commitment to organise regular anatomical classes at S. Maria Nuova, and even then this was by the Accademia del Disegno, as recorded in its statutes of July 1563: 'We wish, moreover, that those consuls who are in office during winter should and must make sure that dissection [*una Anathomia*] takes place in Santa Maria Nuova for the benefit of the young men of the Arte del Disegno, which all must attend by order of the said consuls.'[120] Though no record has so far been found in the archives of the hospital to prove whether such a dissection actually took place, it is important to stress that it was organised for artists and sculptors rather than medical students. After all, by this stage medicine was being taught at Pisa after the Florentine Studio had closed and it is more likely that anatomy for teaching purposes took place in a hospital there rather than in Florence.[121]

Conclusion

Myths are bound to have grown up over the years about an institution such as S. Maria Nuova, which since the Renaissance has played such a central role in the history of medical charity in Florence. To challenge these myths is not to lessen appreciation of the hospital's sizeable contribution, but merely to correct some of the anachronistic assumptions that typify traditional historiography. It is also necessary to divert attention away from over-concentration on S. Maria Nuova, which, after all, shared the burden of looking after the sick poor with the other major medical hospitals of the city.

Avoidance of excessive concentration on S. Maria Nuova is also necessary when assessing the place of hospitals in the careers of doctors working in Florence. It is only too easy to project back onto earlier centuries its much later role as a centre for medical education which developed under the Medici grand dukes. Furthermore, distinctions have to be made between one period and another for, while S. Maria Nuova dominated in the employment of hospital doctors in the Trecento, the following century saw a considerable expansion of the marketplace with the growth of S. Paolo and the foundation of Messer Bonifazio, S. Matteo and the Innocenti. To meet this increased demand, a minimum of eighty-six different practitioners worked for hospitals in the Quattrocento and while S. Maria Nuova employed the largest number, over half worked for other institutions in the city.

Even though S. Maria Nuova may have been the major employer of medical practitioners, it did not have a monopoly on leading physicians if we measure eminence by involvement in guild or communal politics or the Studio. One of the most politically active physicians of his day, Maestro Cristofano di Giorgio Brandaglini, who was elected consul of the guild twenty-two times between 1382 and 1425 and a prior of the commune four times, worked at various times in his career for the hospitals of Messer Bonifazio, S. Matteo and S. Gallo, but never apparently for S. Maria Nuova. Maestro Simone di Cinozzo, who was guild consul ten times and a prior in the late Quattrocento, worked only for S. Matteo. In contrast, a higher proportion of S. Maria Nuova's physicians were members of the College of Physicians. Association with the college was evidently helpful in gaining employment at S. Maria Nuova and vice versa. But when one turns, instead, to the involvement of university physicians in hospital practice, one discovers a different pattern, suggesting that the traditional rivalry between guild and Studio may have transformed itself in the Quattrocento into one between college and Studio. Even if some of those who taught in the Studio were S. Maria Nuova employees, more appear to have chosen to work for S. Matteo and Messer Bonifazio, either together or separately. This was the case with Maestro Bartolomeo di Chambio, who was a reader in surgery at the Studio in 1419–20. Maestro Donato d'Aghostino Bartolini who, as seen above, taught at the Studio between 1431 to 1439, worked exclusively for S. Matteo in 1445.

This chapter has thus shown that the city's major medical hospitals played a crucial role in the development of doctors' careers, providing them with professional, social and political contacts as well as unrivalled experience in treating a wide range of diseases. This was a mutually beneficial relationship. Hospitals also gained prestige through attracting leading doctors to their staff, thus helping the Renaissance hospital to live up to its reputation as providing the best medical treatment available.

CHAPTER 8

'Antechambers of Death'?

Introduction

As has been seen in past chapters, there was a general development in contemporary ideas regarding the proper function of the Italian hospital, broadly characterised as a transition from a medieval to a Renaissance view. On the one hand, the medieval hospital was seen as an unhealthy environment and, as suggested by Giordano da Rivalto, contained thousands of undifferentiated diseases. It was a place where the sick could expect to die rather than recover.[1] On the other hand, the Renaissance hospital was presented as a place of beauty and utility, where the sick were well looked after by teams of devoted servants and expert doctors of the body and soul.

It might be objected that Renaissance commentators had a biased view as they were drawn from among the more affluent members of society and were therefore more likely to have visited a hospital as a beneficent patron than as an inmate. In other words, this perspective on the Renaissance hospital is that of the provider rather than the consumer. The Florentine humanist Cristoforo Landino records in his *Commentary on the Divine Comedy* that 'many foreigners, nobles and very rich men, who travelling [through Florence] and having fallen sick from some illness, have chosen this as the place in which to be looked after'.[2] When evaluating these and similar statements it must be remembered that a hospital like S. Maria Nuova was vast and, as hospitals do today, contained private rooms for the more affluent and for visiting clerics. Whether Florentine patricians, who had the choice of staying at home when sick, would also have elected to be treated in S. Maria Nuova must remain doubtful. Indeed, Landino himself recorded in his *Commentary* that the wish of Violante Gambacorta to die in S. Maria Nuova was opposed by relatives who deemed it inappropriate for a noblewoman to pass her last few hours in a *spedale*.[3]

Previous chapters have examined the physical environment of the ward as well as the role of staff in treating the body and soul. In this chapter I shall look

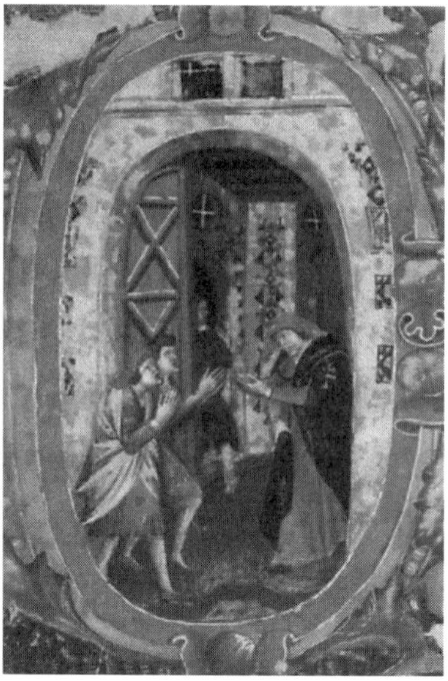

Plate 8.1 Circle of the Master of the S. Giorgio Codex, *Receiving the Poor at the Hospital Door*, Hospital of S. Spirito, Rome, *Liber regulae Sancti Spiritus*, c.1350 (ASR, Ospedale di S. Spirito 3193, f. 131v)

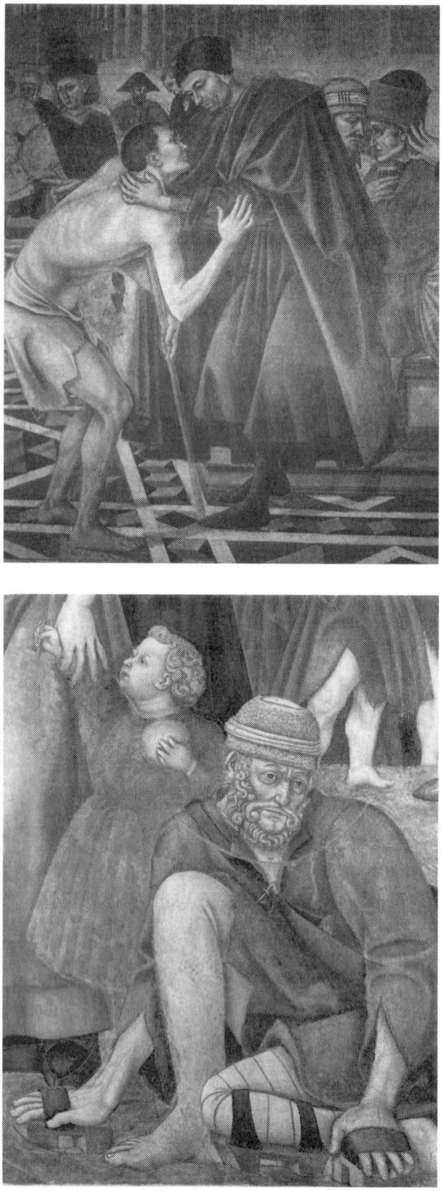

Plate 8.2 Domenico di Bartolo a. A 'Semi-Clad Man' and b. 'A Crippled Beggar', details of *Care of the Sick*, 1440–4, Pellegrinaio ward, Hospital of S. Maria della Scala, Siena

more closely at the patients themselves by assessing the impact of their environment, reconstructing patterns of admissions, mortality and diagnoses as well as by examining the patients' social and occupational profiles in order to determine more exactly the motivation for becoming an inmate.

8.1 'Almost like Christ in their Persons': Admitting the Poor

Plate 8.1, a contemporary image of the poor seeking admission to S. Spirito in Rome, underlines not only the hospital's charitable role, but also the fact that patients came for treatment of their own free will. Unfortunately, little is known about the mechanisms by which patients were accepted into the large hospitals of a Renaissance state. It may very well be that the majority just arrived at the door asking for treatment, while others were brought in by hospital staff on their tours of the city. Smaller institutions may have been more particular, but in any case all hospitals would have applied certain criteria for admission so as to exclude the immoral goats and concentrate on the moral sheep. Some patients may have arrived holding certificates of confession from their parish priests; some hospitals ensured patients were confessed by their chaplain on arrival. Patients were also recommended by their employers; for example, when Lorenzo Strozzi's 'famiglio' arrived in Florence from Rome with a fever in August 1461, Alessandra Strozzi wrote, 'I was pleased that we had arranged that he went to S. Maria Nuova; and we recommended him to the doctor and he lacked nothing there.'[4]

As has been seen in Chapter 5, once patients passed through the door they became small cogs in a vast machine. On admission an initial diagnosis was made by the head of the ward.[5] Patients were then assigned a number for easy identification for treatment and for retrieval of their possessions; they carried this number with them until their eventual exit from the hospital, alive or dead. Once they had been confessed by a doctor of the soul, patients were assigned to a bed to await inspection by the physicians who swept into the ward every morning at a set hour.[6] As has been seen above, they were accompanied by the infirmarer, one of the house doctors and the apothecary, who discussed 'the nature of each patient's illness and its symptoms, his state of mind, and what has been done for him up to that point'. The senior physician 'then carefully prescribes treatment, which the pharmacist's assistant writes down in a book'; the recipe was then made up by the pharmacist, the medicine brought back to the ward and administered to the patient by the nursing staff.

In addition to records of recipes prescribed for the sick, information about each patient was noted in two other types of register, as mentioned in S. Maria Nuova's 'Ordinances':[7]

> the patient's name and patronymic [are recorded] in a book, together with his family or nationality, as well as his bed number and whether he is lying in the upper or lower part. This book is kept in alphabetical order. If the patient should die, there is another book in which the particulars are recorded: when he died, when he left the hospital and when he arrived.

These registers rarely survive; evidently later administrators or archivists decided that records of economic and administrative affairs were of greater importance than those documenting the fate of patients. Even so, it is possible to present a patchwork picture by putting together a few examples: for the fifteenth century the records of S. Matteo (1413–56) and the Misericordia in Prato (1402–78), and for the sixteenth century those of S. Maria Nuova (1512–30) and S. Paolo (1554–68).[8] The most detailed section will be on S. Maria Nuova's 'Books of the Dead', which have never previously been subjected to an in-depth analysis of a sample as substantial as that here of 8,500 patients.[9]

Exact information about total annual admissions is difficult to establish for the vast majority of hospitals over this period, though, as indicated above in Chapter 3, some rough calculations can be made to suggest capacity. In very general terms, it is known that by the early fifteenth century S. Maria Nuova and S. Paolo had 120 and 35 beds respectively, while the newest medical hospitals, S. Matteo and Messer Bonifazio, had 48 and 31 beds.[10] The number of patients that these four hospitals alone could have treated with two per bed was equivalent to about 1.3 per cent of the resident Florentine population of 37,500, though, as will be seen below, a significant proportion of inmates came from outside the city.

What is more difficult to determine from these bed totals is how many people were actually treated in any one year. One of the main problems is the question of bed occupancy. The few sample studies that have been undertaken for this period suggest that this varied between institutions and periods. For example, Paolo Pirillo has shown that beds at the Spedale dei Serristori in Figline in the late sixteenth century were sometimes, though not invariably, used for more than one patient, and occasionally for up to four.[11] Bernice Trexler has concluded of S. Paolo: 'Generally only one patient was in a bed, although there were at least forty-one instances of doubling two patients in one bed for periods lasting from one to eighteen days.'[12] More problematic is the case of S. Maria Nuova, though the assumption in this book has been that normal practice was for there to have been two patients per bed, based on the hospital's 'Books of the Dead', where each patient entry is annotated in the right-hand margin either 'k[ap]o' or 'p[iedi]', head or foot. This suggestion is confirmed by an English visitor to S. Maria Nuova, Henry Piers, who in the late sixteenth century recorded that beds in the male ward held two patients and those in the female ward held three.[13] By 1618, when Grand Duke Cosimo II visited the hospital, the situation had grown worse: four or even six women were forced to share the same bed and this was not even during a crisis caused by food shortage or epidemic disease.[14] Indeed, it was the overcrowding of the female ward that persuaded the grand duke Ferdinando II in 1657 to push for the construction of the new female cruciform ward north of Piazza S. Maria Nuova.[15]

The obvious way to approach the problem of annual admissions is through patient records, but normally only 'Books of the Dead' survive. Extrapolating from the numbers dying at S. Matteo in the first half of the fifteenth century and assuming a 10 per cent mortality rate, the hospital would have admitted about three hundred patients a year.[16] In the same period the Misericordia at Prato admitted only about thirty-eight patients a year.[17] We are on firmer ground with S. Paolo a hundred years later; its surviving admission books record 364 men admitted for the year 1557–8 and suggest a probable annual intake of male and females patients of over six hundred.[18] All these hospitals were dwarfed by S. Maria Nuova, which one contemporary, Cristoforo Landino, claimed treated about three hundred patients each day in c.1470.[19] The records for S. Maria Nuova in the early sixteenth century, which enable one to calculate annual intake from marginal annotations of admission numbers in the male death registers,[20] indicate that between 1512 and 1530 male admissions fluctuated between a low of 3,822 and a high of 4,802. Although no record of the total number of women has survived for these years, by assuming that the sex ratio of those admitted alive was the same for those who died (56 to 44 per cent), combined average admissions would have been about 6,600.

Figures for average admissions inevitably mask seasonal fluctuations due to internal and external factors, and the only hospital where both admission and death registers survive, the Misericordia of Prato, shows just how misleading average figures are over a long period (Figure 8.1). In the first few years the

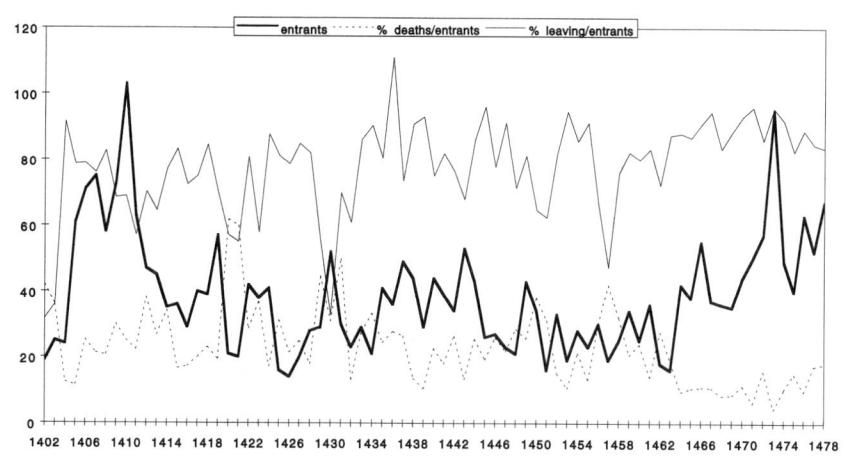

Figure 8.1 Hospital of the Misericordia, Prato: admissions and deaths, 1402–78
Source: G. Paolucci and G. Pinto, 'Gli "infermi"', p.126: Table 4.

hospital admitted the largest numbers of patients (103 in 1410) before falling to a low of sixteen in 1463, after which there was a gradual if rather hesitant growth at a time when standards of living fell.[21] But fluctuations in admissions cannot simply be related to changing economic factors. At S. Maria Nuova there is no significant correlation between changing annual totals in male admissions and the level of real wages in the second and third decades of the sixteenth century (Table 8.1).[22] Ironically it is epidemic disease that helps to explain the fall in admissions to S. Maria Nuova in 1523. In that year many of the hospital's normal clientele, the acute sick, would have been taken directly to lazzarettos as suspected plague cases.

Table 8.1 Hospital of S. Maria Nuova: male patients: admissions and mortality, 1513–28

year	mortality	admissions	% mortality
1513	276	4,111	6.7
1514	300	3,096	9.7
1515	321	3,739	8.6
1516	510	3,625	14.1
1517	469	4,298	10.9
1518	388	4,802	8.1
1519	344	4,611	7.5
1520	318	4,620	6.9
1521	320	4,396	7.3
1522	401	3,945	10.2
1523	285	3,072	9.3
1524	353	2,894	12.2
1525	369	2,822	13.1
1526	304	3,284	9.3
1527	430	3,406	12.6
1528	295	3,196	9.2

Source: SMN 733

8.2 Death and Disease

If there was little obvious correlation between plague incidence and hospital mortality rates in the 1520s, this was not the case for most of the fifteenth century, as can be seen from the experience of S. Matteo in Florence and the Misericordia in Prato.[23]

High peaks in mortality among hospital patients at S. Matteo from 1413 to 1456 correspond to the main outbreaks of plague in the city (Figure 8.2).[24] Over the whole period there was an average of thirty deaths each year, but 1417, 1424 and 1449–50 saw at least a 50 per cent rise. By far the worst

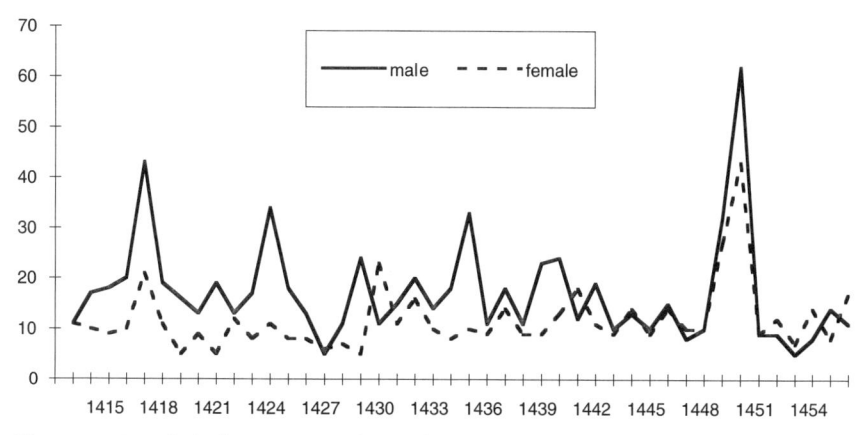

Figure 8.2 Hospital of S. Matteo: male and female deaths, 1413–56
Source: L. Sandri, 'Ospedali e utenti', p. 68: Table 2.

mortality crisis was in 1449–50, when the annual average first doubled and then tripled.[25] Though S. Matteo was not actually used as a lazzaretto, plague evidently broke out there and, as in 1464, it may have been used as a dumping-ground for S. Maria Nuova's patients with 'normal diseases' when the latter in effect became the city's lazzaretto.[26] In Prato, at the Misericordia peaks in mortality also reflected epidemics in the city, with an average mortality in these years of 21 per cent (Figure 8.1).[27]

Just as mortality rates varied between hospitals, so did disease environments between wards in the same institution; for instance, more male patients died at S. Matteo, despite the men's ward having the same capacity as the one for women (Figure 8.2).[28] There were similar rises in mortality for the more severe epidemics of 1417 and 1449–50, but in both 1421–2 and 1440–1 there was a rise in male mortality followed by one among the women. This lagged effect may have been caused by an epidemic having been contained in the male ward in the first year and then spreading to the females in the second year.

The reasons for these differences in mortality between institutions and even between wards remain conjectural, though the more plentiful records of S. Maria Nuova enable one to examine in greater detail the deaths among the patients of a much larger Renaissance hospital. Average male mortality during the period when the available data are sufficiently complete, from 1513 to 1528, was 9.7 per cent,[29] a figure that lies between the rates of the Misericordia at Prato (21 per cent) and S. Paolo (3.5 to 5.2 per cent).[30] Interestingly, historians of the Misericordia consider that even a 20 per cent mortality rate was 'surprisingly low', putting it down to the fact that the hospital catered principally for travellers and pilgrims without life-threatening conditions.[31] The Misericordia's death-rate may appear low when compared with what the prejudices of many general accounts of hospitals in pre-industrial Europe might lead us to expect, but to understand their true significance these figures need to be placed in the wider context of mortality rates within the city as a whole. Thus, the death-rate in Florence among the general population in the first quarter of the fifteenth century was approximately thirty-six to forty per thousand.[32] Even if S. Maria Nuova's rate of a hundred per thousand was still over double that of the city as a whole, this represented a sample of people who were already sick, whereas the figure for the city as a whole was for the total population. Hospitals may not have been places to which the poor were taken to die, but they cannot be depicted as entirely antiseptic environments, especially since, as will be seen below, most patients suffered from acute rather than chronic conditions.

If the average male mortality rate at S. Maria Nuova was about 10 per cent, Table 8.1 shows there was far less variation around the mean than at the Misericordia, which ranged from 10 to 62 per cent. Annual totals mask short-term seasonal variations and a more detailed analysis of S. Maria Nuova's unadjusted monthly death totals – admissions are only known on an annual basis[33] – reflect considerably greater fluctuations during these years.

Figure 8.3 shows that the broad seasonal patterns in male and female mortality were similar between 1513 and 1530. Although the number of females admitted each year is not known, the ratio between male and female deaths remained fairly constant, with an average of 1.22, suggesting that each was subjected in roughly the same proportions to the effects of endogenous and exogenous factors.[34] Each year saw minor monthly variations in deaths, but there was a dramatic interruption to this pattern in the late 1520s, with first a considerable fall and then a high rise. Excluding for the moment the last four years of the period in question, there were four main periods that saw a 50 per cent rise over the monthly average of forty-one: April 1513, April 1516, September to October 1517, and March 1525.

In each case these mortality crises stemmed from outside influences. In April 1513 the apothecary Luca Landucci recorded in his diary that in Florence there had been an exceptionally cold spring 'so that a good number of our people had died, they died within a few days and nobody knows from what sickness'.[35] Presumably the unusually cold weather had led to the spread of some kind of serious chest infection associated with rapid mortality, which may also have been the cause of the rise in hospital deaths in spring 1516, which was very cold and wet. Again seasonal factors may have been at the root of the rises in autumn 1517 and March 1525, but this is far from clear from the sources, especially as during these years there were other months of bad weather not associated with rises in mortality.[36]

'ANTECHAMBERS OF DEATH'? 259

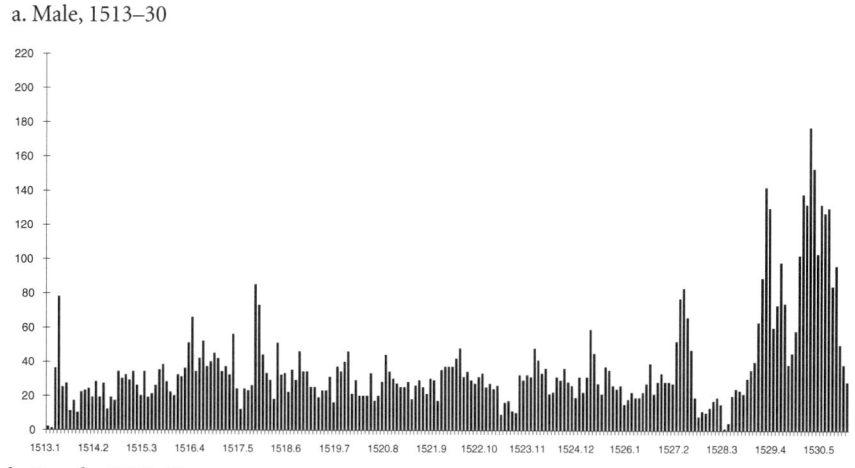

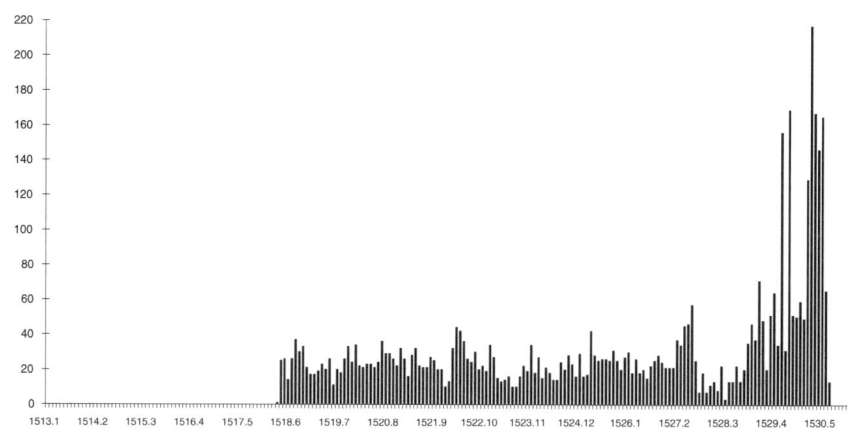

a. Male, 1513–30

b. Female, 1518–30

Figure 8.3 Hospital of S. Maria Nuova: deaths per month
Source: SMN 733–4.

The last four years of this period (Figure 8.4) show a pattern that is significantly different from the previous fourteen years. First, there was an increase in deaths in spring 1527, which was probably related to severe dearth in the city and countryside, which had been exacerbated by the restrictions on the movement of food within the territory since the previous autumn when plague had broken out in the city. By May 1527 the epidemic had returned with renewed virulence, lasting throughout the summer and continuing the following year in parts of Tuscany in what was the worst outbreak of the disease for well over a century. Significantly, as plague mortality rose in Florence, there was a parallel fall in deaths at S. Maria Nuova. The high mortality would have reduced the number of people entering S. Maria Nuova for the treatment of

a. Male

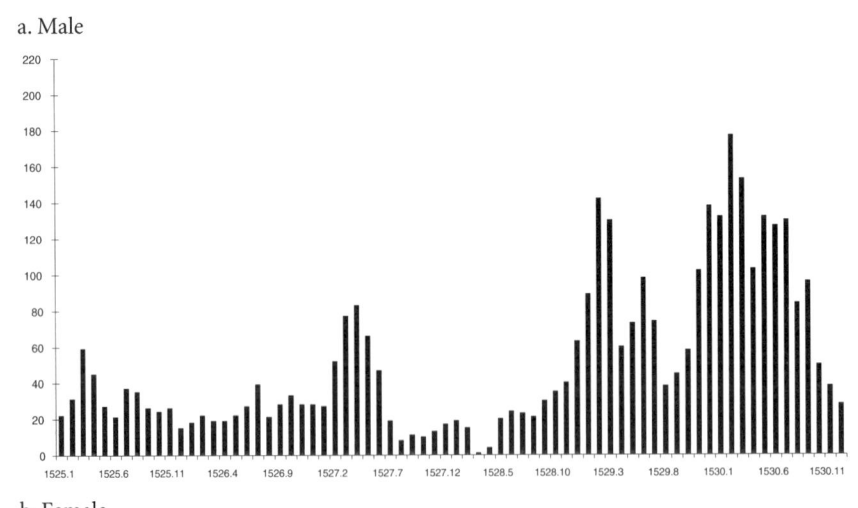

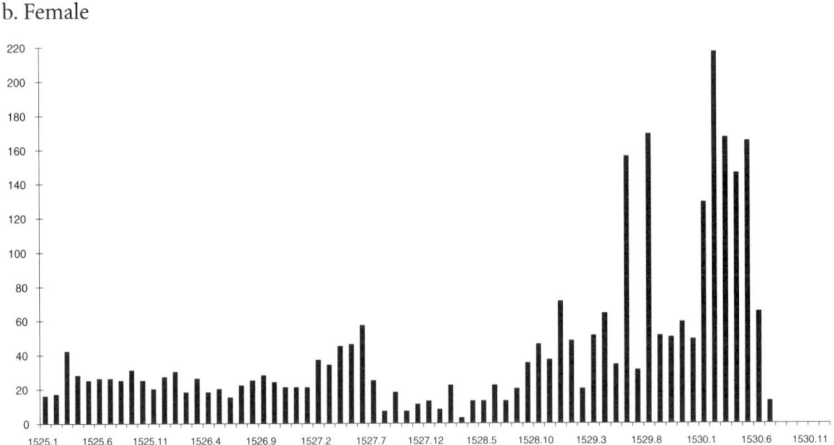

b. Female

Figure 8.4 Hospital of S. Maria Nuova: deaths per month, 1525–30
Source: SMN 733–4

'ordinary sicknesses', as during plague epidemics anybody who displayed symptoms that could even remotely be construed as suggesting plague was sent to a lazzaretto. The reduction in the pool of potential patients is reflected in a fall in the number of male entrants in 1528 (Table 8.1). Furthermore, those who did enter between summer 1527 and summer 1528 were obviously less sick than its normal patients; deaths remained at a very low level and only began to climb in the autumn.

The next two years, 1529 and 1530, reflect a very different pattern: mortality was at its highest during the whole period under observation. Male deaths in these years represented 38 per cent of the total recorded. Mortality was at its worst from November 1529 to August 1530 when Florence was under siege.

Morbidity and mortality rates rose in the city, evidently linked to very high prices and diseases associated with the consumption of poor-quality food. In 1529 the daily real wage of an unskilled labourer was now equivalent to only 16s compared with 28–41s between 1525 and 1526.[37] In February 1529 male deaths jumped to 142, almost double the highest monthly figure in the preceding sixteen years. The price of grain also reached the highest level, at 117s a bushel or over four times the price in more normal times.[38] All charitable institutions played an important part in dealing with the sick and the hungry. The Commissioners for the Poor used hospitals as a central tool in their policy to deal with the emergency. Hospitals served as distribution points for food and, moreover, 'the said most excellent Lords order the directors of these said hospitals … to receive and accept [these poor sick people] in their said hospitals like the other poor sick people under pain of the anger of the Commissioners'.[39] The increase in the number of people weakened by dearth and its associated diseases led to a significant growth in mortality, three-and-a-half times the average annual total of deaths in these years.

A year later, in spring 1530, conditions must have been even worse at S. Maria Nuova. In February there were 177 male and 217 female deaths, which represented respectively a four- and seven-fold increase on the annual average. This was not linked quite so closely to the price of grain, which the government maintained at a lower level than would have been achieved on a free market. Official prices were now double rather than quadruple the normal level, though grain was not the only foodstuff necessary to survival. These two years also saw some significant variations in patterns of male and female mortality: male mortality was higher in spring 1529, and female mortality higher in June and August 1529 and in spring 1530. The exact reasons for these differences were not recorded by hospital administrators but, as with S. Matteo in the previous century, may be explained by epidemics being confined to first one ward and then crossing the piazza to the other.

The decade of the 1520s was a period of crisis not just for the poor of Florence, but also for S. Maria Nuova, which had fallen into considerable debt by the end of the siege.[40] Though mortality was clearly higher in hospitals during epidemics, none of the levels cited for Tuscan hospitals confirms the prejudices of general textbooks. The Foucaultian assumption that hospitals were hell-holes to which the poor were taken to die is based on the idea that they were places of enforced incarceration. If hospitals in Renaissance Italy had had a reputation as 'portails de la mort', they would hardly have been seen by patients as desirable places for treatment or received the support of affluent patrons who wished to advertise their Christian piety in alleviating the sufferings of the poor. To help explain further the policy of the Renaissance hospital towards patients, I shall turn to examine the lengths of their stay and contemporary diagnoses of their ailments.

8.3 'He Could Only Speak like a Wolf':
Patients and their Ailments

Length of Stay

Relatively low mortality figures suggest exclusion of the moribund in favour of short-term patients. This is largely confirmed by the lengths of their stay. At the Misericordia in Prato for most of the fifteenth century patients stayed on average for twenty-nine days, though over time this decreased until by the 1470s it had halved, reflecting the hospital's change in policy from treating chronic to acute conditions.[41]

The drop in the length of stay of patients at the Misericordia may have stemmed from a deliberate change of policy, as at Messer Bonifazio in 1475:

> I record that this day of 24 January the consuls of the Arte di Calimala [the hospital's patrons] together with two syndics of the hospital ... deliberated that from henceforth one must not nor cannot receive any person, whether male or female, in the hospital of Messer Bonifazio for longer than fifteen days ... except those patients and sick people with fever who should remain at the hospital ... as long as they have need.[42]

Admission citeria thus not only changed over time, but also between hospitals, as reflected in different levels of mortality and lengths of stay.

Table 8.2 Hospital of S. Maria Nuova: length of stay of patients who died: male, 1513–28; female, 1518–27

Stay (days)	F	%F of total F	M	%M of total M	F + M	%F + M of total F + M
<1	36	1.3	54	1.6	90	1.5
1–10	759	28.0	1,603	46.5	2,362	38.3
11–20	540	19.9	858	24.9	1,398	22.7
21–30	287	10.6	358	10.4	645	10.5
31–40	180	6.6	182	5.3	362	5.9
41–50	134	4.9	104	3.0	238	3.9
51–60	130	4.8	83	2.4	213	3.5
61–70	84	3.1	54	1.6	138	2.2
71–80	64	2.4	37	1.1	101	1.6
81–90	68	2.5	22	0.6	90	1.5
91–100	50	1.8	17	0.5	67	1.1
>100	382	14.1	76	2.2	458	7.4
Total	2,714	100.0	3,448	100.0	6,162	100.0

Source: SMN 733–4

The close correlation between these two factors is confirmed at S. Maria Nuova, where patients stayed on average twenty-one days and mortality was 10 per cent.[43] This is clearly reflected in Table 8.2, which analyses lengths of stay for those patients who died in the hospital. In the case of men, virtually half died within the first ten days and a massive 83 per cent within the first thirty days. Although these figures represent the length of stay of those who died rather than of the whole population at risk, when we do know the length of stay of those who died, as at S. Paolo, there was little difference (eight and ten days).[44]

A different pattern emerges from an examination of S. Maria Nuova's women patients. Those admitted who died between 1518 and 1527 stayed for well over twice the length of time of their male counterparts, on average fifty days. Table 8.2 shows that though there was also a bunching of female deaths within the first twenty days, greater numbers of women remained in hospital for longer periods. Only 29 per cent of females died within the first ten days, compared to 48 per cent of males, and 60 per cent of women within thirty days compared with 83 per cent of men. As with males who remained at S. Maria Nuova for longer than thirty days, there was a subsequent tailing off, but 14 per cent of women remained over a hundred days compared with only 2 per cent of men.

The difference in lengths of stay for males and females is striking and suggests that the hospital adopted a different strategy towards the two groups. One possible explanation is that male patients were more sick on arrival and therefore died more rapidly, though this is difficult to prove. Another is that it reflected the fact that the Florentine female population was considerably older than the male.[45] The average age at first marriage was thirty for men and seventeen for women, resulting in a larger number of widowed women.[46] Furthermore, given the low rate of female remarriage, elderly women were often seen as particularly worthy of the support of charitable organisations.[47] In the case of S. Maria Nuova, while the higher proportion of long-stay female patients may indicate, as Katharine Park suggests, a more generous policy towards elderly and chronically sick women,[48] as seen in Chapter 6, it also reflects the hospital's specific policy towards *commesse*.

This range of information about both the mortality rates and the lengths of stay of patients indicates that even though hospitals may have adopted different admissions policies, which themselves could change over time, they all shared an underlying philosophy. The aim was to treat short- rather than long-term conditions; in this way patients left quickly rather than outstaying their welcome. But it would be a mistake to view this entirely from the point of view of the institution. Patients, unless they were very poor, were unlikely to want to remain for long periods in an institution full of sick people whose very breath was believed to spread disease. They would also have been aware, as will be seen in the next section, that the majority of the large medical hospitals in a Renaissance city were meant to treat conditions that could be ameliorated or even cured rapidly.

Ailments

Medieval and Renaissance hospitals rarely recorded evidence systematically about the symptoms or conditions of patients. Such information usually has to be pieced together using a variety of sources.[49] These include scattered references in admission or death books, where they survive, normative records such as statutes, records of purchases of medicines for individuals and, as will be seen in the final chapter, recipe collections such as S. Maria Nuova's 1515 lengthy *Ricettario*.[50] Only S. Paolo's admission book in 1567–8 provides consistent descriptions of symptoms.[51]

Even with this dearth of information a general picture does emerge. As has been seen at the Misericordia in Prato, there was a diminution in the admission of people with more chronic long-stay conditions such as the elderly, cripples, and the deaf and dumb, in favour of people with more specific and acute conditions.[52]

S. Matteo's purchases of simples suggest that it treated a wide variety of conditions,[53] ranging from wounds or fractures after a brawl, to the more frequently cited intestinal disturbances such as *pondi* or the generic category of *piaghe* ('sores'). But S. Matteo was also not without chronic inmates. One example was the blacksmith Piero di Giovanni degli Schiatesi from the parish of S. Lorenzo, whose case was recorded by the *spedalingo*:

> He was brought in on 8 May 1464 to our hospital [and] within a few days by the grace of God he was cured from fever, and he was discharged from the hospital by the infirmarer as it is customary in similar hospitals. [However,] seeing that he was old and incapacitated he asked a number of people and his relatives to beg me that I should maintain him as a poor person for the love of God in the said hospital and I, seeing his wretchedness, was moved through compassion to retain him, seeing that he was old, sick and could only speak like a wolf.[54]

Even though there are scattered reference to S. Matteo accepting others with chronic conditions ('old', 'crippled', 'blind, or even mad'),[55] such cases were in the minority. The rather sporadic information about illness in S. Maria Nuova's 'Books of the Dead' can be supplemented with other types of evidence from statutes and account books. The early sixteenth-century 'Ordinances', for example, mention areas where different conditions were treated. The chapter on the duties of the infirmarer in the ward mentions fevers, skin lesions and wounds, while the role of the *medicheria* was to 'treat those with sores and other minor illnesses'.[56]

The hospital contained two extra rooms for patients with bad wounds or skull fractures: 'this ward has no windows, because fresh air is very bad for patients of this sort ... We have set apart another place for those who have lost their minds through illness, where they are kept in chains.'[57] In both cases the rooms where they were treated had obviously been adapted for their treatment. The first had no windows so as to protect those with skull fractures from the dangers of fresh air, and the second had chains to secure the mentally disturbed so that they could not attack themselves or anybody else in the hospital.[58] S. Matteo also provided an area for the mentally disturbed; in the summer of 1434 the hospital constructed a separate 'house' for 'Bartolomea the mad', where she was kept secure with two hundred locks. These special provisions were sometimes paid for by relatives, as in the case of Sandra, the daughter of Ridolfo, a goldsmith from Prato who assigned to S. Matteo the rent from three shops to cover the expense of keeping her, suggesting that families did use hospitals on occasions as convenient places to which to consign the mentally defective.[59]

If hospital records give no indication about how many 'mad' men or women were treated in this period,[60] S. Paolo's patient registers do record that 6.6 per cent of its 346 patients with diagnoses were wounded.[61] People hurt in street fights were brought to S. Maria Nuova, such as Martino di Piero from the parish of S. Frediano, who died 'from a bullet' within a day of his admission on 12 February 1527.[62] Indeed, all those who were listed as wounded only survived a very short time after they had been brought into the hospital. The same was true of seven others who were recorded without names since they were unable to speak; for instance, 'A boy who could not talk came on 13 May 1527 and died on the same day.'[63] Another of S. Maria Nuova's patients, Antonio di Bartolomeo di Nuto, the hospital's baker, was attacked and killed by an inmate: 'on 10 July 1520 he was wounded by a madman from the hospital and was carried to the ward on a stretcher and died immediately.'[64] Such incidents explain the hospital's need for chains for those 'who have lost their minds', although cases of this kind are not likely to have been common. Indeed, this was the only time such an incident was recorded in these eighteen years, although there was also the case of the suicide of Stefano di Giovanni from Piedmont who was also employed in the hospital: 'A house servant and died on 2 March 1515 and killed himself with a knife cutting his throat in the bed during the night.'[65] Evidently these two men were either dead or nearly so on discovery.

Servants of S. Maria Nuova, like those of S. Matteo, also occasionally picked up the dying and dead on the streets,[66] as is suggested by the forty-nine cases in which the scribe annotated the record with 'morì, non si sa il quando' ('died, don't know when'). Curiously this service was provided almost exclusively in summer and early autumn 1517 when there was a small rise in deaths reflecting an epidemic in the city, rather than during the more severe mortality crises in this period.[67]

Table 8.3 Hospital of S. Paolo: diagnoses of male patients, 1567–8

Diagnoses	No.	%
Fevers	220	60.6
Skin diseases	46	12.7
Boils, ulcers, abscesses	16	4.4
French Disease	15	4.1
Pains	12	3.3
Constitutional illnesses	8	2.2
Accidents	23	6.3
For laxatives	6	1.7
Misc.	17	4.7
Total	363	100.0

Source: ASF, Ospedale di S. Paolo 889; summarised by B. Trexler, 'Hospital Patients in Florence: San Paolo, 1567–68', *Bulletin of the History of Medicine*, 48 (1974), p. 4: Chart A.

To put these patients into a wider context, I shall turn briefly to the remarkably detailed admission book of S. Paolo, which was kept by the *infermiere* Benedetto di Lozo Marini, who recorded the description of each patient's condition on admission in the late 1560s[68] when the hospital contained about thirty-five beds and treated on average 343 patients a year.[69] Fever was the most common reason for admission (61 per cent),[70] exemplified by the entry on 20 May 1568: 'Domenicho di Jachopo, a silk weaver, arrived here sick from fever, with his clothes and without any money.'[71] The term 'fever' was probably a catch-all category for acute conditions, which were short-term and from which the individual was likely to recover. The second major group (17 per cent) was represented by those with skin diseases, boils and ulcers, as in the example of Domenicho d'Antonio Polastro, a labourer of Giovanni from Sommaia, who came on 11 June 1568 'sick from scabby itches [*rogna*]'.[72] Others were admitted for work-related conditions, including 6 per cent of accident victims.

Many of the remaining 19 per cent of conditions described in S. Paolo's register were either fairly generic or mentioned only once. An exception was Mal Francese or the French Disease, which did not appear in the fifteenth-century records of the Misericordia or S. Matteo since it did not become epidemic until the mid-1490s. Although twenty-five of S. Paolo's patients had either attended or were intending to visit the Incurabili hospital of SS. Trinita for Guaiacum wood treatment, this did not guarantee that they had the Mal Francese. Indeed, only four were specifically described in these terms, as in the case of the 'auditor [*riveditore*]' Giulio di Francescho, who when admitted in August 1568 had 'pains [*doglie*] of the Mal Francese'.[73] Incurabili hospitals admitted a wide range of people with what were regarded as 'incurable' diseases,[74] and S. Paolo was seen as a short-term stopping-off place either before or after their course of treatment at SS. Trinita. S. Paolo therefore already acted as a convalescent home for some patients before this officially became its main function later in the century.[75]

The range of diagnoses from S. Paolo confirms that most patients had acute rather than chronic illnesses and that they were expected to recover rather than die. This is in stark contrast to the causes of death given in the city's 'Books of the Dead', where the most prominent were plague, old age, long illnesses and conditions whose main symptoms were associated with diarrhoea among young children.[76] As might be expected, many of the main causes of death in the city were not reflected in hospital figures, especially plague. Illnesses that had higher mortality among children than adults, such as intestinal diseases, would also have made less impact on the hospital population given that few children were admitted.

8.4 *The Different Faces of Poverty*

The two men illustrated in the chapter of S. Spirito's *Liber regulae* on admission procedure (Plate 8.1) were dressed simply in cloaks, knee-length undergarments and caps. They represented many hospital patients in Renaissance Italy for they were not from the poorest levels of society, but rather shopkeepers or craftsmen going through a period of temporary financial crisis. Here, as in other such hospital statutes, patients are represented as passive actors; emphasis is placed on the providers rather than the recipients of charity.

This somewhat stereotypical view of hospital inmates can be fleshed out with other types of evidence to provide a more nuanced picture of their socio-occupational status. At the Misericordia, 11 per cent of its c.3,000 patients carried some indication of their occupation.[77] The largest single group (28 per cent of this sample) was made up of the minor employees of the city's main magistracies: servants, messengers and ushers. In common with the servants or slaves employed by private families (14 per cent), many of them were single men who had come from outside Prato and therefore had little chance of direct support from their own families. The other two sizeable categories of patients were artisans, such as tailors, carpenters and smiths (14 per cent) or wool-industry workers (12 per cent), reflecting the fact that wool manufacture was the single largest employer in the city. In contrast, the smaller number of S. Matteo's patients with such data (12 per cent of the 768 male patients who died in the hospital between 1413 and 1456) were scattered thinly across a very wide range of occupations, excepting the forty-three (48 per cent) religious and the eighteen (20 per cent) servants and slaves.[78] S. Matteo was distinguished from the Misericordia by the presence of more religious, although even so they only represented about 6 per cent of total male deaths.

The patients of the Misericordia and S. Matteo – with the exception of the clergy – had much in common with the clientele of confraternities, the other main source of institutional charity in Italian cities. They appear to have been principally made up of the respectable poor, artisans or state employees either living alone or in families. Because their salaries were relatively low they lived at constant risk from the threat of endemic and epidemic poverty caused by both individual misfortune such as sickness or more generalised factors such as famines and epidemics.[79]

This concentration by charitable institutions on the 'respectable poor' is usually taken to have excluded the large numbers of beggars and vagrants who undoubtedly thronged the streets of Renaissance cities in search of a livelihood. Such a focus was partly the result of financial factors (since charities had limited resources they had to restrict their clientele) and partly of religious factors (it was better to be seen to be supporting those who lived 'respectably' according to the social and moral norms of the day). However, this raises the question as to why so few people should have been listed with a trade in the records. Was this entirely random, dependent on the diligence of the scribe, or were there in fact beggars and vagrants among the 90 per cent of hospital patients not recorded with occupations?

Examples of very poor people seeking admission to hospital are shown in Domenico di Bartolo's frescoes in Siena where he represents a semi-clad man dressed in rags and a crippled beggar (Plate 8.2). Indeed, the description of the clothes worn by hospital patients provides a clue to social and economic status: 29 per cent of the men and 8 per cent of women admitted to S. Matteo were described as wearing rags and a further 30 per cent of men and 21 per cent of women were described as being in a very miserable state.[80] A typical example is Antonio di Guglielmo from Arezzo, who died on 25 November 1418 after six days in the hospital and who left behind 'certain rags of clothes of little value'.[81] Clothes of any value were recorded on patients' arrival to be returned to them on exit or, if they died, given to relations or sold. The types of clothes sold by S. Maria Nuova to the second-hand clothes dealer Jacopo on 18 December 1370 are representative:

1 large tunic of coarse undyed woollen cloth for a man
1 doublet in bad condition
1 man's full-length garment with a hood, torn
1 man's ragged cloak of coarse undyed woollen cloth
1 cloak and hood in bad condition
2 torn rags of coarse undyed woollen cloth
1 woman's black skirt [*gonnelluccia*] in bad condition
1 rag of bright blue cloth
1 rag of mixed cloth[82]

Each of these entries underlines the poor condition of the clothes; the majority were in rags, whether a man's ragged cloak or a woman's black *gonnelluccia*. The owners were probably among the poorest patients; their clothes had been sold as they were among the 10 per cent who had died in the hospital and no relative had come forward to claim their goods.

The evidence of socio-economic status presented so far suggests that these hospitals had a preference for treating the respectable poor, including artisans, shopkeepers and servants or their wives, who had fallen on hard times, though some of those without a declared occupation may have been from lower down the social scale. While sharing a common general policy, each of these institutions also appears to have had a preference for helping certain categories of people: the Misericordia for minor government employees, S. Matteo for religious, and S. Paolo for cloth workers. This provides a wider context for interpreting the more limited occupational data of the men who died at S. Maria Nuova (Table 8.4) in the early sixteenth century (this information is given for only 6.3 per cent).

Three main categories stand out among these 384 occupations: services, religious and textiles, together accounting for 60 per cent of the total (Table 8.4). The prominence of 'services' is explained by the fact that over half were the hospital's own servants and *commessi*, a few of whom were described with a specific occupation. These included a stationer, a carrier and a notary; for example, Ser Andrea da Matteo, who before entering S. Maria Nuova as a perpetual servant had been employed by the Buondemonti family.[83] Some had a medical background, as in the case of Francesco di Maestro Antonio Binieri and Francesco di Maestro Gabriello of Milan,[84] while four others were surgeons' assistants.[85]

There were also eighty-two members of the clergy, some of whom worked for S. Maria Nuova, including Ser Antonio di Silvestro from Cerreto who was described as a 'chericho di chasa', Prete Piero who was a 'chapelano di chasa', the priest Batista from Prato, who was the 'confesorio dello spedale', and the friar Ipolito from Colle Valdelsa who had worked as a nurse.[86] The thirty-four friars were drawn from the mendicant orders, although the majority were Augustinians, Carmelites or Franciscans, along with two hermits, including one from Monte Morello, a high and wild area to the north of Florence. Some friars were residents of their orders in the city, while others came from other parts of Italy and from as far afield as England, France and Spain. They would probably have died in the room known as the Sapientia, where Luther would have stayed during his sojourn in Florence on his way to Rome in 1510–11.[87]

Table 8.4 Hospital of S. Maria Nuova: occupational data for male patients who died, 1513–30

Occupation	No.	%
Administration/ professional	30	7.8
Textiles	61	15.9
Leather	21	5.5
Metal	20	5.2
Wood/stone	30	7.8
Food/drink	25	6.5
Service	86	22.4
Labourers	16	4.2
Soldiers	4	1.0
Religious	82	21.4
Misc.	9	2.3
Total	384	100.0

Source: SMN 733

It is not surprising that the occupations of these two most numerous categories should have been recorded given that servants and the clergy would have been known personally to the scribe. In general, the other occupations given were representative of the city, the most prominent of which was the manufacture and distribution of textiles (15.9 per cent). This was the main local employer and significantly nearly half of these men were weavers, the third most numerous occupation listed in the Catasto of Florence.[88] The other categories listed in Table 8.4 are fairly evenly distributed, although significantly two of the more numerous occupations, notaries and cobblers, were also well represented in the Catasto of 1427.[89]

S. Maria Nuova also catered for patients at the other end of the social scale, as was made clear in its 'Ordinances': 'The hospital also has eight rooms with hearths, washbasins, toilets, and other amenities reserved for the sick of higher social class, such as nobles, who have decided to come to us for treatment on account of poverty or a religious vow. We look after them with great care.'[90] But

Table 8.5 Hospital of S. Maria Nuova: patients with surnames, 1513–30

High Status	17
Medium Status	2
Low Status	4
Others	16
Total	39

(For names see below, Appendix 8.1; cf. A. Molho, *Marriage Alliance in Late Medieval Florence* (Cambridge, Mass., 1994), Appendix 8.1 for categories)
Source: SMN 733–4

though few upper-class patients were listed among those who died at S. Maria Nuova – thirty-nine were recorded with a surname – this need not imply that this part of the hospital was not well used, but rather that they returned home to die. If these men were representative of the families who used these facilities, it suggests that the hospital did cater for those at the highest level of society, as can be seen in Table 8.5. This list has been divided into three main social categories, according to Anthony Molho's system of dividing lineages into high, medium and low, along with families that did not appear in any of these lists.[91] It is interesting, if not statistically significant, that of the twenty-three people who fell into these three categories, seventeen were 'high status' and came from some of the leading families who dominated Renaissance Florence. They included the Capponi, Frescobaldi, Machiavelli, Pitti, Serragli and Strozzi. Perhaps not surprisingly, the leaders of these lineages did not themselves die in S. Maria Nuova and the deceased men were probably from minor rather than major branches of these families and, as the 'Ordinances' suggest, came on account of their poverty. Some of these people listed as being among the hospital's dead may have been *commessi*; as has been seen in Chapter 6, in the 1540s only 23 per cent were identified with a surname. A hospital was also used as a place of temporary accommodation by the more affluent. For example, a biographer of Alessandro de' Medici recorded that he was born at S. Matteo, where his parents had been staying temporarily while they were in the process of moving house: 'Ser Alessandro was born [on 2 June 1536] in this place in the rooms that had previously been used by the hospital director'.[92] Other rooms (see Chapter 6) bore the names of particular families where members or their guests may have stayed for short periods or even on retreat.

Until this point I have concentrated on the occupations and social status of male patients since here, as in many other types of contemporary record, the occupations of females were not recorded.[93] Even so, it is possible to piece together a general picture of women patients. It is known that for at least one year, 1528–9, female mortality was higher (26 per cent compared to male at 17 per cent).[94] Furthermore, as seen above, women stayed for much longer periods, on average fifty days compared with twenty-one days for men.[95] It is also possible to calculate their marital status: 28 per cent were widowed, 19 per cent were single and the rest were married (Table 8.6), which in fact reflects the figures of the marital status of women in the city generally.[96] The presence of a large number of married women points to the strain placed on the family budget by the sickness of one of its adult members, particularly in the 1520s, and contrasts with S. Matteo, which had a more specific mission to help widows.[97]

Table 8.6 Hospital of S. Maria Nuova: marital status of female patients who died, 1518–30

	No.	%
Single	561	19.3
Married	1,443	49.7
Widowed	798	27.5
Unknown	101	3.5
Total	2,903	100.0

Source: SMN 734

It is above all the family circumstances of patients that help one to understand why they sought admission. The fact that fewer of the more affluent went to hospitals suggests that people preferred to be treated at home if they could afford it, but this was not a viable option for the many. This was especially true of those who came from outside Florence since they would have left behind them their networks of support. Indeed, the following section, which analyses the provenance of S. Maria Nuova's patients, is an important key to understanding the appeal of this large Renaissance hospital.

8.5 *Cittadini and Contadini*

Once the sick person had been assigned to a bed, he [the sub-infirmarer] … notes his name, father's name, place of origin, family name, and the amount of money he is carrying, if any, and he writes all this on a label attached to the bundle [of clothes].

S. Maria Nuova, 'Ordinances', 1510–11, p. 181[98]

A patient's geographical origins were among the most consistently recorded details in admission and mortality registers. They served as a form of identification since few Italians in this period had surnames. An analysis of the provenance of over eight thousand male and female patients who entered and died in S. Maria Nuova in the early sixteenth century is presented in Table 8.7 and examined in more detail in Maps 8.1 and 8.2.[99]

Table 8.7 S. Maria Nuova: provenance of all patients who died, 1513–30

1. Florence	N*	%
City	1,965	23.4
suburbs +	533	6.4
Total	2,498	29.8
2. *Contado*	3,263	38.9
3. Rest of Tuscany	814	9.7
4. Italy		
North	650	
Centre (excl. Tuscany)	53	
South	45	
Corsica, Elba, Sardinia	15	
Total	763	9.1
5. Outside Italy		
Dalmatia	15	
Flanders	30	
France	92	
Germany (Bassa e Alta)	176	
Spain	19	
Switzerland	18	
Others	19	
Total	369	4.4
6. Unknown total	679	8.1
Overall total	8,386	100.0

* Male and female patients combined
+ Equivalent to the Piviere di San Giovanni, the area within a 9.5-km radius of the city walls.
(I have followed E. Conti, *La formazione della struttura agraria moderna nel contado fiorentino* (Rome, 1965), in adopting the modern administrative divisions for Tuscany and the *contado*).
Source: SMN 733–4

A distinctive picture emerges from this analysis.[100] First, just 23 per cent of patients dying at S. Maria Nuova were identified as being from the city of Florence itself, a figure that increases to 30 per cent if one includes those from the 'suburbs' or the Piviere di S. Giovanni, the area within a 9.5 km radius of the city walls. In other words, S. Maria Nuova exercised a strong attraction over patients who came from further afield, including not just those in Florence on a temporary basis, looking for work or to sell their wares in the markets, but also new arrivals who had already found employment. Some people may have come specifically for treatment, knowing that they would receive more specialised help from the larger general hospitals of the capital than from a local hospital. It was established practice for smaller hospitals outside the capital to send their patients to S. Maria Nuova, as recorded at the Misericordia in Prato and the Serristori hospital in Figline Valdarno.[101]

Given that only 30 per cent of patients were from the city and its environs, it is striking that virtually 50 per cent came from the rest of Tuscany (a total of 4,077). As can be seen from Map 8.1, their distribution was not even; very broadly, the highest concentration in the category of over two hundred

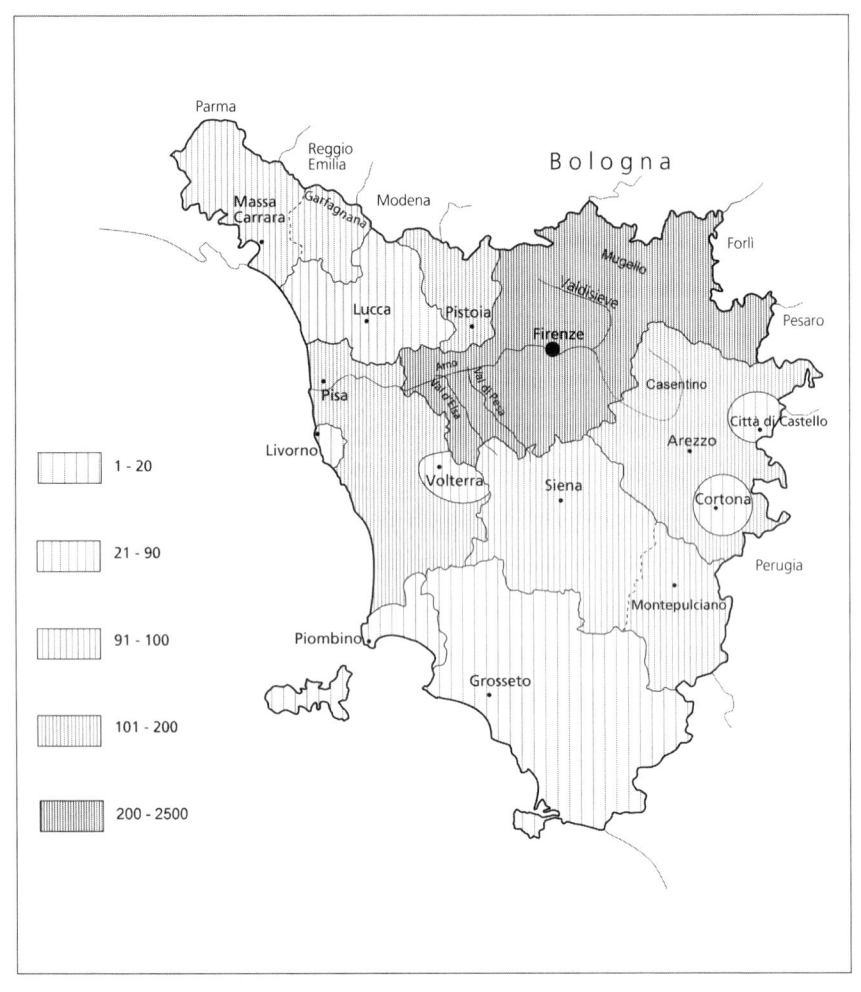

Map 8.1 Provenance of patients who died at S. Maria Nuova, 1513–30: Tuscany
Source: SMN 733–4

patients was in the old Florentine territory (*contado*).[102] The next category, 101–200 patients, was represented by the more recently acquired subject territories, including Pistoia to the north-west, Pisa to the west and Arezzo to the south-east. Those regions that contributed fewer than a hundred patients were ruled over by the independent states of Siena to the south, stretching as far down as the Grossetano on the south-west coast, and Lucca to the north-west. This points to the strength of political barriers between the various Tuscan states. It also underlines the attraction of some of the larger hospitals in regional capitals, such as S. Maria della Scala in Siena and S. Luca della Misericordia in Lucca. A similar explanation may be behind the fact that relatively few patients came from areas within the Florentine territory such as Cortona, Città di Castello and Volterra.

Economic factors would also have played an important role in accounting for the presence of *stranieri* in the city since Florence was one of the largest employers in Italy, with a wide range of commercial, artisanal and industrial activities. The very specific requirements of local industry help to explain the presence of patients who came from outside Tuscany and also reflect changes in the Florentine economy from the second half of the fifteenth century. It is striking that few people came from other parts of south-central Italy – the Marche and Umbria – and even fewer from the southern states. Instead there was a significant presence from north of the Apennines, Emilia Romagna and especially Lombardy.

This suggests that, outside Tuscany, geographical proximity was not the main factor in determining the presence of these northern Italians in the city. It had more to do with the need for skilled workers. The Tuscan construction industry had a long tradition of employing Lombard masons, the number of whom had increased with the building boom in Florence in the second half of the fifteenth century.[103] It was above all the textile industry that attracted the largest number of 'foreigners'. The proportion of non-Tuscan weavers employed in the woollen industry had risen between 1380 and 1480 from 6 to 20 per cent.[104] In the same period there was a significant growth in the manufacture of silk cloth, so that by the late Quattrocento it was almost as important as the woollen-cloth industry, traditionally the largest employer in the city. By the later fifteenth century the woollen industry concentrated on high-quality cloth, which led to a growing demand for specialised workers, as did the silk industry's specialisation in luxury embroidery, neither of which the local labour force had traditionally been trained to produce.[105]

The growth of the silk industry also helps to explain the importance of workers from Low and High Germany (Bassa and Alta Germania). Those from German-speaking areas, including Flanders, alone represented over half of all foreign patients who died in S. Maria Nuova during these years. The majority were probably silk weavers, who had been attracted to the city by a series of tax concessions offered by the Florentine commune in the fifteenth century.[106] The appearance of people from the other countries, even ones as far-flung as Poland, England and Scotland, may also be related to commercial links. This is certainly the case with the significant group of ninety-two who came from France.

The picture that emerges from this general analysis of the provenance of patients broadly confirms the results of other studies of the period: the largest number came from the *contado*, roughly a quarter from the city itself, followed by northern Italy and the German-speaking area of northern Europe. What seems to distinguish S. Maria Nuova in the early sixteenth century from how it was in the Quattrocento is that a larger proportion of patients came from Tuscany.

In order to examine this further I shall look in more detail at the geographical origins of patients within the *contado* (see Map 8.2).[107] Following the practice of recent historians of Florence and its countryside, I have allocated the geographical origins of patients according to the present-day administrative divisions of the *contado*.[108] It is evident immediately that the distribution of patients was far from uniform throughout the area. As seen above, Florence and the Piviere di S. Giovanni, the surrounding area within a radius of about 9.5 km, were the greatest sources, with almost a third coming from the city and this suburban area.[109] If this is not totally unexpected given the physical location of S. Maria Nuova, what is more surprising is that there were hardly any parts of the *contado* that did not contribute patients (shown in white). Even so, the majority of patients did come from within 20 km of the capital and all the areas contributing fifty or more individuals were within this zone. S. Maria Nuova's main catchment area therefore stretched from Empoli in the west (71) and Dicomano in the east (66) to Greve in the south (134) and Barberino di Mugello in the north (193).[110]

The explanation for this pattern of distribution of both patients and areas of settlement lies above all in the physical characteristics of the region. The Florentine *contado* was bounded to the north by the mountain ranges of the Apennines and to the south-east by the Casentino, making a place such as Stia relatively inaccessible, particularly in winter. Hence the vast majority of patients came from along river valleys, as in the case of the River Sieve, which formed an arc at a distance of about 25 km from north to east of the capital, and contained a series of small settlements from S. Piero a Sieve and Borgo S. Lorenzo to Vicchio and Dicomano. The river valley of the Arno which ran west and south-east of Florence also supplied patients from places such as Empoli and Signa in the west to Rignano and Figline in the south-east. Another important contributory factor in the distribution of the provenance of patients, reflecting again the location of urban settlements, was their posi-

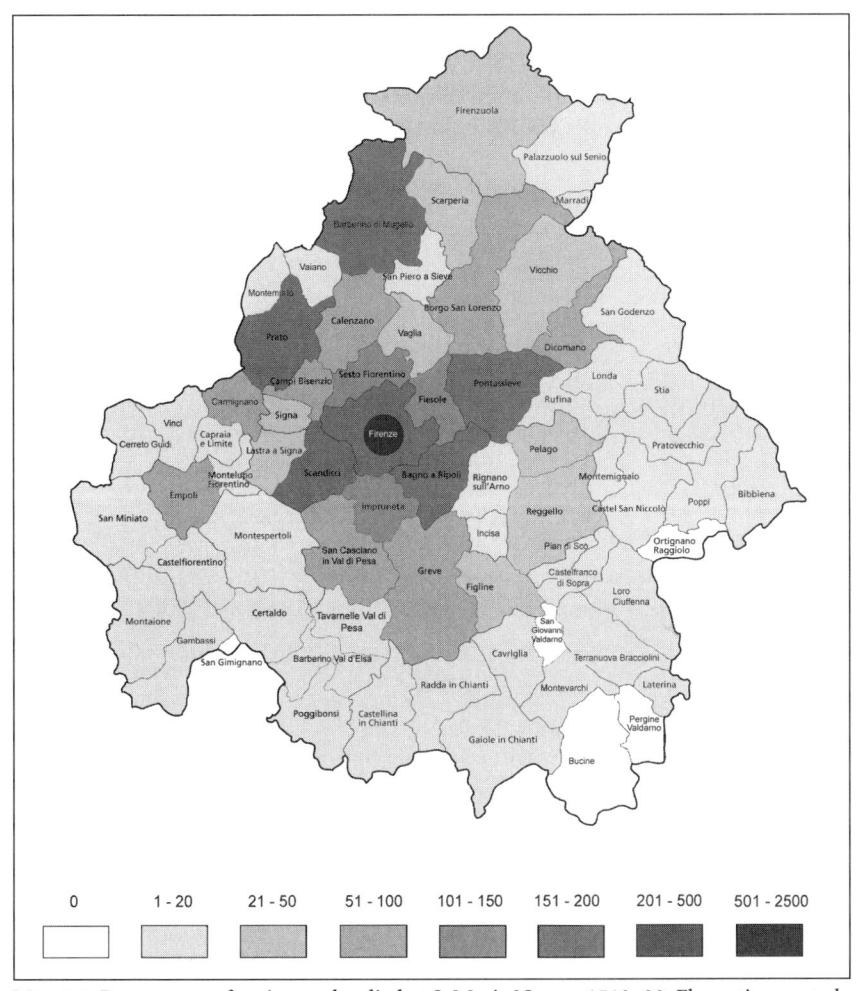

Map 8.2 Provenance of patients who died at S. Maria Nuova, 1513–30: Florentine *contado*
Source: SMN 733–4

tion on axial roads leading out of Tuscany, as in the case of Borgo S. Lorenzo and Firenzuola on the road to Bologna and S. Casciano in Val di Pesa and Tavarnelle on the two roads to Siena.

At the most general level, the pattern of patient provenance reflects the distribution of population within the *contado*. People from very rural areas were more likely to have gone to local medical practitioners, surgeons and women healers than to have travelled long distances to receive treatment in a hospital. This is in contrast to the findings of Philip Gavitt, who concluded that many of the foundlings admitted to the Innocenti in the mid-fifteenth century came from the mountainous areas to the north and east of Florence.[111] The difference is illuminating because it underlines the different roles of these two institutions. Whereas the Innocenti dealt with problems that stemmed from the chronic poverty of *contadini*, S. Maria Nuova instead dealt with acute cases when more immediate treatment was desirable.

Table 8.8 Provenance of S. Maria Nuova's patients in the *contado* within 40 km of Florence, 1513–30*

Distance from Florence	Patients	
	N	%
Band 1 > 10 km		
Bagno a Ripoli	246	8.9
Fiesole	187	6.8
Sesto	192	7.0
Scandicci	220	8.0
Total	845	30.7
Band 2 > 20 km		
Pontassieve (incl. Rignano and Pelago)	276	10.1
Prato and contado	180	6.6
Campi Bisenzio	110	4
Calenzano	98	3.6
Impruneta	108	4.1
S. Casciano Val di Pesa	100	3.7
Vaglia	63	2.3
Total	935	34.4
Band 3 > 30 km		
Borgo S. Lorenzo	125	4.5
Greve	134	4.8
Barberino di Mugello[†]	193	7.0
Scarperia	54	2.0
Carmignano	58	2.1
Pelago	52	1.9
Total	616	22.3
Band 4 > 40 km		
Dicomano	66	2.5
Empoli	71	2.6
Vicchio	58	2.1
S. Miniato	75	2.7
Tavernelle Val di Pesa	78	2.8
Total	348	12.7
Overall total	2,744	100

* only includes areas with over fifty patients
[†] incls. 117 described as from the Mugello, and 2 from Val di Sieci. (I have followed E. Conti, *La formazione della struttura agraria moderna nel contado fiorentino*, Rome, 1965, in adopting the modern administrative divisions for Tuscany and the *contado*)
Source: SMN 733–4

With this general guide to the provenance of S. Maria Nuova's patients from within the Florentine *contado*, I shall now turn to look in more detail at the inter-relationship between numbers and distance.

The attraction of Florence can be well appreciated from Table 8.8, which relates those areas within 40 km that contributed more than fifty patients. Thus, the four areas within 10 km of the city centre contributed 845 patients or almost a quarter of all the *contadini* who died at S. Maria Nuova in these years. While geographical proximity remained a strong influence in the three other zones, it diminished with distance. The next circle (11–20 km from Florence) included more areas and contributed a higher overall number of patients, but the average per locality was lower (136 compared to 211), a pattern also repeated in Bands 3 and 4.

Distance was not the only determinant to affect provenance, as can be seen from the geographical location of patients (Map 8.2 and Table 8.8). It is striking that over half the areas represented in Table 8.8 were to the north of the city (twelve of twenty-two). However, this also changed according to distance and proximity to other urban centres with substantial hospitals. There were fewer patients from places to the west and north-west, like Vaiano and Montemurlo, because they would have fallen into the catchment area of Prato, and Vinci and Cerreto Guidi were closer to Pistoia than Florence. The same was true to the south, with a lower number of patients from, for example, Castellina, Gaiole and Radda; the acute sick from those areas were more likely to have gone to S. Maria della Scala in Siena. More generally, as mentioned above, one of the fundamental factors affecting the distribution of patients was population density within the *contado*, explaining the relatively few people who came to S. Maria Nuova from the mountainous Casentino area between Florence and Arezzo. This is a subject that would benefit from considerably more exploration in relation to patients from all the major hospitals in Tuscany and the ways in which their services interconnected.

Conclusion

There is little doubt that physical incapacity caused by illness was one of the main reasons that patients sought admission to hospitals in Renaissance Italy. Indeed, most general hospitals, apart from normally excluding those sick from chronic or epidemic disease, give the impression of accepting all-comers, 'the poor sick … almost like Christ in their persons'.[112] Even so, this general expression of Christian charity could be misleading, for indications of patients' occupations suggest that hospitals may have been selective. They concentrated on the humble respectable poor, such as shop-keepers and small master-craftsmen or servants, and in towns such as Florence and Prato on those who worked for the government or the main local employer, the textile industry.

Given that even a wealthy institution such as S. Maria Nuova had finite resources which led it to adopt a selective policy, what proportion of the population received treatment? As has been seen, one way of tackling this question is to examine the number of beds per institution, which I have calculated was about 245 for the four main medical hospitals in the city by the early fifteenth century. With a capacity of two patients per bed these four hospitals alone would have provided in-house treatment at any one time for about five hundred patients, equivalent to 1.3 per cent of the city's population at the time of the 1427 Catasto. However, this calculation is a bare minimum; it does not take into account either their out-patient services or the facilities of the many other *spedali*. Furthermore, these figures cannot be more than approximate for they do not tell us anything about turnover and the actual capacities of the majority of hospitals are unknown. Only in the case of S. Maria Nuova is it possible to provide more exact figures; as has been seen, by the early sixteenth century it received on average 6,500 male and female patients every year. This is a very large number of people and would have meant that 9.3 per cent of the city's resident population of seventy thousand could have received in-house treatment over the course of a year, though it has to be remembered that this included many non-resident patients. Contemporaries were well aware of the importance of its services to the sick poor, just as they were of those provided for orphaned children by the Innocenti, which Varchi claimed took care of over a thousand children.

If the picture painted by Varchi of the charitable institutions of Florence is relatively accurate, it is worth comparing it with accounts of hospitals by his contemporaries from other cities. In Milan, for example, Giovanni Giacomo Gilino provided a detailed account of the Ospedale Maggiore in 1508, comparable to the 'Ordinances' of S. Maria Nuova compiled for King Henry VII of England in the same years (see Introduction). Gilino described the medical services and personnel, including physicians, surgeons and nursing staff, and recorded that the number of patients admitted each year was over two thousand.[113] If this figure can be believed, the activities of the Ospedale Maggiore were on a substantial scale, for even though the number of patients was lower than at S. Maria Nuova, it also catered for more than a thousand foundlings.

Though there are few detailed studies of patient records of Italian hospitals for this period, other types of quantitative and qualitative records suggest that most general hospitals admitted or excluded the same categories of patient. At S. Maria della Scala in Siena, emphasis was placed on acute conditions, while those with chronic illnesses such as lepers and cripples were excluded.[114] The same was true at another of the large famous medieval foundations, S. Spirito in Rome, which looked after large numbers of poor and sick people and, in common with the Milanese and Sienese hospitals, took in foundlings. A hospital in Rome that has remarkably detailed admission and exit registers is the Incurabili hospital of S. Giacomo in Augusta. Founded in 1515 to treat the crowds of those sick from the French Disease who had flocked to Rome for charity and medical care, it expanded rapidly over the sixteenth century until by the 1590s it was treating some 2,500 patients a year.[115] Bearing in mind the existence also of a large network of substantial hospitals in the city, the scale of S. Giacomo's activities was impressive for a specialised institution. Here, as in the case of the Tuscan general hospitals, mortality was relatively low; it rarely rose above 12 per cent per annum, except, as at S. Maria Nuova, during epidemics and dearth.[116]

Thus, patient experience at S. Maria Nuova and other Florentine hospitals was not unrepresentative of other general hospitals in Italy, with rapid turnover, concentration on minor acute diseases, except in specialised hospitals, and relatively low mortality *pace* the traditional prejudices of historians. Where S. Maria Nuova and the other major medical hospitals in Florence seem to have been different from some of the hospitals in other major Italian cities is that they specialised exclusively in the acute sick rather than also housing incurables and orphans.

This general characterisation of Italian hospitals should not lead one to conclude that this policy was necessarily typical of other parts of Europe at this time. For example, in mid-fifteenth-century Barcelona the admission registers of the general hospital of Santa Creu record that almost half of the patients were suffering from acute diseases such as fever, but mortality was much higher than in Tuscan hospitals (26 per cent), perhaps owing to the traditional policy of medieval Castilian hospitals to care for the aged.[117] Mortality was even higher at the hôtel-Dieu in Paris in the late fifteenth century (c.33 per cent), reflecting a different policy towards patients and their care. The hospital was an impressive complex, with four large wards containing 279 beds for the sick, but also, in common with many French hôtels-Dieu hospitals, it had twenty-four beds for women giving birth. Though the capacity of the hôtel-Dieu was much greater than that of S. Maria Nuova, normally it treated fewer patients, about 1,500 a year. Higher mortality was explained partly by the fact the hôtel-Dieu accepted more chronic patients than many Italian hospitals and beds were occupied on average by three people.[118]

These examples from cities outside Florence have shown that policies of hospitals changed according to circumstance and geographical location. The evidence of cities such as Barcelona and Paris has suggested a tendency to accept more long-term chronic patients with attendant higher rates of mortality, and the same pattern was true for late medieval England, where the average hospital was on a much smaller scale than its continental counterparts. Even when they were larger, as in London, Norwich and York, there was an increasing tendency for them to become preoccupied with housing more affluent corrodians rather than looking after the sick poor.[119]

The wider implications of these regional and national differences and similarities concerning the treatment of the sick cannot be properly appreciated before further studies of patient records have been published and before these results have then been examined within the wider demographic contexts in relation to changing systems of social and welfare services available for the poor. What is clear, however, from even a brief comparison between hospitals in Italian urban centres and their counterparts in many areas of northern Europe is that the former experienced a much earlier and more widespread development of their medical services and therefore a precocious concentration on the sick poor. In Florence, as seen above, this process was reflected in the growing number of doctors employed by hospitals and in their treatment of a wide variety of ailments. The next chapter will examine this process of medicalisation in greater depth by looking at the practice of medicine and in particular at the recipes prescribed by hospital doctors.

Appendix 8.1

S. Maria Nuova's Patients with Surnames

High Status

Benci, Pagolo di Niccholò ('scrivano in Fondacetto di S. Maria Nuova')
Bini, Bino di Pasquino da Pistoia
Chaponi, Francescho di Bernardo
Ciaia, moglie di Giuliano
Corsini
Freschobaldi, Lorenzo di Tomaso
Lapi
Machiavegli, Nicholò di Bernardo
Martelli (Martegli), Domenicho di Domenicho
Pazzi, Ghaleazzo de'
Pitti: Neri di Buonachorso di Neri (popolo di S. Maria a Chastello); Bonaccorso di Luca
Salviati, Prete Timoteo di Lionardo
Serragli, Lorenzo di Giuliano di Firenze
Strozzi: ? di Alessandro; Lionardo di Stagio d'Antonio; Piero di Nicholo
Total: 17

Medium Status

Del Bene, Antonio di Zanobi
Riccardi, Ricciardo di Bernardo
Total: 2

Low Status

Borghini
Buonacorsi (Buonacoliti), Buonacholito di Piero
Buoninsegni, Giovanni di Charlo
Toregli (*commesso*)
Total: 4

Others Surnames

Attavanti, Lorenzo di Domenicho
Banchelli, Piero di Giovanni (Partereno)
Binieri
Borghese, Piero do Pagolo
Buonaiuto
Busaragli, Biagio d'Antonio da Piano di Ripoli
Cacci, Raffaello di Giovanni
Chonsigli, vedova di Pietro
Della Valle, Franciescho d'Antonio da Scharperia
Dalla Volta, Jachopo
Di Pace, Rinieri di Franciescho
Forchoni, Lorenzo di Franciescho di Matteo
Lanfranchi, Giampiero da Riccho Pisano
Mechini, Lorenzo d'Antonio da Settignano
Panini, Antonio di Bartolommeo d'Andrea
Razzini, Ser Tonino di Giannotto
Total: 16
Overall Total: 39
Source: SMN 733–4

Appendix 8.2

Provenance of Patients from S. Maria Nuova: Florence and Contado

Location	Total
a. **Florence & suburbs**	2,499
b. *Contado*	
201–500	
Pontassieve	276
Bagno a Ripoli	246
Scandicci	220
151–200	
Sesto Fiorentino	192
Barberino di Mugello*	193
Fiesole	187
Prato	180

*Incl. 117 described as from the 'Mugello' and two from the 'Sieci'

101–50
Greve	134
Borgo S. Lorenzo	125
S. Godenzo	117
Campi Bisenzio	110
Impruneta	108

51–100
S. Casciano Val di Pesa*	100
Calenzano	98
Tavarnelle Val di Pesa*	78
S. Miniato al Tedesco	75
Reggello	73
Empoli	71
Dicomano	66
Vaglia	63
Carmignano	58
Vicchio	58
Scarperia	54
Pelago	52

21–50
Signa	43
Montelupo Fiorentino	43
Londa	39
Certaldo	39
Firenzuola	37
Lastra a Signa	35
Figline Valdarno	34
Castelfiorentino	34
Poggibonsi	27
Cerreto Guidi	24
Incisa	21

1–20
Castelfranco di Sopra	20
S. Piero a Sieve	20
Montespertoli	18
Rufina	17
Montevarchi	15
Terranuova Bracciolini	15
Gaiole in Chianti	14
Barberino Val d'Elsa	13
Vinci	13
Poppi	10
Radda in Chianti	9
Pratovecchio	8
Montemurlo	8
Castellina	7

*Incl. 50 from 'Val di Pesa'

Stia	7
Bibbiena	7
Montaione	6
Marradi	6
Laterina	5
Cavriglia	5
Loro Ciuffenna	5
Castel S. Niccolò	5
Gambassi	3
Capraia e Limite	2
Palazzuolo sul Senio	2
Montemignaio	2
Pian di Scò	1

0
S. Giovanni Valdarno
Bucine
Ortignano Raggiolo
Source: SMN 733–4

CHAPTER 9

TREATING THE POOR: APOTHECARIES, PILLS AND POTIONS

Introduction

Earlier chapters have traced the process of the 'medicalisation' of some of the city's larger hospitals through their concentration on treating the sick poor. This led to the employment of a growing number of professional medical staff, among whom were some of the leading practitioners of the day who were attracted by security and prestige. Another hallmark of 'medicalisation' was the employment of an apothecary, who played a crucial role as intermediary between practitioner and patient. Indeed, a brief discussion of the role of the apothecary (*speziale*) and the hospital pharmacy provides an essential introduction to the main focus of this chapter, an analysis of the comprehensive collection of recipes contained in S. Maria Nuova's early sixteenth-century recipe book. This study, the first of its kind for pre-industrial Italy, is important because it enables one to examine the implementation of medical theory in the practice of medicine in one of the largest medical institutions in Europe.

9.1 'To Make the Medicines and Syrups that Need to Be Made Up for our Patients': Apothecaries and Pharmacies

Apothecaries

The duties of a hospital apothecary were laid out in the contract between S. Matteo and Girolamo di Ser Nicholaio di Neri in 1507:[1]

> [he]is obliged to do everything that appertains to [the duties of a *speziale*] in the pharmacy and to make the medicines and syrups that need to be made up for our patients and to help the servants when our patients are fed, and to take care not to make mistakes at the times when [a patient's] fever is increasing and [to help] with all their other necessities. With this [contract] he is not obliged to undertake guard duties by night more than is needed,

except in cases of necessity, since he does not have the right of board and lodging in our hospital.

This contract was subject to the judgement of the prior in office at the time.

As was also the practice at another medium-sized hospital, Messer Bonifazio, the apothecary combined his office with the duties of an infirmarer; only S. Maria Nuova needed and could afford to employ one full time. The apothecary's primary responsibility was to prepare the medicaments prescribed for the treatment of the sick. At S. Matteo he also helped feed patients, since diet, as one of the six non-naturals, was seen as being as important as simple or compound medicines. But the *speziale* was credited with more responsibility than an ordinary nurse, as can be seen from the injunction to take special care when a patient's fever was rising. Mistakes had evidently been made in the past in the treatment of fever patients, who predominated among people admitted to general medical hospitals.[2]

The final clause of Girolamo's annual contract stipulated a salary of 96 lire and that these conditions of employment were subject to the judgement of the prior or *spedalingo*, which suggests that they could be changed according to circumstances, whether relating to the hospital's finances, the number of patients or the demands of the apothecary himself. For example, though Girolamo did not live in the hospital, the contract of one of his predecessors, Maestro Giovanni di Marcho Nuti, specified that 'he must be resident and stay continuously in our hospital'.[3] Enforcing the authority of the *spedalingo* was also necessary if an apothecary misbehaved, as in September 1496 when the *spedalingo* of S. Matteo discovered that Piero di Capo had 'created many scandals', although what sins he committed were not recorded.[4]

S. Maria Nuova's early sixteenth-century 'Ordinances' laid down the relationship between the apothecary and his staff and their interaction with physicians.[5] The pharmacist's assistant would record in a notebook the treatment prescribed by the physician on his daily ward round and, after he left, 'the pharmacist makes up all the prescriptions and gives them back in order to the infirmarer'. Care was taken so that each patient received the correct treatment: 'The name of the sick person for whom these remedies are prescribed is written on a scrap of paper; the bed number also serves to identify the flasks or trays used to bring the patient his medication.' These medical recipes were then copied into a book, as will be seen in the discussion below of a late fifteenth-century register of the Misericordia in Prato.[6]

Girolamo's contract and the 'Ordinances' together provide a clear idea of the duties of an apothecary in a Renaissance hospital. However, this picture represents the culmination of a long process. In their initial periods of growth hospitals contracted one or more independent apothecaries to supply them. In the mid-1320s, for example, S. Maria Nuova paid two *speziali*, Ser Baldo and Naldo of the Mercato Vecchio, for simple and compound medicines, candles and wax as well as sweetmeats, including white sugar, *penidi* (a sort of sugared cake) and crystallised fruit, which was a regular part of a patient's diet.[7] This arrangement continued after the Black Death; in 1351 the hospital purchased various kinds of medicines, including rose-water and 'herbs to make medicines, pills and unguents', which were made up by an apothecary, Francesco di Gerino, in his workshop on the orders of its physician, Francesco Noli.[8]

Such associations point to the close links between physicians and apothecaries. It was standard practice for doctors to see and treat patients in an apothecary's workshop. All medicines would then be bought directly from the apothecary, although it was prohibited by law for physicians to share the profits in order to prevent them from prescribing expensive recipes to increase their profit.[9] These professional links were often reinforced through family bonds or marriage, as in the case of the Florentine diarist and apothecary Luca Landucci, who was related to both *speziali* and physicians.[10] These ties would also have had important implications for those doctors and apothecaries employed by hospitals for, as in so much of Florentine society, hospitals would have built up connections with particular professional families and suppliers. S. Maria Nuova's *speziale* Piero di Giovanni Fruosino may have been related to the miniaturist Bartolommeo di Fruosino, who was employed by the hospital in this period, and also to the *spedalingo* Michele di Fruosino (1413–43).[11]

The purchase of simple and compound medicines did not preclude hospitals from having an area for storage and preparation, as suggested by S. Maria Nuova's order in June 1351: 'we pay on the said day for herbs to make medicines 4s and for a *mezzetta* of white wine for the sick 3s 6d'; 'for materials in order to make unguents for the sick, 15s.'[12] Over the following twenty years S. Maria Nuova clearly developed this facility, as is reflected in this substantial order in 1373:

> We pay to Ugholino di Bonsi apothecary and companions, on 4 November 1373, 100 gold florins, which sum he has as part payment for sugar and powdered sugar, candied fruit, turpentine, cassia, honey, pills, incense, aniseed, saffron, sugar cake, wax, candles, tapers and small tapers, cotton, plaster, lead and other spices that we have had from them … between 17 April 1372 and 8 December 1373.[13]

This combination of supplies points to the range of products sold by apothecaries. The business of a *speziale* was not restricted to medicines, but also included spices and herbs for cooking, perfumes and cosmetics, paints, dried fruit and sweets, as well as wax, candles, oil, soap and products for lighting the hospital's premises.[14] Three years later S. Maria Nuova's first surviving inventory contained a detailed account of what was in its pharmacy workshop. This included long lists of simple and compound substances and also receptacles and containers, such as retorts and pestles and mortars for the preparation of medicines.[15]

Thus, Florentine medical hospitals had a range of contractual arrangements with apothecaries. If S. Maria Nuova began by purchasing made-up medicines and then established its own pharmacy, one hundred years after its foundation it employed a full-time apothecary.[16] In contrast, the new medical hospitals were conceived with a pharmacy and an in-house apothecary. Hence, S. Matteo placed a large order for simple and compound medicines in 1409, a year before the hospital actually began to admit patients.[17] Contractual arrangements with the apothecary were flexible and might be for anything from daily visits to a full-time live-in member of staff with full board and lodging, the differences being reflected in the salaries on offer.[18] At Messer Bonifazio, Agnolo di Luca da Cortona was contracted on 7 December 1412 'to stay with us as apothecary and infirmarer in the hospital with a salary of 15 gold florins a year'.[19] Thus, as in the case of Giovanni di Francesco Machi, who was employed as surgeon and apothecary, Angnolo di Luca also fulfilled two roles.[20]

Any *speziale* living and working in a hospital would have had a humbler lifestyle than that associated with the owner of even a modestly successful apothecary's shop, given that this was one of the wealthiest professions in Florence in 1427.[21] However, as with hospital doctors, there are a number of factors that have to be taken into account when comparing the salaries of hospital apothecaries with their colleagues working in their own workshops. First, a part-time apothecary would have worked for other institutional or private clients, or so one would assume from their hospital salaries, which were almost derisory for professional men. When Agnolo di Luca da Cortona was employed by Messer Bonifazio in 1408 he was paid only 15 gold florins a year. Even taking into account free board and lodging, which has been estimated as worth about 14 gold florins a year, this was still only about half the amount an unskilled labourer might receive a year in full-time employment.[22] A hundred years later the annual stipend of Girolamo di Ser Nicholaio di Neri at S. Matteo was also only 14 gold florins, again considerably less than the annual stipend of an unskilled labourer.[23]

Part of the explanation for low salaries may be that hospital apothecaries came from the lower echelons of the spice and drug trade or belonged to the poorer branches of wealthier families. Two of those employed by S. Maria Nuova between 1430 and 1441 were recorded as having no taxable wealth in the Catasto, after allowable deductions had been taken into account.[24] A former employee, Jacopo d'Ugolino, was estimated at a value of 389 florins, but he had since built up an independent practice. Lucca di Nanni Mini was the only *speziale* at S. Maria Nuova who can be identified with an affluent family of apothecaries. Although the head of the family, Pagolo di Ser Giovanni Mini, had an estimated wealth of 4,915 florins, Lucca himself was not listed in the tax records.[25] Finally, when considering these levels of payment it is important not to forget that, as in the case of hospital doctors, a number of other factors might have compensated an apothecary for the lack of a more substantial salary: a regular income, the prestige of working for a charitable institution and personal piety.

This brief survey has traced a gradual professionalisation of the process by which hospitals in Florence provided medicines to their patients. In the first half of the Trecento S. Maria Nuova and S. Paolo were supplied with medicines in an already made-up form by apothecaries in the city. Then followed the development of the infirmarer's role 'to care for the sick', which involved nursing and participation in the preparation of medicines.[26] Finally, by the middle to late Quattrocento all of these hospitals employed full-time apothecaries who lived and worked on the premises. This evolution of the role of the apothecary was also linked to the evolution of the medical role of the hospital and to the growth of the physical premises of the pharmacy itself.

Pharmacies

The presence of a pharmacy was one of the main features that served to distinguish a 'medical' hospital from one that simply provided hospitality. There is no evidence that other types of institutions calling themselves *spedale*, such as the Innocenti, set aside a separate area for a pharmacy, even if their activities had important medical components.[27]

By the early fifteenth century each of the major medical hospitals had pharmacies in which medicines were stored and prepared for distribution to patients according to the instructions of physicians. General advice for the placing of a *spezeria* was provided by the Florentine College of Physicians' official *Nuovo riceptario*, compiled in 1499 to provide guidelines for good practice:[28]

> We say that every diligent apothecary must choose a location and place for his workshop, which should be suitable to preserve all the simple and compound medicines. This location must have [all] these characteristics or the majority: that is, it should be distant from wind, from dust, from sun, from dampness and from smoke.

If these general principles were taken into account when hospital pharmacies were built, no specific instructions have survived from either the founders or their medical advisors as to their placement and layout.[29] Even so, the location of these spaces can be reconstructed from building accounts, inventories and later plans. For example, the 1376 inventory of S. Maria Nuova records that the pharmacy was sited to the right of the lowest section of the male ward, and was therefore readily reached from the piazza (Plate 9.1: 6). In this way it could be accessed easily by both physicians and infirmarers when they prescribed recipes for those treated in the wards and for the many out-patients who came to the hospital for advice, treatment and the purchase of medicines.[30] The importance of an out-patient service is also evident at the hospital of S. Fina in San Gimignano which in the sixteenth century provided medicines to its patients and to 'poor people and to the shame-faced poor medicines as much as they need, as well as to poor pregnant women and to other poor women chickens and other things according to their needs'.[31]

By the early fifteenth century, therefore, each of the major medical hospitals in Florence had pharmacies run by trained personnel. The centrality of the role of the pharmacy in S. Maria Nuova's new image in early Renaissance Florence was symbolised by its expansion in 1429–30 to occupy three interconnecting rooms (Plate 9.1).[32]

Though no Renaissance pharmacies survive in Florence, a useful guide to their probable appearance is an anonymous fresco of c.1500 painted in one of the lunettes in the portico of the castle of Issogne in Valle d'Aosta (Plate 9.1).[33] This shows a room divided into two distinct spaces by a wooden counter, described variously in hospital inventories as a 'large table' (S. Matteo) and a 'counter of walnut', measuring some 3 metres in length (S. Fina, San Gimignano).[34] The counter marked the boundary between the public space and the more private space of the apothecary. In the foreground the fresco shows a woman purchasing medicines. She also may possibly have come to the pharmacy to consult a physician.[35]

The apothecary is shown working with his assistants to prepare, measure out and sell medicines. One of the men weighs out the simples, while the scribe notes down a recipe or prepares a bill for the waiting customer. The walls of the pharmacy are lined with shelves on which are arranged containers for the simple and compound medicines. S. Maria Nuova's 1376 inventory lists a series of bookcases and cabinets for storage, some of which could be locked to prevent the theft of valuable medicines: 'A small wooden cupboard, two wooden cupboards in bad condition, five wretched wooden benches on top of which are kept goods, one large cupboard with chests, a desk with a lock, a desk with two locks.'[36]

The Issogne fresco, which shows shelves and cabinets for storing a wide range of glass and terracotta jars, echoes the advice of Andrea Mattioli for the preservation of simple and compound medicines in his translation and commentary on Dioscorides' *De materia medica*:[37]

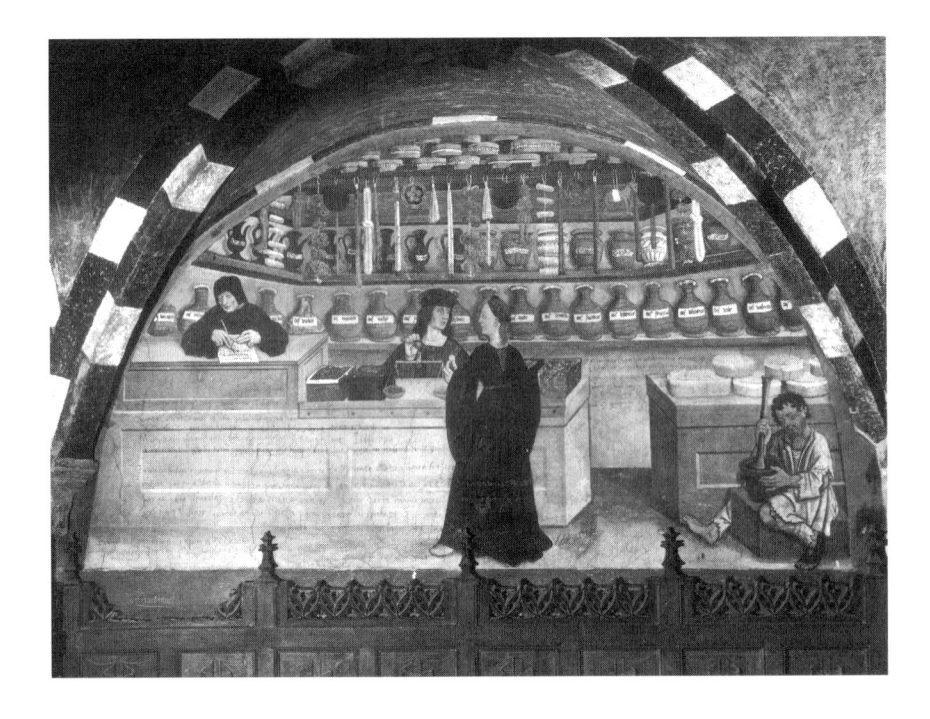

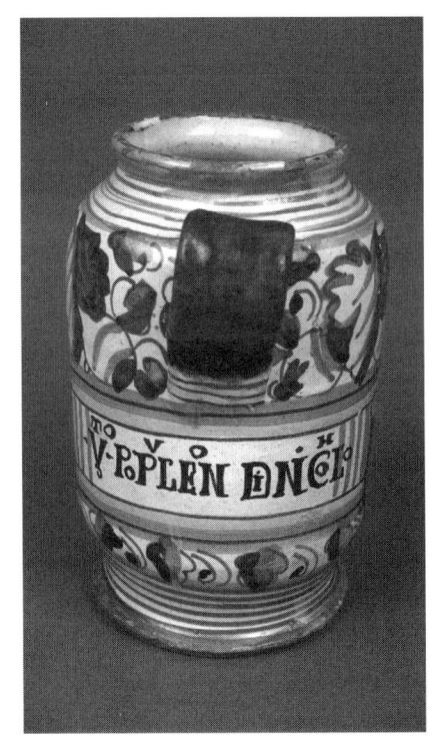

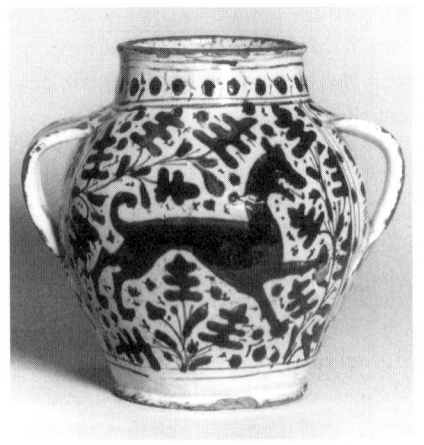

Plate 9.1 Anon., *Interior of a Pharmacy*, c.1500, Castle of Issogne, Valle d'Aosta

Plate 9.2 Late sixteenth-century Tuscan albarello from Montelupo (private collection)

Plate 9.3 A two-handled pharmacy jar from S. Maria Nuova (Fitzwilliam Museum)

In order to preserve the strength of properties of herbs and likewise roots there is no better thing to do than keep them in well-closed boxes or in terracotta vases, as Hippocrates wrote to Crateva in these words: 'All medicines that are like juices and liquors should be kept in glass vases and the herbs, flowers and roots in new terracotta vases in such a way that neither the wind nor air can diminish their strength.'

S. Maria Nuova's inventory lists containers made from a variety of materials.[38] Copper cauldrons were used to store syrups and medicines; 36 large and small glazed jugs for syrups; 15 more terracotta jugs for oils, 10 of which were glazed; 4 large copper and 42 glass vases for distilled water; an earthenware bowl for plasters and a large lead one for unguents; a quart lead vase for the wonder-drug theriac; and finally 57 *albarelli*, the cylindrical jars common to all Renaissance pharmacies. In the case of the *albarelli*, as with the two-handled jugs known as *orcioli*, the scribe was careful to distinguish those which were glazed: '15 very large glazed earthenware *albarelli*; 30 earthenware *albarelli*, large and small; 12 *albarelli* for keeping unguents.' Clearly additional purchases were made as pots were broken, but a particularly large order for around a thousand jars was placed in 1430–1 for the new pharmacy,[39] followed three years later by another of two hundred glazed small *albarelli*, two large *albarelli* and three small white *albarelli* which cost £55.16s.[40] These earthenware pots have survived in museum collections around the world and are easily recognisable because they were covered with a white tin glaze and often decorated with vivid designs.

These orders and hospital inventories make it clear that the albarello was one of the dominant forms of drug jar. Plate 9.2 provides a good idea of the appearance of a late sixteenth-century albarello, which is characterised by its cylindrical shape, though this one is unusual in also having a handle. The decoration here is the relief-blue pigment (*zaffera a rilievo*) with an oak-leaf motif that is characteristic of the production of central Italy and in particular of Montelupo. Furthermore, the obvious feature of a pharmacy jar was that it was labelled on the front with the ingredients stored inside, as in the case of this yellow cartouche with the words 'Unguento di Populeon di Niccholao', a well-known remedy listed in the 1499 *Nuovo Riceptario* and named after one of its ingredients, the buds of poplar trees.[41]

Some pharmacy jars can be identified with institutions such as hospitals and convents through the presence of their emblems. For instance, a S. Maria Nuova crutch can be seen clearly on an *orciolo*, a bulbous jar, in the Fitzwilliam Museum in Cambridge (Plate 9.3). This two-handled jar in manganese and relief-blue is decorated on each side with playful images of running hounds which provide a striking contrast with the simple and restrained green crutches on each handle.⁴² Other examples include the ladder associated with S. Maria della Scala or the 'SF' within a cartouche on the side of the jars ordered by S. Fina in 1505–6.⁴³

As the inventories show, *albarelli* were far from being the only type of container to be found in pharmacies. The two-handled orcioli containing syrups and oils are listed in S. Maria Nuova's inventory and can be seen on the lower shelf of the Piedmontese fresco. Other surviving examples in relief-blue, like the Fitzwilliam jar, feature lively designs of a wide variety of animals, including rabbits, as well as fish, birds such as cranes and eagles, fleur de lis and the familiar oak leaves of pharmacy jars made in Montelupo.⁴⁴ The Issogne fresco shows many other types of containers and jugs of wood, glass and metal including flat, round storage boxes that were used for keeping and serving medicaments,⁴⁵ while S. Maria Nuova's inventory lists both copper pans for the preservation of sweetmeats and a perforated copper mug for quince jam, as well as glass containers for distilled water.⁴⁶

What remains just as unclear from the iconographic evidence as from S. Maria Nuova's inventory is exactly how the different activities were distributed over the pharmacy. The fresco shows processes for the preparation of medicines as being carried out in the same room in which customers were served. In the foreground a ragged, partly shod assistant vigorously grinds simples with a pestle and mortar while the apothecary himself weighs medicines. All these elements would certainly have been present in an apothecary's shop, but the artist did not paint a direct representation of the premises.

In reality most hospital apothecary shops would have had two separate areas. The first, that shown in the fresco, represented the public face of the business and was where the simple and compound medicines were sold and distributed. The second area was the more private space of the workshop, also sometimes known as the *cucina*, where medicines were prepared or 'cooked up'.⁴⁷ At S. Maria Nuova this room was contiguous and behind the main *spezieria*, as it was at S. Fina in San Gimignano when it was rebuilt in the early sixteenth century.⁴⁸

The importance of the workshop to the medical function of a hospital was proudly underlined in S. Maria Nuova's early sixteenth-century 'Ordinances':⁴⁹

> we have built a large and well-equipped workshop to store the herbs and spices used by our salaried pharmacist to make up medicines and ointments … The room has twenty-two vessels for distilling things needed for medicines. Two are used to prepare drop by drop the extract of chicken and capon that we give to the seriously ill both in the hospital and outside it.

They are in continual use, and we use eight or ten capons every day in this way. The assistants prepare all the medicines using only the best ingredients. Each year we consume 4,000lb of cane sugar and as much again of honey, 2,000lb of native wax, 800lb of white wax, 2,000lb of cassia, 20lb of rhubarb, 12lb of manna, and other things of this sort. The total cost comes to between 1,500 and 2,000 gold florins.

The workshop was also an important storage area for the very substantial number of ingredients used in making up the medicines prescribed by hospital doctors. Already by the late Trecento, S. Maria Nuova's inventory suggests that it possessed a large collection of simple and compound medicines in the pharmacy even before its expansion in 1428–30.[50] In the 1370s the contents of the pharmacy were distributed over two main areas. The first contained some 220 products including forty different oils and waters, while the second was home to 180 simple and compound medicines such as unguents, powders and pills.

The *cucina* can be identified in the inventory because it contained large vessels and instruments for the various stages in the production of medicines. First, individual simples were ground to a fine powder using 'three stone mortars and four wooden pestles' as well as 'two small bronze mortars and two iron pestles'. S. Matteo's inventory of 1456 also lists '1 medium mortar of bronze to grind spices', '1 small mortar (*mortaiuzzo*) of bronze for pills and recipes', and '2 iron pestles, 1 big and 1 little'.[51] The presence of various types of pestle and mortar indicates the two processes involved in the preparation of medicines: the first was rougher grinding in the bronze pestles and mortars, followed by a finer grinding using stone mortars for the production of electuaries and pills.[52]

Another process involved extraction, for which S. Maria Nuova possessed containers made from copper and iron in which ingredients were heated on a tripod over a fire.[53] The aim was to reduce substances such as plant roots, animal and human bones, and minerals to a fine dust or even to burn them, as with 'burnt alum'. Distillation was an important way to extract the essences from plants and flowers. Ingredients were put in water in a metal alembic, a container shaped like a bell, then placed over a fire and the vapour drained off. As Mattioli explained, these containers were made of lead because 'This metal through its cold nature should be more apt than all the others to condense the vapour of the plants heated by the fire and convert it into liquid', though in fact usually only the upper part, the *campana*, was made of lead and the rest was copper or iron.[54]

In the 1370s S. Maria Nuova used 'two lead bells for distilling',[55] which suggests a relatively limited operation, as remained true at S. Matteo in the

PRIMA FORNACE.

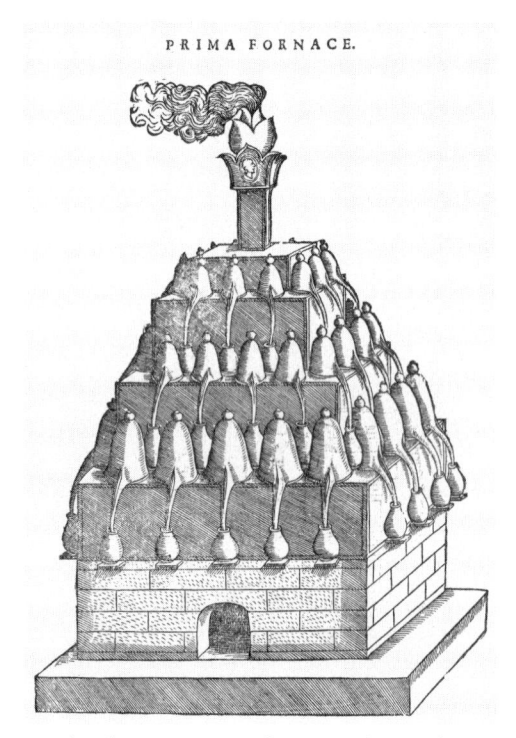

Plate 9.4 Andrea Mattioli, *The First Furnace*, from *De i discorsi di M. Pietro Andrea Mattioli Sanese* (Venice, 1585)

early sixteenth century when the hospital's inventory lists three bells, 'two large and one small'.[56] In time, as Mattioli records, a furnace was created that contained ever more alembics, 'so that with just one fire and with much less expense and work it proved possible to produce a much larger quantity of liquid every day'.[57] The logic of this argument was evidently understood by S. Maria Nuova for by 1510 the number of *campane* for distillation in the *spezeria* had increased from two to twenty-two, reflecting how much the hospital's operations had grown over the past 130 years.[58] The probable appearance of S. Maria Nuova's oven can be seen in an illustration entitled 'The First Furnace' in Mattioli's *Discorsi* (Plate 9.4)

Grinding, heating and distillation were, then, some of the main ways that a wide range of simple and compounds were prepared in the pharmacies of Florence's major medical hospitals. To examine how these medicines were used I shall turn to the main task of this chapter, an analysis of S. Maria Nuova's lengthy *Ricettario*.

9.2 'A Universal Book of Many Things, All Recipes Tried and Tested': S. Maria Nuova's Medical Recipes and their Authors

S. Maria Nuova's *Ricettario* is an exceptionally useful guide to the practice of medicine in one of the largest Renaissance hospitals in Europe, partly because the collection is so extensive (over a thousand recipes) and partly because the recipes themselves are so informative.[59] Its wider value lies in the fact that it throws light on the relationship between medical theory and practice; an examination of these simple and compound medicines brings us closer to understanding why they were used to treat specific disorders.

The practice of keeping a *ricettario* evolved over time, as part of an on-going process to record and standardise the more successful and commonly used recipes.[60] The prologue to S. Maria Nuova's *Ricettario* records that it 'was written by me, Hectorre di Lionello di Francesco Baldovinetti, at the request of the doctor Maestro Pagholo, today, this day of 17 October 1515';[61] Maestro Pagholo was most likely the 'house doctor', Maestro Pagholo di Maestro Giovanbatista.[62] Its compilation probably reflects pressure from the College of Physicians, which in 1499 had published the *Nuovo riceptario* – also known as the *Ricettario fiorentino* – to standardise recipe preparation in the city, *contado* and district. In its preface the College justified this move on the grounds that the 'diversity of recipe books' and apothecaries' practices in making up preparations meant that the sick incurred 'many dangers' from prescriptions that were prepared incorrectly.[63] As is clear from the records of the College later in the century, members were concerned to enforce standards in apothecary workshops and institutional pharmacies, principal among which were those in hospitals and religious houses.[64] The long-term effect of this policy is reflected in the 1695 inventory of the apothecary's shop of S. Fina in San Gimignano, which includes two *ricettari* and a copy of Mattioli's *Discorsi*, one of the most influential collections of recipes in early modern Italy and Europe.[65]

S. Maria Nuova's new *Ricettario* was described by Baldovinetti as a 'universal book of many things, all recipes tried and tested, indeed obtained and taken from S. Maria Nuova'.[66] There are a number of references that make it clear that Maestro Pagholo was present when recipes were prescribed to particular patients. For example, there was the 'Electuary that was made for Francesco our accountant according to a recipe that he gave me for his sight' or another that 'marvellously liberated the women who suffered from suffocation as I have seen and this is proven'.[67] In other cases Maestro Pagholo recorded his instructions as given to an apothecary: for instance, 'leave it to dry as I said above.'[68]

The *Ricettario*, then, represents the end of a process that began when the physician prescribed treatment for patients on the ward. The intermediate stage was the notebook kept by the pharmicist of recipes for individuals, an example of which has survived from the Pratese Spedale della Misericordia. On 31 November 1492 we find written:

For a baby girl
R: white sugar: 1oz
Make a very fine powder from it to use according to the given method
Item oil from Cologne: 1oz
To rub on the stomach

For an old man of the hospital
R: Electuary [of Mesué] health-giving and expert 2oz
To hold in the mouth once an hour

For Stephano
R: lavender oil: 1oz
To rub on the stomach, evening and morning before meals

For Frate Antonio
R: grated liquorice: 3oz
Sieved Corinthian grapes: 3oz
Borage: no. 8
Plums: no. 6
Saffron crocus: no. 20
Barley: 1 handful
To make water for the chest

For Maria
R: compound of syrup of endive
Ordinary vinegar
Hop water: 2oz
Maidenhair fern: 2oz
Violets: 2oz
Mix two times

For Giovanni the nurse
R: Plaster for wounds: 4oz
To put on top of the wound[69]

These examples of simple recipes for minor complaints coincide, as will be seen below, with the more straightforward examples of those recorded as 'tried and tested' at S. Maria Nuova. The *Ricettario* also included more complex recipes, which may have been copied from existing collections, such as the 'ricettario per la spezaria' bought in 1406 for £12 from the apothecary

Benedetto di Miniato.[70] It likewise contained recipes from well-known Arab and classical authorities common to collections belonging to medical men and faculty libraries, as well as remedies attributed to more recent practitioners, such as doctors working for Florentine hospitals. It was written in Italian rather than in Latin to make it easier and faster to consult for apothecaries and surgeons, who may have been more at home reading their mother tongue. The importance of the vernacular is underlined by the inclusion in this volume of Peter of Spain's *Tesoro dei poveri*.[71] Indeed, it may have been this work that was bought by S. Paolo in February 1349, only a few years after the hospital had begun to specialise in treating in-patients – 'a book of remedies for the good health of the poor'.[72]

The authors of the recipes named in S. Maria Nuova's *Ricettario* are listed in Table 9.1, along with the number of recipes attributed to each writer. The table represents 197 of the 1,035 recipes (19 per cent) that were identified with a named individual, whether a recognised medical authority or a practitioner working for one of the main Florentine hospitals.

Table 9.1 S. Maria Nuova's *Ricettario*, 1515: recipes and their authors

Named practitioner	No.	%
Aghostino, maestro, medicho di casa	18	9.1
Alberto di Messer Simone, maestro	1	0.5
Alessandro	3	1.5
Angniolo, maestro, medicho di casa	2	1.0
Antonio di Francesco da Cagli, maestro	2	1.0
Banducci, Bandino di maestro Giovanni, maestro	1	0.5
Benedetta, medica di casa	2	1.0
Bino, maestro	1	0.5
Bonino, maestro	2	1.0
Caterina, medica di casa	3	1.5
Cierretani, Giovanni, maestro	1	0.5
Dino francioso, maestro	1	0.5
Domenico, maestro	2	1.0
Ficino, Diotifeci d'Agnolo, maestro, medicho di casa	30	15.2
Francesca, medica di casa	1	0.5
Francesco da Ghamberaia, maestro	3	1.5
Francesco dal Ponte, maestro, medicho di casa	1	0.5
Francesco, maestro	1	0.5
Fruosino, maestro, barbiere	5	2.5
Ghaletto, maestro	2	1.0
Ghottifredi, maestro	1	0.5
Giovanni da Luccha, maestro	1	0.5
Giovanni Francioso, maestro	3	1.5
Giuliano da Pavia, maestro	1	0.5

Table 9.1 continued

Named practitioner	No.	%
Iachopo di Dino de' Pecori	1	0.5
Iachopo di Monte Chalvo, maestro	1	0.5
Iachopo, coiaio	1	0.5
Lodovicho, maestro	1	0.5
Matteo barbiere, maestro	2	1.0
Michele da Pescia, maestro, medicho di casa	19	9.6
Michele di Mariano, maestro, che medicha a San Paolo	6	3.0
Niccholò, maestro	4	2.0
Paolo	1	0.5
Piero, maestro, medicho di casa	7	3.6
Santi Putavino, catelano, maestro	1	0.5
Taddeo de' Pechori	1	0.5
Tommaso	3	1.5
Total	**136**	**69.0**
Medical Authorities		
nostri autori; secondo alchuni	10	5.1
Agrippa, re di Giudei	2	1.0
Alberto Magno	2	1.0
Avicenna	9	4.6
Dino del Garbo, maestro	2	1.0
Galeno	8	4.1
Ippocrate	1	0.5
Mesué	11	5.6
Niccholaio [*Antidotarium*]	6	3.0
Rasis	9	4.6
Serapione	1	0.5
Total	**61**	**31.0**
Overall total	**197**	**100.0**

The vast majority of the named recipes (69 per cent) were attributed to Florentine practitioners, in contrast to the *Ricettario fiorentino*, where most were derived from the medical canon.[73] Significantly, of the few recipes of contemporary physicians appearing in the *Ricettario fiorentino* two were those of Maestro Cristofano di Giorgio Brandaglini, who, as seen above in Chapter 7, was one of the most eminent doctors in early Quattrocento Florence.[74] The connections between S. Maria Nuova's recipe collection and the *Ricettario fiorentino* are reflected by the inclusion in the latter of an electuary of Dyasena, 'which is a sovereign remedy [*magistrale*] and is used in S. Maria Nuova'.[75] Evidently the attribution of a recipe to a famous Florentine physician or to the city's main medical centre added lustre and authority, in the same way as citing the medical canon or leading scholars such as Dino del Garbo.

In contrast to the *Ricettario fiorentino*, only about a third of the named recipes in S. Maria Nuova's collection were attributed to medical authorities. In both, the most common names mentioned were the great Arab physicians, Avicenna (nine), Mesué (eleven) and Rhazes (nine), along with the most obvious Western classical authority, Galen (eight). Recipes were also drawn from well-known collections, such as the eleventh-century Salernitan *Antidotarium Nicolai* (six), and, as mentioned above, it was prefaced by Peter of Spain's *Tesoro dei poveri*. S. Maria Nuova's collection also included a wider range of recipes from medical authorities. While the College's was dominated by Mesué (53 per cent of recipes were attributed to him),[76] S. Maria Nuova's also contained recipes by Dino del Garbo, one of the most illustrious and widely cited university physicians in fourteenth-century Italy, as well as vague references to authorities, 'nostri autori' and 'secondo alchuni' (ten).

Most of the thirty-seven contemporary practitioners who contributed recipes to the *Ricettario* worked for S. Maria Nuova.[77] Doctors from other Florentine hospitals were included as specialists in particular conditions, such as Maestro Michele di Mariano of S. Paolo who was known for treating diseases associated with legs.[78] Maestro Fruosino, who was probably the Fruosino d'Andrea *barbiere* employed by S. Matteo in 1468, specialised in mouths, which he treated with *acquaforte*, as in the case of a woman whose mouth was 'all cancerous'.[79]

The largest number of recipes attributed to a single practitioner was to Maestro Diotifeci d'Agnolo Ficino (thirty). Most probably, as with Cristoforo di Giorgio cited in the *Ricettario fiorentino*, Maestro Diotifeci was well represented in part for reasons of prestige, though the large number of recipes also reflected the fact that he had been employed by the hospital over a twenty-year period.[80] Maestro Diotifeci was well connected in Florentine society, as Cosimo de' Medici's family doctor and as father of the famous Neoplatonic philosopher Marsilio Ficino, who was associated closely with Lorenzo de' Medici. His social success also reflected his popularity as a practitioner; in one of his letters Ficino described his father as 'a surgeon in Florence and outstanding amongst his contemporaries'.[81] Maestro Diotifeci brought to S. Maria Nuova his reputation as a skilled practitioner and the right social connections. Another of S. Maria Nuova's doctors, Maestro Michele di Maestro Michele da Pescia, who was also particularly well represented in this recipe collection (nineteen), was similarly well connected. He shared with Maestro Diotifeci the experience of having well-known children: both his sons, Niccolò and Francesco, became priors of the commune in the late fifteenth century.[82]

The relatively large number of recipes in the *Ricettario* attributed to contemporary doctors at S. Maria Nuova underlines the compiler's claim that the collection reflected practices within the hospital. This is borne out further by the inclusion of recipes from three women practitioners, Benedetta, Caterina and Francesca, each described as a 'medica di casa' in the female ward. The practical nature of the collection is also emphasised by the inclusion of Peter of Spain's *Tesoro dei poveri*, which had a wide circulation in medieval Europe, specifically because it provided a simplified account of diseases and treatment. Such recipes would have been more understandable to the average surgeon and apothecary at S. Maria Nuova, who would have had less knowledge than a physician of some of the more sophisticated distinctions in diagnosis and treatment. The *Ricettario fiorentino*, in contrast, depended more heavily on traditional authorities, whose works formed the staple of the curriculum of the medical faculties of Italian universities.[83]

Before analysing S. Maria Nuova's *Ricettario* in general, I shall begin by examining the recipes prescribed by two of the hospital doctors, who were especially well represented, the surgeon Maestro Diotifeci and the physician Maestro Michele, to establish what types of recipe were associated with these two different types of practitioner. As might be expected, Diotifeci's recipes were mostly to treat external conditions and included seventeen unguents, two plasters and nine poultices (see Table 9.2).

Table 9.2 S. Maria Nuova's *Ricettario*, 1515: recipes of Diotifeci d'Agnolo Ficino

Head wounds	5
Head: bruised without wound	1
Headache	1
Eyes	1
Hands	1
Feet: corns and cracked skin	2
Bones	8
Boils	1
Scrofula (*scrofe mangnio*)	1
Poultices: constricting	1
: *capitale istiricho*	1
Powder, constricting	1
Unguento di calci d'Avicenna	1
Unguent of Pietro d'Abano (*unguento del conciliatore*)	2
Unguento di Gratia Dei	1
Unguent (*unguento difensivo rosso*)	1
Nitric acid (*acqua forte*)	1
Total	30

It is significant that when Marsilio Ficino proudly described his father's medical skills in a letter in 1474 to Francesco Marescalchi of Ferrara, he cited the treatment of the son of a *contadino* named Tommaso 'whose head had been most gravely wounded'.[84] Though the purpose of Ficino's story was to emphasise the miraculous intervention of the Virgin Mary and the power of prayer in healing, the choice of an example featuring a patient with a damaged head reflected one of his father's specialisations. S. Maria Nuova's *Ricettario* included five of his recipes for unguents or poultices for *capirotti*, literally 'broken heads', but probably meaning more general head wounds. Other recipes include a poultice for a head wound without bruising and an unguent for a wound causing head pains. He was also a bone specialist, with eight recipes for broken or ulcerated bones, as well as offering treatments for skin complaints that included unguents and poultices for the hand, hard and cracked skin on the foot, a boil (*rogna*) and scrofula (*scrofe mangnio*).

Maestro Diotifeci's recipes were for the treatment of both patients and members of the residential staff whom he knew personally. These included one of the hospital's chaplains, Ser Giovanni, for a boil and a certain Ghabriello for a fracture. He also prescribed unguents of litharge for the hand of Paghola, 'a servant of the house', another for a corn on one of Monna Caterina's feet, and an Arabic recipe from Mesué – an ointment of *sieffi bianchi* – for one of Dorotea's eyes.[85] Mention of Mesué reminds us that while Maestro Diotifeci may have devised many of these recipes himself, important sources for treatment were also the classics of the medical curriculum. He was clearly familiar with Rhazes' *Ad Almansorem* since he cited it as his source for the poultice for a bruised head, likewise Avicenna (for an unguent of calcium) and the famous early fourteenth-century professor of medicine at Padua Pietro d'Abano (for the 'ointment of the Conciliator').[86]

The majority of the nineteen recipes attributed to S. Maria Nuova's physician Maestro Michele di Maestro Michele da Pescia were, as might be expected, for internal rather than external use, though he did prescribe four plasters and two unguents for new and old pains and head wounds. Other recipes included pills made of incense for a consumptive condition known as *tisicho*, a mixture of barley water, sugar, dragon's blood, a syrup and oil of roses, and egg yolk to treat intestinal disorder (*mal di pondi*), an electuary for a chest condition, and syrups made of quince and cordials for coughs.[87]

The recipes of both Maestro Diotifeci and Maestro Michele were to treat those external and internal conditions familiar from Chapter 8's analysis of the ailments of hospital patients. More generally, Table 9.1 suggests that the recipes used at S. Maria Nuova came from a wide range of sources, including the well-known medical authorities that formed the backbone of the libraries of doctors and universities. It is striking that a significant proportion derived from doctors working in Florentine hospitals. The *Ricettario* is further personalised by the inclusion of the names of individuals associated with S. Maria Nuova who had been prescribed specific treatment. For example, a member of the patronal family, Bernardo Portinari, is recorded as having been given two recipes. The first was a powder to treat his gout and the second was a plaster 'for pain in one of his knees, according to the recipe of Maestro Aghostino'.[88] There were also two recipes that were mentioned in connection with the long-standing *spedalingo*, Bonino Bonini. The first was an electuary prepared for 'a friend of our Benino' to treat his head and stomach, while the second was a recipe for 'Imperial pills according to the recipe of Maestro Aghostino given and made for our Benino of the house, tried and tested'.[89]

Many of these recipes did reflect medical practice at S. Maria Nuova, as will become increasingly apparent in the next section, which examines the whole *Ricettario* in relation to treatment of ailments of specific parts of the body. It should be noted that all treatment was based on an imagined imbalance of the humours. Humoral theory was fundamental to medical treatment in this period. Disease was seen as having been created by the imbalance of the complexional qualities within the body (hot, wet, cold, dry) and the humours. The latter were divided into four categories: blood, phlegm, choler, which was equivalent to red or yellow bile, and melancholy, or black bile. Each of these substances was also seen as equivalent to one of four actual bodily fluids and it was the maintenance of their correct balance according to the proper complexional make-up of an individual that was the aim of much Renaissance medicine. This balance was achieved through following a regime of blood-letting and the proper balancing of the six non-naturals, those physical and environmental factors that affected health, among which the most important were exercise, diet, excretion and the passions. When treating the sick the aim was to return the individual to the proper balance of health and humours through the administration of simple and compound medicines.[90]

Other recipes in the *Ricattario*, such as for beautification – *decorso del corpo* – may seem extraneous to hospital medicine. However, cleanliness was an important contemporary preoccupation and was a traditional part of advice literature and recipe collections, such as Taddeo Alderotti's *Consilia* and collections of *materia medica* like Mattioli's *Discorsi*.[91]

9.3 'We Begin First of All with the Ailments of the Head, Descending as Far as the Feet'[92]

S. Maria Nuova's *Ricettario* will be analysed in terms of two interrelated themes: symptoms and recipes. Symptoms will be discussed in relation to the parts of the body, the data having been organised from head to toe, in line with contemporary discussions of diseases (Table 9.3). This follows a well-established tradition in practical manuals, from Book IX of Rhazes' *Ad Almansorem* to Peter of Spain's *Tesoro dei poveri*, to Mattioli's *Discorsi*.[93]

Table 9.3 S. Maria Nuova's *Ricettario*, 1515: body parts and symptoms

	Body Parts		Symptoms N	%
1. Head	mouth		44	5.2
	head		99	11.8
	throat		15	1.8
	nose		5	0.6
	eyes		58	6.9
	ears		12	1.4
		sub-total	233	27.7
2. Torso	heart		6	0.7
	breast		4	0.5
	chest		21	2.5
		sub-total	31	3.7
3. Abdomen	liver		11	1.3
	spleen		11	1.3
	posterior		14	1.7
	digestive organs		102	12.1
	urogenital			
	female		25	3.0
	male		16	1.9
	bladder & kidney		51	6.1
		sub-total	230	27.4
4. Limbs	limbs		99	11.8
		sub-total	99	11.8
5. General	body		21	2.5
	named diseases		61	7.3
	pains		21	2.5
	bites & poisons		14	1.7
	beauty		29	3.5
	fevers		10	1.2
	wounds, etc.		31	3.7
	nerves		12	1.4
	ulcers, boils, etc.		48	5.7
		sub-total	247	29.4
	Total		840	100.0

Indeed, Mattioli is central to this chapter. Though his edition of Dioscorides was first published in 1544, thirty years after the hospital's *Ricettario* was compiled, the *Discorsi* are an invaluable source on the theory and practice regarding the use of specific medicines and recipes. Mattioli is an ideal guide; as a Sienese citizen he had a detailed knowledge of the identity and use of local Tuscan simples. He also had an enviable knowledge of the works of both classical and medieval writers that underlay the use of traditional simple and compound medicines as well as knowing about those from the New World and chemicals increasingly available in the sixteenth century.[94]

I shall begin by examining in general terms all those symptoms and body parts mentioned in S. Maria Nuova's *Ricettario*. Although it cannot be assumed that the number of recipes in each category was proportional to the prevalence of that particular condition in the hospital, inclusion provides an overall idea of treatment. Indeed, given that 872 body parts or symptoms are mentioned in these 1,036 recipes, this analysis will constitute a substantial addition to our knowledge of the reasons for which people were admitted to Tuscan hospitals.[95] Other types of evidence examined above, in Chapter 8, from financial records to books of admissions and deaths, only provided general disease labels and gave little specific information about patients' illnesses.

There is no space here to examine in detail the symptoms and recipes for each part of the body. I shall begin, therefore, with diseases of the whole body and then concentrate on the three most numerically significant areas represented in Table 9.3 (head, abdomen and general diseases), ignoring the torso and limbs. In this way it will be possible to discuss a wide variety of internal and external conditions affecting the head, three of the most important internal organs – stomach, liver, spleen – and reproduction.

Three broad categories stand out when looking at the distribution of symptoms between the various parts of the body: the head, the abdomen and general ailments of the whole body (28, 27 and 29 per cent of recipes respectively). This pattern was not uncommon, as reflected in Mattioli's *Discorsi*: head 22 per cent; abdomen 27 per cent; the whole body 38 per cent.[96] The greatest difference is that 9 per cent more of Mattioli's recipes were for the 'whole body'.

The recipes for 'general conditions' fall into two parts: those prescribed by physicians to treat diseases of the whole body, such as plagues and fevers, and a substantial number of cases in which a condition was applicable to any part of the body, such as boils and ulcers, bites and poisons, and wounds and burns. A discussion of plagues and fevers will serve as an introduction to the detailed analysis of S. Maria Nuova's *Ricettario*.

9.4 Plagues, Pestilences and Fevers

Plagues and Pestilences

This period saw a growing tendency among medical men to begin to think in ontological terms, that is, in disease categories, especially in relation to illnesses of the whole body. This developed an existing tradition in which named conditions were identified with specific parts, such as melancholy or epilepsy with the head or hysteria with the womb. It has been argued that this new emphasis on disease categories resulted from the emergence in late medieval Europe of a series of epidemics, the most obvious of which was plague, which had first swept through Europe in 1347–9 and then had remained endemic, reappearing roughly every ten to fifteen years. Even if plague itself came to be identified with a discrete set of symptoms, the broad terms of *morìa*, *mortalità*, *peste* and *pestilenzia*, which appear in this recipe collection, were applicable to any epidemic, though sometimes a distinction was made between summer and winter 'pestilences'. To confuse the issue further, contemporaries often elided these categories in their discussions of 'pestilential fevers', underlining the undesirability for the historian to impose disease categories too rigidly. S. Maria Nuova's recipe collection is a good example of contemporaries putting into practice Arnold of Villanova's dictum that it is not necessary to distinguish disease from symptom unless it is helpful for treatment.[97]

Both more and less problematic than plague was the other epidemic disease typical of early modern Europe, the Mal Francese. It was less problematic because its symptoms were quite well defined. However, for contemporaries it was also more problematic because these symptoms could not be identified with those diseases described in the medical corpus taught at universities. Consequently, this led to public disputations in the 1490s in both Italy and southern Germany centring on debates about whether this was a 'new' or an 'old' disease, though in the end it was generally accepted as new.[98]

It is no surprise that there should not be even one recipe for the Mal Francese in Table 9.3 since, as seen above in Chapter 3, specific 'Incurabili' hospitals were established for the *mal franciosati*. As a general medical hospital S. Maria Nuova would normally have excluded those suffering from chronic epidemic diseases. Consequently St Anthony's Fire and smallpox are only represented by one recipe each in its recipe book and their inclusion either points to rare cases of in-house treatment of these conditions or suggests that these recipes had been taken from other collections and copied into the *Ricettario*. The inclusion of recipes to treat plague is more understandable since S. Maria Nuova continued to house plague victims until the late 1470s.

Recipes for 'plagues' were for internal rather than external use and were in the form of pills, cordials or powders. Two were attributed to Maestro Piero, 'doctor of the house', and a third to Albertus Magnus, who had died over sixty years before the Black Death.[99] Of these recipes only that of Albertus Magnus included theriac, the wonder-drug which Marsilio Ficino in his plague tract cites, on the authority of Galen, as the best remedy for plague: '[because] the plague is a dragon with a body of air that blows poison against man, and theriac is a purgative that purges the said poison and kills the dragon.'[100] If theriac was not available then Ficino advised his reader to take mithraditum, which appears in another of these recipes against plague, the 'Electuary or true pills for the pestilence, but they are very hot'.[101]

The warning added to the title of this last recipe points to one of the main properties of these ingredients, which was to combat the humidity and the putrefaction of the humours that were caused by plague. All four recipes for pills to treat plague contained two simples well known for their drying qualities – aloe and Armenian bole – as well as myrrh and saffron for their heating action.[102] The simples included in Albertus Magnus' powder were also recommended for similar qualities. In addition to theriac, he recommended Armenian bole and red sandalwood, endive water and white dittamo, known for drying, as well as camphor to preserve patients from putrefaction.[103]

Many of these ingredients were standard in any recipe against plague, as is confirmed by Ficino in his tract. Pills taken to 'preserve [a patient] from the plague' included simples to 'open and heat and greatly resolve the spirits', though he also added that 'some wash the aloe and add terra sigillata or Armenian bole or camphor' in order to mitigate their effects by drying and cooling.[104] This is some indication of the complexity behind the use of different simples in recipes that not only had varying degrees of strength, but that when used in combination also had different effects. The same complexity was true of recipes for fevers, which since antiquity had been the subject of even more numerous tracts written by leading medical authorities.[105]

Fevers

Fevers represented the second major category of diseases of the whole body and were one of the most common reasons patients were admitted to general medical hospitals. Following medical treatises of the time, the fevers listed in the *Ricettario* were distinguished by the periodicity of their occurrence: daily, tertian and quartian, as well as 'ephemeral fever' (*febbre frematicha*). Two recipes for fever were attributed to medical authorities; the first was a powder that Avicenna had prescribed for ephemeral fever. It was composed of Indian jalap plant, white ginger, mastic and white sugar, which were finely ground up together and given to the patient in the morning with chicken soup and a decoction of maidenhair fern, grape juice and aniseed. The second recipe was a lotion of colocynth, scammony and rock salt, attributed to the fourth-century Roman physician Serapion and described by the compiler of the *Ricettario* as 'proven'. The function of all these simples was to treat heat, which all writers give as the cause of fever, and in particular innate heat, which Galen had characterised as 'heat contrary to nature'.[106]

Most of these recipes for fevers were beverages though there were also two ointments, one of which was a 'fine oil of mandrake', a powerful plant with an almost human-shaped root and to which were attributed semi-magical properties.[107] Together with opium it was included in the ointment for its cooling and drying properties as well as its soporific effect.[108] Inducing sleep was the effect of another ingredient, storax or 'storacie cholamita', while two species of endive were included because of their drying action to counter the danger of putrefaction associated with fevers.[109] The method of preparation also provides an idea of its main uses:[110]

> *To make fine mandrake oil*
> Leave the juice in the oil for ten days and place it in the sun and mix it and then cook it so that the juice is consumed and when it is cooked take it from the fire and when it is cold add the opium and storax.
>
> The medicament should be well mixed and stored in a vase and it is good for acute fevers when the pulses of the feet and hands are anointed with it and it sends the patients to sleep and combats the heat of the liver when it is anointed. It is also good for many great pains of the head and is good for delirium; to induce sleep put it into the nostrils of the nose and anoint the pulses of the hands and of the feet and the temples and there will be no problems with sleep and [the effects of] this oil have been proven by many people.

As with all these recipes, the basis of the treatment was complexional: that is, it aimed to combat the heat generated by the fever. It was particularly important to treat the liver if it became overheated as a result of fever; according to Galenic theory, the liver played a vital role in the physiological system as the main blood-making organ of the body. It is also worth noting that this recipe, in common with many others in the *Ricettario*, had a very practical bent; some simples included in these recipes, such as opium and poppy seeds, were intended to dull the pain associated with high temperatures and to induce sleep.

9.5 'The Head of our Body Is Made like the Chimney in the House'

A similar combination of theory and practice underlay treatment for the head (Tables 9.4 and 9.5), which constituted the largest number of recipes for a single part of the body. The head was more prominent here than in Mattioli's *Discorsi* (28 per cent compared with 22 per cent), probably reflecting actual practice at S. Maria Nuova, especially as an unusually high proportion of these recipes were attributed to named hospital doctors. Indeed, the importance of the head in contemporary medical theory is underlined in Maestro Ugolino's 'Consiglio' to Averardo de' Medici: 'The head of our body is made like the chimney in the house made to receive the smoke and vapours.'[111]

Table 9.4 S. Maria Nuova's *Ricettario*, 1515: general symptoms associated with the head

	No.	%
Head	99	42.5
Ears	12	5.1
Eyes	58	24.9
Nose	5	2.1
Mouth	44	18.8
Throat	15	6.4
Total	233	100.0

Table 9.5 S. Maria Nuova's *Ricettario*, 1515: specific symptoms associated with the head

General	
Head (*capo*)	13
Internal	
Apoplexy	5
Bewitched	1
Brain (*cerebro*)	1
Catarrh (*catarro/ghocciola*)	13
Choler (*collera*)	2
Convulsions (*mal maestro*)	6
Dampness (*umidità da ristorare*)	3
Dizziness (*capogirli*)	5
Epilepsy (*mal caduco*)	2
Headache/migraine (*magrana*)	4
Headache/pain (*doglia*)	11
Heated (*rischaldato*)	1
Humours (*omore*)	2
Insomnia (*dormire*)	22
Meloncholy (*malincholia*)	6
Paralytic	1
Passions (*contro a molto passione*)	1
Phlegm (*flemma/ flemmatico*)	2
Total internal	88
External	
Bruised without wounds (*ammacchatura senza ferite*)	1
Fractures (*capirotto*)	15
Wounds (*ferite*)	3
Total external	19
Overall total	120

The single largest number of recipes in Table 9.4 are in the first general section (ninety-nine of 233) and are included either because the recipe mentions the head but no specific organs or because it follows contemporary practice in linking the head to what we would call 'psychological' conditions such as melancholy.

Before passing on to more obvious external conditions, such as fractures, it should be noted that I have followed contemporary categorisation by including under 'head' those recipes to treat conditions associated with the naturals and non-naturals and above all to balance the humours. It is in this context that one can best understand the inclusion of recipes under 'head' for the general category of humour, two for treating choler, red or yellow bile, and six for melancholy or black bile. The first, the 'Pills of Niccolaio' – the eleventh-century *Antidotarium Niccolai* from the medical school of Salerno – is a general recipe appropriate for the 'head and any bad humour that is created in the body', made from eighteen different simples of which the main ones are aloe and diagridium. Aloe is one of the most common ingredients in recipes, for, as Mattioli says, it 'completely purges the body'. Quoting the authority of Galen and Mesué, he claims that when mixed with cinnamon it 'opens the tracts of the stomach and is a substance that diminishes the coarse and sticky humours that one finds there'. Furthermore, aloe 'dissolves the choler and the phlegm and cleanses the head of them and also the stomach and is good for all pains'.[112]

As with Mattioli's account of simples, many in S. Maria Nuova's *Ricettario* for the head derived from a combination of classical authorities and more recent writers. One recipe said to be by Albertus Magnus (d. 1280) was for balsamic oil which was 'good against many passions', that is, the passions or 'accidents of the soul,' one of the non-naturals.[113] The compiler of S. Maria Nuova's *Ricettario* cites other authors on the miraculous effects of various recipes, including a specific reference to the third part of Raymond's book on distillation and Arnold of Villanova's treatises on 'acquavite and compound waters'.

It is some measure of the practical bent of the *Ricettario* that the two other humours, blood and phlegm, were not discussed in theoretical terms but as physical substances. The recipes devoted to blood were to stop its flow from wounds, while those for phlegm were designed literally to dry it up: 'whoever is phlegmatic having pain in the chest or in the mouth of the stomach should take aromatic rose-water early in the morning and also a good broad bean and then fast for one or two hours, and this recipe has been demonstrated.'[114] 'Aromatico rosato', composed of about twenty ingredients including roses, had cleansing properties to help clear phlegm from the chest.[115] Fasting for an hour or two was aimed to help this work, while the bean purified the stomach. As Maestro Ugolino explains in his 'Consiglio' to Averardo de' Medici, catarrh is caused by vapours 'that are generated by indigestion in the stomach'. He stresses that the most common form of catarrh is caused by the 'rising of vapours' from the stomach to the head because the head is 'the chimney in the house' which 'receives the smoke and vapours'. Furthermore, he explains that 'when these vapours are in the brain, which is cold by its very nature, they condense there and then fall from there to one place or another, as one can see in the case of the stove where the vapours and smoke rise to the sky and then fall as rain'.[116]

Mental Imbalance

Cleansing and purging were also among the main elements in the treatment of mental disturbances.[117] These ranged from passive conditions such as lethargy and melancholy, for which there were six recipes, to more violent forms of madness, such as *mal caduco* or epilepsy (two), and frenzy.[118]

The two recipes for *mal caduco* contained few ingredients. The first lists senna leaves, which are laxatives and, according to Mattioli, comfort the brain; the latter cites Serapione as saying that they are good for those who 'speak out of place'.[119] Also included were cloves, which Mattioli says are 'good for many things which are hot and dry', and primrose or *erba paralisis* for its drying qualities.[120] The second recipe contained only sage and purple bettony infused in white wine, following Galen's recommendation.[121]

In contrast to the *Ricettario*'s two straightforward recipes made from plants, Peter of Spain's treatment for *mal caduco* was completely dominated by animal ingredients, including goat's horn, wolf's brain, bear's bile, horse's milk and 'a red stone that one finds in the stomachs of swallows when they are sitting on their nests'.[122] He also recommended the parents of a child with *mal caduco* to take him to church to hear Mass on Wednesday and Friday through Sunday and then 'the priest says over his head that passage from the Gospels in which it says "hec generatio demoniorum" '.[123] This linked treatment of the physical and spiritual and reflects not just the dual role of the Renaissance hospital, but also specifically Peter of Spain's clerical office.

Contemporaries recognised various degrees of mental disturbance as having different causes. Melancholy at its mildest was believed to begin at the entrance to the stomach with black bile descending, while at its most severe it began in the stomach with an excess of black bile which mixed with the other three humours and then ascended to the brain, creating an infection of the central ventricle.[124] Both aloe and squirting cucumber were important ingredients in S. Maria Nuova's recipe for 'pills of wild cucumber that purge choler and melancholy', while aloe 'purges through vomiting and equally below the choler and phlegm'.[125] Three more recipes were included to treat melancholy. One was a general recipe for 'aquavita' which was described as a 'cosa preziosa', a 'precious thing', reflected in its exotic character, as it was alleged to have been used at the courts of the emperor of Constantinople and of the kings of India,

Armenia and Egypt. It was used for a wide range of conditions – indeed, it seems to have been something of a general panacea – including for 'sadness of the heart and against melancholy'.[126] A recipe designed specifically to treat melancholy was for pills containing a series of purgatives: a fern called polypody, dodder, black hellebore and lavender. The latter, according to Mattioli's citation of Mesué, 'dissolves melancholy and phlegm'.[127]

The *Ricettario* also included two recipes for the mad, though because treatment of *pazzi* was not a high priority, these were placed among recipes to help people sleep. In fact, S. Maria Nuova, in common with other hospitals of this period, tended to avoid admitting the mad along with other patients with chronic conditions. The reference to its 'place for those who have lost their minds through illness, where they are kept in chains',[128] suggests these patients were not admitted already 'mad', but became so subsequently. The use of chains was common practice in this period to prevent the mad harming themselves.[129] S. Maria Nuova's room for madmen would have been cool and well ventilated since madness was associated with those with a hot and dry complexion and was thought to be caused by an excess of bile heating the blood, which when mixed together produced a hot vapour which rose to the brain.[130]

The main aim in treatment of the mad was to calm these symptoms and bring the patient back to sanity by attacking the cause of madness, as reflected in the two recipes in S. Maria Nuova's *Ricettario*. The first was a suppository prescribed by one of the hospital's own doctors, Maestro Agostino, which was designed 'to send a madman to sleep'. The ingredients included a base of honey with finely ground turbit, colocynth and rock salt.[131] The first two simples were purgatives; colocynth, according to Mattioli, was used 'to move the body'.[132] The violence of this treatment may have had more to do with purging the humours, since madness was seen as stemming from their imbalance,[133] than with sleep, though patients may have been so exhausted that they fell asleep at the end of the treatment. The second recipe for inducing madmen to sleep was an external treatment:[134]

> *To send a madman to sleep*
> Put the following ingredients into a chicken or into the lung of a castrated ram, which is [then] placed on top of the head, [which] should be shaved, so that it covers the whole head: white poppies and black poppies, henbane, skin of mandrake root, violets and lettuce seeds and seeds of purslane, camomile flowers and dill.
>
> Grind all the ingredients and put them in the cock which has been split into two and heated and put it on top of the head and leave it there for a day and a night and once this is done you should remove it and use other remedies.

At first sight this may seem a rather extraordinary method of treatment, but the use of a small animal or the lungs of a larger one such as a ram was not uncommon. Both Bartholomeus Anglicus and Thomas of Cantimpré recommended this treatment for frenzy, the latter suggesting as an alternative a 'little dog or a cock opened through its back'. Whichever animal or fowl was used, the aim was to ensure maximum contact with the head, the seat of madness, by ensuring that the patient was shaved and the whole surface was covered.[135] Many of the simples involved have been encountered above in relation to headaches and were active ingredients that were natural soporifics.[136]

The preference for rams also underlines the importance of astrology in explaining madness and the condition's specific association with Capricorn. Evidently using the ram alone was sufficient for some conditions, as in the recipe to treat people who not only could not sleep, but 'who [also] speak nonsensically': 'Take the warm ram's lung and place it on the shaved head and leave him in a dark place without light and repeat this three times.'[137] This repetition, associated with the Trinity, again underlines the close association between physical and spiritual healing.

Headaches

Many of the recipes for aches and pains of the head tended to be simple and directed towards immediate relief of an observable symptom rather than linked to a complex theoretical background: four were for *magrana* or migraine and eleven were to treat 'pains' or headache. Remedies for *magrana*, ranging from the gentle to the more violent, include a liquid and three unguents. The liquid, a mixture of rosemary, sage, figs and currants, was drunk and 'liberated' the patient from the pains.[138] Both rosemary and sage have heating properties, which they shared with figs which were also purgative.[139] The two unguents were made from a simple in a liquid. The first consisted of euphorbia or spurge and water, which were boiled together and then 'when the pain comes place two drops on the nose'. The other involved poplar and pig fat 'mixed together on a low heat to create a thick mixture which was then spread on the head'.[140] Spurge was a simple that had been respected by writers since the time of Galen because of its heating and caustic qualities; indeed, Mattioli recommended that apothecaries should get a 'porter or other vile people and labourers' to grind it up since it was able to 'penetrate with air into the nostrils of the nose and induce there an unbearable burning sensation'.[141] The final unguent, containing alabaster and called 'Alabastro Nardi Prezioso', was a complex remedy of twenty-three ingredients that was a cure-all for a large number of conditions involving aches and pains. The recipe was supposed to have had an ancient origin, for 'the Romans brought [it] from Jerusalem at the time of Jesus Christ's crucifixion and Mary Magdalene anointed the body of

Jesus with this'. The association with Mary Magdalene's ointment had made it doubly 'prezioso'.[142]

The majority of recipes for the more generic 'headaches' or 'head pains' were as straightforward as most of those for migraine. Many claimed that when used each 'takes away the pain immediately'.[143] One was a drink made from white wine which, boiled up with white ginger, was 'heating';[144] another was a solution used to wash the head and was made from 'good vinegar' boiled up with tips of willow branches, which had a drying quality good for pains and any impediments;[145] while a mixture of purslane juice and onion was held above the nose to clear the head, for, according to Galen, it was good for 'head pains caused by heat for it [purslane] was cold in the third degree'.[146] Other recipes included heating ointments applied to the head, such as minced garlic with crushed beans,[147] and breadcrumbs and juice of coriander, well known for its cooling properties.[148] As in the case of migraine, there were also more complex recipes, as with Maestro Diotifeci Ficino's mixture of the oils of waterlily, violets, henbane and dill with opium and saffron in a base of wax.[149]

This long series of remedies for the same conditions appears bewildering since many seem to have had different effects. The main simples in each remedy were supposed to change the temperature of the patient. That some had opposite effects – some heating, some cooling – is explained by Mattioli as arising from the fact that some pains of the head were caused by heat and others by cold. He lists simples he considers to be most suitable for treating headaches stemming from either heat or cold on the first page of his 'Table of the Remedies of all the Illnesses of the Human Body'.

Insomnia

The single most frequent condition associated with the head in S. Maria Nuova's *Ricettario* is insomnia (twenty-two). The corresponding recipes may have been designed for members of staff and patients who found it difficult to sleep through pain or fever or following a surgical intervention. There were eight different types of recipe to treat sleeplessness divided between external and internal treatments. External treatments included ointments, a plaster, baths and, as seen above, one for an insomniac madman, placing the warm lungs of a ram on his head. Baths involved immersion in warm water in which had been boiled up a series of simples, including poppies, barley, violets, red roses and mandrake.[150] The latter was particularly powerful for, as Mattioli says, 'it takes away the energy of the whole body and therefore leads to the deepest of sleep'.[151]

Internal treatments for sleep can be sub-divided into liquids, pills and suppositories. These would have been prescribed by a physician and, indeed, two of these recipes were attributed to one of the hospital's doctors, Maestro

Agostino, who was responsible for a wide range of recipes in the hospital's *Ricettario*. The liquids contained ingredients that would have caused drowsiness. The first was headed 'To induce sleep; this recipe is most efficacious'.[152] It included the leaves and seeds of poppy and opium, of which Mattioli remarks, 'one grain of opium eases pains, matures, helps sleep ... but taken in larger quantities it is poisonous'.[153] Other ingredients include wild thyme, known to be good for headaches; styrax oil (*isquarmi storicie*), which is 'most excellent for heating and acts as an emollient, but causes pain and heaviness of the head and leads to sleep'; and, finally, incense, which, according to Galen, heats and dries and when mixed with the other medicines increases their potency.[154] The other two internal recipes for sleep included the suppositories examined above and Pills from Thebes for madmen, containing only three ingredients: cinnamon, saffron and the soporific opium.[155]

Head Wounds

In addition to recipes associated with internal conditions, Table 9.5 reflects the importance of treatments for patients with wounds and injuries to the head, often administered in special rooms without windows to avoid the dangers of fresh air. *Capirotti* – literally broken heads – were the most frequently mentioned condition (fifteen) associated with the head and reflect the brawls and fights typical of city street life, as reflected in contemporary court records. S. Maria Nuova would also have treated the wounds of members of the Florentine militia returning home from campaigns and of mercenaries passing through the city.

These conditions were treated externally with unguents and plasters by surgeons like Maestro Diotifeci Ficino or, in the case of women patients, by the nursing staff. The recipes enable us to compare the types of ingredients used by Marsilio Ficino's father and the *commesse*. The most obvious difference is that the women's recipes contain fewer simples than Maestro Diotifeci's (sixteen compared to twenty-six), but it is worth examining how far this might also imply a qualitative difference.

> *Unguent for fractured heads when gone green, an unguent which we have from Monna Francesca and Monna Caterina, doctors of the house, and from them we have the recipe which works marvellously*[156]
> Honeysuckle and wild sage: 2lb each
> Betony: 1lb
> Aconite or erba San Cristofano, rosemary, salad-burnet ½lb each
> Purslane, nightshade: 1lb each
> Aura: 4oz
> Paleo (dog-grass) and domestic sage: 1 piece each

Laurel oil: 4oz
Common oil: 6lb
Turpentine, pine resin, yellow wax: 4lb each
Ordinary wax: 2lb
Pig fat: 4 drams
Red wine

Method
Put the said herbs into red wine as long as necessary and add 4 drams of pig fat and keep stirring.

The first ingredients formed the base of Francesca and Caterina's recipe: oils, turpentine, pine resin, wax and pork lard, a cheap fat found in the kitchen. They were binding agents with therapeutic properties; laurel oil, for example, was heating, while pine resin was especially designed to treat inflammation of wounds[157] and wax was recommended to take away the strong smell of pork.[158]

All the active ingredients were herbs suitable for the treatment of wounds that were readily available in the hospital's own garden.[159] Honeysuckle, for example, was recommended by the well-known surgeon Giovanni di Vigo for leg ulcers, as were wild and domestic sage, which 'purifies malign and sordid ulcers' and blocks the flow of blood from wounds. Rosemary was particularly good for treating inflammations and bringing out apostemes, and betony was described by Mattioli as having a more general application: 'Betony is truly a herb which is universally known by everyone and is full of infinite virtues, from which is born the proverb: "You have more virtues than betony." Used as a plaster on head wounds it heats with marvellous rapidity.'[160]

Maestro Diotifeci Ficino's recipe for head fractures is more complex:[161]

Plaster for fractured heads
We have the recipe from Maestro Ficino doctor of the house and it works miraculously; Neri di Gino Capponi had it from Maestro Michele.
Fat of bear, wild ass and beaver: 4oz each
Oil of fine bay, mastic, sweet almonds, lavender, rose: 3oz each
Oil of camomile, dill: 2oz each
Gum, incense, myrrh, finely ground cinnamon: 3oz each
Dragon's blood: 1½oz
Aloe, wild olive: 1oz
Washed turpentine: 8oz
New wax, pine resin, wild sage, salad burnet: 7oz each
Vervain, marjoram, thyme: 7oz each

Method
Boil all these ingredients, that is, the herbs, in white wine so they are reduced to half the volume and to this mixture add the turpentine, fats, resin, wax and oils. Place this on a low flame and when it has been boiled for an eighth of an hour put it in a large clean basin and allow to cool. When it is cool throw away any wine which remains and then put it on a low flame and leave it until it is consumed, slowly stirring it with a stick, and when it is liquefied so that it is very hot add the other ingredients which have been finely ground, always stirring with the stick until it is cool and when it is done store it and use it for plasters when needed.

The base for the recipe consisted of three different types of animal fat: bear, beaver and wild ass,[162] less readily available than pork fat. Mattioli tells us that while 'all fats are hot, soft or emollient and dilute the humours', there was a reason for using more than one because each had slightly different qualities, being more or less constrictive or hot.[163]

Some of the simples in Maestro Diotifeci's recipe were also contained in the women's, most notably turpentine, wax, pine resin, wild sage and salad burnet. These and some of the other plants or herbs in his recipe, such as lavender, camomile, dill and bay, could be found in the hospital's garden. Other ingredients were more expensive and less common and so would have been supplied by the hospital's pharmacist. Myrrh, for example, is a gum resin from trees in the Middle East, especially Arabia and Egypt, recommended because it 'heals head wounds'.[164] Incense also boasted exotic origins since it was imported from Africa and India and had appropriate qualities for treating wounds: 'filling deep ulcers and equally joins and reinforces fresh wounds, stems all bloody fluxes ... heals malign ulcers.'[165] A substantial additional benefit of these two ingredients was their religious associations which were thought to add greatly to their efficacy. Another exotic ingredient was 'dragon's blood', which Mattioli says was 'most efficacious for stanching blood'. He identifies it with Dioscorides' cinnabar, or red mercuric sulphide, which had been imported from Africa. However, he records that the latter was rarely used because of its 'grandissimo prezzo' ('enormous price'). Instead the dragon's blood found in most apothecaries' workshops was made from 'sulphur and mercury cooked together for a long time on the fire'.[166]

Maestro Diotifeci's recipe for *capirotti* was, then, differentiated from that of the women practitioners because it included more expensive and exotic ingredients. Many of these had classical authority behind them, including Avicenna, Dioscorides, Galen and Hippocrates. If Maestro Diotifeci was more aware of their classical pedigree and of the sophisticated theory of qualities that underlay many of these ingredients,[167] in practice this made little difference;

the simples included by the women had similar properties to those used by this eminent surgeon.

Eyes

After the more general category of 'capo' or head, it is the eyes and mouth that stand out in Table 9.4.[168] This reflects the practice noted above, in Chapter 2, that from the first half of the Trecento the hospital employed empirics, specialised in cataract removal as well as the treatment and drawing of 'sad teeth'. However, it is significant that of the fifty-eight recipes for eyes only one specifically mentioned cataracts, presumably because the majority were treated surgically (Table 9.6). This followed the tradition of other recipe books; neither Peter of Spain nor Mattioli's *Discorsi* included treatments for cataracts. The one recipe for cataracts described in the *Ricettario* as 'provata' (tested) was a complex powder made up of fifty-two different simples, an expensive preparation available only to institutions or surgeons with access to large, well-equipped pharmacies.[169]

Table 9.6 S. Maria Nuova's *Ricettario*, 1515: symptoms associated with the eyes

Eyes (general)	31
sick / pain	4
red	3
swollen	3
ruptured	3
stung	1
cataract	1
Improve sight	8
Tears: staunch	3
Colour blue	1
Total	58

Just over half of the fifty-eight recipes associated with eyes are generic, simply listing ingredients without describing the symptoms they are intended to treat. Others are more specific and designed to make sight 'clearer' or stop tears, treat pain or inflamed eyes, or deal with ruptured eyeballs, as in:[170]

Poultice for the rupture of the flesh of the eye
Red roses, broad-leaved plantain, willow leaves, pomegranate flowers: a handful of each
Saffron: 2 drams
Broadbean flour, lentil flour: 1oz

Method
Cook the above-mentioned ingredients in plantain water and make up a poultice with this mixture without any grease.

The majority of these ingredients had drying and cleansing properties. Mattioli says of pomegranate flowers that they 'constrict, dry, knit and strengthen fresh wounds',[171] while willow leaves 'heal fresh and bloody wounds'.[172] He cites Galen's explanation for the use of plantain water as a drying and astringent agent: it 'has a mixed temperament, since one finds in it a certain watery and cold faculty as well as sourness. This is because it has the cold and dryness of the soil and as such cools and dries in the second degree.'[173] The inclusion of these simples was thus justified from both a practical point of view, as understood by readers of Peter of Spain's *Tesoro dei poveri*, and from a more intellectual and theoretical standpoint.

Mouths

Table 9.7 S. Maria Nuova's *Ricettario*, 1515: symptoms associated with the mouth

Mouth	1
pain	3
cancerous	1
smell	2
	7
Teeth	7
pain	6
pull	1
worms	1
secure	1
set on edge	1
preserve	1
	18
Gums	3
strengthen	1
black	1
broken	1
	6
Lips	1
broken or cracked	8
	9
Tongue	1
swollen	2
wounded	1
	4
Total	44

The practical and theoretical also underlay the forty-four recipes for the treatment of the mouth, the second-most numerous category of recipes among those for head injuries (Table 9.7). They included a recipe for bad breath – 'puzzo della bocca' – which consisted of a mouthwash of mint cooked in white vinegar.[174] Others were for swollen tongues. For example, when a patient's tongue was so large that he was unable to talk, ground pepper was 'placed in the mouth and after a few hours he is cured'.[175] Another eight recipes were designed to treat cracked or 'chapped lips'.[176]

The hospital surgeon Maestro Fruosino's treatment for a woman whose mouth was 'tutta incancherita', cancerous or full of ulcers, contained two active metallic ingredients, alum and verdigris.[177] These were added to white wine and vinegar, which when boiled together produced a concentrated solution to be placed on the infected area. Alum from mines in Egypt or Sardinia and the more common verdigris had corrosive properties. The main qualities of the former were to 'heat, constrict and clean' and it was recommended to stop the growth of putrid and corrosive ulcers and to dry the humidity of gums created by infections such as gingivitis.[178] Verdigris reinforced these qualities because it too was known to 'corrode and liquefy flesh'.[179] Mattioli recommended that this ointment should be applied 'in small quantities with the tip of a pen onto the swollen ulcers, and the following day they will be smaller'. However, he warns that 'if one applies a larger quantity of the ointment the ulcer will be found not so much reduced as completely corroded and eaten up'.[180] Once again Mattioli cites classical authorities for the use of these ingredients, including Galen, and records that this recipe was in common use in Western Europe.

Problems with teeth were the most numerous symptoms associated with the mouth. There were twenty-four separate recipes for treating teeth and gums, including: black teeth with a mixture of barley and salt; broken teeth; worms, to be treated with leek and mistletoe in wax; and gum problems leading to loss of teeth. All recipes for toothache, the most common ailment, were simples. For instance:[181]

Recipe for toothache
Opium from Thebes
Celery seeds
St John's wort
Ginger
Mustard
Mastic
Roses

Method
Boil [together] in a pint of wine until it is reduced to half, then leave it to cool and hold it in the mouth.

This dense liquid, which once heated and cooled may have created quite a solid substance not unlike chewing gum – depending on the quantity of mastic – was to be held in the mouth to reduce toothache. The ingredients included a number that were well known for the treatment of pain. Opium from Thebes was also used to aid sleep, but as Mattioli warned it should not be taken in too large a quantity for otherwise it would poison the patient, leading to lethargy and even death. The second ingredient, celery seeds, when included in a compound medicine was also known to reduce pain in teeth, as was the third, St John's wort, and was recommended by both Galen and Dioscorides, while mustard, according to Mattioli, was used 'universally for all painful spots'.[182]

These simples were well known for treating pain in general and toothache in particular. All produced heat, an important quality in humoral theory in combating the frigidity associated with pain. With certain ingredients Mattioli was moved to include a health warning. One such was stavesacre, a species of larkspur: three seeds were put inside a piece of linen cloth which was then placed against the aching tooth 'and immediately the pain will disappear'. It was not to be put into the mouth unprotected, 'for it is dangerous and should not be allowed to cut or burn the throat'.[183] Another was euphorbia, which took away the pain when boiled up in wine but should be used only once a month as a mouthwash for it 'burns all the day'.[184] Finally, ground-up stag's horn was heated until it produced a white powder, which was then applied to the tooth in question from which it 'takes away the pain'.[185]

Recipes to treat toothache were clearly a mixture of medical theory inherited from classical sources and empirical evidence gathered from the experience of treating hospital patients. But it should not be forgotten that supernatural cures were as important as natural cures, as in the following advice given for the extraction of teeth:[186]

To pull teeth, ask the name of the person whose tooth you want to extract and then say 'In Nomine Patris et Filii et Ispiritus Sancti. Amen' or 'Lord Jesus Christ, living Son of God, you who freed St Apollonia allow me to pull this tooth out, as Nicodemus pulled out the nails from Christ' or 'Tooth come out through the virtues of Christ and of St Apollonia the Virgin. In Nomine Patris Filii et Spiritus Sancti. Amen.' Who wishes to do this should fast the Vigil of St Apollonia, the night before 8 February.

The relevance of St Apollonia to the cure would have been clear to contemporaries. She was a deaconess in Alexandria who had lived in the third century at the time of the persecution of the early Christians. She was invoked frequently against toothache and all dental diseases since following her arrest her tormentors had knocked out her teeth before burning her at the stake.[187]

The link between natural and supernatural remedies also underlay remedies to treat the abdomen, the area of the body that attracted the third-largest number of recipes (Table 9.8).

9.6 Digestion, Excretion and Sex

Table 9.8 S. Maria Nuova's *Ricettario*, 1515: recipes for the abdomen

Liver	11
Spleen	11
Digestive organs:	
stomach	53
belly and gut	49
Posterior	14
Urogenital:	
female	25
male	16
Bladder and kidneys	51
Total	230

It is necessary to return to humoral theory to understand how contemporaries saw the interrelationship between the main internal organs. According to Galenic medicine, the functions of the stomach, liver and spleen were complementary. The stomach was seen as essential in the production of humours. Through the digestive process it converted food into chyle, from which it then extracted what goodness it needed and sent the residue to the intestines. There, the food was further sorted into useful chyle, which was sent on to the liver, and the useless, which was eliminated through excretion. The liver, meanwhile, began to convert the chyle into blood with which to nourish the rest of the body. During this process the liver further cleansed the blood of the red or yellow bile, which went via the gall duct to the gall bladder. The black bile went to the spleen, to which it provided nourishment, and eventually travelled back to the stomach to aid digestion. At this point the purified chyle became blood and flowed from the liver to the other parts of the body.[188] The four humours were therefore regarded as real bodily fluids, each with a natural origin and location within the body.

It is hardly surprising, given the central role of the stomach in Galenic theory, that a large number of recipes in the *Ricettario* were for the digestive organs. I shall begin with the treatment of ailments associated with the stomach, liver and spleen since this was believed to lead to the proper balancing of the humours, and conclude with the urogenital area.

Stomach

Many of the recipes for the stomach were either recommended by named practitioners who worked for the hospital or were drawn from other well-known recipe collections. For example, ointments for pains in the stomach were prescribed by Maestro Aghostino and Maestro Dino the Frenchman, while recipes for stomach electuaries came from Maestro Michele da Pescia, Maestro Santi *pitavino* from Poitou and Maestro Giovanni da Lucca. There were also prescriptions for specific patients, such as the electuary for the head and stomach of a friend of 'Bonino nostro', the *spedalingo* of S. Maria Nuova, and an ointment to treat the 'cold stomach' of Nastasia, one of the *commesse* of the hospital. Other recipes came from more exotic sources and were associated with famous people in the past, such as an unguent for gripe, which was said to have derived from Agrippa, king of the Jews. An exceptionally complicated recipe was said to have been made up by the 'abbot of the court' for Duke Ruberto Ghuglielmo, while the *pillole istomatiche* were taken from one of the standard medical textbooks, the *Ad Almansorem* of Rhazes.

There were both internal and external recipes for the treatment of stomach disorders. Internal medicines included electuaries, medicinal powders mixed with honey (nine); syrups (one); pills (three); a laxative; aquavita; and a powder. Half merely stated that they were remedies for the stomach without indicating a particular ailment. Others were more specific, including recipes for conditions that sound familiar today, such as pains, hardness, gripe, wind and indigestion. Yet others remind one of the role of the stomach in the overall humoral theory of physiology: coldness, humidity, phlegm and blockage of humours. Thus, aquavita was prescribed for both a 'weak' stomach and more generally for 'cold sickness', an electuary for drying the 'humidity' of the stomach, and pills (*pillole istomatiche*), prescribed by 'some of our authors', were recommended for drying the phlegm in the stomach. Laxatives were also prescribed for removing superfluities or bad humours in the stomach, including one, 'very strong', which was good for treating tertian fever. The same principles lay behind the recipes for external treatments, mostly by surgeons, with ointments (nine) and plasters (ten). There were also three recipes using small sacks containing simples, which through their heating properties provided comfort to the stomach.

Recipes for the stomach were often designed as a general aid to digestion, as can be seen in Maestro Benedetto Reguardati da Norcia's *De conservatione sanitatis* (1477), probably written for the duke of Milan, Francesco Sforza:[189]

And when you feel weakness of the stomach in digestion, put on the stomach a plaster of simple gum mastic, that is, made up just from powdered gum mastic, placing in a small tin receptacle an ounce of powdered mastic with three drops of oil of mastic, keeping it on a low flame until it is melted, and then, immediately before it becomes solid, pour it on a thin tissue in the shape of a shield and place it on the stomach.

These recipes can be understood in terms of humoral theory, that is, as treating heat or cold or as freeing blockages, but also in terms of their practical and pragmatic effects. They can be plotted along a continuum, from the more theoretical and abstruse to the more simple and practically straightforward. This reflects the wide variety of sources on which this hospital *Ricettario* was based, from the more sophisticated ones drawn from the books of medicine taught in medical faculties to the simpler ones devised by the *commesse*. However, it is a mistake to distinguish too rigidly between learned, theoretical medicine and an unlearned, practical approach because all practitioners shared the same Galenic world-view.

Liver and Spleen

Table 9.9 S. Maria Nuova's *Ricettario*, 1515: recipes for the liver and spleen

Liver	
liver	4
pain	1
hardness	4
blockage	2
	11
Spleen	
spleen	2
pains and hardness	2
sick	4
swollen	1
blockage through frigidity	2
	11
Total	22

According to this system, the stomach was closely related to the liver and spleen, which themselves were seen as inter-dependent. As such, many of the conditions associated with these organs had shared recipes (Table 9.9). Pain and hardness and the feeling of being 'liverish' were easily identified as being purely physical sensations, but it would take the physician to interpret what this meant in terms of humoral theory and to decide on the appropriate remedy. As has been seen, the liver was central to the Galenic physiological system for it was believed to be the main blood-making organ of the body. It was here that one of the two main sorts of blood originated, the venous, which fed the body and ensured its growth. Arterial blood originated in the heart and carried life to the rest of the body.[190]

The vast majority of the treatments for 'hardness' or pains in the liver and spleen used plasters; a 'small winter sack' was recommended for somebody who felt liverish ('feghatoso'). Two were derived from medical textbooks, as in the case of the 'liver poultice [which] is good for the hardness of the liver, according to Mesué at chapter xxxiiii'.[191] This was a complex recipe involving thirteen different simples, as was another cited for hardness of the liver 'according to our authors', which included three different sorts of sandalwood (white, yellow and red), hepatic aloe, juice from absinthe and endive, saffron, barley flour, juice from deadly nightshade, and spodium.[192] Spodium, according to Mattioli, has 'very subtle qualities, much aids digestion and cleansing, so that it heats and dries almost to the third degree, such that it dries more than it heats'.[193]

Medicines to treat blockage tended to be taken internally. The ingredients of a 'ferrous electuary' to combat blockage of the liver caused by 'frigidity'[194] had heating properties and included iron filings as well as white and black pepper, white ginger, cinnamon, cardamom, saffron and galanga, all in a base of honey to make it less unpleasant to swallow. Galanga, according to Mattioli, 'heats in the third degree and, moreover, helps the stomach to digest and counters the pains generated by those who have cold humours or flatulence'.[195]

There was also a number of less complex recipes associated with medical authorities. Three involved animal products and two vegetable products. The basis of the first two were the spleens of other animals, used on the principle of treating like with like. Thus, a goat's spleen has to be taken 'as it is removed from the goat and then place it on your spleen and tie it there … and repeat it two or three times'.[196] For an ox spleen: 'split it and place it on the head like a garland … and do this three times, then hang that spleen above the fire and when it is dried out he will be cured.'[197] The third was a snail cooked as fritters; when it was eaten, 'you will be cured'![198]

The two plant recipes were also to be consumed but in different ways. The first was a mixture of camomile flowers and roses cooked together and inhaled so that you 'receive those vapours through the nostrils'.[199] The second consisted of a mixture of bryony, strawberry plant and honey:[200]

> Bryony given to eat makes the patient urinate and consumes the sickness that contaminates the spleen and to increase its virtue it is put into theriac

and it is drunk in infusions. If you carry bryony in your belt or on your head you should know that no disease can affect you, as has already been said. And if you drink strawberry plant and its juice together with honey it cures the liver.

These more straightforward recipes for diseases of the spleen were based on a combination of animal and vegetable simples easily obtainable from the wild or the hospital's gardens, though the last recipe also included the wonder-drug theriac. This mixture of animal and vegetable simples was also the basis for the treatment of diseases of the urogenital tract, though usually combined with minerals.

The Urogenital Tract

Treatments for diseases of the urogenital tract also represent a significant proportion of the 840 recipes identified with a symptom or body part (11 per cent). I have divided these complaints into three: those associated particularly with women, those linked to men, and common conditions of the bladder and kidney.

Table 9.10 S. Maria Nuova's *Ricettario*, 1515: recipes for female urogenital conditions

Womb	4
hot and hard	1
pains	2
sick	4
hysteria or suffocation of the womb	3
Menstruation	
bringing on	3
Bloody flux	2
Pregnancy	
testing for	1
Giving birth	
if unable	1
to induce it early	2
a dead baby	2
Total	25

When dealing with women's illnesses it is useful to remember the standard Galenic line about the basic differences between men and women, as formulated in the Trotula treatise the influential collection of three works on women's medicine from twelfth-century Salerno.[201]

> He [God] made the nature of the male hot and dry and that of the female cold and wet so that the excess of each other's embraces might be restrained by the mutual opposition of contrary qualities… Since then women are by nature weaker than men it is reasonable that sicknesses more often abound in them, especially around the organs involved in the work of nature.

There were a large number of recipes for the 'organs involved in the work of nature', a logical corollary of the weakness of women, whose genitals were regarded as an imperfect imitation of men's (Table 9.10).

Menstruation was the most obvious sign of the weakness of women and their potential for physical problems. This regular expulsion of blood was explained by the idea that women, being cold and wet by their very nature, did not have enough heat within themselves to consume the moisture that collects within them. The monthly 'curse' was therefore seen as nature's way of expelling corrupt humours, which if left inside the body could cause putrefaction and sickness.[202] Five different recipes related specifically to the problems of the menses, as relevant for treating *commesse* as female patients. Two are for women who have excessive flows of blood, three for those who have 'lost' their periods and two to 'provoke' their return.

The Trotula treatise ascribes a number of reasons for an excessive flow of blood:[203]

> This happens because the veins of the uterus are large and open, or because the patient breaks wind and thence blood flows in great quantities. The flowing blood appears bright and red. Because too much food and drink has generated too much blood and since it cannot be contained within the blood vessels, it bursts forth outside. Sometimes it happens on account of excessive heat of the blood. Yellow bile pouring back from the gall bladder makes the blood feverish to such an extent that it cannot be contained in the veins. Sometimes a salty phlegm is mixed with the blood and thins it and makes it burst forth outside. If the blood that comes becomes yellowish or inclines to a yellow colour, it is due to the bile. If it is inclined towards a whitish colour, it is due to phlegm. If to a red colour, it is from the blood. Sickness of this kind comes about on account of bad moistures internally and nature disdains to maintain it.

The first of S. Maria Nuova's recipes dealing with menses is for 'when the woman has her period outside the normal time and with over-much flow of blood',[204] and the second is simply 'Against women's flow of blood, tested'. The instructions for the first are: 'Take pimpernel root and carry it around the neck and then grind it up with warm white wine and then drink it.' The second instructs the doctor to take 'the woman's hair and tie it to a tree and the woman will be freed and the tree will dry up'.[205] Obviously both these recipes contained an element of sympathetic magic. This was especially true of the second, with its link between the woman's hair and the tree, although even if the author of the hospital's *Ricettario* assures us that the recipe was 'provata' he does not indicate how long the patient has to remain tied to the tree before the treatment will work! The active ingredient in the first recipe was root of pimpernel, probably *solbastrella*, the type most common in Tuscany.[206] The first type, which he described as 'hot and dry to the second degree', was used to combat the cold and wet nature of women and more specifically what the Trotula treatise called the 'bad moistures', the cause of excessive menstrual blood. According to Mattioli, the second type of pimpernel was employed 'to congeal and to block' and was therefore 'extremely efficacious in menstrual flows'.[207]

Other recipes were designed to treat various conditions of the womb including aches and pains.[208] A 'hot and hard' womb was rare given women's predisposition to coolness and wetness,[209] although the Trotula does recognise that 'It happens sometimes that the womb is deranged in temperature to such an extent that great burning and heat are felt there'.[210] The hospital recipe was a wax poultice and the three main ingredients were finely ground white wax, lead white and rose oil. These were heated together until they turned black, then were allowed to cool before being applied to the affected area and left to 'mature for as long as possible'.[211] The two active drying ingredients were the lead white and rose oil. The Trotula recipe, on the other hand, consisted of opium, goose fat, wax, honey, oil, egg white and woman's milk, which were mixed together and 'injected on a tampon'.[212]

Three other recipes treated a condition frequently associated with women, 'hysteria' or 'suffocation of the womb', which was well described in the Trotula treatise:[213]

> *On suffocation of the womb*
> Sometimes the womb is choked; sometimes it is lifted upwards and there results a subversion of the stomach and a loss of appetite due to a weakening of the circulation. Sometimes women faint and the pulse seems to vanish if it is not felt for deeply. Sometimes the woman is convulsed, her head is brought to her knees, she lacks sight and cannot speak; her nose is twisted, her lips are compressed, she grits her teeth, and her breathing is shallower than normal.

It was believed that when the womb moved upwards it had a knock-on effect on the other organs such as the stomach which might lead to fainting or convulsions. Another cause of hysteria related to the belief that women also produced semen; indeed, one of the roles of the monthly period was seen as the evacuation of superfluous seeds from the womb. If these were not evacuated, they could become corrupted and a 'certain cold substance is formed which ascends to certain parts, which by common use are called collaterals because they are neighbours to the heart, the lungs and vocal organs, whence an impediment to the voice is wont to happen'.[214] Trotula's remedies for this condition include the rubbing of the woman's hands and feet with oil of laurel and the application to the nostrils of simples with 'a heavy odour', including oil of laurel, galbanum, opoponax, beaver and 'birch, burnt wool, burnt linen cloth, burnt skin and asafoetida'. Many of these ingredients were known from the time of Galen onwards as being hot and dry and would have been used to combat the 'certain cold substance'. More prosaically, strong smells were designed to shock the patient out of her fainting fit or convulsion.[215]

The *Ricettario* had its own recipe for the suffocation of the womb: 'place inside [her] crushed nettle, therefore immediately if it [the womb] falls it will be returned to its place and the same thing is also achieved by drinking parsnip seed.'[216] Nettle was well known for stanching the flow of blood and relaxing the womb, and was particularly appropriate because it was dry and hot, 'although not so hot that it can sting'.[217] Another recipe, of theriac together with cloves and garlic 'prepared warm with good wine and given to drink', was recommended because it 'marvellously frees the women who suffer from suffocation [of the womb], as I have seen and this is tested'.[218] The final recipe, a 'Capital Poultice', was for external treatment and was supplied by the hospital's surgeon, 'Maestro Ficino medico'.[219] The main ingredients shared the same qualities as those in the recipes above, namely heating and drying: myrtle, pomegranate flowers and skin, musk, aloe wood, sweet calamus, barley flower, sour and aromatic red wine.[220]

Treatments contained in the hospital *Ricettario* did not confine themselves to physical problems relating to the sexual organs, but also tackled those caused by the non-physical. This can be seen in the following recipe, appropriate for out-patients if not for the serving staff who were supposed to be celibate:[221]

Medicine if any man or woman should be bewitched so that they cannot have sexual union
They should go into a field where there are hanging blackberry bushes and find one that is well grown and long enough so that it is possible to get underneath and then kneel there and say together three Pater Nosters and three Ave Marias in honour of God and of the Virgin Mary and of the Holy Trinity and each of them must say 'Jesus of Nazarus son of David: Miserere

Mei' and say this three times. And if the wife and husband say this three times and enter underneath the blackberry bush and go against the sun, then the wife goes to the master [the doctor] and he takes her by the right hand from outside the bush and leads her back along the same way and walks around the bush three times and then goes to running water and they [wife and husband] embrace each other until they see her shadow, and then the master who accompanies them takes the water three times from behind her shadow and they put the water in a little vase and return home in the evening and when they go to bed, each of them drinks the water three times and done in this way every spell would be undone.

This recipe appears to represent folk medicine rather than that taught to aspiring doctors in universities at the time. It is a combination of Christian and pre-Christian rituals and medical lore. While blackberry may have been chosen partly because its bushes were substantial enough for somebody to crawl inside, there was also a medical reason for its selection. According to Mattioli, the various parts of the blackberry acted as a general panacea for many ills, including women's fluxes.[222] The inclusion of this recipe in the hospital's *Ricettario* also confirms my earlier assumption that this manuscript was a compilation of a series of collections from a number of sources. They were intended to treat not just in-patients, but also Florentines who had come to the *medicheria* for treatment and even for advice on sexual matters.

It would be easy to dismiss this type of recipe as untypical in its inclusion of religio-magical elements, but this would be to miss the point. Many recipes were based not simply on a narrowly defined 'medical' tradition, but more broadly on a world of symbols, which were seen as being particularly efficacious through their association with divine figures and members of the ecclesiastical and secular elite. This was as true of problems associated with men as with women, as can be seen in relation to the eighteen recipes relating to the male sexual organ. Table 9.11 shows that the vast majority of conditions were associated with the penis: swollen, smelly, heated, weak, livid and with warts. These may have been sexually transmitted diseases, a subject about which there had been growing concern with the recent epidemic of the Mal Francese,[223] though general hospitals like S. Maria Nuova specifically excluded those suffering from this disease.

Many of these recipes were simple and intended to provide gentle relief from symptoms. For example, when a penis appeared swollen and livid three ingredients were mixed together into an ointment and placed onto the infected part. These included juice from absinthe or wormwood, powdered cumin and honey, all of which were used as specifics to treat both male and female sexual problems.[224] The recipe to treat a 'heated penis', described as 'provata', was a mixture of bitter almonds and dried figs which 'heals perfectly'.[225] The two recipes to cure the smell of the penis both involved baths: 'wash it with wine which has been cooked with sage and you will be cured soon', and a 'hot bath with wine in which olive leaves have been cooked cures you'.[226]

Table 9.11 S. Maria Nuova's *Ricettario*, 1515: recipes for male urogenital conditions

Penis	3
heated	1
inflamed	3
smell	2
weak	1
warts	1
to open	1
lack of sperm	2
bewitched so unable to have sex	1
Testicles	
swollen and big	1
	16

Treatment was somewhat less anodyne for warts. The 'Powder to dry up the warts of the penis or in another place, tested', included orpiment, black pepper and a corrosive substance, vitriol, all of which had to be ground together before being heated over a flame until the mixture became fine and grey.[227] The poultice for a man with 'swollen and big testicles' was more complex and used simples from vegetables rather than minerals, including flour made from broad beans and chickpeas, together with fenugreek, cumin, seeds of the chaste-tree, camomile flowers, currants, a bunch of rue, combined with the fat of a female goat and of a goose, and finally oil of camomile and elder.[228] Many of these ingredients (broad beans, chickpeas, oil of camomile) were to reduce inflammation; others (fenugreek) were well known for acting as an emollient.[229] The poultice, then, was aimed to calm and reduce the swelling of the testicles, a swelling that would probably have been seen as derived from a blockage of humours that created heat, which was also true of conditions associated with the bladder and kidneys (Table 9.12).

At their more generic, these consisted of pain and weakness, inflammation and inability to urinate. Kidney stones were the most common complaint and there were twelve recipes for it. One of the simplest was by a certain 'Maestro D.' and consisted of the 'cooling seeds' of cucumber and melon mixed with pumpkin to relieve the symptoms by cooling the pain and inflammation which created heat.[230] Another simple recipe was an electuary made by boiling in malmsey the dung of a hen that had not yet mated with a cock; once it had reduced to half the quantity, a powder was added consisting of dried betony, horse-radish, white ginger and honey and the resulting mixture was then taken with warmed malmsey or a good Trebbiano wine.[231]

Table 9.12 S. Maria Nuova's *Ricettario*, 1515: recipes for the bladder and kidneys

Bladder	16
pain with inflammation	1
constricted	1
Kidneys	3
constricted	1
weakness	1
pain	4
purge	1
Stone	2
pain	6
break	2
against	2
Urine	
retention	1
cannot	3
affare	2
burning	1
constricted	1
Pain and stinging	1
during sleep	2
	51

Two other named recipes were much more complex and were probably copied from other collections. One was the 'Duke's Electuary' mentioned above, prepared by the 'abbot of the court', which in contrast to Maestro D.'s recipe included fifty-nine ingredients.[232] The other recipe, attributed to Avicenna, was especially 'strong to break the stone'. The main ingredients were the ashes produced through heating sodium nitrate, scorpions, the heads of cabbages, hares and eggshells collected after the birth of chicks. These were mixed together with the dried blood of an old goat, *lapis judaici* or the fossilised spines of sea urchins, a specific against stones, and 'pietra di spungnia', the small moluscs that live in sponges, gum from walnuts and sweet sedge in equal parts.[233]

While some recipes were designed specifically for kidney stones, others were made to treat a series of conditions of the urogenital tract, as with the 'diuretic syrup' used to 'purge the kidneys and the bladder of the coarse humours'.[234] Ingredients were renowned for their purgative, heating and drying qualities: saxifrage, celery, parsley, Macedonian parsley and asparagus. The following simples were then added to make a syrup: anise, lovage, dill, cardamom, lynx stone (*lapis lyncis*)[235] and agaric fungus – the latter, according to Mattioli, was good for 'crude humours and kidney pains'.[236] Finally, goat's blood, clove leaves and cinnamon were added, together with dried cicadas, without heads and wings, for, according to both Mattioli and Galen, 'eaten roasted in food they help the pains of the bladder'.[237]

Conclusion

Recipes to treat problems of the urogenital tract, in common with other sections of the *Ricettario*, reflect as wide a range of conditions as those found in works of both contemporary and Classical medical writers. Many aimed to correct a complexional imbalance within the patient's body; hence the emphasis on prescribing simple and complex medicines with specific heating, drying or cooling properties. However, recipes in each of the sections discussed above reflect the combined importance of theory and practice and treatments could often be justified in terms of both internal and external medicine.

The foregoing discussion of S. Maria Nuova's *Ricettario* has also shown that, in contrast to the modern custom of dividing diseases into neat nosological categories, the separation in the Renaissance between symptoms and diseases was elastic. Indeed, although the authors and compiler of this *Ricettario* do mention a wide range of ailments, these labels are often vague and illnesses are usually described in terms of the dysfunction of a particular part of the anatomy.

The elasticity of terminology also helps to explain what may ostensibly seem a curious feature of S. Maria Nuova's collection of medical recipes, that is, the inclusion of a section on beautification or *decorso del corpo*. In fact, this follows a well-established tradition, for similar recipes, were included in many of the major collections, including Avicenna and Peter of Spain and Mattioli's *Commentaries* on Dioscorides' *Discorsi*.[238] Indeed, recipes collected here reflect eternal human preoccupations that would not be unfamiliar to a beauty consultant today. Treatments include recipes for loss of hair, changing its colour to white, blond or black, and removing hair growing on hands. Recipes for the complexion include making the face 'bella' or a 'good colour'. Six other treatments for skin might have had both a medical and cosmetic function, for they involve removing or increasing growth of skin and getting rid of warts.

More generally, the combination of medical and religious elements in recipes for treating problems of the urogenital area, reminds us of the need to avoid thinking simply in terms of physical cures. For contemporaries, the effectiveness of medieval and Renaissance medicine was linked as much to belief in the power of spiritual medicine as in the inherent virtues of the combinations of plants, animals and minerals. It is for this reason that the image of Christus Medicus remains so powerful for the Renaissance hospital, with the spiritual doctor playing as essential a role as the physical doctor in the treatment of a wide range of illnesses of both natural and supernatural origins.

Conclusion

Part III has shown that the scale of the medical activities of the hospitals in Renaissance Florence goes some way to justify the proud claims of writers such as Benedetto Varchi, whose account of the charitable institutions of his native city rings with *campanilismo*. Indeed, one of the main aims of this book has been to examine those features identified by contemporaries which made the major Florentine hospitals into prime examples of what we think of as the 'Renaissance hospital'.

Thus Part I, 'Hospitals and the Body of the City', concentrated on the evolution of the leading medical hospitals and on their role in treating the sick poor and maintaining the health of Florentines during epidemics and periods of severe shortage. It has been seen that this became an important part of the republic's self-image as a *buon comune* which provided for the less fortunate members of society and at the same time gained spiritual merit through the implementation of the imperatives of the Seven Works of Mercy. This image was reinforced by the Renaissance idea of the ideal city with its emphasis on health and hygiene and rational organisation of its parts. Indeed, the Quattrocento saw the emergence of the Renaissance 'system of care', in which the various components of the sanitary structure of the city came to be seen as a whole, whether they dealt with the sick poor, orphans or those affected by chronic conditions such as leprosy and later the Mal Francese. However, even though Florence saw itself as 'above all others copiously provided with hospitals', by the mid-Quattrocento even the Signoria recognised that its system had an inherent defect because it lacked a lazzaretto for plague victims whose presence in the major hospitals infected those with ordinary diseases.

The rulers and citizens of Renaissance Florence thus shared with other states a sense of pride in their health service as in many other aspects of their political and cultural life. Even so, Florence's system of care had a different pattern of evolution from that of other large cities such as Milan, Rome and Siena, which by the thirteenth century all had hospitals – the Brolo, S. Spirito, S. Maria della Scala – on a very substantial scale. Florence instead had a large network of smaller *spedali* in this period, whose roles need further investigation. Indeed, the chronicler Giovanni Villani was particularly impressed by the number of hospitals in the city in 1388 (thirty-three) rather than their size to which contemporaries would typically draw attention a hundred years later. Though S. Maria Nuova and S. Paolo already provided substantial services to the poor and sick, it was the very complexity of the intermeshing system of smaller institutions that impressed the chronicler. Before the Black Death Florentines tended instead to draw attention to the great company of Orsanmichele, which provided wide-ranging support for the poor throughout this period, especially appreciated by the commune during famines and plagues. One also has to take into account the wider charitable system of the city, from the Church to the trade guilds and the numerous smaller confraternities, and especially the informal support of relatives, friends and neighbours, who in turn depended on the patronage networks of the city.

If the pride of Florentines before the Black Death was expressed in their descriptions of Orsanmichele and the numerousness of small *spedali*, by the mid-Quattrocento the picture had been reversed. Many of the large traditional charitable confraternities were in decline and Florentines concentrated their patriotic fervour instead on the substantial hospitals, many of them new. These hospitals were distinguished from those of many other large Italian cities by their specialisation, from treating the sick poor to looking after foundlings or providing accommodation for poor widows. In contrast the leading hospitals of Rome, Siena and Milan were all multi-functional and provided accommodation for the sick and foundlings under the same roof. Indeed, S. Spirito in Rome and S. Maria della Scala in Siena had been founded in or before the thirteenth century with a wide remit to respond to the demands of their position on major pilgrim routes. By the fifteenth century multi-functionality was also part of the movement for hospital reform in Lombardy, a key element of which was the institution of the Great Hospital such as the Ospedale Maggiore in Milan. Here the aim was to combine the charitable systems of the city into a rational whole as part of the increasing centralisation of the Renaissance state. In Tuscany this process was not undertaken until the mid-sixteenth century by the Medici duke Cosimo I. In a sense, though, Renaissance Florence had less need to reform its charitable system because it already had the two main elements of the Lombard movement: the 'Great Hospital' of S. Maria Nuova and an integrated system of care. If this charitable system conformed to the ideals of the Renaissance city, contemporaries realised that it was also open to threat from epidemic disease. The second half of the fifteenth century therefore saw Florence influenced by the wider movement in Italy towards the establishment of specialised hospitals for victims of the two new major diseases, plague and the Mal Francese, leading to the foundation of a lazzaretto and the Incurabili. Rulers now not only exchanged administrative and architectural models for large hospitals for the acute sick, but through their health magistrates actively corresponded about the problems generated by epidemics and developed common strategies to cope with these threats.

The sixteenth century also saw wider changes in Church and society impacting on the development of hospitals. As has been seen, the new 'redemptive charity' of the Counter-Reformation inspired a series of initiatives to 'save' abandoned boys and girls from immoral exploitation and marginal groups like prostitutes and beggars from a life of ignorance and sin. It is well known that this led to the establishment of new hostels for these groups, but the impact of this new moral climate on the atmosphere of existing hospitals is less often recognised, especially when the new orders of the Counter-Reformation took an active role in the way they were run. If the Counter-Reformation added a new moralistic tone, intolerant attitudes towards beggars which are so often seen as characteristic of the early modern period were hardly new. It should be stressed that many of the initiatives that were regarded as innovative in fact grew out of existing ideas, as seen in Alberti's strictures against the lazy poor. Measures such as the establishment of the Ospedali dei Mendicanti grew out of temporary expedients to deal with crises caused by natural disasters and their subsequent history had more to do with the responses of the Renaissance state to provide for the life-cycle poverty of the poorer strata of society than a policy of social control.

Thus, during the three hundred years covered by this book Florence gradually evolved the main features of a Renaissance hospital system that played a significant role in realising the contemporary concept of the ideal city with its emphasis on rational organisation of health provision and the relationship of beauty to functionality. Indeed, *bellezza*, the underlying theme of Part II, provided the second recognisable feature of the Renaissance hospital, reflected in both architectural and artistic terms. Vast new buildings were constructed and existing ones were expanded so that hospitals came to form important parts of the renewed fabric of the Renaissance city. In the process the hospital came to fuse many elements of Renaissance culture for, as Alberti underlined, the design of a building was an expression of civic and familial pride, reflecting honour and magnificence on patrons and city alike. I have argued that in general their structures grew in response to demand, but their design and construction would repay considerably more attention. For example, detailed reconstructions of building phases would enable one to test how far these spaces were adapted and expanded in response to changing medical and spiritual ideas, whether concerning the circulation of diseased air or the requirements of the Counter-Reformation.

CONCLUSION

Part II stressed that *bellezza* did not just play an aesthetic role, but was an essential expression of the religious character of the Renaissance hospital, reflected in the commissioning of devotional programmes by leading artists. Just as parish and conventual churches became important centres for the commissioning of Renaissance art, so did the hospital. However, by definition the role of altarpieces and frescoes and sculptural cycles had an extra dimension in a medical context, one that would repay further investigation. The physical environment of the church and ward chapel within the hospital needs to be better explored in relation to the role of spiritual medicine and to the contemporary understanding of disease and its causation and treatment.

The medical role gave the Renaissance hospital its third major characteristic and provided the theme of Part III. Here I considered the question raised in the Introduction, whether the reality of the pre-modern hospital bore more relation to the positive picture presented by contemporaries or to the negative Foucaultian view of them as 'antechambres de la mort'. On the positive side it has been shown that the Renaissance hospital was far from being a place of confinement; indeed, the fact that such numbers of people sought admission voluntarily suggests that the poor saw these institutions as likely to have beneficial effects on their health. The large trained medical and nursing staff and plentiful and well-stocked pharmacy enabled the Renaissance hospital to treat a wide variety of conditions, an area of investigation that could be developed much further in future research. Mortality rates of 5–10 per cent suggest that relatively few people died in hospital – *pace* Foucault – partly because the vast majority were admitted with relatively minor acute conditions such as fevers. However, one also has to take into account prevailing attitudes towards death – again underlining the importance of religion – in particular, the contemporary emphasis on the Good Death which meant dying at home with friends and family. Clearly, though, one should not be taken in by the patriotic praise of well-shod writers who spent more time dwelling on the *bellezza* of the buildings than on the actual conditions within the hospital. From the perspective of the twenty-first century it is difficult to judge the latter. Even if we would not paint Renaissance hospitals as entirely antiseptic environments, at the same time they have to be considered within the wider context of normal living conditions of the poor, which would probably have been much dirtier, colder and smellier than in these institutions. Writers during the Renaissance rarely noted the sanitary conditions within the city itself, except during epidemics when their perception of the relationship between their physical environment and disease was heightened and the ambience of hospitals was simply taken as symptomatic of a more universal problem.

The patient lies at the heart of all this but in this period he or she was principally recorded as a passive rather than an active agent, at least in the surviving documentation. In the future, however, it should be possible to learn more about how patients arrived by reconstructing the networks of recommendations from patrons, landlords and local parish priests and discovering whether hospital tenants enjoyed preferential treatment. The new bureaucracy of the Medici grand dukes, for example, should provide the opportunity to examine these issues through the large numbers of surviving petitions to the duke and his administrators from both individuals and corporations. It is this type of documentation in particular that will enable future historians to delve more deeply behind the façade of the Florentine hospital to examine the connections between the patrons, personnel, patients and property in these fundamental institutions of the Renaissance and early modern state.

In sum, then, the image that has emerged from this study provides another dimension to our understanding of the Renaissance. This book recognises that the hospital and indeed the diseased bodies within it represent a microcosm of the interplay of the many facets of the city. It is also true that the hospital presents a microcosm of the interplay of the many facets of the city. While the physical structure of the hospital added *bellezza* to its fabric, the emphasis on rational organisation and the functionality of the buildings and administration formed a part of the ideal of the state. If Leonardo da Vinci presented a vision of the ideal city with carefully zoned areas of rich and poor, the Renaissance hospital treated large numbers of the sick so that they could return well to the community and continue to make a useful contribution to society. But behind the carefully crafted vision of the Renaissance city of theorists such as Alberti and Leonardo there lay more intolerant attitudes towards the poor sick. Indeed, these ideas were developed further over the course of the sixteenth century when a more divisive idea of the relationship between the social classes emerged. The body of the city came to be seen as a physical body, with the nobler organs being identified with the rich, while the poor were associated with the weaker organs which became the depository of poisons and therefore the cause of disease. These topics will lead the investigation forward in time to the relationship between hospitals and the city in periods that showed a greater sensitivity to the links between sickness and the physical urban environment and debates about the hospital as a healthy or unhealthy place to treat the sick.

APPENDIX

Provisional List of Hospitals Founded in Florence, 1000–1550

This appendix represents a working summary of hospitals established in Florence in the period 1000 to 1550. In common with other recent lists of Florentine hospitals, my starting point has been Passerini, *Storia degli stabilimenti di beneficenza* and Davidsohn, *Forschungen* and *Storia*. Where possible all sources have been checked and updated and supplemented by the inclusion of references in other archival sources, such as the various redactions of the Catasto and the Decima in the fifteenth century. This list includes the majority of hospitals active in the city in this period, although it is hoped that future historians will be in a position to make additions and corrections through further archival research.

Recent lists of Florentine hospitals include R. Stopani, ed., *Firenze e i primi Giubilei. Un momento di storia fiorentina della solidarietà* (Florence, 1999), pp. 63–89, and Fondazione Michelucci, *L'Ospedale e la città. Dalla fondazione di S. Maria Nuova al sistema ospedaliero del 2000*, ed. A. Aleardi, G. Germano, C. Marcetti and N. Solimano (Florence, 2000), pp. 92–117.

Sources (abbreviations)

(See Bibliography for full references)
Davidsohn = R. Davidsohn, *Storia*
Fanelli = G. Fanelli, *Firenze*
Paatz = W. and E. Paatz, *Die Kirchen von Florenz*
Passerini = L. Passerini, *Storia degli stabilimenti di beneficenza*

KEY
1. **Fields**
a. Title
b. Date of foundation, unless otherwise stated
c. Last date when known to have been active

d. Location
e. Function
f. Founder
g. Source
h. Capacity
i. Miscellaneous

NB fields have been omitted when data are unknown

2. Functions

1 = Pilgrims and travellers
2 = Poor
3 = Sick
4 = Old
5 = Foundlings
6 = Women
7 = Artisans
8 = Religious
9 = Unknown

1. a. Spedale della Badia Fiorentina (S. Niccolò)
   b. 2.xi.1031
   c. At least 1273
   d. Opposite entrance to Badia Fiorentina
   e. 1: Pilgrims and travellers
   f. Abate Pietro
   g. Davidsohn, VII, p. 87; Paatz, IV, p. 357; *Firenze e i primi Giubilei*, p. 65; Fanelli, pp. 256–7 lists this hospital as 'presso il Bargello'.

2. a. Spedale di S. Giovanni Evangelista (Hospital Canonice Florentine)
   b. 1040
   c. 1296 demolished
   d. Between S. Reparata and the Baptistery: 'Iuxta ecclesiam et domum S. Johannis Baptiste'
   e. 1 & 2: Poor and pilgrims
   f. Rolando, Proposto of S. Reparata, and Canon Orlandino
   g. Davidsohn, VII, pp. 89–91; Passerini, p. xxv; *Firenze e i primi Giubilei*, p. 65.
   i. Listed in the papal Decima of 1276–7: *Tuscia: Decima*, p. 13

3. a. Spedale di S. Paolo a Pinti or Spedale di Pinti or Spedale di S. Pier Maggiore
   b. 28.x.1065
   c. 1751
   d. Via Pinti, near church of S. Pier Maggiore; belonged to Vallombrosan monks
   e. 1 & 2 & 4: Accommodation for poor and travellers and by 1300 for old and sick
   f. Fiorenzo detto Barone Donati
   g. Catasto 185.II, f. 412v (1429); Passerini, pp. 197–200; Davidsohn, VII, pp. 87–8; Fanelli, p. 154; Paatz, IV, p. 609; listed in the papal Decima for 1276–7 and 1302–3: *Tuscia: Decima*, p. 10
   i. In 1438 the Monache di Santa Apollonia became their patrons.

APPENDIX 343

4. a. Spedale di S. Sepolcro al Ponte Vecchio
   b. Pre-1068
   c. Damaged during 1333 flood and certainly ceased to exist by 1542
   d. Ponte Vecchio
   e. 1 & 3: pilgrims and sick
   f. Knights of St John of Jerusalem
   g. Passerini, pp. 142–5; Davidsohn, VII, p. 104; *Firenze e i primi Giubilei*, pp. 72–3
   i. Administered successively by the Order of the Templars and the Knights of St John of Jerusalem

5. a. Spedale di S. Miniato del Ponte or Spedale di Folco
   b. From 1068
   c. 1333 – destroyed during flood
   d. 'iuxta pontem veterem'
   e. 1 & 3: pilgrims and sick
   f. 'Florentius qui Fulco vocatur', who gave it to Benedictine monks of S. Miniato al Monte
   g. Davidsohn, VII, p. 88; Paatz, II, pp. 120–1; *Firenze e i primi Giubilei*, p. 66

6. a. Spedale di San Lorenzo
   b. First documented: 1117
   c. Listed in Decima of 1495
   d. Between church of S. Lorenzo and the second city walls
   e. 2 & 3: poor and sick
   f. Chiesa di S. Lorenzo
   g. Davidsohn, I, p. 1091; Davidsohn, VII, p. 89, 501; Decima 67, f. 184v

7. a. Spedale di S. Jacopo a San Eusebio, or Spedale di S. Sebio
   b. 1186
   c. Stopped functioning in 1780
   d. (i) Popolo di Santa Lucia d'Ognissanti in sul Prato
      (ii) In 1533 transferred to 'Campoluccio', near Ponte a Rifredi
   e. 3: sick: leprosarium
   f. Vinciguerra dei Donati
   g. Passerini, pp. 125–31; Davidsohn, vii, pp. 91–3; *Firenze e i primi Giubilei*, pp. 76–7; listed in the papal Decima for 1276–7 and 1302–3: *Decima*, p. 11; Catasto 190, ff. 25v–32v; 291, ff. 16v–23v; 292, f. 235r; 293, f. 10r
   h. By 1428 there were seven resident lepers: Catasto 190, ff. 25v–32v; it had 24 beds in 1562, by which time it also housed those sick from other diseases
   i. Administered by the Arte di Calimala

8. a. Spedale di S. Paolo dei Convalescenti
   b. 1208
   c. 1780 suppressed
   d. Piazza di S. Maria Novella
   e. 1–3: initially pilgrims and out-relief to poor of city; from 1345 came to concentrate progressively on the sick poor and in late sixteenth century came to house convalescents

f. By 1224 taken over by the Franciscan Third Order or *pinzocheri*: Paatz, iv, 602
g. Henderson, ' "Splendide case di cura" ', pp. 32–7; Passerini, pp. 163–88; Davidsohn, *Forschungen*, IV, p. 391
h. 34 beds by c. 1400: This number is cited in a petition contained in a Provv. Reg. 93, f. 116r: 9.ii.1404: Passerini, p. 169

9. a. **Spedale di S. Gallo**
   b. 1218
   c. 1529: destroyed during preparations for the siege of Florence
   d. Just outside Porta S. Gallo along the Mugnone
   e. 1, 2 & 5: founded for poor men and women and pilgrims, by 1294 it had also become an orphanage, a function for which it became best known. In 1463 it was united with the Ospedale degli Innocenti
   f. Guidalotto di Volto Dell'Orco
   g. AOIF, ser. II.I, ff. 1r–6r; Davidsohn, *Forschungen*, IV, pp. 389–91, and *Storia*, VII, pp. 93–5; Passerini, pp. 659–75; 1495 Decima 70, f. 122v
   h. In 1428 it had '30 letta dove alberghano e poveri' as well as paying for 35 to 40 infants at wet-nurse and 5 children in-house: Catasto 194.II, f. 379v
   i. From 1294 it was administered by the silk guild of Por Santa Maria

10. a. **Spedale di S. Pancrazio**
    b. First documented 1219
    d. Near church of S. Pancrazio: Fanelli, p. 154
    e. Two small related *ospizi*, one for sick monks and the other for travellers
    f. 1 & 2: Travellers and poor and presumably monks of the Vallombrosan Order which owned the church
    g. Davidsohn, *Forschungen*, IV, p. 391; Davidsohn, VII, p. 88
    i. Appears in 1276–7 Decima: *Tuscia: Decima*, p. 11.

11. a. **Spedale di San Niccolò**
    b. c.1229
    c. Early Trecento absorbed by Hospital of S. Paolo
    d. Borgo di S. Maria Novella
    e. 9: unknown
    f. Founded by the Spedale di S. Nicola in Fontemanzina, Firenzuola
    g. Davidsohn, VII, pp. 95–6

12. a. **Spedale dei Templari**
    b. c.1242
    d. Fuori della Porta S. Francesco
    e. 1: pilgrims
    f. Order of Templars
    g. Davidsohn, *Forschungen*, IV, p. 165 n. 2
    i. 1361 given to the Compagnia di S. Maria della Croce al Tempio

13. a. **Spedale dei Serviti**
    b. 1250 founded; 1255 opened
    d. SS. Annunziata
    e. 8: for the friars

APPENDIX

   f. Servite Order
   g. O. Andreucci, *Il Fiorentino istruito nella chiesa della Nunziata di Firenze. Memoria storica* (Florence, 1857), pp. 32, 213–14

14. a. **Spedale di Buonamico**
    b. First documented 1252
    d. Borgo S. Frediano, near where Porta S. Frediano was built
    e. 1: pilgrims and travellers
    g. Davidsohn, *Forschungen*, IV, p. 392; Davidsohn, VII, p. 105; Fanelli, p. 154; *Firenze e i primi Giubilei*, p. 75
    i. Patrons: first bishop of Florence; by 1277 the Hospitallers of St John of Jerusalem

15. a. **Spedale di S. Trinita**
    b. First documented 1256
    d. 'siti prope ecclesiam Sancte Trinitatis in capite pontis novi de Sancta Trinitate'; 1277 moved to Via Parione; by 1393 moved to Via de' Fossi
    e. 9: unknown
    g. AOIF, ser. II.I, ff. 1r–6r; Richa, III, p. 149; Davidsohn, *Forschungen*, IV, p. 393, and *Storia*, VII, p. 88; Paatz, V, p. 39

16. a. **Spedale di S. Giorgio dello Spirito Santo**
    b. First documented 1273.
    d. Church of S. Giorgio, Costa S. Giorgio
    e. 9: unknown
    g. Davidsohn, VII, pp. 88–9; *Storia della solidarietà a Firenze*, pp. 12–13

17. a. **Spedale di S. Pier Gattolino**
    b. First documented 1273
    d. Church of S. Pier Gattolino
    e. 9: unknown
    g. Davidsohn, VII, pp. 88–9; Paatz, IV, p. 628

18. a. **Spedale di S. Onofrio or S. Nofri de' Tintori**
    b. 1280
    c. 1720
    d. 'In su' Renai': between Porta S. Francesco and S. Croce
    e. 7: artisans: for retired dyers; orphans of guild members; temporary accommodation for poor
    f. Confraternity of S. Onofrio dei Tintori
    g. Catasto 185, ff. 627r, 628r; Passerini, pp. 98–104; *Firenze e i primi Giubilei*, p. 80; Carrara, Sebregondi and Tramonti, *Gli istituti di beneficenza*, p. 37.
    h. V. Vannucci, *Istituzioni fiorentine* (Florence, 1902), pp. 93–4 says it was a 'ricovero di 12 poveri vecchi'
    i. By c.1550 it had become a hostel for poor girl orphans

19. a. **Spedale di S. Lucia de' Magnoli**
    b. 1283
    c. In the late eighteenth century the building was incorporated into Palazzo Bardi-Canigiani

    d. Via de' Bardi, next to church of S. Lucia de' Magnoli
    e. 3: one hospital for sick (?) men and another for women ('per uso di ritenere [uomini e donne]')
    f. Compagnia Maggiore della Vergine Maria; by 1428 administered by the Bigallo
    g. Catasto 194, f. 654r, 194.I, f. 671r, 194.II, ff. 610r–v; 293, f. 35r; Passerini, p. 14; Paatz, II, p. 600; Fanelli, p. 154; *Firenze e i primi Giubilei*, pp. 74–5
    h. Total capacity of male and female hospitals in 1428 Catasto: 21 beds

20. a. **Spedale di S. Candida**
    b. First documented 14.iii.1284/5
    c. Destroyed in 1325 to create Porta alla Croce
    d. Site of Porta alla Croce
    e. 9: unknown
    f. Frati Crociferi dell'Osmannoro
    g. Davidsohn, VII, p. 97

21. a. **Spedale di S. Maria Nuova**
    b. Founded in 1286; opened in 1288
    c. Still exists
    d. Piazza S. Maria Nuova
    e. 3: poor sick
    f. Folco di Ricovero Portinari
    g. Passerini, pp. 284–395
    h. Opened with 17 beds; by early sixteenth century it was treating up to 6,500 patients annually (see above, Chapter 8)

22. a. **Spedale di S. Spirito (after S. Spirito in Sassia, Rome) or S. Sebastiano dei Bini**
    b. By 1288
    c. 1563
    d. Via Romana, between nos 8 and 10
    e. 1: pilgrims
    f. Messer Gianni degli Amidei; renamed in early sixteenth century following a substantial legacy from Sebastiano Bini
    g. Passerini, pp. 146–7; Davidsohn, VII, pp. 98–9; Paatz, V, pp. 90–6; Fanelli, p. 154; *Firenze e i primi Giubilei*, p. 73
    i. This may have dated from the eleventh century, as the hospice of the monastery of S. Felice in Piazza

23. a. **Spedale di Giamboni**
    b. First documented 1293
    e. 9: unknown
    g. Davidsohn, *Forschungen*, IV, p. 395

24. a. **Spedale dell'Ospizio del Servante**
    b. First documented 1295
    d. Popolo di S. Felice in Piazza
    e. 9
    g. Davidsohn, *Forschungen*, IV, p. 395

APPENDIX

25. a. Spedale di S. Bartolomeo al Mugnone
    b. 1295
    c. By 1441 at latest
    d. Porta al Prato: 'iuxta portam novam civitatis Florentie'
    e. 2 & 3: poor and sick
    f. Bennuccio Senni Del Bene
    g. Davidsohn, *Forschungen*, IV, pp. 395–6; *Storia*, vii, pp. 100–1; Paatz, I, p. 332
    h. '20 letta alberghano poveri': Catasto 194.I, ff. 390v–392r (1428)

26. a. Spedale di San Giovanni Battista Decollato or Casa di Misericordia del Beato Messer Giovanni Battista o Spedale dei Portatori
    b. 1297
    c. Closed in c.1542; transferred to Via Santa Caterina in 1565 until 1754
    d. Via S. Gallo, opposite today's Via di Camporeggi
    e. 7: artisans: old and sick porters
    f. Compagnia dei Portatori di Norcia
    g. Catasto 185.I, f. 599r; Davidsohn, VII, pp. 102–3; *Firenze e i primi Giubilei*, p. 67
    h. '13 lecta … per aloghare i poveri': Catasto 185.I, f. 599r

27. a. Spedale di SS. Jacopo e Filippo della Porcellana e dei Michi
    b. Pre-1300
    c. Suppressed in 1504
    d. Via della Scala, corner of Via Porcellana
    e. 1: pilgrims
    f. Michi family
    g. Catasto 194.II, f. 172v; Passerini, pp. 160–2; Paatz, I, p. 483; II, pp. 97–100
    h. 1428 Catasto: 13 beds
    i. Appears in Decima 68, f. 162r; 1504 property passed to the Ospedale di S. Paolo

28. a. Spedale di San Bernardino degli Uberti
    b. 1300–50
    c. 1510
    d. Via della Scala near Spedale di S. Maria della Scala
    e. 1
    f. Founded by Vallombrosan monks of S. Pancrazio
    g. Passerini, p. 685; Fanelli, p. 257: App. 10

29. a. Spedale di S. Jacopo in Campo Corbolini
    b. 1311
    c. Possibly ceased to exist by 1367
    d. Via Faenza
    e. 2: poor
    f. Lippo Forese detto Lippo del Soldato; run by Order of the Templars and then by Knights of St John of Jerusalem
    g. Passerini, pp. 145–6

30. a. Spedale di Gesù Pellegrino della Compagnia dei Pretoni (Hospital Clericorum)
    b. 1312

- c. Late seventeenth century
- d. Via S. Gallo
- e. 8: looked after poor and old priests and lodged priests on pilgrimage
- f. Compagnia di Gesù Pellegrino of priests
- g. Catasto 185.II, ff. 618r–619r; Davidsohn, VII, pp. 103–4, 419; Passerini, pp. 519–29; *Firenze e i primi Giubilei*, pp. 66–7; W.M. Bowsky, 'The Confraternity of Priests and San Lorenzo of Florence: A Church, a Parish and a Clerical Brotherhood', *Ricerche storiche*, 27 (1997), pp. 53–92

31.
- a. Spedale di S. Maria della Scala
- b. 1316
- c. 1530 when taken over by the nuns of SS. Bartolomeo e Martino
- d. Via della Scala
- e. 1 & 5: poor travellers and pilgrims, and looked after abandoned children
- f. Founded by the Siennese hospital of S. Maria della Scala and first major benefactor was Maestro Cione di Lapo di Gherardo Pollini legnaiolo
- g. Catasto 185, ff. 528r–585v; Passerini, pp. 675–85; Davidsohn, vii, pp. 101–2; *Firenze e i primi Giubilei*, p. 85
- h. In 1428 Catasto: 71 babies at wet-nurse and 85 in the hospital
- i. 1351 came to be administered by the Arte della Seta in conjunction with Siennese hospital

32.
- a. Spedale di S. Giovanni fra l'Arcora
- b. 1317
- c. Demolished during siege of Florence in 1529
- d. Outside city walls on the old Via Cassia
- e. 3: sick poor, male and female
- f. Frate Jacopo di Bartolino, a Knight of Jerusalem
- g. Davidsohn, VII, pp. 104–5, 451; Passerini, p. 142.
- i. Run by the Knights of St John of Jerusalem

33.
- a. Spedale dell'Arcangelo Michele e dei Broccardi
- b. 1329
- c. 1751
- d. Via S. Gallo, near today's Via Bonifazio Lupi
- e. 1: male and female travellers and pilgrims
- f. Pietro di Francesco di Simone Broccardi
- g. Passerini, pp. 201–2; *Firenze e i primi Giubilei*, pp. 67–8; Catasto 190, f. 13r (1428)
- i. In c.1380 came to be administered by Arte di Calimala and was linked to the hospital of Messer Bonifazio after its foundation. In 1542 it began to look after orphaned boys and from 1593 orphaned girls

34.
- a. Spedale di S. Spirito della Madonna Santa Maria del 'Piccione'
- b. 1332
- c. 1752
- d. (i) Via S. Chiara, 'allato alle Convertite'; (ii) 1460 transferred to Via Romana, popolo di S. Pier Gattolino
- e. 2: 'si dà ricietto e albergo a poveri'
- f. Compagnia dei Laudesi di S. Spirito

APPENDIX

    g. Catasto 185, f. 612r; Passerini, pp. 120–1; Davidsohn, VII, p. 99; Decima 70, f. 385r
    h. Passerini says 12 beds (some of which slept 2–3), though unclear if this was in the Trecento or in 1853!

35. a. Spedale di S. Antonio
    b. 18.v.1333
    c. Destroyed in 1534
    d. Near Porta a Faenza
    e. 3: Fuoco di S. Antonio
    f. Order of S. Antonio: Fra Guido d'Orlando
    g. Passerini, pp. 133–41
    i. Run by the Canons of S. Antonio

36. a. Spedale di S. Maria delle Stinche
    b. From 1333
    d. Prison of the Stinche
    e. 3: sick prisoners
    g. Davidsohn, vii, p. 104; *Firenze e i primi Giubilei*, pp. 80–1; mentioned in 1428 Catasto: Catasto 190, f. 670r
    i. Prison of Stinche was built 1299–1301 (Fanelli, p. 63)

37. a. Spedale di San Niccolò della Misericordia detto dei Fantoni
    b. 1338
    c. 1751
    d. Via Romana, opposite Via del Campuccio
    e. 2: short-stay accommodation for female beggars: max. three nights
    f. Lapo di Baldo Fantoni; foundation administered by Compagnia del Bigallo
    g. Passerini, pp. 107–8; Paatz, IV, p. 399
    h. Ten beds for women

38. a. Spedale di S. Trinita dei calzolai
    b. 1342
    c. 1542
    d. Near church of S. Simone
    e. 7: two beds for elderly members of the cobblers' guild
    f. Banco di Ser Puccio
    g. Passerini, p. 110

39. a. Spedale di SS. Gherardo e Clemente
    b. c.1345
    c. 1808
    d. Via S. Gallo
    e. 2: poor
    f. Company of Orsanmichele
    g. Fanelli, p. 256: App. 10

40. a. Spedale di S. Piero Novello dei Ridolfi
    b. 1349
    c. 1751

d. Via Romana, opposite the Annalena
e. 2: overnight accommodation for poor
f. Piero di Cione Ridolfi
g. Passerini, pp. 121–2; *Firenze e i primi Giubilei*, p. 74
h. Ten beds (according to Passerini, p. 122)

41. a. **Spedale di S. Caterina dei Talani**
    b. Founded in 1349; opened in 1370
    c. 1751
    d. Via S. Gallo, near the Porta S. Gallo
    e. 3: poor sick
    f. Alessandro di Talano dei Filipetri
    g. Catasto 989 (1478); Passerini, pp. 648–58
    h. 1527 census of city mentions 14 beds: BNCF, NA 987 (under Quartiere di S. Giovanni)

42. a. **Spedale di S. Lò or SS. Eligio e Lorenzo dei maniscalchi**
    b. 1361
    c. suppressed in 1751
    d. Via S. Gallo near Via di S. Caterina
    e. 1: pilgrims for a max. of three days
    f. Compagnia dei Maniscalchi (farriers)
    g. Catasto 185.II, ff. 617r–v; Passerini, p. 106; Paatz, II, p. 463
    h. Capacity in 1428 Catasto: 'sei letta dove s'albergha poveri per Dio'

43. a. **Spedale di S. Giovanni Battista della Calza**
    b. 1362
    d. Piazza della Calza, inside Porta Romana
    e. 2 & 3: poor and sick
    f. Knights of Jerusalem or Knights of Malta
    g. Paatz, II, pp. 272–3; *Firenze e i primi Giubilei*, pp. 12–17

44. a. **Spedale di S. Giuliano a Colombaia de' Vettori**
    b. 1363
    d. Via Senese, before ex-Convento di S. Gaggio
    e. 1 & 2: 'alberghare poveri pellegrini di passaggio': Catasto 185, f. 615r
    f. Messer Pagholo Boccucci dei Vettori
    g. Catasto 185.II, ff. 615r–v; Catasto 425, f. 9v; Decima 68, f. 145r; *Firenze e i primi Giubilei*, pp. 13–14
    h. The 1428 Catasto records 24 beds
    i. In 1371 administration passed to Arte della Lana

45. a. **Spedale dell'Orbatello**
    b. 1372
    c. Nineteenth century (?)
    d. Via della Pergola
    e. 6: housing elderly widows
    f. Niccolò di Jacopo degli Alberti
    g. Passerini, pp. 639–48; Paatz, IV, 474; Trexler, 'A Widows' Asylum', pp. 119–49

APPENDIX   351

    h. Between 1511 and 1562 housed between 154 and 259 people: Trexler, 'A Widows' Asylum', p. 126
    i. In 1400 administration passed to Capitani di Parte Guelfa when Alberti family exiled from Florence

46. a. **Spedale di Messer Bonifazio e di S. Giovanni Battista**
    b. 1377; open by 1388
    c. 1886
    d. Via S. Gallo
    e. 3: sick poor
    f. Bonifazio Lupi da Parma
    g. Catasto 190, ff. 43r–53r; 291, ff. 25r–34r; 292, ff. 230v–232v; Passerini, pp. 156–228; Lombardi, *Messer Bonifacio Lupi da Parma*
    h. In 1428 Catasto it looked after 35 'infermi'
    i. After Bonifazio Lupi's death in 1389 it was administered by Arte di Calimala

47. a. **Spedale di S. Maria dell'Umiltà o dei Vespucci; later S. Giovanni di Dio**
    b. 1380; open by 1388
    c. Still active
    d. Borgo Ognissanti
    e. 3: sick poor: 'per ritenere uomini' and 'povere femine'
    f. Simone di Piero Vespucci
    g. Catasto 194, ff. 654v, 656r; 194.I, f. 671r; 293, f. 35v; Passerini, pp. 395–8; see Sandri, ed., *L'Archivio dell'Ospedale di San Giovanni di Dio di Firenze*, pp. 1–15
    h. The 1428 Catasto recorded 18 beds
    i. 1588 taken over by the Order of S. Giovanni di Dio

48. a. **Spedale di S. Matteo di Lemmo Balducci**
    b. 1385; opened 1410
    c. 1784
    d. Piazza S. Marco/Via Ricasoli
    e. 3: sick poor
    f. Lemmo Balducci
    g. Catasto 185.II, ff. 601r–607r; Passerini, pp. 149–60
    h. In 1428 Catasto: 45 male and female patients

49. a. **Spedale di San Lorenzo a S. Pier Gattolino**
    b. c.1390
    c. 1547
    d. Popolo di S. Pier Gattolini, La Cella
    e. 6: poor women: 'per uso di ritenere povere femine'
    f. Maffeo di Michele di Bartolino
    g. Catasto 194, ff. 654v, 656r; 293, f. 35v; Passerini, p. 16
    h. In 1428 Catasto: 12 beds
    i. Cf. Fanelli, pp. 256–7

50. a. **Ospizio delle vedove di Sant'Agnese or Spedale delle Divote della Vergine Maria**
    b. 1403
    c. 1785

d. Piazza del Carmine; later in Borgo S. Frediano
　　　e. 6: to house six poor honest widows
　　　f. Filippo di Gardo *Orpellai*; administered by the Laudesi di S. Agnese
　　　g. Catasto 185.II, ff. 626r–626b r; Passerini, pp. 112–15
　　　h. In 1428 Catasto housed seven women

51. a. Spedale di SS. Jacopo e Filippo or Ceppo delle Sette Opere della Misericordia
　　　b. 1414–17
　　　c. By 1530 no longer received pilgrims
　　　d. 'Popolo di S. Jachopo tra le fosse, luogho detto di Renaio della Torricella': Catasto 185.II, ff. 633r–634v; this is now Via Tripoli
　　　e. 1 & 2: housing pilgrims and poor: 'ricevere e ricettare e poveri ispirituali che arivono'
　　　f. Compagnia delle Sette Opere della Misericordia
　　　g. Catasto 185, ff. 633r–634v; Catasto 194.I, ff. 155v–158r; Passerini, pp. 188–97

52. a. Spedale di S. Maria degli Innocenti
　　　b. 1419; opened in 1444
　　　c. 1875
　　　d. Piazza SS. Annunziata
　　　e. 5: abandoned babies and children: function described in 1428 Catasto as 'per ricettare e povere fanciulli gittatelli abandonati'
　　　f. Francesco di Marco Datini
　　　g. Catasto 190, ff. 80r–83v; Passerini, pp. 685–724; Gavitt, *Charity and Children*, ch. 1
　　　h. Census of hospital inmates on 17.i.1483: 151 children resident and 20 being weaned: Gavitt, *Charity and Children*, p. 169
　　　i. In 1421 the silk guild, the Arte di Por San Maria, became the patron

53. a. Spedale di S. Niccolò
　　　b. 1420
　　　c. 1531 was given over to the confraternity of S. Maria della Croce al Tempio
　　　d. Near Porta la Croce
　　　e. 1: sick pilgrims for three nights
　　　f. Niccolò di Lotto Aliotti; administered by Bigallo
　　　g. Catasto 194, f. 653v: it was still being built in 1428; Passerini, pp. 16–17
　　　h. Six beds for women and ten for men

54. a. Spedale di S. Salvadore
　　　b. First documented 1428 Catasto
　　　d. Via Chiara
　　　e. 6: to house poor women
　　　g. Catasto 194.1, ff. 663v; 194.II, f. 646v

55. a. Spedale di S. Giuliano in Verzaia
　　　b. First documented 1428
　　　d. Near Porta di S. Frediano/S. Maria in Verzaia
　　　e. 2: 'per ricettare i poveri di Dio'
　　　g. Catasto 185, f. 614r; 194.I, f. 147v; Catasto 425, f. 9v
　　　h. In 1428 Catasto: ten beds

APPENDIX

56. a. Spedale delle Donnucce or Donne Spagnole
    b. First documented 1428
    d. Piazza di S. Maria Maggiore
    e. 6: Spanish women
    g. Catasto 185, ff. 616r–v; Decima 67, f. 356v

57. a. Ospizio delle vedove in Via Chiara
    b. 1430
    c. Still functioning in 1851
    d. Began in Via della Scala and then moved to Via Chiara
    e. 6: to house four honest poor widows aged over 55
    f. Lisa di Ranieri Paganelli, wife of Gentile di Vanni degli Albizzi, left a house to be administered by the Arte dei Medici e Speziali
    g. Passerini, pp. 115–16; C. Arrigoni, *Istituti di beneficenza fiorentini* (Florence/Rome, 1882), p. 127
    h. Four widows

58. a. Spedale di SS. Salvi e Michele
    b. Pre-1431
    c. 1751 suppressed
    d. Via del Sole: 'allato a San Pancrazio'
    e. 2: poor
    f. Manetti family
    g. Catasto 425, f. 11r (1431); Passerini, p. 203
    i. This is not to be confused with the *ospizio* at the monastery of S. Salvi mentioned by Davidsohn, VII, p. 88. Cf. *Firenze e i primi Giubilei*, p. 83

59. a. S. Stefano e S. Martino (spedale e cappella)
    b. First documented 1431 Catasto
    d. Badia di Firenze
    e. 9: unknown
    g. Catasto 425, f. 11r (1431)

60. a. Spedale di S. Sebastiano degli ammorbati
    b. 1479 begun to be built; opened for 1495 plague epidemic
    c. 1529
    d. 'In sul Prato della Giustizia'
    e. 3: lazzaretto for plague victims
    f. Florentine republic
    g. Henderson, 'Peste, Mal Francese e gli Ospedali di Firenze nel Rinascimento', pp. 18–19; F. Carrara, 'Montedomini', in Carrara, Sebregondi and Tramonti, *Gli istituti di beneficenza*, pp. 72–3
    h. Twenty-six beds in 1496
    i. Knocked down during siege of Florence in 1529 and then it subsequently became the site of two communities of nuns, the Clarisse of Monticelli and Montedomini

61. a. Spedale di S. Maria degli Angioli dei battilani
    b. 1489
    c. Probably seventeenth century

        d. Via del Campaccio (today: Via S. Reparata)
        e. 7: for elderly wool-beaters (*battilani*)
        f. Compagnia dei Battilani
        g. Passerini, pp. 108–10
        h. Six beds

62. a. **Spedale di S. Lodovicho**
    b. First documented 1495
    d. Via S. Gallo
    e. 9: unknown
    g. Decima 70, f. 161v: 1495

63. a. **Spedale di S. Angniolo della Povertà dei Chapponi**
    b. First documented 1495 Decima
    d. Legnaia: fuori dalla Porta a S. Frediano
    e. 9: unknown
    f. Capponi family
    g. Decima 67, f. 26v; 69, f. 48v.

64. a. **Spedale di S. Giovanni**
    b. First documented Decima of 1495
    d. 'Al canto alla Porta a S. Friano'
    e. 9: unknown
    g. Decima 68, f. 145r
    i. Linked to the Bigallo

65. a. **Spedale di S. Giuliano**
    b. 1508
    c. Suppressed in 1750
    d. Near Porta di S. Niccolò
    e. 2: accommodation for homeless men and women
    f. Ser Alberto di Ser Rucco da Rondinaia and administered by Arte dei Mercatanti
    g. Passerini, pp. 148–9
    h. Nine beds: four for men and five for women

66. a. **Spedale di S. Rocco**
    b. 1508
    c. Suppressed in 1751
    d. Via S. Gallo, next to Porta
    e. 1: pilgrims: max. three days
    f. Company of S. Rocco
    g. Passerini, p. 110
    h. Four beds for men and six for women
    i. Used in 1520 as a temporary place for incurables: Henderson, 'Ospedali ed epidemie a Firenze', p. 21

67. a. **Spedale di SS. Trinita degli Incurabili**
    b. 1520
    c. 1781

APPENDIX

   d. Via S. Gallo
   e. 3: to treat sick from incurable diseases, especially the Mal Francese
   f. Compagnia della SS. Trinita
   g. Passerini, pp. 203–16; Henderson, 'Peste, Mal Francese e gli Ospedali di Firenze', pp. 20–1

68. a. **Spedale di San Dionisio**
   d. Via S. Gallo, opposite Sant'Agata
   e. 9
   g. *Firenze e i primi Giubilei*, p. 69
   i. Belonged to the Frati della Certosa until 1558 and then passed to the Monache del Ceppo

NOTES

Abbreviations

AOIF: Archivio dell'Ospedale degli Innocenti di Firenze
ASF: Archivio di Stato di Firenze
ASP: Archivio di Stato di Prato
ASI: *Archivio Storico Italiano*
BNCF: Biblioteca Nazionale Centrale di Firenze
BON: Ospedale di Messer Bonifazio
MKIF: *Mitteilungen des Kunsthistorischen Institutes in Florenz*
SE: Ospedale di S. Eusebio
SM: Ospedale di S. Matteo
SMN: Ospedale di S. Maria Nuova
SP: Ospedale di S. Paolo

SMN, 1376 inventory: L. Chiappelli and A. Corsini, 'Un antico inventario dello spedale di Santa Maria Nuova in Firenze (1376)', *Rivista delle Biblioteche e degli Archivi*, 32 (1921), pp. 13–22.

SMN (1330) and SMN (1374): S. Maria's statutes of 1330 and 1374, published in *Il reggio arcispedale di S. Maria Nuova. I suoi benefattori, sue antiche memorie* (Florence, 1888).

SMN (1510–11): K. Park and J. Henderson, ' "The First Hospital among Christians": The Ospedale di Santa Maria Nuova in Early Sixteenth-Century Florence', *Medical History*, 35 (1991), pp. 164–88.

S. Maria Nuova, *Ricettario*: BNCF Magl. XV.415.

G. Villani, *Cronica: Cronica di Giovanni Villani: a miglior lezione ridotta coll'aiuto de' testi a penna* (Florence, 1823; Rome, 1980 reprint), 8 vols (cited by book and chapter numbers)

M. Villani, *Cronica: Cronica di Matteo e Filippo Villani: a miglior lezione ridotta col'aiuto de 'testi a penna* (Florence, 1825–6; Rome, 1980 reprint), 4 vols (cited by book and chapter numbers).

Introduction

1. R. Davidsohn, *Storia di Firenze*, trans. G.B. Klein (Florence, 1972), Vol. 7, p. 89.
2. For a discussion of this topic see L. Franchini, ed., *Ospedali Lombardi del Quattrocento. Fondazioni, trasformazioni, restauri* (Como, 1995), esp. introduction on cruciform wards.
3. ASF, SMN 1, under 'Life of Buonafé, f. 5r; cf. also SMN 74.11, f. 64v: 'Leonardo Buonafede, già spedalingho di questo spedale et monacho di Certosa e al presente governatore dignissimo dello spedale di Sancto Spirito di Roma.'

4. E. Chaney, ' "Philanthropy in Italy" ': English Observations on Italian Hospitals, 1545–1789', in T. Riis, ed., *Aspects of Poverty in Early Modern Europe* (Stuttgart, 1981), pp. 183–217.
5. There are two versions of the original manuscript: Bodleian Library, Oxford, MS 488, and British Library, Additional MS 40077. They were transcribed, with errors, by L. Passerini, *Storia degli stabilimenti di beneficenza e d'istruzione elementare gratuita della città di Firenze* (Florence, 1853), pp. 851–67. The manuscript can be dated to 1510–11, but not to 1527 since the 'Ordinamenti' were addressed to King Henry VII and not to Henry VIII, as suggested by Passerini. They have been edited and translated by K. Park and J. Henderson, ' "The First Hospital Among Christians": The Ospedale di Santa Maria Nuova in Early Sixteenth-Century Florence', *Medical History*, 35 (1991), pp. 164–88.
6. Park and Henderson, ' "The First Hospital" ', pp. 165–8.
7. See M. Holmes, *Fra Filippo Lippi. The Carmelite Painter* (New Haven and London, 1999), pp. 44–5, 253 n. 74; B. Buhler Walsh, 'The Fresco Painting of Bicci di Lorenzo' (Unpublished Ph.D. thesis, Indiana University, 1981), pp. 21ff.; J.H. Beck, 'Masaccio's Early Career as a Sculptor', *Art Bulletin*, 53/2 (1971), p. 181. See the hospital's 'Quaderno di cassa' for the years 1422 to 1424: SMN 5051, f. 113v: 'Le dipinture di fuori della chiesa dea dare a dì iii d'ottobre ad Andrea sta col Bicci per l sacco di chalcina per le dipinture di fuori della chiesa.'
8. The actual dedication of the church had been performed earlier in the day by the cardinal of Bologna: Holmes, *Fra Filippo Lippi*, p. 45. The early eighteenth-century historian of the hospital erroneously has Martin V consecrating rather than confirming the consecration: SMN 10, ff. 8r–v, 11r.

    On the renovations see SMN 10, f. 8r: 'A dì 5 di settembre 1418 si cominciò a cavare et fare i fondamenti per la nuova chiesa di Santo Egidio al tempo di Ser Michele di Fruosino spedalingo di detto spedale'; W. and E. Paatz, *Die Kirchen von Florenz* (Frankfurt-am-Main, 1954), Vol. 3, 1952, pp. 5, 10, 15–16, 84; A. Rensi, 'Interventi architettonici del primo Quattrocento nello Spedale di Santa Maria Nuova', in C. De Benedictis, ed., *Il patrimonio artistico dell'Ospedale Santa Maria Nuova di Firenze. Episodi di committenza* (Florence, 2002), pp. 63–77.
9. Cf. Holmes, *Fra Filippo Lippi*, pp. 44–6.
10. 'Diario fiorentino di Bartolommeo di Michele del Corazza, anni 1405–1438', G.O. Corazzini, ed., *Archivio storico italiano*, 5th ser., 14 (1894), p. 272.
11. On the ceremony see the communal decree of 16.x. 1420 transcribed in SMN 4, ff. 27v–28v; described by G. Richa, *Notizie istoriche delle chiese fiorentine divise nei quartieri* (Florence, 1754), vol. 8, p.198. See also Holmes, *Fra Filippo Lippi*, pp. 44–6.
12. A useful recent summary of the historiography of the Renaissance is J.J. Martin, 'Introduction: The Renaissance: Between Myth and History', in J.J. Martin, ed., *The Renaissance: Italy and Abroad* (London, 2003), pp. 1–23; for a perceptive survey of hospital history see P. Horden, ' "A Discipline of Relevance": The Historiography of the Later Medieval Hospital', *Social History of Medicine*, 1 (1988), pp. 359–74; and for recent approaches in history of medicine see W.F. Bynum and R. Porter, eds, *Companion Encyclopaedia of the History of Medicine* (London, 1993), 2 vols.
13. See, for example, T. Verdon and J. Henderson, eds, *Christianity and the Renaissance* (Syracuse, NY, 1990).
14. For a very useful survey of trends in the historiography of Italian hospitals see M. Garbellotti, 'Ospedali e storia nell'Italia moderna: percorsi di ricerca', in J. Henderson and A. Pastore, eds, *Medicina dell'Anima, Medicina del Corpo: l'Ospedale in Europa tra Medio Evo ed Età Moderna*, in *Medicina e storia*, 6 (2004), pp. 115–38.
15. P. Biller and J. Ziegler, eds, *Religion and Medicine in the Middle Ages* (York, 2001); J. Ziegler, *Medicine and Religion, c.1300. The Case of Arnau de Vilanova* (Oxford, 1998); D. Gentilcore, *From Bishop to Witch: The System of the Sacred in Early Modern Terra d'Otranto* (Manchester, 1992).

16. A. Hayum, *The Isenheim Altarpiece. God's Medicine and the Painter's Vision* (Princeton, 1989); C. Rawcliffe, *Medicine for the Soul. The Life, Death and Resurrection of an English Medieval Hospital* (Stroud, 1999).

17. Rawcliffe, *Medicine for the Soul*; A. Saunier, 'Le pauvre malade' dans le cadre hospitalier médiéval. France du nord, vers 1300–1500 (Paris, 1993); J.W. Brodman, *Charity and Welfare: Hospitals and the Poor in Medieval Catalonia* (Philadelphia, 1998). More generally see L. Brockliss and C. Jones, 'Introduction. Towards a New Medical History of Early Modern France', in *The Medical World of Early Modern France* (Oxford, 1997); C. Jones, 'The Construction of the Hospital Patient in Early Modern France', in N. Finzsch and R. Jütte, eds, *Institutions of Confinement: Hospitals, Asylums and Prisons in Western Europe and North America, 1500–1950* (Cambridge, 1996), pp. 55–74; and P. Horden, 'A Non-Natural Environment: Medicine without Doctors and the Medieval European Hospital', in B. Bowers, ed., *The Medieval Hospital and Medical Practice* (Aldershot, forthcoming).

18. G. Pomata, *Contracting a Cure. Patients, Healers and the Law in Early Modern Bologna* (Baltimore and London, 1998); M. Pelling and F. White, *Medical Conflicts in Early Modern London. Patronage, Physicians and Irregular Practitioners, 1550–1640* (Oxford, 2003).

19. On this theme see P. Horden, 'A Non-Natural Environment'. I am most grateful to Peregrine Horden for allowing me to read this important article before its publication.

20. E.S. Welch, *Art and Authority in Renaissance Milan* (New Haven and London, 1995); C. Stevenson, *Medicine and Magnificence: British Hospital and Asylum Architecture, 1660–1815* (New Haven and London, 2000).

21. For a detailed discussion of this process in relation to Florence see J. Henderson, *Piety and Charity in Late Medieval Florence* (Oxford, 1994).

22. Cf. D. Balestracci and G. Piccinni, 'L'Ospedale e la città', in D. Gallavotti Cavallero, ed., *Lo Spedale di Santa Maria della Scala in Siena. Vicenda di una committenza artistica* (Siena, 1985), pp. 21–2; G. Albini, *Città e ospedali nella Lombardia medievale* (Bologna, 1993), p. 72, on the history of the Brolo in Milan; Saunier, 'Le pauvre malade', pp. 128–43; M.R. McVaugh, *Medicine before the Plague. Practitioners and their Patients in the Crown of Aragon, 1285–1345* (Cambridge, 1993), pp. 3, 190–1, 200–1, 225–9.

23. J. Henderson in J. Arrizabalaga, J. Henderson and R. French, *The Great Pox: The French Disease in Renaissance Europe* (New Haven and London, 1997), chs 2, 3, 8.

24. D. Lombardi, *Povertà maschile, povertà femminile. L'ospedale dei Mendicanti nella Firenze dei Medici* (Bologna, 1988).

25. S. Woolf, *The Poor in Western Europe in the Eighteenth and Nineteenth Centuries* (London, 1986); S. Woolf, ed., *Domestic Strategies: Work and Family in France and Italy, 1600–1800* (Cambridge, 1991); S. Cavallo, *Charity and Power in Early Modern Italy. Benefactors and their Motives in Turin, 1541–1789* (Cambridge, 1995); P. Horden and R. Smith, eds, *The Locus of Care* (London, 1998); P. Gavitt, *Charity and Children in Renaissance Florence. The Ospedale degli Innocenti, 1410–1536* (Ann Arbor, 1990).

26. See, for example, the influential essay by M. Becker, 'Aspects of Lay Piety in Renaissance Florence', in C. Trinkaus and H. Oberman, eds, *The Pursuit of Holiness* (Leiden, 1974), pp. 177–99.

27. Cf. A. Pastore, 'Strutture assistenziali fra Chiesa e Stati nell'Italia della Controriforma', in G. Chittolini and G. Miccoli, eds, *La Chiesa e il potere politico dal medioevo alla'età contemporanea*, in *Storia d'Italia, Annali*, 9 (Turin, 1986), pp. 431–65; Garbellotti, 'Ospedali e storia nell'Italia moderna'.

28. Henderson, *Piety and Charity*.

29. H.W. van Os, *Vecchietta and the Sacristy of the Siena Hospital Church. A Study in Renaissance Symbolism* (Maarssen, 1974); Gallavotti Cavallero, *Lo Spedale di Santa*

Maria della Scala in Siena; F. Scharf, *Der Freskenzyklus des Pellegrinaios in S. Maria della Scala zu Siena: Historienmalerei und Wirklichkeit in einem Hospital der Frührenaissance* (Hildesheim, 2001). Most recently see: A. Whitley, 'Concepts of Ill Health and Pestilence in Fifteenth-century Siena' (unpublished Ph.D. thesis, University of London, 2004). On S. Spirito see E. Howe, *The Hospital of Santo Spirito in Sassia* (New York, 1978) and V. Cappelletti and F. Tagliarini, eds, *L'antico Ospedale di Santo Spirito dall'istituzione papale alla sanità del terzo millennio* (Rome, 2001–2), 2 vols.

30. Cf. most recently J.I. Miller, 'Miraculous Childbirth and the Portinari Altarpiece', *Art Bulletin*, 77:2 (1995), pp. 249–61; R.J. Crum, 'Facing the Closed Doors to Reception? Speculations on Foreign Exchange, Liturgical Diversity and the "Failure" of the Portinari Altarpiece', *Art Journal*, 57 (1998), pp. 5–13.

31. R.A. Goldthwaite and R.W. Rearick, 'Michelozzo and the Ospedale di San Paolo in Florence', *MKIF*, 21 (1977), pp. 221–306; A. Rensi, 'L'Ospedale di San Matteo a Firenze', *Rivista d'arte*, 39 (1987), pp. 83–145; and various articles on S. Maria Nuova in De Benedictis, ed., *Il patrimonio artistico*. See also F. Carrara, L. Sebregondi and U. Tramonti, *Gli Istituti di beneficenza a Firenze. Storia e collezioni* (Florence, 1999). For the Innocenti: H. Saalman, *Filippo Brunelleschi. The Buildings* (London, 1993); L. Sandri, ed., *Gli Innocenti e Firenze nei secoli. Un ospedale, un archivio, una città* (Florence, 1996). Cf.: Milan: Franchini, ed., *Ospedali Lombardi del Quattrocento*; Welch, *Art and Authority*. Venice: B. Aikema and D. Meijers, eds, *Nel regno dei poveri. Arte e storia de grandi ospedali veneziani in età moderna, 1474–1797* (Venice, 1989); Siena: Gallavotti Cavallero, *Lo Spedale di Santa Maria della Scala*: conceived as a more integrated project. See also on Prato: F. Carrara and M.P. Mannini, *Lo Spedale della Misericordia e Dolce di Prato. Storia e collezioni* (Prato, 1993).

32. See, for example, C. Rawcliffe, 'Hospital Nurses and their Work', in R. Britnell, ed., *Daily Life in the Late Middle Ages* (Stroud, 1998), pp. 43–64, 202–6; Saunier, '*Le pauvre malade*'; Brodman, *Charity and Welfare*, pp. 50–60. For Italy see A. Benvenuti Papi, '*In Castro Poenitentiae*'. *Santità e società femminile nell'Italia medievale* (Rome, 1990). Examples of studies of the Order of the Holy Spirit: Rome: Cappelletti and Tagliarini, *L'antico Ospedale di Santo Spirito*; U. Mayer and R. Steffens, *Die Spätmittelterlichen Urbare des Heiliggeist-Spitals in Mainz* (Stuttgart, 1992).

33. Martin Luther, *Table Talk*, in *Luther's Works*, ed. and trans. T.G. Tappert (Philadelphia, 1967), Vol. 54, p. 296.

34. G. Pinto and G. Paolucci, 'Gli "infermi" della Misericordia di Prato (1401–1491)', and L. Sandri, 'Ospedali e utenti dell'assistenza nella Firenze del Quattrocento', in G. Pinto, ed., *La società del bisogno. Povertà e assistenza nella Toscana medievale* (Florence, 1989), pp. 101–29, 61–100; K. Park, 'Healing the Poor: Hospitals and Medical Assistance in Renaissance Florence', in J. Barry and C. Jones, eds, *Medicine and Charity before the Welfare State* (London, 1991), pp. 26–45; and J. Henderson, ' "Splendide case di cura." Spedali, medicina ed assistenza a Firenze nel Trecento', in A.J. Grieco and L. Sandri, eds, *Ospedali e città. L'Italia del Centro-Nord, XIII–XVI secolo* (Florence, 1997), pp. 15–50.

35. See Gavitt, *Charity and Children*. For Turin see Cavallo, *Charity and Power*.

36. See, for example, M.T. López Díaz, 'La botica del Hospital del Amor de Dios de Sevilla', *Boletín de la Sociedad española de historia de la farmacia*, 37 (1986), and M.T. López Díaz, *Estudio histórico-farmacéutico del Hospital del Amor de Dios de Sevilla (1655–1755)* (Seville, 1987). The most innovative recent work on the subject in Italy is G. Silini, *Umori e farmaci. Terapia medica tardo-medievale* (Bergamo, 2001). For Tuscany see also *Una farmacia preindustriale in Valdelsa. La spezieria e lo spedale di Santa Fina nella città di San Gimignano, secc. XIV–XVIII* (San Gimignano, 1981), and V. Vestri, *Malati, medici e terapie all'Ospedale della Misericordia di Prato nel secolo XIV* (Prato, 1998).

37. See E. Garin, 'La cité idéale de la renaissance italienne', in *Les Utopies à la Renaissance* (Brussels and Paris, 1963), pp. 13–37; Stevenson, *Medicine and Magnificence*, pp. 12–16.

Chapter 1

1. Archivio Vaticano, Rome, Cod. Vaticano-Urbinate, n. 227. See A. Mori and G. Boffito, *Firenze nelle vedute e piante. Studio storico cartografico* (Florence, 1926), pp. 8–12, and T. Frangenberg, 'Choreographies of Florence. The Use of City Views and Plans in the 16th Century', *Imago Mundi*, 46 (1994), p. 42.
2. G. Fanelli, *Firenze. Le città nella storia d'Italia* (Rome and Bari, 1981), pp. 76–7.
3. For the number of confraternities in Florence in this period see J. Henderson, *Piety and Charity* (Oxford, 1994), ch. 2.
4. E. Fiumi, 'La demografia fiorentina nelle pagine di Giovanni Villani', *ASI*, 108 (1950), pp. 105–18, and 'Fioritura e decadenza dell'economia fiorentina', *ASI*, 116 (1958), p. 465. See also C.-M. de La Roncière, *Prix et salaires à Florence au xive siècle, 1280–1380* (Rome, 1982), p. 676, and D. Herlihy and C. Klapisch-Zuber, *Tuscans and their Families: A Study of the Florentine Catasto of 1427* (New Haven and London, 1985), pp. 68–9, 74.
5. On the population of Florence see de La Roncière, *Prix et salaires*, p. 676, and Herlihy and Klapisch-Zuber, *Tuscans and their Families*, pp. 68–9, 74.
6. For a consideration of this theme see Henderson, *Piety and Charity*, esp. ch. 9.
7. For population levels see de La Roncière, *Prix et salaires*, p. 676, and Herlihy and Klapisch-Zuber, *Tuscans and their Families*, pp. 68–9, 74.
8. Henderson, *Piety and Charity*, pp. 279–96.
9. For a detailed summary of these factors in this period, especially as they related to fluctuating standards of living and the response of charities to the needs of the poor, see Henderson, *Piety and Charity*, ch. 7.
10. Ibid., on the developing policy of the largest charitable fraternity in the city, the company of Orsanmichele.
11. See again ibid., and G. Pinto, ed., *Il libro del Biadaiolo. Carestie e annona a Firenze dalla metà del '200 al 1348* (Florence, 1978), pp. 107–30.
12. Cited by G. Paolucci and G. Pinto, 'Gli "infermi" della Misericordia di Prato', in G. Pinto, ed., *La società del bisogno* (Florence, 1989), p. 127 n. 131; cf. I. Naso, *Medici e strutture sanitarie nella società tardo-medievale. Il Piemonte dei secoli XIV e XV* (Milan, 1982), p. 21 n. 15.
13. For a comprehensive survey of the building of the city walls see Paula Spilner,' "Ut Civitas Amplietur." Studies in Florentine Urban Development, 1282–1400' (Unpublished Ph.D. thesis, Columbia University, 1987), chs 1, 3.
14. P. Skinner, *Health and Medicine in Early Medieval Southern Italy* (Leiden, 1997), p. 103.
15. For a general discussion of their development see Davidsohn, *Storia di Firenze*, Vol. 7, pp. 87–104. Cf. also A. Benvenuti Papi, *'In Castro Poenitentiae'*, pp. 635–65. This is an aspect that would repay investigation, especially given the recent positive re-evaluation of monastic charity in England in this period. See N. S. Rushton, 'Monastic Charitable Provision in Tudor England: Quantifying and Qualifying Poor Relief in the Early Sixteenth Century', *Continuity and Change*, 16:1 (2001), pp. 9–44.
16. B.Z. Kedar, 'A Twelfth-Century Description of the Jerusalem Hospital', in *The Military Orders*, Vol. 2: *Welfare and Warfare*, ed. H. Nicholson (Aldershot, 1998), pp. 3–26; S. Edgington, 'Medical Care in the Hospital of Jerusalem', in ibid., pp. 27–33.
17. The hospitals of S. Sepolcro and S. Miniato were damaged during the great flood of November 1333, not surprisingly given their proximity to the river; they had ceased

to exist by the mid-sixteenth century (see Appendix I). L. Mencacci, 'L'assistenza sanitaria nello spedale di Altopascio', in A. Cenci, ed., *L'ospitalità in Altopascio. Storia e funzioni di un grande centro ospitaliero. Il cibo, la medicina e il controllo della strada* (Lucca, 1996), pp. 130–48.

18. F. Sznura, *L'espansione urbana di Firenze nel Dugento* (Florence, 1975), pp. 70–91; cf. also Spilner, ' "Ut Civitas Amplietur" '.
19. Davidsohn, *Storia*, Vol. 7, pp. 87–8.
20. Ibid., p. 89.
21. See Paolucci and Pinto, 'Gli "infermi" della Misericordia di Prato', pp. 120–3.
22. AOIF, ser. II.I, ff. 2r–3r: Guidalotto re-established the hospital in October 1218; f. 6r: privilege from Boniface VIII on 1 February of the fourth year of his reign as pope.
23. D. Moreni, ed., *Prediche del Beato Fra Giordano da Rivalto dell'Ordine dei Predicatori recitate in Firenze dal MCCCIII al MCCCVI* (Florence, 1831), Vol. 1, p. 55.
24. AOIF, ser. II.1, ff. 9r–13v, esp. f. 9r. Undated but certainly before 1338 since a donation of piece of land is recorded on f. 19r (25.iv.1338).
25. Giordano da Pisa, *Prediche inedite (dal ms. Laurenziano, Acquisti e Doni 290)*, ed. C. Iannella (Pisa, 1997), pp. 166–7.
26. Davidsohn, *Storia*, Vol. 1, pp. 995, 1155; Vol. 7, pp. 91–3.
27. ASF, Capitoli 40, f. 63v.
28. G. Villani, *Cronica*, VIII, 2.
29. ASF, Capitoli 40, ff. 62r–72v. See also Passerini, *Storia*, pp. 128–30, repeated in R. Stopani, ed., *Firenze e i primi Giubilei. Un momento di storia fiorentina della solidarietà* (Florence, 1999), pp. 76–7.
30. P. Giusti and P. Guidi, eds, *Rationes Decimarum italiae nei secoli XIII e XIV. Tuscia* (Città di Vaticano, 1932–42), p. 11; ASF, Capitoli 40, ff. 67r–72v.
31. Passerini, *Storia*, p. 130.
32. There is considerable confusion in the literature about the exact location of the hospital. Davidsohn, *Storia*, Vol. 7, pp. 91–3 suggests that from the twelfth century it was 'accanto la chiesa dei Santi Michele ed Eusebio, presso al luogo over poi gli Umiliati edificarano il convento d'Ognissanti'. This church was demolished in the thirteenth century (Passerini, *Storia*, p. 128). Cf. Sznura, *L'espansione*, pp. 79–84.
33. ASF, Capitoli 40, ff. 64r.
34. R. Caggese, ed., *Statuti della Repubblica Fiorentina*, Vol. 2: G. Pinto et al, eds, *Statuto del Podestà dell'anno 1325*, new edn (Florence, 1999), p. 63.
35. Cf. Horden, ' "A Discipline of Relevance" ', p. 367.
36. S.K. Cohn Jr, *Death and Property in Siena, 1205–1800* (Baltimore, 1988), ch. 5.
37. Cf. J. Henderson, 'Charity in Late-Medieval Florence: The Role of the Religious Confraternities', in S. Bertelli. N. Rubinstein and C. H. Smyth, eds, *Florence and Milan. Acts of Two Conferences at Villa I Tatti, Florence* (Florence, 1988), Vol. 2, pp. 147–63.
38. Spilner, ' "Ut Civitas Amplietur" ', ch. 4. Cf. Fanelli, *Firenze*, p. 49; L. Sandri, 'Aspetti dell'assistenza ospedaliera a Firenze nel xv secolo', in Centro Italiano di Studi e d'Arte, Pistoia, *Città e servizi nell'Italia dei secoli XII–XV* (Pistoia, 1990), pp. 241–6.
39. See A. Rubio Vela, *Podreza, enfermedad y asistencia hospitaria en la Valencia del siglo XIV* (Valencia, 1984), p. 26; M. Mollat, 'La vie quotidienne dans les hôpitaux medievaux', in J. Imbert, ed., *Histoire des hôpitaux* (Toulouse, 1982), p. 100; G. Giordanengo, 'Les hôpitaux arlésiens du xiie au xive siècle', *Assistance et charité* (Cahiers de Fanjeaux, 13) (Toulouse, 1978), pp. 190–3. Cf. De La Roncière, *Prix et salaires*, pp. 661–78.
40. Benvenuti Papi, '*In Castro Poenitentiae*', pp. 629–32.
41. P. Fanfani, ed., *Capitoli della Compagnia dei Portatori o S. Giovanni Decollato* (Bologna, 1858), pp. 9–10, 6–7.
42. Further up the road two hospices for the poor and pilgrims were founded in this

period: the Arcangelo Michele established by Pietro di Francesco di Simone Broccardi in 1329 (33) and SS. Gherardo e Clemente, which was apparently set up by the large charitable confraternity of Orsanmichele in c.1345(39). Though their normal role may have been to provide accommodation to pilgrims, they may actually have been founded to help the poor, given that both were founded during two of the worst dearths in the first half of the Trecento. See Henderson, *Piety and Charity*, pp. 279–96.

43. Richa, *Notizie istoriche delle chiese fiorentina*, Vol. 5, pp. 293–301.
44. Cf. B. Rano, 'Ospitalieri di Santo Spirito', in G. Pelliccia and G. Rocca, eds, *Dizionario degli Istituti di Perfezione* (Rome, 1974–88), Vol. 6, pp. 994–1006.
45. Via della Scala had been completed in 1299: Spilner,' "Ut Civitas Amplietur" ', p. 232. Two smaller hospitals were also founded in this period in Via della Scala: SS. Jacopo and Filippo, established by the Michi family around 1300 and better known as the Porcellana because it was situated on the corner of Via Porcellana (27), and S. Bernardino degli Uberti, founded by the monks of the Vallombrosan Order from their Florentine base in S. Pancrazio (28).
46. See Henderson, *Piety and Charity*, ch. 7.
47. Passerini, *Storia*, pp. 937–41 prints both the Florentine bishop's permission to convert Pollini's two houses into a hospital (30.vi.1316) and the record of the guild in which are summarised two laws of the commune concerning Por S. Maria's position as administrator of the hospital (Oct. 1351, June 1373).
48. AOIF, ser. III, no. 16, f. 242v.
49. Passerini, *Storia*, pp. 141–6 discusses the various hospitals established in Florence by this order.
50. Though it was demolished during the siege of Florence in 1529, some idea of its appearance in the late fifteenth century is provided by the 'Catena' map of the city of c.1471–80.
51. G. Vasari, *Le vite de più eccellenti pittori, scultori e archittetori*, in *Le opere di Giorgio Vasari* (hereafter Vasari-Milanesi), ed. G. Milanesi (Florence, 1906; 1973), Vol. 1, p. 516.
52. Cf. I. Ruffino, 'Canonici regolari di Sant'Agostino di Sant'Antonio di Vienne', in Pellicia and Rocca, *Dizionario degli Istituti di Perfezione*, Vol. 2, pp. 134–41.
53. M. Villani, *Cronica*, VIII. 110; cf. Passerini, *Storia*, p. 139.
54. Location discussed by: Goldthwaite and Rearick, 'Michelozzo and the Ospedale di San Paolo in Florence'; Saalman, *Filippo Brunelleschi*, p. 33.
55. On the history of S. Paolo see Passerini, *Storia*, pp. 163–88; Goldthwaite and Rearick, 'Michelozzo', pp. 221–306; B.J. Trexler, 'Hospital Patients in Florence, San Paolo, 1567–68', *Bulletin of the History of Medicine*, 48 (1974), pp. 41–59. For S. Maria Nuova: Passerini, *Storia*, pp. 284–395; G. Pampaloni, *Lo spedale di S. Maria Nuova* (Firenze, 1961); F. Brasioli and L. Ciuccetti, *S. Maria Nuova. Il tesoro dell'arte nell'antico ospedale fiorentino* (Florence, 1989); *S. Maria Nuova in Firenze. Memorie, testimonianze, prospettive* (Florence, 1991); and most recently, De Benedictis, ed., *Il Patrimonio Artistico*.
56. For the topographical location of S. Paolo see Goldthwaite and Rearick, 'Michelozzo', pp. 222–3.
57. On the early history of S. Paolo see Passerini, *Storia*, pp. 163–88; R. Franci, 'L'Ospedale di S. Paolo in Firenze e i Terziari Francescani', *VII centenario del Terz'Ordine Francescano, Studi francescani*, n.s. 7 (18) (1921), pp. 52–70; G.G. Meersseman, *Dossier de l'Ordre de la Pénitence au XIIIe siècle* (Freiburg, 1961); Goldthwaite and Rearick, 'Michelozzo', pp. 221–306; Benvenuti Papi, '*In Castro Poenitentiae*', pp. 15–57.
58. ASF, SP 975, ff. 15r, 31v.
59. SP 976, f. VIv: 'Due spedali posti in Borgho San Paolo, l'uno per albergare ilgli uomini e l'altro le femine.'

60. Sznura, *L'espansione*, p. 80.
61. Passerini, *Storia*, doct. G: p. 835. The statutes of S. Maria Nuova from 1330 and 1374 are published in *Il Reggio Arcispedale di S. Maria Nuova. I suoi benefattori, sue antiche memorie* (Florence, 1888): cited as SMN followed by the date. The original manuscript of the 1330 statutes is in the Biblioteca Corsiniana, Rome, though it has not been traced by the present librarian, while a copy of those of 1374 is in SMN 1, ff. 14v–26v. For this reference see SMN (1330), p. 41.
62. SMN (1330), pp. 44–5, and in Passerini, *Storia*, p. 836.
63. Pampaloni, *Lo spedale di S. Maria Nuova*, pp. 5–6. 14–17; ASF, SMN 10, f. 4r; Davidsohn, *Storia*, Vol. 3, pp. 604–5; Vol. 7, pp. 79–80; Richa, *Notizie*, Vol. 8, pp. 191–2.
64. SMN (1330), p. 56. Passerini, *Storia*, pp. 354–5: 'La costruzione di questo cimitero data pure dal secondo decennio del secolo decimoquarto.'
65. Pampaloni, *Lo spedale di S. Maria Nuova*, pp. 19–20, based on SMN 1.
66. Historians usually rely on and take at face value the manuscript history of S. Maria Nuova written in 1662: SMN 1.
67. Pampaloni, *Lo spedale di S. Maria Nuova*, p. 19 gives the early fourteenth century, though without providing any evidence.
68. Ibid., pp. 18–19.
69. SMN 1, ins. 2, ff. 6r–v; ff. 5r (1324); ff. 6r–v (1329); f. 3v (1330s).
70. SMN (1330), p. 57: 'lato delle femine servigiali.'
71. SMN 4390: 1325–7: f. 3r (1325): 'nele decte ricopertura dele case dele femine che si rimesono tucte quelle teta per mano e spedale nuovo dele femine e ricopritur lo spedale degli uomini; il legniame del palcho ch'è sopra la sagrestia'; f. 5r (1325): 'per lo spedale nuovo dele femine quando si murava'; ff. 13r–v (1327): 'in dodici pezi d'assi per le finestre delo spedale dele femine; in bandelle e aghuti per le finestre; per mezane da matonare lo spedale dele femine' (cf. also f. 20r); f. 15r: 'in sete assi d'olmo per la porta grande delle femine' (cf. also f. 20v); f. 21r: 'lengnio d'olmo per le graticole della capella dele femine'; f. 23v: 'a due maestri che lavoravano nela capella delo spedale dele femine'; f. 22r: '7 bordoni d'albaro per fare il palcho delo spedale vecchio dele femine; in pietre per l'agio de' refetorio dele femine'; f. 28r (30.v.1328): 'per ricoprire il tetto del chiostro, 20 soldi.'
72. Passerini, *Storia*, p. 356; Pampaloni, *Lo spedale di S. Maria Nuova*, p. 80 n. 47, based on SMN 1, ins. 3.
73. Cf. SMN 4392 (1335–44): 1340–1: many expenses for building; SMN 4393 (1345–7); 4398, f. 1v: year from July 1348: 'tecto dello spedale degli uomine e delle donne'; 'dormentorio delle donne'; 'chiesa di S. Egidio'; 4398, f. 10v: building the *infermeria*, began in Aug. 1348.
74. SMN 10, f. 13r: 'La cappella dello spedale da lato degli huomini, secondo che si vede per lettere intagliate nella pietra la quale è posta dal lato dinanzi all'altar di detta cappella, fu edificata e fatta del mese di maggio 1369, al tempo di Ser Guido spedalingo e rettore di detto spedale.'
75. SMN 1, f. 3v: ins. 3: 'nella testata della corsia era l'altare, quale era posto sotto una cupoletta, però coperto di legname e embrici.'
76. G. Villani, *Cronica*, VIII.2.
77. Davidsohn, *Storia*, Vol. 7, pp. 89–91. Although a new hospital dedicated to the Evangelist was built in what is now Via Martelli, little is known about its activities and it appears to have ceased functioning within a short time.
78. Davidsohn, *Storia*, Vol. 3, pp. 286, 569–70; Vol. 1, pp. 286, 958, Vol. 4, p. 551; Vol. 2, p. 61.
79. For discussion of this process see McVaugh, *Medicine before the Plague*, pp. 190–1, 200–1, 225–9.
80. On S. Paolo: Passerini, *Storia*, pp. 163–88; Franci, 'L'Ospedale di S. Paolo', pp. 52–70;

Meersseman, *Dossier*; Goldthwaite and Rearick, 'Michelozzo', pp. 221–306; Benvenuti Papi, '*In Castro Poenitentiae*', pp. 15–57.
81. On the role of nursing staff and *conversi* see below, Chapter 7; and O. Redon, 'Autour de l'Hôpital S. Maria della Scala à Sienne au XIIIe siècle', *Ricerche storiche*, 15:1 (1985), pp. 17–34; Benvenuti Papi, '*In Castro Poenitentiae*', p. 629.
82. Statutes of Sept. 1325 in SP 976: cap. viii: fol. 108v. For a full discussion of this process see Henderson, ' "Splendide case di cura" '.
83. SP 977, f. 1r: 'adì xxiiii di novembre proximo si cominciaro a ritenere l'infermi nello spedale de' poveri l'anno predecto [1345], il quale si compie del detto mese di novembre al tempo de'detti frati Piero Bindi et Giovanni Lozi ministri.'
84. For example, 15 April to 20 May 1347 as recorded in SP 661, which also included payments to the 'Poor of Christ'.
85. SP 661, f. 5v: 'le quali erano molto utili et necessarie ai detti frati per li poveri di Cristo.'
86. SP 661 (unpaginated), under 20.iv.1347, 13.vi.1347, 19.viii.1347, 24.viii.1347, 9.xii.1347, 13.i.1348.
87. SMN (1330), p. 41; cf. Passerini, *Storia*, doct. G: p. 835.
88. SMN (1330), p. 53 (24.ii.1329 according to the Florentine year).
89. Ibid., p. 56.
90. Ibid., p. 53.
91. ASF, SMN 4390, f. 25r.
92. Ibid., ff. 23v, 38v.
93. Ibid., ff. 34v, 41r.
94. K. Park, *Doctors and Medicine in Early Renaissance Florence* (Princeton, 1985), p. 68; A. Feigenbaum, 'Early History of Cataract and the Ancient Operation for Cataract', *American Journal of Opthamology*, 49 (1960), pp. 305–26.
95. ASF, SMN 4390, ff. 2r, 7v, 11r, 33r, 38v, 46v.
96. See, for example, D. Jacquart, *Le milieu médical en France du XIIe au XVe siècle* (Geneva, 1981); C. O'Boyle, 'Surgical Texts and Social Contexts: Physicians and Surgeons in Paris, c.1270 to 1430'; D. Jacquart, 'Medical Practice in Paris in the first half of the fourteenth century', in L. Garcia-Ballester et al., eds, *Practical Medicine from Salerno to the Black Death* (Cambridge, 1994), pp. 156–85 and 186–210.
97. I. Naso, *Medici e strutture sanitarie*, chs 4, 6; Park, *Doctors*, pp. 58–9.
98. ASF, SMN 4390, f. 39v (Simone *barbiere*).
99. ASF, Provvisioni Registri 34, ff. 135r–v.
100. Henderson, *Piety and Charity*, Part 2.
101. For this theme in Florence cf. De La Roncière, *Prix et salaires*, Vol. 1, pp. iii–iv; R.A. Goldthwaite, *The Building of Renaissance Florence. An Economic and Social History* (Baltimore and London, 1980), ch. 6; and in relation to the clientele of charities see C.-M. de La Roncière, 'Pauvres et pauvreté à Florence au xive siècle', in M. Mollat, ed., *Etudes sur l'histoire de la pauvreté* (Paris, 1974), pp. 661–745; Henderson, *Piety and Charity*, Part 2.
102. McVaugh, *Medicine before the Plague*, pp. 200–1.
103. R. Ciasca, *L'Arte dei medici e speziali nella storia e nel commercio fiorentino dal secolo xii al xv* (Florence, 1927; repr. 1977), pp. 10–16.
104. Ibid., pp. 267–8; Park, *Doctors*, pp. 15–21; Davidsohn, *Storia*, Vol. 6, pp. 314–15.
105. Park, *Doctors*, pp. 99–109.
106. Cf. ibid., pp. 87–99; Naso, *Medici e strutture sanitarie*, pp. 32–55, 97–101, 193–201; McVaugh, *Medicine before the Plague*, pp. 3, 190–1, 225–9; V. Nutton, 'Continuity or Rediscovery? The City Physician in Classical Antiquity and Medieval Italy', in A.W. Russell, ed., *The Town and State Physician in Europe from the Middle Ages to the Enlightenment* (Wolfenbüttel, 1981), pp. 9–46.
107. Davidsohn, *Storia*, Vol. 2, pp. 630–1.

108. Passerini, *Storia*, p. 676.
109. For the legislation relative to S. Maria Nuova: SMN 4; summarised in SMN 10, ff. 26v–27r. The communal privileges to the company of Orsanmichele were published (with some erroneous transcriptions) by S. La Sorsa, *La compagnia d'Or San Michele, ovvero una pagina della beneficenza in Toscana nel secolo XIV* (Trani, 1902), pp. 209–23, and discussed by Henderson, *Piety and Charity*, chs 6, 7.
110. See Henderson, *Piety and Charity*, pp. 273–9.
111. In general on the 1340s see ibid., pp. 279–92; on the petition see Passerini, *Storia*, p. 295.
112. *Decrees of the Ecumenical Councils*, Vol. 1: *Nicaea I to Lateran V*, ed. N.P. Tanner (London and Georgetown, 1990).
113. AOIF, ser. II.I, ff. 2r–3r.
114. Passerini, *Storia*, pp. 662–6.
115. SMN 1, f. 1r; SMN 10, f. 1v.
116. SMN 1, f. 2v; SMN 10, f. 2v.
117. SMN 1, ff. 2v–3r.
118. See also the conflicts which typified the hospitals of twelfth- and thirteenth-century Milan: Albini, *Città e ospedali*, ch. 1.
119. Provvisioni Registri 4, f. 8r: 19.v.1294: Passerini, *Storia*, pp. 935–7.
120. L. Sandri, 'La gestione dell'assistenza a Firenze nel XV secolo', in *La Toscana al tempo di Lorenzo il Magnifico. Politica, economia, cultura, arte* (Pisa, 1996), Vol. 3, pp. 1363–80.
121. See Davidsohn, *Storia*, pp. 91ff.
122. Cf. Henderson, *Piety and Charity*, pp. 16–20.
123. Passerini, *Storia*, pp. 519–24.
124. Davidsohn, *Storia*, Vol. 7, pp. 91ff.
125. SMN 1, f. 1r; SMN 10, f. 1v.
126. Cohn, *Death and Property in Siena*, ch. 5.
127. Albini, *Città e ospedali*, pp. 34–46.
128. A. Esposito, 'Gli ospedali romani tra iniziative laicali e politica pontificia (secc. XIII–XV)', in *Ospedali e città*, ed. A.J. Grieco and L. Sandri (Florence, 1997), pp. 234–5, based on the text of the *Regola* published by P. De Angelis, *L'Ospedale di S. Spirito in Sassia* (Rome, 1960–2), Vol. 1, pp. 381–4.
129. Gallavotti Cavallero, *Lo Spedale di Santa Maria della Scala in Siena*, pp. 55–7; D. Balestracci and G. Piccinni, 'L'ospedale e la città', in ibid., p. 21.
130. A. Cenci, ed., *L'ospitalità in Altopascio* (Lucca, 1996), pp. 130, 135.
131. G. Piccinni and L. Vigni, 'Modelli di assistenza ospedaliera tra Medioevo ed Età Moderna. Quotidianità, amministrazione, conflitti nell'Ospedale di S. Maria della Scala di Siena', in Pinto, ed., *La società del bisogno*, pp. 131–74, esp. pp. 145–58; G. Piccinni, 'L'Ospedale di S. Maria Scala di Siena. Note sulle origini dell'assistenza sanitaria in Toscana (xiv–xv secolo)', in *Città e servizi sociali nell'Italia dei secoli XII–XV* (Pistoia, 1990), pp. 297–324; Balestracci and Piccinni, 'L'ospedale e la città', p. 21 date the medicalisation of S. Maria della Scala as having taken place between the redaction of their 1305 and 1318 statutes.
132. Cenci, ed., *L'ospitalità in Altopascio*.
133. For France see: the chapters written by M. Mollat in J. Imbert, *Histoire des hôpitaux en France* (Toulouse, 1982), pp. 35–47, 78–9; J. Chiffoleau, *La comptabilité de l'au-delà. Les hommes, la mort et la religion dans la région d'Avignon à la fin du moyen-âge (vers 1320–vers 1480)* (Rome, 1980), pp. 314–21; Saunier, 'Le pauvre malade'. Cf. also C. Marchesini and G. Sperati, *Ospedali genovesi nel medioevo. Atti della società ligure di storia patria*, n.s. 21 (1981), pp. 60–2; G. Albini, *Guerra, fame, peste. Crisi di mortalità e sistema sanitario nella Lombardia tardomedioevale* (Milano, 1982), pp. 63–78; Albini, *Città e ospedali*.

Chapter 2

1. Cf. N. Orme and M. Webster, *The English Hospital, 1070–1570* (New Haven and London, 1995), pp. 127–9.
2. Rawcliffe, *Medicine for the Soul*, p. 65.
3. Henderson, *Piety and Charity*.
4. Ibid., ch. 7.
5. Ibid., pp. 318–20.
6. On the Orbatello see Passerini, *Storia*, pp. 639–48; R.C. Trexler, 'A Widows' Asylum of the Renaissance: The Orbatello of Florence', in P.N. Stearns, ed., *Old Age in Pre-Industrial Society* (New York, 1982), pp. 119–49; C. De Benedictis, 'Vicende e trasformazioni dell'Ospedale di Santa Maria di Orbatello', *Antichità viva*, 26 (1987), pp. 28–34. On the Innocenti: Gavitt, *Charity and Children in Renaissance Florence*; Sandri, ed., *Gli Innocenti e Firenze nei secoli*.
7. On S. Matteo see E. Lucas-Lybor, 'The Spedale di S. Matteo in Florence' (unpublished Ph.D. thesis, University of Essex, 1988); Sandri, 'Ospedali e utenti nella Firenze del Quattrocento'; and most recently E. Diana, *San Matteo e San Giovanni di Dio: due ospedali nella storia fiorentina* (Florence, 1999). On Messer Bonifazio: E. Coturri, 'L'ospedale cosidetto "di Bonifazio" in Firenze', *Pagine di storia della medicina*, 3:2 (1959), pp. 73–8; E. Lombardi, *Messer Bonifacio Lupi da Parma e la sua fondazione in Via San Gallo in Firenze* (Florence, 1992); A.M. Zandri, C. Acidini Luchinat and S. Francolini, *Lo Spedale di Messer Bonifazio* (Florence, 1989).
8. Goldthwaite and Rearick, 'Michelozzo', pp. 223–4; Park, 'Healing the Poor: Hospitals and Medical Assistance in Renaissance Florence', pp. 27–32; and cf. McVaugh, *Medicine before the Plague*, pp. 228–35.
9. 23.xii.1377: Passerini, *Storia*, p. 825.
10. See S.K. Cohn Jr, *The Cult of Remembrance and the Black Death* (Baltimore and London, 1992), pp. 45–6.
11. M. Villani, *Cronica*, I.8.
12. SMN 4398, f. 5r.
13. SMN 4398, f. 3v: 'medichare gli infermi dello spedale, gli uomini e le femine.'
14. SMN 4398, ff. 143v–145v: 1350.
15. SP 662, ff. 1r–2v: 5.ii.1349–18.i.1350.
16. SP 662 under 9.ii.1349 and 24.vii.1349.
17. SP 676 under 23.iv.1359 and 17.iii.1359, and SP 677 under 18.iii.1358. Before this date no physician is recorded in these fragmentary accounts except Maestro Ambrogio, who received a salary in January 1348 and, like Sennuccio, may have survived the plague: SP 661 under 13.i.1348.
18. It has been suggested that one of the reasons for its great enrichment in this period is that it had been made the 'mandatory final substitute heir to all Florentine estates' by the commune, though no convincing evidence is provided for this statement: R.C. Trexler, *Public Life in Renaissance Florence* (New York, 1980), p. 134.
19. For a detailed discussion of Orsanmichele see Henderson, *Piety and Charity*, pp. 175–95. The hospital's books of testaments which purport to cover the Black Death are: SMN 59 (listed in the inventory as 1300 to 1500, but mostly from the fifteenth century); SMN 60 (1340–79, though clearly only a partial record); SMN 62 (a mixture of records, including inventories and testaments, for 1320–85); SMN 63 (1345–51, though incomplete); SMN 64 (1348: incomplete: summary of sums paid out under bequests).
20. This is discussed in detail in Henderson, *Piety and Charity*, chs 6, 8.
21. SMN 4398, f. 41r: 'Item paghamo [10 lire] adì v d'aghosto quando Ser Guido fu sostenuto da' Priori che stette sostenuto xii dì nelle Stinche per non volere dare i denari de' poveri a Priori e puoi non pagha nulla lodato sia Idio.'

22. See, for example, that recorded for the friars of S. Maria Novella: S. Orlandi, *'Necrologio' di Santa Maria Novella* (Florence, 1955); cf. J. Henderson, 'The Parish and the Poor in Florence at the Time of the Black Death: The Case of S. Frediano', in J. Henderson, ed., *Charity and the Poor in Medieval and Renaissance Europe*, in *Continuity and Change*, 3:2 (1988), pp. 247–72.
23. SMN 4390, f. 1r; SMN 4400, f. 3r: 'la maggiore parte della famiglia anticha.'
24. SMN 10, f. 58v. No exact date is given here for his death. Confusingly SMN 1.iii, f. 2r gives 1347 as the year of his death, though this may simply suggest that he died in the spring, before 25 March, when the Florentine year changed.
25. SMN 4400, f. 3r.
26. SMN 10, f. 58v.
27. SMN 4409: 'A voi Sengnori capitani dela Compagnia dela Vergene Maria d'Ortosanmichele, lo spedalingo e quelli che servono agl'infermi delo spedale di Santa Maria Nova vi se mandano molto racomandando e pregando per l'amore di Dio e dela Vergene Maria che voi facciate al loro limosena per fornire gli decti infermi, però ch'ano molti infermi e anno molto bisogno e lo Spirito Santo v'alumini in ciò ch'avete affare. Amen.' This is an undated loose piece of paper in the front cover of the hospital's account book for 1355–6; I have assumed that the letter also dates from this time.
28. Provv. Reg. 51, f. 7r: 21.viii.1363. Discussed in Henderson, *Piety and Charity*, pp. 190–1, and R.C. Trexler, ' "Florence by the Grace of the Lord Pope …" ', *Studies in Medieval and Renaissance History*, 9 (1972), pp. 168–9. How far the commune availed itself of this self-granted privilege can only be determined through a detailed analysis of the financial records of these institutions.
29. Cohn, *The Cult of Remembrance*, pp. 44–6.
30. Will of Messer Bonifazio Lupi cited in Lombardi, *Messer Bonifacio Lupi*, p. 191.
31. The discrepancy between the total in Table 1.1 (seventeen) and the total in Table 2.1 can be accounted for by the fact that the latter includes 1349 when two hospitals were founded.
32. See C. Klapisch-Zuber, *Women, Family and Ritual in Renaissance Italy* (Chicago and London, 1985).
33. B. Varchi, *Storia fiorentina*, ed. L. Arbib (Florence, 1839–41), Vol. 2, IX, pp. 100–1; his statistics may have been based on the 1527 census of the city of Florence in Biblioteca Nazionale Centrale di Firenze, NA 987.
34. Herlihy and Klapisch-Zuber, *Tuscans and their Families*, p. 74: Table 3.5.
35. Goldthwaite, *The Building*, pp. 13–22; S.K. Cohn Jr, *The Laboring Classes in Renaissance Florence* (New York and London, 1980), ch. 5, which argues for the displacement of the *popolo minuto* from central to larger suburban parishes within the early fourteenth-century walls.
36. On the Innocenti see Saalman, *Filippo Brunelleschi*, p. 33.
37. Passerini, *Storia*, pp. 121–2; R. Stopani, ed., *Firenze e i primi Giubilei. Un momento di storia fiorentina della solidarietà* (Florence, 1999), p. 74.
38. The Spedale di S. Jacopo in Campo Corbolini in the northern part of the city was also under its administration.
39. Passerini, *Storia*, pp. 142–5.
40. Catasto 185, f. 615r.
41. Passerini, *Storia*, pp. 395–6; Catasto 194, ff. 654v, 656r; 194.I, f. 671r; 293, f. 35v; L. Sandri, ed., *L'archivio dell'Ospedale di San Giovanni di Dio di Firenze (1604–1890)* (Milan, 1991), pp. 1–15.
42. The Catasto of 1427–30 includes the returns of thirty-five religious corporations termed *spedali* in Florence in the following volumes: Catasto 185.I–II; 190; 194.II; 195; 291–3. At the end of the century the 1495 Decima records thirty-two *spedali* in the city: Decima della Repubblica 66–77.
43. There were a few notable gaps in these records, such as the return of the Spedale di

S. Paolo and the *incarichi* or debit side of the account of S. Maria Nuova. In addition, I cannot find the returns of the following: S. Trinita dei Calzolai; Ospizio di Orbatello; S. Caterina dei Talani; and the Spedale delle Stinche (though the last is mentioned in a bequest to another hospital: Catasto 190, f. 670r). For discussion of confraternity Catasto returns see Henderson, *Piety and Charity*, chs 3, 4.

44. Catasto 185.II, f. 615r; 194.II, ff. 610r–v.
45. S. Giuliano de'Vettori: Catasto 185.II, ff. 615r–v; S. Lucia de' Magnoli: Catasto 194, ff. 654r, 662v, also Passerini, *Storia*, p. 14; S. Maria dell'Umiltà: Catasto 194, f. 656r.
46. Catasto 194, ff. 654r, 656r.
47. Catasto 185, f. 614r; 194, f. 663v; 185, f. 633r.
48. Catasto 190, f. 13r; 185, ff. 616 r–v.
49. SMN (1330); BON 5, f. 7v: 24.i.1475: patients restricted to a stay of fifteen days.
50. Although the Florentine republic was traditionally suspicious of organisations of people from the same trade: see Henderson, *Piety and Charity*, ch. 9.
51. Wellcome Institute Library, London, Wellcome Western MS 275, f.15v: 'sonci ventotto lectiere usate e ventotto sacconi usati; otto carpite tra buone e cattive; otto matterasse cattive; cinque paia di lenzuola usate; uno paio di lenzuola buona e tre casse vecchie; una tavola de duo trespoli; una imagine di legno di S. Giovanni Batista.'
52. Catasto 185, ff. 616r–v.
53. Passerini, *Storia*, p. 115.
54. Catasto 185, f. 626r: 'Monna Maria, donna che fu d'Andrea d'Antonio da Firenze, d'anni 80 ed è inferma e non escie di letto; Monna Sandra, figlia di Maso da Firenze, d'anni 25, è stata inferma un'anno o più e da infermità da non ghuarire mai sennone quando si morrà di quello.'
55. Ibid.: 'Monna Nicholosa, figlia che fu di Giovanni da Chasentino, d'anni 50, iscianchata e inferma.'
56. Details from Passerini, *Storia*, pp. 641–2; see also Trexler, 'A Widows' Asylum'.
57. Catasto 190, f. 80r: 'Anchora fa la detta arte [Por San Maria] fare e edifichare uno spedale presso alla Piazza de' Servi di Firenze per ricettare e poveri fanciulli gittatelli abandonati.'
58. For S. Maria della Scala see Catasto 185, ff. 584r–585v; S. Gallo: Passerini, *Storia*, p. 669; and the Innocenti: Provv. Reg.161, f. 255v; Passerini, *Storia*, p. 704.
59. Catasto 185, ff. 528r–585v, though the 'incharichi' (ff. 576r–585v) provide the majority of information for this discussion.
60. Cf. R.C. Trexler, 'The Foundlings of Florence: New Sources and First Results', *History of Childhood Quarterly*, 1 (1974), pp. 259–84.
61. Cf. Gavitt, *Charity and Children*, p. 209: Table 6.
62. Catasto 185, f. 581r.
63. Ibid.
64. Gavitt, *Charity and Children*, pp. 155–7.
65. Catasto 194.II, f. 379v: 'per mantenere 30 letta dove alberghano e poveri e chonperare lenzuole e altre chose necessarie, l'anno fior. 30'; 'pannilini e lani per gli infermi.'
66. Passerini, *Storia*, pp. 133–41; Park, *Doctors*, pp. 103–4 n. 58.
67. Catasto 184, f. 112r: 'In prima la chiesa, spedale, et magione di S. Antonio di Firenze, chon l'orto overo giardino et due casecte tucte insieme chontigue poste nel popolo di Sancto Lorenzo di Firenzo, luogo decto a S. Antonio.'
68. Provv. Reg. 137, ff. 116r–117r: 29.vi.1446: Passerini, *Storia*, p. 139, where he also cites a law of 28.iv. 1450.
69. See Catasto 190, ff. 25v–32v; 291, ff. 16v–23v.
70. Passerini, *Storia*, pp. 125–33.
71. See Catasto 291, f. 23v; and 1527 census of the city: BNCF, NA 987, under Quarter of S. Maria Novella.
72. ASF, Ospedale di S. Eusebio 2, f. 1r: 'In prima l'abitazione dello spedalingho del detto

hospidale con chiesa, corte, volta e sala, camera, orto e pratello posta in Firenze nel popolo di Santa Lucia d'Ognessanti in sul Prato.'
73. Ibid., f. 6r: 'Una abitatione in modo di spedale colle case e abituro per lo spedalingo e chiesa principiata dove stanno e ritengosi l'infermi infetti fuori della città di Firenze.'
74. See Catasto 190, ff. 25v–32v; 291, ff. 16v–23v.
75. ASF, Ospedale di S. Eusebio 2, f. 6r.
76. Cf. also Paatz, *Die Kirchen von Florenz*, Vol. 1, pp. 395–405; Vol. 4, pp. 148–57.
77. M. Villani, *Cronica*, XI. 2.
78. Provv. Reg. 57, f. 153r: 25.i.1370; ASF, Diplomatico dell'Ospedale di Messer Bonifazio, 19.ix.1380: Lombardi, *Messer Bonifacio Lupi*, pp. 99–100, 183.
79. Provv. Reg. 65, ff. 241r–243r: 23.xii.1377: Passerini, *Storia*, p. 825.
80. On restitution by usurers see R.C. Trexler, 'Death and Testament in the Episcopal Constitutions of Florence (1327)', in A. Molho and J.A. Tedeschi, eds, *Renaissance Studies in Honor of Hans Baron* (Florence, 1971), pp. 42–3.
81. Cf. Passerini, *Storia*, pp. 149–50.
82. Diplomatico dell'Ospedale di S. Matteo, 5.xi.1381; Passerini, *Storia*, pp. 819–22, esp. p. 820.
83. See discussion in Gavitt, *Charity and Children*, ch. 1.
84. See ibid., pp. 39–40.
85. Ibid., p. 37.
86. Ibid., pp. 45–9, 51–6.
87. Act of Florentine bishop, 4.iv.1385: Passerini, *Storia*, p. 817. For Messer Bonifazio see Provv. Reg. 65, ff. 241r–243r: 23.xii.1377: Passerini, *Storia*, p. 825: 'quoddam hospitale seu quasdam domos pro peregrinis et pauperibus receptandis … pro consolatione et refrigerio pauperum et infirmorum ibi degentium.' His will is cited in Lombardi, *Messer Bonifacio Lupi*, p. 191; papal bull of 5.xi.1389: Passerini, *Storia*, p. 820.
88. Thus Bonifazio Lupi founded his hospital only three years after the severe epidemic of 1374, while Lemmo Balducci established his institution two years after another episode of plague: Herlihy and Klapisch-Zuber, *Tuscans and their Families*, p. 191. Cf. Goldthwaite and Rearick, 'Michelozzo', pp. 223–4.
89. Gavitt, *Charity and Children*, p. 44. On Datini's participation in the Bianchi movement see Henderson, *Piety and Charity*, p. 53.
90. See the 'ordinances' in Wellcome Institute Library MS 453, and Lombardi, *Messer Bonifacio Lupi*, ch. 25, citing the testament.
91. Passerini, *Storia*, p. 129.
92. Cf. Sandri, 'La gestione dell'assistenza a Firenze nel XV secolo'.
93. Gavitt, *Charity and Children*, pp. 51–5.
94. Messer Bonifazio: Catasto 291, f. 34r; SM 326, f. 90r (1409–12); Catasto 185.II, f. 606v (1428).
95. Catasto 190, f. 52r includes 'uno speziale in casa' under the heading 'Bocche che sono di continuo in casa'.
96. SM 180, ff. 6v–85: 12.iv.1409. See also the discussion of these entries in Sandri, 'Ospedali e utenti', pp. 86–9.
97. Catasto 185.II, f. 606v; Catasto 291, f. 34r; Provv. Reg. 93, f. 116r: 9.ii.1404: Passerini, *Storia*, p. 170.
98. See Henderson, *Piety and Charity*, chs 7, 8.
99. See SP 675 for 1370–1; and in general for the subsequent development of the hospital in these years see Passerini, *Storia*, pp. 168–74.
100. Benvenuti Papi, 'In Castro Poenitentiae', p. 629.
101. Although it did not actually submit a Catasto return, the 'Spedale delle Stinche' was mentioned in a bequest to S. Maria Nuova: Catasto 190, f. 670r.

102. Park, *Doctors*, pp. 89–90.
103. S. Matteo: SM 108, ff. 9v, 12r; Catasto 185.II, f. 606r; Messer Bonifazio: Catasto 291, f. 34r; cf. Passerini, *Storia*, pp. 156, 228; S. Paolo: Provv. Reg. 93, f. 116r: 9.ii.1404: Passerini, *Storia*, p. 169.
104. For this and information about patients see below, Chapter 8.
105. Cf. Sandri, 'Aspetti dell'assistenza', pp. 238–41; A. Patetta, 'Gli ospedali a Pisa nel medioevo', in *Strutture sanitarie a Pisa. Contributi alla storia di una città, secc. XIII–XIX* (Pisa, 1986), pp. 49–75; Albini, *Città e ospedali*. The most recent studies of the hospitals of medieval Pisa are E.P. Rothrauff, 'Charity in a Medieval Community: Politics, Piety and Poor-relief in Pisa, 1257–1312' (Unpublished Ph.D. thesis, University of California at Berkeley, 1994), and A. Patetta, *La storia dell'Ospedale di S. Chiara in Pisa: dalle origini fino al 1771* (Pisa, 1994); for Milan: G.C. Bascapé, 'L'assistenza e la beneficenza a Milano dall'alto medioevo alla fine della dinastia sforzesca', Fondazione G. Treccani degli Alfieri, *Storia di Milano* (Milan, 1957), Vol. 8, pp. 387–419.
106. Albini, *Città e ospedali*, p. 72.
107. Cf. Horden, ' "A discipline of relevance" ', p. 367.
108. Varchi, *Storie fiorentine*, Vol. 2, IX, pp.101–2.
109. For figures for wage rates and prices of consumables: de La Roncière, *Prix et salaires*; Goldthwaite, *The Building of Renaissance Florence*.
110. A year later Paolo Soldini paid 'per minatura delle chonstituzioni nostre': SMN 4428, f. 30r: 26.x.1375. SMN statutes of 1374, p. 63; SMN 4426: Entrata e Uscita (1373–4); SMN 1, 'Inventario', ff. 7r–9v: SMN, 1376 inventory, pp. 13–22.
111. Total expenditure for the year 2.xi.1325–1.xi.1326 was £2,921; calculated from SMN 4390, ff. 5r–11r.
112. C.-M. de La Roncière, 'Indirect Taxes or "Gabelles" at Florence', in N. Rubinstein, ed., *Florentine Studies: Politics and Society in Renaissance Florence* (London, 1968), p. 176: Table II.
113. Marchionne di Coppo Stefani, *Cronaca fiorentina*, ed. N. Rodolico, *Rerum Italicarum Scriptores*, n.s. 31: 1 (Città di Castello, 1903), 745; Herlihy and Klapisch-Zuber, *Tuscans and their Families*, p. 191.
114. SMN 4427, f. 99r: 'Entrata delle limosine manualmente fatte e delle oblationi della chiesa e degl'altari e di ceppi delgli spedali delgli huomini e delle femine'; f. 101r: 'Traemo dì xxiii d'ottobre del ceppo che allato dell'uscio del chiostro dello spedale delgli huomini £8.3.3. e del ceppo della porta dello spedale delgli uomini e del ceppo dello spedale delle femine £3.8.7 somma £22.1.2.'
115. SMN 4426, ff. 239r–240r, 243r–v.
116. Ibid., f. 237r.
117. See, for now, A.J. Grieco, 'Il vitto di un ospedale: pratica, distinzioni sociali e teorie mediche alla metà del Quattrocento', in L. Sandri, ed., *Gli Innocenti e Firenze nei secoli: un ospedale, un archivio, una città* (Florence, 1996), pp. 85–92.
118. SMN 4426, ff. 267r–268v.
119. SMN (1376), f. 25r; SMN 4426, ff. 267r–268v.
120. SMN 4426, ff. 248r–v.
121. Ibid. for the specific ingredients. A useful guide to contemporary terminology is C. Masino, *Voci di spezieria dei secoli XIV–XVIII*, ed. D. Talmelli and G. Maggioni (Padua, 1988).
122. SMN 1, 'Inventario', ff. 7r–9v.
123. SMN 1, f. 19r.
124. SMN 4426, ff. 285r, 286r.
125. SMN 4453, ff. 43r, 44v, 46v, 47r. His employment by the city's major hospital may seem surprising given that only four years before he had been declared a virtual indigent; in 1369–70 his name had been cancelled from the rolls of the city's Prestanza,

or forced loan, as too poor to pay tax: see Park, *Doctors and Medicine*, p. 55 n. 25.
126. G.A. Brucker, *Florentine Politics and Society, 1343–1378* (Princeton, 1962), pp. 94, 233, 248, 255; G.A. Brucker, *The Civic World of Early Renaissance Florence* (Princeton, 1977), pp. 104, 131–2.
127. It is some measure of the esteem in which S. Maria Nuova was held that these individuals should entrust such considerable sums to the hospital. All were local inhabitants: Lucha di Pagno from the parish of S. Simone; Francesco Battagluzzi from S. Lorenzo; and Monna Vaggia, the widow of a prominent patrician, Francesco di Filipozzo dei Bardi. Although the size of these three individual bequests did skew the importance of this category of expenditure, even when they are removed from the equation, testamentary expenses still represent 10 per cent of all outgoings. This was in part spent on paying the gabelle or indirect tax on testaments (£156), but largely on 'testaments, codicils and last wishes' (£1,873).
128. SMN 4408, f. 50r: 13.viii.1354: 'A cierti preti per dire messe quando si fecie la rinovale di morti di Portinari, soldi 12.'
129. SMN 10, f. 13r.
130. SMN 4465, f. 28r: 'A Filippo di Tomaso e compagni speziali adì xvi di novembre [1413] per la cera e coltri e drappi e panche per la sepoltura del nostro padre spedalingho Ser Piero Mini che morì adì 29 d'ottobre prossimo passato, per tutto fior. 30 d'oro'; f. 28v: 'A Michele di Jacopo setaiolo adì xxx di novembre [1413] per iiii mappe di seta avemo da lui per lo ghuanciale per la coltre si fece, £10.'
131. SMN (1374), ch. 1, pp. 63–4.
132. Ibid., p. 63.
133. Ibid.: SMN 1, f. 15r.
134. Cf. Henderson, *Piety and Charity*, ch. 3.
135. SMN, 1376 inventory, pp. 1–37. It is no coincidence that the inventory was drawn up on 6 July. The statutes required this to be done before a new *spedalingo* was installed and Paolo di Piero Torri took office on 9 July. The contents of all occupied spaces were listed and the only areas omitted were those such as cloisters and the cemetery which at this stage apparently did not contain movable objects.
136. SMN, 1376 inventory, pp. 7–12; SMN 4426, ff. 253v, 254r, 255r, 256r.
137. The 'infirmary' was a separate area for members of the staff who had fallen sick: see SMN (1374), p. 73, and the 1376 inventory, p. 23. The total spent at this time on these two projects was £730 and £496 respectively: SMN 4398, ff. 10v–12r.
138. SMN 4398, f. 13r: Sept. 1349.
139. SMN 4424, f. 4v: 191 gold florins paid for 'lo lavorio del acrescimento dello spedale delli uomini'. The exact area to be extended was clarified in another payment, to the stonemason Marcho da Fiesole for the stone 'for the chapel that is being made in the men's ward'.
140. SMN 4424, ff. 3r–17v; f. 16v: 'Paghamo adì xvi di maggio [1369] a Zanobi di Vinci per 18 cavretti de' quali mandamo tre a Messer lo Vescovo quando facemo consegrare l'altare di Messer S. Lucha.'
141. SMN 4426, ff. 251r–256r: 'lavoro dal lato delle donne.'
142. Ibid. This total included 'spese dell'edifichationi e reparationi dello spedale e delle chase e delle lettiere, panche, deschi e di tutti ferramenti'.
143. SMN 1, ff. 13v–15r: SMN, 1376 inventory, pp. 28–30.
144. See Holmes, *Fra Filippo Lippi*, pp. 26–7 for a reconstructed plan of S. Maria del Carmine.
145. SMN 1, ff. 15r–16v: SMN, 1376 inventory, pp. 31–2.
146. D. Herlihy, *Medieval and Renaissance Pistoia. The Social History of an Italian Town* (New Haven, 1967), pp. 247–8; Catasto 190, f. 83r; Catasto 185, ff. 612r, 619r.
147. Herlihy, *Medieval and Renaissance Pistoia*, pp. 247–8.
148. G.A. Brucker, 'Urban Parishes and their Clergy in Quattrocento Florence: A

Preliminary "Sondage" ', in *Renaissance Studies in Honor of Hugh Craig Smyth*, ed. A. Morrogh et al. (Florence, 1985), p. 27 n. 21: 36,441 florins.
149. Catasto 195, f. 271v; 194.II, f. 380r; 292, ff. 230v–232v.
150. Catasto 291, ff. 72r, 68r.
151. Catasto 195, f. 262r; 185.II, ff. 601r–606r; Brucker, 'Urban Parishes', p. 27 n. 21.
152. Varchi, *Storia fiorentina*, Vol. 2, IX, pp. 101–2.
153. Catasto 194.II, f. 172v; 195, f. 280v (1430); 194.II, ff. 646v, 610r–v; on confraternities see Henderson, *Piety and Charity*, ch. 2, Table 3.
154. See, for example, the property owned by S. Maria Nuova: Catasto 185.II, ff. 640r–699r; and below for a discussion of the assets of S. Matteo.
155. See G. Pinto, *La Toscana nel tardo Medioevo. Ambiente, economia rurale, società* (Florence, 1982), pp. 247–329.
156. The shares of Florentine hospitals in the communal debt are listed among the assets in their Catasto returns, as for S. Matteo (Catasto 185.II, ff. 601r–606r) and the Innocenti (Catasto 190, ff. 80r–82v).
157. Passerini, *Storia*, p. 355; R.A. Goldthwaite, 'Local Banking in Renaissance Florence', *Journal of European Economic History*, 14 (1985), pp. 44–5; and most recently Rab Hatfield, *The Wealth of Michelangelo* (Rome, 2002).
158. R. De Roover, *The Rise and Decline of the Medici Bank* (Cambridge, Mass., 1963), pp. 355–6.
159. SMN 30, f. 6v: 'Memoria che Curado Tedescho da Norberghe, cioè un huomo grande con barba rossa, diè i'servanza 1362, xii d'aprile, fior. 64 d'oro e disse in presenza di Ser Jacopo d'Arezzo e di Nastagio di Nino che se non tornasse per gli decti 64 fiorini d'oro di qui adì xvii d'aprile 1363 che volea che i decti denari fossono di poveri infermi delo spedale di Santa Maria Nuova e anche ci lasciò per sengniale uno grosso d'ariento che ha dal uno lato due santi e dal'altro lato uno santo, e uno ne tenne per se simigliante a quello. Currado decto riebe i decti denari 1362 dì iii di maggio, presente Nastagio e Ser Jacopo d'Arezo decto dì sopra.'
160. Hatfield, *The Wealth of Michelangelo*, p. 55.
161. On S. Maria della Scala see S.R. Epstein, *Alle origini della fattoria toscana. L'Ospedale della Scala di Siena e le sue terre (metà '200–metà '400)* (Florence, 1986); and, most recently, G. Piccinni and L. Travaini, *Il libro del Pellegrino (Siena, 1382–1446). Affari, uomini, monete nell'Ospedale di Santa Maria della Scala* (Naples, 2003).
162. Provv. Reg. 35, ff. 135r–v. The legislation concerning Orsanmichele and inheritance is discussed by Henderson, *Piety and Charity*, pp. 176–93.
163. A law of 13 Aug. 1348 extended to S. Maria Nuova all the privileges that had been granted to Orsanmichele over the previous decades. The texts of these laws were then copied down by its notary and can be found in SMN 10; they were then summarised in Italian in SMN 10, ff. 26v–27r. The text is printed by La Sorsa, *La compagnia d'Or San Michele*, pp. 226–9, though the actual law has not been traced in the *fondo* of the Provvisioni Registri.
164. Income in 1373–4: 6,065 gold florins = £22,137 at an exchange rate of 1 florin = 73s; cf. Tables 2.2 and Table 2.3.
165. SMN 4476, f. 63v.
166. Catasto 185.II, ff. 604v–605r.
167. Herlihy, *Medieval and Renaissance Pistoia*, pp. 247–8; Catasto 190, f. 83r; Catasto 185, ff. 612r, 619r.
168. Catasto 185.II, f. 606v; 'spesa di mangiare e bere di 36 boche tra maschi e femine sani che stanno al servigio delli infermi e l'ortolano e dei preti e un cherico e un fattore.' The hospital of S. Bartolomeo al Mugnone instead calculated that its staff consumed 15 florins-worth of food each year: Catasto 194, f. 381r.
169. Catasto 194.II, f. 379v. A *moggio* was equivalent to 8 bushels, while a *cogno* was a measurement in numbers of barrels.

170. BON 291, f. 34r: 'mantenere lecta, chamicie e foderi: 50 fl.'; 185.II, f. 606v: 'vestimenti, chalze, scharpette di 25 persone che stanno al servigio delli infermi tra donne e huomeni fl. 50.' Cf. for S. Eusebio: Catasto 291, f. 23v: 'el vestimento de' lebbrosi.'
171. For example, S. Lorenzo a San Piero Gattolino: 'per buchati ale lenzuola di letta 12' (Catasto 194, f. 656r; also 293, f. 35v).
172. Catasto 190, f. 166r: 'E in detto spedale trenta letta a uso de' poveri e forestieri, coltrici picchole e vecchie copertoi vecchi e rotti e lenzuola rotte e straciate.'
173. Catasto 291, f. 34r.
174. See the unpublished study of Francesca Carrara, 'Ospedale di S. Maria Nuova. Analisi delle fasi di crescita dello Spedale', Table 4.
175. See SMN 10, f. 8r: 'A dì 5 di settembre 1418 si cominciò a cavare et fare i fondamenti per la nuova chiesa di Santo Egidio al tempo di Ser Michele di Fruosino spedalingo di detto spedale'; f. 8v: 'A dì xxvii d'agosto 1422 per detto Ser Michele spedalingo fu cominciato a fare edificare il chiostro primo del detto spedale e il cimitero delle ossa e il granaio al lato al cimiterio detto et il secondo cimiterio et il fondachetto et più altri muramenti di detto spedale, li quali furno per lui successivamente finiti.' See Passerini, *Storia*, p. 357; SMN 10, f. 8v.
176. See expenses recorded in SMN 4479 for 1428–9 and SMN 5817 for 1437–41.
177. S. Matteo (Catasto 185.II, f. 606v): '3 preti stanno continuivi in chasa: 36 flor.; 1 chiericho che serve nella chiesa: 5 flors.'; S. Gallo (Catasto 194.II, f. 379r): '3 preti, due cherici'; Messer Bonifazio (Catasto 291, f. 34r): '2 chappellani e 2 cherici.'
178. S. Eusebio (Catasto 292, f. 235r): 'di spesa ordinaria e obrighi di testamenti, in piatanze e ufici a certe chiese e altre spese l'anno: grano st.158; contanti 140 fl.'
179. Spedale dei Preti: Catasto 185, f. 619r; see also Messer Bonifazio: Catasto 185.II, f. 606v: 'la spesa bisognia in chiesa: cera, olio, ecc., 10 fiorini.'
180. S. Nofri de'tintori (Catasto 185, f. 628r): 'Festa di S. Nofri e'l palio che vi spende £140 e più'; S. Maria dei poveri de' laudesi (Catasto 185, f. 612r): 'Festa di Nostra Donna di Marzo, £4.' See also S. Bartolomeo al Mugnone: 'per fare la festa di Santa Maria della Neve di San Bartolomeo spendono 7 fiorini' (Catasto 194, f. 381r).
181. The records have not been traced in the 1427–8 Catasto records and indeed the absence of its totalled assets in the summaries of their capital for the years 1428 and 1430 suggests a return may not have been submitted (Catasto 195, f. 262r).
182. The texts of the relevant bulls and *provvisioni* are in SP 978, and summarised in SP 616, 'Relazione dell'antico istituto dello Spedale dei Convalescenti' by the eighteenth-century *spedalingo* of the hospital, Giovanbattista Seratti; Passerini, *Storia*, pp. 168–74 relied on both in his discussion of these episodes.
183. These passages are contained in the introduction to S. Paolo's new constitutions of 6.xi.1425: SP 978 (ff. 66r–67r: Latin version; ff. 68r–70v: Italian translation), f. 68r. Quoted by Passerini, *Storia*, pp. 172–3.
184. SP 978, f. 68r.
185. Passerini, *Storia*, p. 171.
186. For a useful discussion of this issue in relation to the status of hospitals as a 'locus pius', especially the Innocenti, see Gavitt, *Charity and Children*, ch. 2.
187. For a full discussion of this subject see Henderson, *Piety and Charity*, ch. 8.
188. Provv. Reg. 87, ff. 295r–296r: 23.x.1398; cf. Passerini, *Storia*, pp. 226–7, and Gavitt, *Charity and Children*, pp. 61, 66. S. Maria Nuova and then the Innocenti followed suit, with their petitions being granted in 1425 and 1430 respectively: Provv. Reg. 115, ff. 143v–144v: 30.viii.1425, and Provv. Reg. 121, ff. 78v–79v: 29.x.1430; cf. Gavitt, *Charity and Children*, pp. 66–7.
189. Passerini, *Storia*, pp. 678–9.
190. Messer Bonifazio: 1377, 1388, 1398: Passerini, *Storia*, 226–7, 221–2, Doct. D: pp. 831–2; S. Maria della Scala: 1388, 1395: Passerini, *Storia*, p. 682; S. Matteo: 1414 and 1449 on the same grounds as S. Maria Nuova, Messer Bonifazio and S. Eusebio (Passerini, *Storia*, p. 152); S. Paolo: Passerini, *Storia*, pp. 169, 171

191. Passerini, *Storia*, p. 682.
192. Gavitt, *Charity and Children*, p. 78.
193. Provv. Reg. 137, ff. 116r–117r: 29.vi.1446: Passerini, *Storia*, p. 139.
194. H.W. van Os, *Vecchietta and the Sacristy of the Siena Hospital Church*, pp. 4–5.
195. During the 1448–9 epidemic it was S. Maria Nuova that housed the *appestati* and the commune granted it 200 gold florins to purchase the chickens to make soup to distribute to the poor in its houses: Provv. Reg. 139, f. 125r: 3.x.1448: A. Corsini, *La Morìa del 1464 in Toscana e l'istituzione dei primi Lazzaretti in Firenze ed in Pisa* (Florence, 1911), pp. 31–3.

Chapter 3

1. Published in Corsini, *La Morìa del 1464 in Toscana*, p. 34.
2. G. Dati, *Istoria di Firenze*, ed. L. Pratesi (Florence, 1904), cited in C. Gilbert, 'The Earliest Guide to Florentine Architecture', *MKIF*, 14 (1969–70), p. 46.
3. U. Middeldorf, 'Dello Delli and *The Man of Sorrows* in the Victoria and Albert Museum', *Burlington Magazine*, 456, Vol. 78 (1941), pp. 77–8; Beck, 'Masaccio's Early Career as a Sculptor' attributes this to Masaccio.
4. Cf. S. Avery-Quash's catalogue entry no. 68 in G. Finaldi, ed., *The Image of Christ. The Catalogue of the Exhibition Seeing Salvation* (London, 2000), pp. 176–7; M. Meiss, *Painting in Florence and Siena after the Black Death* (New York and London, 1973 ed.), pp. 123–4.
5. A. Schiaparelli, *La casa fiorentina e i suoi arredi nei secoli XIV e XV* (Florence, 1908), Vol. 1, pp. 67–72; F.W. Kent, 'The Rucellai Family and its Loggia', *JWCI*, 35 (1972), pp. 397–401; A. Rensi, 'L'Ospedale di San Matteo a Firenze', pp. 105–6; Gavitt, *Charity and Children*, pp. 141–3.
6. Davidsohn, *Storia*, Vol. 3, p. 672, Vol. 7, p. 87 on the Spedale di S. Lorenzo, and Vol. 1, pp. 267–8, 1098–9, and Vol. 7, pp. 89–91 on the Spedale di S. Giovanni Evangelista. See also Stopani, ed., *Firenze e i primi Giubilei*, pp. 9–46. A tenuous case has been made for the appearance of the latter based on a seventeenth-century drawing of a lost fresco in S. Croce, which purports to show its façade. If true, this would be an important record, given that both the hospital and fresco have disappeared; the hospital itself was demolished in 1296 to make way for the extension of the Piazza di S. Giovanni.
7. Most recently on the building of this complex see Saalman, *Filippo Brunelleschi*, pp. 32–81.
8. Goldthwaite and Rearick, 'Michelozzo', p. 242; for new documents belonging to S. Paolo and discovered recently by Richard Goldthwaite see his 'Michelozzo and the Ospedale di San Paolo in Florence: Addendum', *MKHIF*, 44 (2000), pp. 338–9.
9. L. Ciuccetti, 'Un grandioso progetto di Bernardo Buontalenti', in De Benedectis, ed., *Il patrimonio artistico dell'Ospedale Santa Maria Nuova*, pp. 94–100.
10. SM 1.A, ff. 32r–33r: 'Ancora siano tenuti e debbiano i decti Romolo e Sandro ... hedificare, fare e murare in colonne uno portico dinanzi alle porte di sopra detti due spedali nella forma e modo che è facto hedificato e murato in colonne il porticho che è dinanzi alle porte di detti spedali di Messer Bonifazio Lupo in Firenze nella via di S. Gallo col muro dinanzi e parapetto grosso quanto bisogna e alto alla guisa del parapetto del detto portico di Messer Bonifazio': cf. P. Sanpaolesi, 'Alcuni documenti sull'Ospedale di San Matteo in Firenze, *Belle Arti*, 2 (1946–8), p. 80; N. Bemporad and D. Mignani Galli, *L'Ex-ospedale di San Matteo – la loggia. Restauro dell'aula di scenografia nell'Accademia di Belle Arti* (Florence, 1979), pp. 55–8; discussed also by Rensi, 'L'Ospedale di San Matteo', p. 86, and Lucas-Lybor, 'The Spedale di S. Matteo in Florence'.

11. SM 1A, ff. 32r–33r: 'tanto debbiano essere bene e delicatamente intonacati a guisa dello intonico dello Spedale di Messer Bonifazio in Via S. Gallo.'
12. On this hospital see Saalman, *Filippo Brunelleschi*, pp. 34–5.
13. For a discussion of the Innocenti's loggia see Gavitt, *Charity and Children*, pp. 141–3; and Saalman, *Filippo Brunelleschi*, pp. 39–40, 48.
14. Gavitt, *Charity and Children*, pp. 54–5; L.H. Heydenreich, *Architecture in Italy, 1400–1500* (Harmondsworth, 1974, New Haven and London, 1996), pp. 153–4 n. 21.
15. Goldthwaite and Rearick, 'Michelozzo', pp. 279–80.
16. L.B. Alberti, *On the Art of Building in Ten Books*, trans. J. Rykwert, N. Leach and R. Tavernor (Cambridge, Mass., and London, 1988), p. 129.
17. *Antonio Averlino detto il Filarete. Trattato di Architettura*, ed. A.M. Finioli and L. Grassi (Milan, 1972), Vol. 1, p. 139; Welch, *Art and Authority*, p. 153.
18. Cited in Gavitt, *Charity and Children*, p. 142.
19. Van Os, *Vecchietta and the Sacristy*, p. 4; H. Saalman, *The Bigallo: The Oratory and Residence of the Compagnia del Bigallo e della Misericordia in Florence* (New York, 1969), pp. 19–24.
20. L. Cavazzini, 'Dipinti e sculture nelle chiese dell'Ospedale', in L. Sandri, ed., *Gli Innocenti e Firenze nei secoli. Un ospedale, un archivio, una città* (Florence, 1996), pp. 118, 146 n.16.
21. Goldthwaite and Rearick, 'Michelozzo'.
22. F. Gurrieri and A. Amendola, *Il fregio robbiano dell'Ospedale del Ceppo a Pistoia* (Pistoia, 1982). On the history of the hospital see *Contributi per la storia dello Spedale del Ceppo a Pistoia* (Pistoia, 1977).
23. 'Diario fiorentino di Bartolommeo di Michele del Corazza', p. 272.
24. For the latest discussion of Martin V's stay in Florence and for the events surrounding both the consecration of S. Egidio and S. Maria del Carmine see Holmes, *Fra Filippo Lippi*, pp. 42–50.
25. Corrazza, 'Diario fiorentino', pp. 271–2.
26. Ibid., p. 256.
27. Although S. Maria Nuova was the largest hospital complex in Florence, we still only know about its architectural development in general terms, except for building programmes in the early fifteenth and the late sixteenth and seventeenth centuries. The most recent summary of the status quo is the sadly unpublished series of plans of S. Maria Nuova by Francesca Carrara; I am most grateful to her for her generosity in allowing me to consult them. They carefully reconstruct the development of the hospital site north of the piazza century by century from its beginnings until 1870, summarise the present state of our knowledge about the architectural development of S. Maria Nuova in the later Middle Ages and point to the real need for further detailed research to establish each stage of its building history.

    For both the earliest and later periods see G. Pampaloni, ed., *Lo Spedale di S. Maria Nuova e la costruzione del loggiato di Bernardo Buontalenti ora completata dalla Cassa di Risparmio di Firenze* (Florence, 1961); F. Gurrieri, 'L'architettura dello "Spedale di S. Maria Nuova", 1288–1988', in *Lo Spedale di S. Maria Nuova, 1288–1988* (Florence, 1988), pp. 29–46; and in addition on the later period see L. Ciuccetti, 'Profilo architettonico del complesso di S. Maria Nuova', in F. Brasioli and L. Ciuccetti, *S. Maria Nuova. Il tesoro dell'arte nell'antico ospedale fiorentino* (Florence, 1989), pp. 9–17. Most recently De Benedictis, ed., *Il patrimonio artistico*, which contains a series of articles of varying quality, some of which even provide contradictory hypotheses. See L. Ciuccetti, 'Lo Spedale di Santa Maria Nuova e la sua evoluzione attraverso settecento anni di storia', pp. 13–46; 'Lo sviluppo architettonico dello Spedale di Santa Maria Nuova dalla sua fondazione al XV secolo', pp. 47–62; and 'Un grandioso progetto di Bernardo Buontalenti: scoperte, ipotesi e conferme', pp. 79–106. See also Rensi, 'Interventi architettonici del primo Quattrocento', pp. 63–78, and G. Leoncini,

'L'Arcispedale di Santa Maria Nuova e la sua storia architettonica', pp. 107–18. Expenses for 1428–9 are recorded in SMN 4479.
28. SMN, 1376 inventory, pp. 12, 36; SMN (1510–11).
29. SMN 4461 (1409–11); cf. also Ciuccetti, 'Lo sviluppo', pp. 55, 60 n. 42.
30. Ciuccetti, 'Lo sviluppo', p. 55 provides two hypotheses for this building: that it represented either an extension of the height of the eastern section of the ward or the beginnings of the northern section, in line with her overall idea for the development of the hospital. Neither of these seems very likely and the most probable explanation is provided by Giovanni Leoncini, 'L'Arcispedale di Santa Maria Nuova', pp. 111–12, that this merely represented the first phase of the western wing.
31. See discussion in J. Henderson, 'Healing the Body and Healing the Soul: Hospitals in Renaissance Florence', *Renaissance Studies*, 15 (2001), pp. 188–216, and below, Chapter 5.
32. Ciuccetti, 'Un grandioso progetto', pp. 79–105.
33. SMN 5817, cc. 93, 95: 'Spese fatte nel muramento dal lato delle donne infino dell'anno 1437 d'andare a dì xxiv d'ottobre 1441.'
34. SMN (1510–11), p. 186.
35. As noted in 1977 by Goldthwaite and Rearick, 'Michelozzo', pp. 267–77. Neither of the two more recent studies of Messer Bonifazio examines in detail the hospital's architectural development: Zandri, Acidini Luchinat and Francolini, *Lo Spedale di Messer Bonifazio*, and E. Lombardi, *Messer Bonifazio Lupi*. The only guide is Paatz, *Die Kirchen*, Vol. 1, pp. 395–405, which summarises the information contained in earlier histories by such as Del Migliore, Richa and Passerini.
36. On the changes from the sixteenth to the late eighteenth centuries see Rensi, 'L'Ospedale di San Matteo a Firenze', pp. 83–145, 94–7; Bemporad and Mignani Galli, *Ex-Ospedale di S. Matteo*; Paatz, *Die Kirchen*, Vol. 1, pp. 395–405.
37. SM123, ff. 5r–6v; SM 123, ff. 7r–v; as in Rensi, 'L'Ospedale di San Matteo a Firenze', pp. 122–5, 128–33, and Lucas-Lybor, 'The Spedale di San Matteo', pp. 17–22. For the inventories of S. Matteo see SM 108, ff. 1r–114r; 328, ff. 302v–305r (1454); 196, ff. 136v–138r (1508 with addition in 1528).
38. Rensi, 'L'Ospedale di San Matteo a Firenze', p. 140.
39. See Davidsohn, *Storia*, Vol. 7, pp. 79–80.
40. Discussed by Rensi, 'L'Ospedale di San Matteo'.
41. Much less is known about the internal disposition of Messer Bonifazio than that of S. Matteo, partly reflecting the fact that virtually nothing survives of the physical structure. Cf. for S. Paolo the exemplary 1977 study of Goldthwaite and Rearick, 'Michelozzo', which combines the skills of an archivally based economic historian with those of an architectural historian.
42. The contemporary views normally cited are Pietro del Massaio's map of Florence of 1472 and the three manuscript copies of Ptolemy's 'Geography' which shows the top of these three buildings (see Plate 1.1: bottom right-hand corner). Goldthwaite and Rearick, 'Michelozzo', pp. 230–3 consider these views in relation to S. Paolo.
43. This is not made clear by Goldthwaite and Rearick, 'Michelozzo'.
44. B. Geremek, 'Il pauperismo nell'età preindustriale (secc. XIV–XVIII)', in *Storia d'Italia*, Vol. 5: *I documenti* (Turin, 1973), pp. 678–84, esp. pp. 683–4.
45. C. Landino, *Scritti critici e teorici*, ed. R. Cardini (Rome, 1974), Vol. 1, p. 116.
46. R. Friedenthal, *Luther: His Life and Times* (London, 1970), p. 78.
47. See below, Chapter 8; Landino mentions that 'molti uomini esterni, e nobili et ricchissimi, oppressi in viaggio da alcuna malatia, hanno eletto tale domicilio alla sua cura' (*Scritti critici*, Vol. 1, p. 116).
48. Park and Henderson, ' "The First Hospital among Christians" ', p. 76.
49. Varchi, *Storia fiorentina*, Vol. 2, IX, pp. 101–2.
50. Alberti, *L'Architettura*, Vol. 1, pp. 366–8.

51. Cf. Albini, *Città e ospedali*.
52. See Welch, *Art and Authority*, ch. 6.
53. B. Pullan, 'Support and Redeem: Charity and Poor Relief in Italian Cities from the Fourteenth to the Seventeenth Century', *Continuity and Change*, 3:2 (1988), pp. 190–3; Albini, *Città e ospedali*, ch. 5.
54. Three were probably founded earlier in the century since their existence is first recorded in the Decima tax of 1495 (see Appendix I).
55. The tax returns for hospitals in Florence can be found in Catasto 185.I–II, 190, 194.II, 195, 291, 292, 293; Decima della Repubblica 66–70; the 1527 census is in BNCF, NA 987.
56. O. Fantozzi Micali and P. Roselli, *Le soppressioni dei conventi a Firenze. Riuso e trasformazioni dal sec. XVIII in poi* (Florence, 1980), pp. 12–21.
57. See Henderson, *Piety and Charity*, ch. 10.
58. Passerini, *Storia*, pp. 148–9, 106–7.
59. See Goldthwaite, *The Building of Renaissance Florence*, pp. 317–50, esp. pp. 318–19.
60. For a discussion of standards of living and population levels see Herlihy and Klapisch-Zuber, *Tuscans and their Families*, pp. 73–8.
61. Gavitt, *Charity and Children*, p. 209: Table 6; P. Gavitt, ' "Perché non avea chi la governasse" ', in J. Henderson and R. Wall, eds, *Poor Women and Children in the European Past* (London, 1994), p. 66: Table 3.1; cf. Passerini, *Storia*, p. 704.
62. G.C. Romby, 'Le vicende architettoniche nei secoli', in Sandri, ed., *Gli Innocenti e Firenze*, p. 25.
63. S. Matteo, for example, was granted the same privileges in 1449 as S. Maria Nuova over inheritance: Passerini, *Storia*, pp. 152–3.
64. For example, in 1413 S. Matteo was given the same tax privileges as S. Maria Nuova, S. Eusebio and Messer Bonifazio; in 1450 it obtained the same rights as S. Maria Nuova over inheritance; and from 1480 the commune granted it 6 bushels of salt every six months. Passerini, *Storia*, p. 152; SM 189, f. 104v. For privileges relating to Messer Bonifazio see Passerini, *Storia*, pp. 226–8.
65. Passerini, *Storia*, pp. 333–4; cf. Gavitt, *Charity and Children*, pp. 95–6.
66. Ibid.
67. Varchi, *Storia fiorentina*, Vol. 2, IX, pp. 101–2.
68. Passerini, *Storia*, pp. 333–4: 27.ii.1445.
69. Passerini, *Storia*, p. 669, citing a law of 23.iii.1448/9.
70. Passerini, *Storia*, pp. 699, 704; Gavitt, *Charity and Children*, pp. 86–7.
71. Passerini, *Storia*, pp. 295–301 discusses the role of S. Maria Nuova and the lazzaretto during plagues from 1448 to 1531. Cf. also Corsini, *La Morìa*. On 1448 see Provv. Reg. 139, f. 125r: 3.x.1448, as in Corsini, *La Morìa*, pp. 31–3.
72. Provv. Reg. 157, f. 58r: 12.vi.1464; Passerini, *Storia*, pp. 297–8; Corsini, *La Morìa*, pp. 33–40.
73. Provv. Reg. 155, f. 58r; Corsini, *La Morìa*, p. 34: 12.vi.1464.
74. Provv. Reg. 158, ff. 212r–v: 15.ii.1468; cf. Passerini, *Storia*, pp. 156–7.
75. Provv. Reg. 155, f. 58r: 12.vi.1464; cf. Corsini, *La Morìa*, p. 34.
76. R.J. Palmer. 'L'azione della Repubblica di Venezia nel controllo della peste. Lo sviluppo della politica governativa', in Comune di Venezia, *Venezia e la peste, 1348–1797* (Venice, 1979), p. 104.
77. Provv. Reg. 157, f. 58r: Corsini, *La Morìa*, p. 36.
78. Provv. Reg. 157, f. 58r: Corsini, *La Morìa*, pp. 34–5.
79. Provv. Reg. 157, f. 58r: Corsini, *La Morìa*, p. 37.
80. Provv. Reg. 163, f. 126v: Corsini, *La Morìa*, p. 42; SMN 4512: 1472–4; Provv. Reg. 167, f. 75v: 21.viii.1476.
81. Provv. Reg. 170, f. 16r: Corsini, *La Morìa*, p. 49.
82. Carrara, Sebregondi and Tramonti, *Gli Istituti di beneficenza a Firenze*, pp. 72–3.

83. Provv. Reg. 170, f. 32r: 9.vi.1479.
84. MAP XXXVII.457: 5.vi.1479: Passerini, *Storia*, pp. 336–8.
85. Provv. Reg. 170, f. 32r: 9.vi.1479.
86. MAP XXXVII.457: 17.vi.1479.
87. MAP XXXVII.488: 5.vii.1479: Passerini, *Storia*, pp. 338–9. There is no evidence in the hospital's 'Ricordanze' of 1469–1507 of extra payments for plague in 1479 (AOIF, ser. III, no. 17), either because the funds were paid directly by S. Maria Nuova or because these expenses were recorded in another set of account books.
88. MAP XXXVII.594: 30.vii.1479: cf. Passerini, *Storia*, p. 300.
89. Passerini, *Storia*, p. 337 n. 1.
90. Cf. also the 1478 Catasto return of the Monache del Monastero di S. Jacopo di Ripoli dentro alle mura di Firenze: Catasto 989, f. 377v: 'Preghiamo le vostre charità Signori Ufficiali che noi vi siamo racomandate perchè noi siamo qua giù abandonate da ogni persona per rispecto della guerra e della morìa. Noi no[n] guadagnamo più niente perché le botteghe non ce ne vogliono dare per rispetto di questa morìa che abbiamo all'uscio cioè la Schala. Non ci parrebe faticha pagare se noi guadagnassimo saracci forza d'andare achattare ellimosinare. Fateci meno male che voi potrete.' (I am grateful to Kate Lowe for this reference.)
91. Cf. N. Rubinstein, *The Government of Florence under the Medici, 1434–1492* (Oxford, 1966), Part II.
92. Albini, *Guerra, fame, peste*, p. 81.
93. Provv. Reg. 170, f. 82v: 21.xii.1479: Corsini, *La Morìa*, pp. 50–1.
94. For a brief summary of these problems see Henderson, *Piety and Charity*, ch. 10.
95. Otto di Guardia e Balìa 102, c. 236; M.S. Mazzi, 'La peste a Firenze nel Quattrocento', in R. Comba, G. Piccinni and G. Pinto, eds, *Strutture familiari, epidemie, migrazioni nell'Italia medievale* (Naples, 1984), p. 111 n. 76.
96. J. Nardi, *Istorie della città di Firenze*, ed. L. Arbib (Florence, 1842), Vol. 1, p. 115.
97. L. Landucci, *Diario fiorentino dal 1450 al 1516, continuato da un anonimo fino al 1542* (Florence, 1883; repr. 1985), p. 150.
98. Ibid., pp. 150, 152.
99. For S. Maria Nuova in 1497 see SMN 5875, c. 122: payments to Bartolomeo di Gherardo 'chi governa e morbati'; for S. Matteo see SM 193, ff. 51r, 74r. Cf. also A.G. Carmichael, *Plague and the Poor* (Cambridge, 1986), pp. 102–7, on the 1490s and the lazzaretto in Florence.
100. See J. Henderson, 'Epidemie nella Firenze del Rinascimento: teoria sanitaria e provvedimenti governativi', in A. Pastore and P. Sorcinelli, eds, *Sanità e Società. Emilia Romagna, Toscana, Marche, Umbria, Lazio, secoli XVI–XX* (Udine, 1987), pp. 49–60.
101. Landucci, *Diario*, p. 141, under 5.xii.1496.
102. Cf. A. Malamani, 'Notizie sul Mal Francese e gli spedali degli incurabili in età moderna', *Critica storica*, 15 (1978), pp. 193–216; A. Foa, 'Il nuovo e il vecchio: l'insorgere della sifilide (1494–1530)', *Quaderni storici*, 19 (1984), pp. 11–34; Arrizabalaga, Henderson and French, *The Great Pox*, ch. 2.
103. On S. Giacomo in Augusta in Rome see A. Cavaterra, 'L'Ospedalità a Roma nell'età moderna. Il caso di San Giacomo (1585–1605)', *Sanità, scienza e storia*, 2 (1986), pp. 87–123; Henderson in Arrizabalaga, Henderson and French, *The Great Pox*, ch. 8; Henderson, 'The Mal Francese in Sixteenth-Century Rome: The Ospedale di San Giacomo in Augusta and the "Incurabili" ', in E. Sonnino, ed., *La popolazione di Roma dal medioevo all' età contemporanea. Fonti, problemi di ricerca, risultati* (Rome, 1999), pp. 483–523.
104. For descriptions of these events see Richa, *Notizie istoriche delle chiese fiorentine*, Vol. 8, pp. 317–27, and Passerini, *Storia*, pp. 203–16.
105. An extract of Giulio's bull of 25.iii.1521 appears in Richa, *Notizie*, Vol. 8, p. 319.

106. Arrizabalaga, Henderson and French, *The Great Pox*, pp. 158–9.
107. *Salvatoris Nostri Domini Jesu Christi*, 15 Aug. 1515, in A.M. Cherubino, ed., *Bullarium Romanum a B. Leone Magno usque ad S.D.N. Clementem X* (Lyon, 1892), Vol. 1, pp. 567–71, esp. p. 567; Ospedale di S. Trinita detta degli Incurabili 102, cc. 13–14.
108. Passerini, *Storia*, pp. 648–50, 106–7.
109. L. Polizzotto, *The Elect Nation. The Savonarolan Movement in Florence, 1494–1545* (Oxford, 1994), pp. 397, 409.
110. Passerini, *Storia*, pp. 208–11; Paatz, *Die Kirchen*, Vol. 5, p. 394. For Rome see Arrizabalaga, Henderson and French, *The Great Pox*, ch. 8.
111. Ospedale degli Incurabili 102, cc.1, 9, 17.
112. Ibid., c. cxvii.
113. Ibid., c. 14; Richa, *Notizie*, Vol. 8, pp. 322–5.
114. Senato dei Quarantotto 1, c. 91; A. D'Addario, *Aspetti della Controriforma a Firenze* (Rome, 1972), pp. 80, 461.
115. The legacies to the hospital are listed in Incurabili 9; Passerini, *Storia*, p. 211; Paatz, *Die Kirchen*, Vol. 5, p. 394.
116. Incurabili I, ff. 5r–v.
117. Incurabili I, ff. 5r–v.
118. Alberti, *L'Architettura*, Vol. 1, pp. 367–8.
119. See Albini, *Città e ospedali*.
120. See C.M. Cipolla, *Public Health and the Medical Profession in the Renaissance* (Cambridge, 1976).
121. On this see Henderson, 'Epidemie nella Firenze del Rinascimento'. In 1522–3, S. Maria Nuova was involved in some expenses for plague victims 'spese per gli amorbati', which involved providing 'granate per le case': see SMN 5093.
122. Cf. B. Pullan, 'The Famine of Venice and the New Poor Law, 1527–1529', *Bollettino dell'Istituto di Storia della Società e dello Stato Veneziano*, 5–6 (1963–4), pp. 141–202.
123. Signori e Collegi, Deliberazioni, ordinaria autorità 131, f. 36r: 28.iii.1529: 'attesa la multiplicatione de'poveri rispecto alla insolita penuria e carestia la quale … va crescendo in modo è cosa miserabile e crudele a vedere e udire tutto di querele e voce di quelli nella città che periscono di fame.'
124. Ibid., f. 36v: 'Et perchè molti di decti poveri sono e truovonsi malati per le vie per la debolezza della fame [i Commissionari per li Poveri] di potere mandare decti poveri così malati alli spedali di S. Maria Nuova, Lelmo, San Pagolo et Bonifazio di Firenze … e prefati excellentissimi Signiori comandono alli spedalinghi di decti spedali … ricevere e acceptare [tali poveri infermi] in decti loro spedali come gli altri poveri infermi sotto pena della loro indigniatione.'
125. R. A. Goldthwaite, 'I prezzi del grano a Firenze dal XIV al XVI secolo', *Quaderni storici*, 28 (1975), p. 36.
126. Gavitt, *Charity and Children*, pp. 298ff., and ' "Perché non avea chi la governasse" ', pp. 84–5.
127. Cf. Varchi, *Storia fiorentina*, Vol. 2, IX, p. 137; C. Roth, *The Last Florentine Republic* (London, 1925), pp. 197, 269–70. Another example is the Misericordia: F. Niccolai, ed., *La Misericordia di Firenze: memorie, curiosità, tradizioni* (Florence, 1984), p. 76.
128. Roth, *The Last Florentine Republic*, pp. 190–1.
129. Varchi, *Storia fiorentina*, Vol. 3, XIII, pp. 30–1. Cf. Magistrato Supremo 1, f. 52v.
130. Recorded in SMN 4, ff. 73v–74r: 21.iii.1533; Senato dei Quarantotto 48, ff. 56v–57v: 31.iii.1533 provided additional privileges to help its finances. Cf. Passerini, *Storia*, pp. 340–2, and D'Addario, *Aspetti*, pp. 81–2.
131. SMN 4, ff. 73v: 21.iii.1533.
132. SMN 4, f. 73v. Cf. Varchi, *Storia fiorentina*, Vol. 3, III, p. 31; Passerini, *Storia*, pp. 335–6, 340–1; cf. also Hatfield, *The Wealth of Michelangelo*.
133. Magistrato Supremo 1, ff. 29v–30r; Senato dei Quarantotto 1, ff. 56v–57r (also in SMN 4, ff. 74v–75r).

134. SMN 4, ff. 73r–74r: 21.iii.1533; ff. 75v–76r: 5.iv.1533.
135. Ibid., ff. 76v–77r.
136. D'Addario, *Aspetti*, p. 78.
137. Passerini, *Storia*, pp. 308–10; D'Addario, *Aspetti*, pp. 77–8. Cf. also SMN 10, ff. 29v–30r.
138. See Passerini, *Storia*, pp. 306–10; D'Addario, *Aspetti*, pp. 77–8.
139. SMN 10, ff. 29v–31v, discussed by Passerini, *Storia*, pp. 306–10, and D'Addario, *Aspetti*, pp. 77–8.
140. Passerini, *Storia*, pp. 810–12; D'Addario, *Aspetti*, pp. 89–90; D. Lombardi, *Povertà maschile, povertà femminile*, p. 71.
141. Passerini, *Storia*, pp. 689–91; D'Addario, *Aspetti*, p. 78.
142. Passerini, *Storia*, p. 177.
143. On S. Paolo see Passerini, *Storia*, pp. 176–9; D'Addario, *Aspetti*, pp. 76–7; cf. also SP 912 on the reforms of the hospital in 1571.
144. C. Bresnahan Menning, *The Monte di Pietà of Florence. Charity and the State in Late Renaissance Italy* (Ithaca and London, 1993), p. 187.
145. Ibid., p. 186.
146. SMN 10, ff. 29r–v.
147. SP 640, 889, 893.
148. SP 912, f. 18r: ch. XLVII: 'Essendo stata la principale intentione di chi fondò questo luogo pio che effettualmente ci si exerciti, et principalmente la carità inverso li poveri infermi.'
149. D'Addario, *Aspetti*, p. 75; cf. ASF, 'Uffici e Stato della città di Firenze': Archivio Mediceo del Principato 663, as in A. D'Addario, 'Burocrazia, economia e finanze dello Stato Fiorentino alla metà del Cinquecento', *ASI*, 121 (1963), pp. 385–456; '1561. Magistrati e ufizi della città di Firenze': Archivio della Guardaroba 50; App., n. 35.
150. Bresnahan Menning, *The Monte di Pietà*, ch. 6.
151. The text of the law is in Bigallo 1669.2, ff. 3r–6v. See also F. Diaz, *Il Granducato di Toscana. I Medici* (Turin, 1976), ch. 2; A. D'Addario, 'Testimonianze archivistiche, cronistiche e bibliografiche', in *La comunità cristiana fiorentina e toscana nella dialettica religiosa del Cinquecento* (Florence, 1980), pp. 165–6.
152. Senato dei Quarantotto 5, ff.13v–15v: 19.iii.1542. Cf. Passerini, *Storia*, pp. 27–31, 799–800, and D'Addario, *Aspetti*, pp. 464–9, which discusses and publishes the final version of the document, dated 17.xi.1542.
153. G. Parenti, *Prezzi e mercato del grano a Siena (1546–1765)* (Florence, 1942), pp. 76–7; B. Licata, 'Il problema del grano e delle carestie', in G. Spini, ed., *Architettura e politica da Cosimo I a Ferdinando I* (Florence, 1976), p. 336.
154. Senato dei Quarantotto 5, ff. 13v–15v: 19.iii.1542. Cf. Passerini, *Storia*, pp. 27–31, 799–800; D'Addario, *Aspetti*, pp. 464–9. Confirmed by Pope Paul III: Diplomatico del Bigallo: under 4.vii.1543: Passerini, *Storia*, pp. 802–5.
155. The text of the Senate's deliberation is in Senato dei Quarantotto 5, ff. 13v–15r: 17.xi.1542 and published by Passerini, *Storia*, pp. 807–9 and, with corrections, by D'Addario, *Aspetti*, pp. 465–7.
156. D'Addario, *Aspetti*, pp. 465–7.
157. Bigallo 1360; cf. N. Terpstra, 'Competing Visions of the State and Social Welfare: The Medici Dukes, the Bigallo Magistrates and Local Hospitals in Sixteenth-Century Tuscany', *Renaissance Quarterly*, 54 (2001), pp. 1319–55.
158. Cf. Terpstra, 'Competing Visions'; D. Lombardi, 'Poveri a Firenze. Programmi e realizzazioni della politica assistenziale dei Medici tra cinque e seicento', in G. Politi, M. Rosa and F. Della Peruta, eds, *Timore e carità. I poveri nell'Italia moderna* (Cremona, 1982), p. 166 and n. 4; D'Addario, *Aspetti*, p. 92.
159. Senato dei Quarantotto 5, f. 13v; D'Addario, *Aspetti*, p. 465.
160. D'Addario, *Aspetti*, pp. 88–9; Lombardi, 'Poveri a Firenze', pp. 166–7.

161. Passerini, *Storia*, p. 31.
162. Ibid., pp. 802–5, and discussed on pp. 28–31. The two briefs of 1542 and the papal Bull of 1543 are in Bigallo 1669.4, ff. 6r–10v, 14r–16r.
163. Bigallo 1669.2, ff. 9r–25r, quoted by D. Lombardi, 'Poveri a Firenze', pp. 167–8.
164. The Monastero di S. Maria e S. Niccolò was founded by Francesco di Giovanni Rosati.
165. D'Addario, *Aspetti*, p. 51.
166. D. Lombardi, 'Poveri a Firenze', pp. 167–8, 172; SMN, Monastero di Santa Caterina 7, f. 2r lists their names.
167. Monastero di S. Maria e S. Niccolò del Ceppo 1 bis, f. 1r; SMN, Monastero di S. Caterina 7, f. 1r.
168. Diaz, *Il Granducato*, p. 134; Licata, 'Il problema del grano', pp. 333–71.
169. Monastero di S. Maria e S. Niccolò del Ceppo, 1 bis, f. 12r. See also D'Addario, *Aspetti*, pp. 51–4; D. Lombardi, 'Poveri a Firenze', pp. 166–8.
170. Monastero di S. Maria e S. Niccolò del Ceppo, 1 bis, ff. 14r ff: chs vii–ix.
171. See S. Cohen, *The Evolution of Women's Asylums since 1500. From Refuges for Ex-Prostitutes to Shelters for Battered Women* (New York and Oxford, 1992).
172. The statutes as reflected in Cardinal Pucci's brief: Passerini, *Storia*, pp. 29–30, 802–5, on which the following discussion is based. In general on the problem of beggars see D. Lombardi, '"L'ondata di pauperismo", *Il XVII secolo: la dinamica di una crisi*', in R. Romano, ed., *Storia d'Italia* (Milan, 1989), pp. 169–92.
173. Passerini, *Storia*, pp. 803–4.
174. For the Spedale dei Mendicanti in Florence see D. Lombardi, *Povertà maschile, povertà femminile*.
175. See Henderson, *Piety and Charity*, pp. 244, 403–4.
176. Alberti, *L'Architettura*, Vol. 1, 367.
177. See Pullan, 'Support and Redeem', pp. 190–3; Pastore, 'Strutture assistenziali fra Chiesa e Stato nell'Italia della Controriforma', pp. 435–8.
178. On this period see H.C. Butters, *Governors and Government in Early Sixteenth-Century Florence, 1502–1519* (Oxford, 1985); J.N. Stephens, *The Fall of the Florentine Republic, 1512–1530* (Oxford, 1983).
179. Incurabili I, ff. 14r–v.
180. For Florence see Cohen, *The Evolution of Women's Asylums since 1500*.

Chapter 4

1. R. Arbesmann, 'The Concept of "Christus Medicus" in St. Augustine', *Traditio*, 10 (1954), pp. 19–20, 26.
2. Ibid., p. 20. Cf. the discussion of this theme by C. Rawcliffe, 'Medicine for the Soul: The Medieval English Hospital and the Quest for Spiritual Health', in J. Hinnells and R. Porter, eds, *Religion, Health and Suffering* (London, 1999), pp. 321–3.
3. J. Pope-Hennessey, *Catalogue of Italian Sculpture in the Victoria and Albert Museum* (London, 1964), Vol. 1, pp. 64–5; Avery-Quash's catalogue entry no. 68 in Finaldi, *The Image of Christ*, pp. 176–7 convincingly throws doubt on this attribution.
4. Pope-Hennessey, *Catalogue of Italian Sculpture*, Vol. 1, pp. 64–5.
5. Cf. Avery-Quash in Finaldi, *The Image of Christ*, p. 176; Meiss, *Painting in Florence and Siena*, pp. 123–4.
6. In general see Hayum, *The Isenheim Altarpiece*, Plate 7: the *Crucifixion*.
7. Domenico Cavalca, *Lo specchio della croce*, ed. Tito Sante Centi (Bologna, 1992), pp. 288–97. For the secondary title see BNCF, Conventi Soppressi G2, a manuscript of 1410 which came from S. Maria degli Angeli, the convent contiguous with S. Maria Nuova. Cf. also Rawcliffe, 'Medicine for the Soul', pp. 316–38, esp. pp. 320–4; *Medicine for the Soul*, pp. 103–5.

8. Cf. Rawcliffe, 'Medicine for the Soul', pp. 123–4; M. Warner, *Alone of All her Sex. The Myth and Cult of the Virgin Mary* (London, 1978), pp. 192–205. Mary's healing powers continued to be transmitted for centuries after her death through contact with her surviving possessions and the miraculous appearance of her milk.
9. Cf. the discussion of the theme of the *Coronation of the Virgin* in relation to Fra Filippo Lippi's picture of the same subject in E. Borsook, 'Cults and Imagery at Sant'Ambrogio in Florence', *MKIF*, 25 (1981), pp. 167–70.
10. As also noted by C. Seymour Jr, *Sculpture in Italy: 1400–1500* (Harmondsworth, 1966), p. 120. The payments to Bicci di Lorenzo are recorded in SMN 4474, f. 99r, though the colour of the paint was not specified. See Beck, 'Masaccio's Early Career as a Sculptor', p. 180.
11. Beck, 'Masaccio's Early Career as a Sculptor', p. 190.
12. Cf. Paatz, *Die Kirchen*, Vol. 4, p. 13.
13. See M. Holmes, 'Giovanni Benci's Patronage of the Nunnery Le Murate', in P. Rubin and G. Ciappelli, eds, *Family, Memory and Art* (Cambridge, 1999), p. 117.
14. De Roover, *The Rise and Decline of the Medici Bank*, p. 233.
15. F. Ames-Lewis, 'Domenico Veneziano and the Medici', *Jahrbuch der Berliner Museen*, 21 (1979), pp. 68–9.
16. D. Kent, *Cosimo de' Medici and the Florentine Renaissance* (New Haven and London, 2000), pp. 107, 337–8, 356–7.
17. De Roover, *The Rise and Decline*, p. 233.
18. On S. Paolo see Goldthwaite and Rearick, 'Michelozzo'; for S. Matteo: Rensi, 'L'Ospedale di San Matteo'; Lucas-Lybor, 'The Spedale di S. Matteo'. For a more detailed study of the artistic commissions of a hospital church see Cavazzini, 'Dipinti e sculture nella chiesa dell'Ospedale'.
19. These measurements have been derived from those in the 1780 plans.
20. See Goldthwaite and Rearick, 'Michelozzo', pp. 264–7.
21. SMN 24: dated 1780, according to Rensi, 'L'Ospedale di S. Matteo', p. 94.
22. SMN 1, ff. 2v–5r: SMN, 1376 inventory, pp. 7–12. In common with most inventories, only movable objects and permanent decorative features were included.
23. SMN (1374), p. 73.
24. SMN 4392, f. 2v: 28.vi.1335: 'in pesce e in ciriege per la vigilia di S. Piero: 21s'; f. 26v: 30.viii.1336: 'in polli per la festa di S. Gilio: £4.17s.10d'; SMN 4400, f. 17r: 'Anche paghamo la Vigilia d'Ognisanti per vii libre di pescie, 14s'; f. 18v: 'Anche paggamo adì 18 di novembre per la festa di S. Lisabeta per carne di vitella e di bue, 10s'; cf. also SMN 4424, f. 16r: 'Paghamo detto dì [8.v.1369] a più preti che ci furono a dire messa per la festa di Sa' Michele per l'amore di dio £1.5s.'
25. SMN 1, ff. 2v, 3v: SMN 1376 inventory, pp. 7, 9.
26. One of these missals may have been commissioned in 1351; it was illuminated by 'Paulo da Santa Maria Novella': SMN 4398, f. 36v: 25.ii.1351.
27. L.B. Kanter et al., *Painting and Illumination in Early Renaissance Florence, 1300–1450* (New York, 1994), pp. 287–93; M. Levi-D'Ancona, *Miniatura e miniatori a Firenze dal XIV al XVI secolo: Documenti per la storia della miniatura* (Florence, 1962), p. 451.
28. SMN, 1376 inventory, pp. 11–12. Another image that may very well have come from S. Maria Nuova is the *Madonna Lactans* attributed to Lorenzo di Niccolò Gerini which contains the Portinari coat of arms. Until it was stolen in 1987, this picture was in the church of S. Maria delle Grazie near Stia of which the hospital was the principal patron. See M. Holmes, 'Disrobing the Virgin. The *Madonna Lactans* in Fifteenth-Century Florentine Art', in G. Johnson and S. Matthews Grieco, eds, *Picturing Women in Renaissance and Baroque Italy* (Cambridge, 1997), pp. 192, 289 n. 67.
29. SMN 1, ff. 2v, 5v: SMN, 1376 inventory, pp. 7, 12.
30. Jacobus de Voragine, *The Golden Legend. Readings on the Saints*, trans. W. Granger Ryan (Princeton, 1993), Vol. 1, pp. 101–4; see also *Butler's Lives of the Saints*, ed. H. Thurston and D. Attwater (London, 1956), Vol. 1, pp. 133–4.

31. Bargello A67; see SMN 5817 (under 2.vii.1474); Levi-D'Ancona, *Miniatura*, p. 451.
32. On representations of this scene see M. Rubin, *Corpus Christi: The Eucharist in Late Medieval Culture* (Cambridge, 1991), pp. 131–4.
33. Vasari-Milanesi, Vol. 1, pp. 674–5, Vol. 1, p. 655; Richa, *Notizie*, Vol. 8, p. 191. Paatz, *Die Kirchen*, Vol. 4, p. 23 is based on these passages by Vasari and Richa. Cf. also M.A. Jack Ward, 'The Accademia del Disegno in 16th-Century Florence. A Study of an Artists' Institution' (unpublished Ph.D. thesis, University of Chicago, 1972), pp. 6–16.
34. As pointed out recently by Anna Padoa Rizzo, 'Luca della Robbia e Verrocchio. Un nuovo documento e una nuova interpretazione iconografica del tabernacolo di Peretola', *MKIF*, 38 (1994), p. 49. The statutes of the company are in ASF, Accademia del Disegno 1; see f. 1r for the reference to their meeting place: Z. Wazbinski, *L'Accademia medicea del Disegno a Firenze nel cinquecento: idea e istituzione* (Florence, 1987), Vol. 2, p. 419. The choir of S. Egidio was referred to as the 'Cappella Maggiore della chiesa di Sancto Gidio di questo spedale' or the 'Cappella dell'altare magiore': SMN 5059, cc. 134, 185; SMN 5060, f. 94v; SMN 5817, ff. 35v, 58v; 5818, f. 53v.
35. J. Gardner, 'Altars, Altarpieces, and Art History: Legislation and Usage', in E. Borsook and F. Superbi Gioffredi, eds, *Italian Altarpieces, 1250–1550. Function and Design* (Oxford, 1994), pp. 5–40, esp. pp. 10–11.
36. SMN, 1376 inventory, p. 7; SMN 4426, f. 256r: 'A Francescho dì Vanni orafo dì decto [30.x.1374] per chompimento di paghamento d'uno tabernachollo d'ariento che fece per le reliquie di Sancto Egidio ... 35 fiorini d'oro, lire 28.9s.0d.'
37. C. Rawcliffe, *The Hospitals of Medieval Norwich* (Norwich, 1995), pp. 95–6.
38. See Jacobus de Voragine, *The Golden Legend*, Vol. 2, pp. 147–9.
39. Van Os, *Vecchietta and the Sacristy*, pp. 4–16; Gallavotti Cavallero, *Lo Spedale di Santa Maria della Scala in Siena*, pp. 80–107, esp. p. 80.
40. On which see Van Os, *Vecchietta and the Sacristy*.
41. Paatz, *Die Kirchen*, Vol. 4, pp. 5, 10–11, 23–25.
42. Ibid., pp. 10–11; H. Wohl, *The Paintings of Domenico Veneziano, ca. 1410–1461. A Study of Florentine Art of the Early Renaissance* (Oxford, 1980), p. 200.
43. Bargello A67; see SMN 5817 (under 2.vii.1474); Levi-D'Ancona, *Miniatura*, p. 451.
44. Monte's dates were 1448–1529 and his brother, c.1444–97: J.J.G. Alexander, ed., *The Painted Page. Italian Renaissance Book Illumination, 1450–1550* (London and Munich, 1994), p. 70.
45. R.W. Muncey, *A History of the Consecration of Churches and Churchyards* (Cambridge, 1930), ch. 7: pp. 67–76.
46. 'Diario fiorentino di Bartolommeo di Michele del Corazza', pp. 270–1.
47. Vasari-Milanesi, Vol. 2, p. 66 n. 5; Middeldorf, 'Dello Delli and *The Man of Sorrows*', p. 77. Payment for the painting and gilding is recorded in SMN 4474, f. 99r; Beck, 'Masaccio's Early Career', p. 180. Vasari notes that this commission took place after the ceremony, but the terracotta statues may have been designed for the consecration.
48. 'Diario fiorentino di Bartolommeo di Michele del Corazza', pp. 270–1.
49. On consecration crosses see Muncey, *A History of the Consecration*, pp. 44–7.
50. SMN 4471, f.126v: 'da fare la grillanda alla chiesa d'alloro ... e di poi per dipignere l'arme de' padroni e per dipigniere le viti e per oro per le viti e per le manifattura delle viti.'
51. See Wohl, *Paintings of Domenico Veneziano*, pp. 206–7; cf. F. Brasioli, 'Una Collezione da Riscoprire e Rivalutare', in F. Brasioli and L. Ciuccetti, *Santa Maria Nuova. Il tesoro dell'arte nell'antico ospedale fiorentino* (Florence, 1989), p. 21, which gives instead a possible attribution to Andrea del Castagno.
52. Cf. also Kanter et al, *Painting and Illumination*, p. 306 n. 3. See M. Eisenberg, *Lorenzo Monaco* (Princeton, 1989), pp. 118–20, 214–15.
53. SMN 5049, ff. 11r, 217r; SMN 5050, ff. 3r, 53r, 120v, 170r, 218v, published in

Eisenberg, *Lorenzo Monaco*, pp. 214–15, docts 16A to 16G. There remains some doubt whether this was intended for the church's main altar since it is argued that 182 gold florins was too high a price for a single altarpiece, given that an average in this period was about 40 to 70 gold florins. Cf. also Kanter et al., *Painting and Illumination*, p. 306 n. 3.

54. See Paatz, *Die Kirchen*, Vol. 4, p. 49 n. 92; J. Pope-Hennessey, *Fra Angelico* (London, 1974), pp. 18, 195 gives c.1435; S. Orlandi, *Fra Angelico* (Florence, 1964), pp. 30–1 gives 1441–3; see also J.T. Spike, *Fra Angelico* (New York and London, 1997), pp. 235–6, cat. nos 79 A–C.

55. The provenance has been based on the prominence of St Giles in the picture and remarks by two near-contemporaries, Antonio Billi and Antonio Manetti, that the altarpiece was in S. Egidio: *Il libro di Antonio Billi*, ed. F. Benedettucci (Rome, 1991), p. 77; P. Murray, 'Art Historians and Art Critics:4.14: Uomini Singhulari in Firenze', *Burlington Magazine*, no. 655, vol. 99 (1957), p. 335.

56. Pope Hennessey, *Fra Angelico*, p. 195 bases his statement (that it was 'Painted for the nuns' choir in S. Egidio') on Vasari-Milanesi, Vol. 2, p. 516 (cf. Paatz, *Die Kirchen*, Vol. 4, p. 49n). Historians have rarely stopped to consider the implications of this idea for the appearance of the church and the spatial and liturgical relationship between the different elements in the decorative programme, whether sculpture, panel painting or fresco, nor has anybody thought of examining its size, type or placement. An even more fundamental question is exactly when the choir-screen or Tramezzo was built. It has been assumed that it was constructed some time between the enlargement of the Cappella Maggiore and the date of the commissioning of Fra Angelico's *Coronation*. There is little evidence except for a payment of 4 lire 16s in January 1420 to a certain 'Giuliano d'Antonio, maestro di legniame' for 'work done a number of times, including making the *ponte* and other things', though the 'ponte' may simply have been scaffolding (SMN 4471, f. 122r: 'Giuliano d'Antonio, maestro di legniame per opere vi lavorò tra più volte tra fare ponte ed altre cose'). If there had indeed been a tramezzo it would have been no more than a small wooden screen since at this time there was no resident female monastic staff to necessitate a more substantial barrier of privacy.

57. Paatz, *Die Kirchen*, Vol. 4, p. 49 n. 92; Pope-Hennessey, *Fra Angelico*, p. 195.

58. See, for example, the payments to Castagno recorded in S. Maria Nuova's account book on 11.i.1450: 'Andrea di Bartolomeo di Chastagnio dipintore inchominciò a dipingnere la cappella maggiore dela chiesa di Santo Gidio di questo spedale': SMN 36, f. 468r, and M. Horster, *Andrea del Castagno* (Oxford, 1980), p. 205, doct. 11. More recently on Castagno's relationship with S. Maria Nuova: J.R. Spencer, *Andrea del Castagno and his Patrons* (Durham, NC, and London, 1991), pp. 81–4, 124–5, though he adds little new. See also payments to Domenico Veneziano and others for painting the frescoes: SMN 5059, c. 185; 5060, f. 94v; 5817, ff. 35v, 58v, as in Wohl, *Paintings of Domenico Veneziano*, pp. 341–2. The choir was also referred to in these documents as 'La chappella dell'altare magiore di Sancto Gidio': SMN 5059, c.134; SMN 5817, f. 35v: Wohl, *Paintings of Domenico Veneziano*, pp. 341–2.

59. Borsook, 'Cults and Imagery at Sant'Ambrogio in Florence', p. 168.

60. SMN 1, f. 2v: SMN, 1376 inventory, p. 7.

61. J. Hook, *Siena: A City and its History* (London, 1978), pp. 139–41.

62. According to Orlandi, *Beato Angelico*, pp. 30–1 n. 1, there is no reference to the painting in the surviving Registri dell'Uscita, 1423–50, and therefore it is likely that it was commissioned in the period for which the registers are missing, 1442–9. He suggests that it is possible that the painting was commissioned by Messer Girolamo di Bernardo dei Bardi. Orlandi's case is based on the fact that Bardi deposited 1,000 florins in the Monte Comune in favour of the hospital in 1441 and that St Jerome is a prominent figure in the altarpiece. Most other writers on Fra Angelico argue for an earlier date for the commission, of about 1435.

63. De Roover, *The Rise and Decline*, p. 233, repeated by Ames-Lewis, 'Domenico Veneziano', p. 72.
64. De Roover, *The Rise and Decline*, p. 262.
65. Having completed the *Annalena Altarpiece* (c.1434–5), probably for the Medici family chapel in the church of S. Lorenzo, and in the years to which the *Coronation* has been dated, Fra Angelico painted the *Virgin and Child with Saints* for the Medici chapel in the Franciscan convent at Bosco ai Frati on their estates in the Mugello: Hood, *Fra Angelico*, pp. 102–7; D. Kent, *Cosimo de' Medici*, pp. 144–5.
66. Paatz, *Die Kirchen*, Vol. 4, pp. 15–16, 24–5; Wohl, *Paintings of Domenico Veneziano*, pp. 200–7; Horster, *Andrea del Castagno*, pp. 13–14, 37, 47. SMN 5059, cc. 134, 185; SMN 5060, f. 94v; 5817, f. 35v, 58v; 5818, f. 53v: 'La chappella grande di San Gilio' (as in Wohl, *Paintings of Domenico Veneziano*, pp. 341–3); SMN 36, f. 468r (as in Horster, *Andrea del Castagno*, p. 205).
67. Wohl, *Paintings of Domenico Veneziano*, docts 2–7.
68. Horster, *Andrea del Castagno*, pp. 13–14, 37, 47.
69. SMN 37, c.57, as in Wohl, *Paintings of Domenico Veneziano*, pp. 347–8: doct. 7.
70. Horster, *Andrea del Castagno*, p. 37.
71. Vasari-Milanesi, Vol. 2, pp. 676–9; see Wohl, *Paintings of Domenico Veneziano*, pp. 206–7; Ames-Lewis, 'Domenico Veneziano'. For discussion of the question of Vasari's identification of portraits in fifteenth-century frescoes see Holmes, *Fra Filippo Lippi*, pp. 42–50.
72. Ames-Lewis, 'Domenico Veneziano', pp. 69–70.
73. Ibid., p. 72.
74. SMN 5059, c.134: 13.vi.1439: as in Wohl, *Paintings of Domenico Veneziano*, p. 341.
75. SMN 4477, f. 34r.
76. SMN 5053, f. 157r: 'Chosimo e Lorenzo de' Medici e compagni banchieri deono avere levati in questo ad c. 146 flor. 745 £1.9s.11d' (i.e., this was the total paid for the period 18.iii.1427–3.vii.1427: f. 146v).
77. SMN 5059: for S. Maria Nuova's financial dealings in 1438–9 with the Monte Comune and 'Cosimo dei Medici e compagni'.
78. De Roover, *The Rise and Decline*, pp. 338–50. See also L.A. Waldman, 'New Documents for Memling's Portinari Portraits in the Metropolitan Museum of Art', *Apollo*, Feb. 2001, pp. 28–33.
79. SMN 10, f. 13v.
80. B. Hatfeld Strens, 'L'arrivo del Trittico Portinari a Firenze', *Commentari. Rivista di critica e storia dell'arte*, 19 (1968), pp. 315–19: SMN 4515, f. 123r; SMN 5875, c. 332.
81. For discussion of the influence of Flemish on Italian art see K. Christiansen, 'The View from Italy', in M.A. Ainsworth and K. Christiansen, eds, *From Van Eyck to Breugel: Early Netherlandish Painting in the Metropolitan Museum of Art*, exh. cat., Metropolitan Museum of Art (New York, 1998), pp. 39–62; P. Nuttall, 'Early Netherlandish Painting in Florence: Acquisition, Ownership and Influence, c.1435–1500' (unpublished Ph.D. thesis, University of London, 1990).
82. De Roover, *The Rise and Decline*, pp. 338–9.
83. E. Dhanens, *Hugo van der Goes* (Antwerp, 1998), pp. 257, 263.
84. Hayum, *The Isenheim Altarpiece*, p. 16.
85. Discussed by Dhanens, *Hugo van der Goes*, pp. 270–3.
86. Crum, 'Facing the Closed Doors to Reception?'.
87. Miller, 'Miraculous Childbirth, pp. 257–8. For a detailed discussion of this altarpiece see Dhanens, *Hugo van der Goes*, pp. 250–301.
88. Miller, 'Miraculous Childbirth', pp. 258–9.
89. Cf. ibid., pp. 258. Miller is uncertain about the existence of this chapel.
90. E. Panofsky, *Early Netherlandish Painting: Its Origins and Character* (Cambridge, Mass., 1953), pp. 333–4; cf. also Dhanens, *Hugo van der Goes*, pp. 280–6.

91. ASF, SMN 4480, f. 31v. See also G. Cora, *Storia della maiolica di Firenze e del contado: secoli XIV e XV* (Florence, 1973), Vol. 1, pp. 273, 231; T. Wilson, *Ceramic Art of the Italian Renaissance* (London, 1987), p. 32.
92. R.A. Koch, 'Flower Symbolism in the Portinari Altarpiece', *Art Bulletin*, 46 (1964), pp. 76–7.
93. Miller, 'Miraculous Childbirth', p. 257; Hatfield Strens, 'L'arrivo del Trittico Portinari a Firenze', p. 316.
94. Hayum, *The Isenheim Altarpiece*, pp. 20–1, Plate 8.
95. See C. Knorr, 'The Coming of the Shepherds', *Art Bulletin*, 78 (1996), pp. 370–1.
96. Gallavotti Cavallero, *Lo Spedale di Santa Maria della Scala in Siena*, pp. 153–65.
97. Vasari-Milanesi, Vol. 2, p. 676 and n. 1.
98. Ibid., p. 592.
99. SMN (1374), pp. 69, 73. The 1510–11 'Ordinances' indicate the time of the Mass in the wards: SMN (1510–11), p. 180.
100. SMN 10, f. 11v.
101. Copy of *provvisione* of 16.x.1420 in SMN 4, ff. 27v–28v; cf. also Trexler, *Public Life*, p. 3.
102. SMN 4477, f. 109r: 'A banditori del comune a dì iii di settembre [1428] per bandire la sagra di Sancto Egidio ch'è adì 9 di questo mese £2.'
103. SMN 5878: c. 88: 'E a dì 24 d'aghosto [1493] 37s 1d paghamo a Ser Franceschо d'Antonio per 70 San Gili. (6 sett.: 50 vergine Maria); Biagio di Michele da Maiano da Fiesole per some 4 di mortina ... per la sagra: 3.12.0'; 7 sett.: 'per messe e pel vespro per la festa di San Gilio e per la sagra: 7.18.0; e adì 2 di set. [1494] £8.4.4 ... per dare a 9 preti al predicatore e a xi clerici e per 103 San Gili e per some ii d'alloro tutto per la nostra festa di San Gilio'; 10 sett.: '£7.2.4 ... per dare a preti e cherici che vennono alla nostra festa della sagra.'
104. SMN 5817, ff. 38v, 228v: 'A frate Antonio di Niccolò di Pierozzo £26.8s. I quali danari li si danno per Dio per rimuneratione che ci predichò questa quaresima passata.'
105. See in general for Florence Trexler, *Public Life*, and in relation to confraternities that organised many of the religious festivities in the city see Henderson, *Piety and Charity*, chs 3, 4, 10.
106. Listed in SMN, 1376 inventory: p. 11. The main collection is in the Museo del Bargello; others are in the hospital of S. Maria Nuova itself and the Biblioteca Laurenziana.
107. See discussion in J.J.G. Alexander, ed., *The Painted Page. Italian Renaissance Book Illumination, 1450–1550* (New York and Munich, 1994).
108. MAP 37.436: 17.vi.1479: Passerini, *Storia*, pp. 336–7.
109. Cf. SMN 60: Testamenti, 1340–79; SM 23: Testamenti; SMN 10, ff. 13v–14r, though many wills that involved hospitals did not lead to commemorative Masses in the hospital but rather in testators' own parish churches or friaries.
110. SMN 1, ff. 1r, 1v: printed version: *Il regio arcispedale*, pp. 42, 44.
111. SMN 1, f. 1r; Pampaloni, ed., *Lo Spedale*, pp. 6, 18; Richa, *Notizie*, Vol. 8, p. 191.
112. SMN (1374), pp. 69, 73.
113. De Roover, *The Rise and Decline*, pp. 356–7.
114. SMN 5076, c. 357: 6.viii.1490: 'Spese che si farano nel mortorio di Folcho d'Ado[a]rdo Portinari ... £2.10s ... paghati a preti achompangnorono il corpo che si seppellì in San Gilio'; De Roover, *The Rise and Decline*, pp. 93, 387.
115. Provv. Reg. 65, ff. 241r–3r: 23.xii.1377: Passerini, *Storia*: Doct. B, pp. 825–8.
116. Passerini, *Storia*, p. 223.
117. Mass for Bonifazio: BON 5, f. 2r (1474): 'Abbiamo a ffare nella chiesa overo chappella del nostro spedale uno uficio solenne chon dodici preti che dichano la messa, fornito el choro di falchole e chandele onorevoli ogni anno adì xxi di gennaio per l'anima di Messer Bonifazio Lupo da Parma.' On Bonifazio see J. Richards, *Altichiero. An Artist and his Patrons in the Trecento* (Cambridge, 2000), pp. 138–44.
118. BON 5, f. 184r: 23.i.1476/7: 'Alla chiesa per l'uficio de M. Bonifazio, lib. trentaquattro infra falchole, chandele per appichare et per dare in mano a preti, lib. 34.'

119. BON 6, f. 17r: 3.viii.1475: 'nostro sonatore d'orghani nella nostra chiesa, sonare tutte domeniche, feste chomandate, pasque o altre feste si facessino in chiesa.' His salary was £16.0.0 p.a.
120. Other pictures associated with the hospital include Cenni di Francesco's *Madonna and Child* (1375–8), now at the Innocenti, and Lorenzo di Bicci's *Madonna of Humility and Saints* (c.1405), now in the church of S. Maria Assunta in Loro Ciuffena. There is some disagreement about whether Cenni di Francesco's *Madonna and Child* came from Messer Bonifazio or from the Innocenti. A. Padoa Rizzo, 'Cenni di Francesco', in *Dizionario biografico degli Italiani* (Rome, 1979), Vol. 23, p. 536, and Brasioli, 'Una collezione', p. 30 opt for Messer Bonifazio, while Bellosi's Innocenti catalogue claims it for the Innocenti: *Il museo dello Spedale degli Innocenti* (Milan, 1977), p. 233 n. 33. On Cenni see also L.B. Kanter, et al., *Painting and Illumination in early Renaissance Florence, 1300–1450* (New York, 1994), pp. 177–86.
121. B. Deimling, 'Tommaso del Mazza (Master of Santa Verdiana)', in S. Pasquinucci and B. Deimling, 'Tradition and Innovation in Florentine Trecento Painting: Giovanni Bondi-Tommaso del Mazza', in M. Boskovits, *A Corpus of Florentine Painting*, Section 4, Vol. 8 (Florence, 2000), pp. 228–9 nn. 90 bis, 104–5, 108 a, b, c. Cf. on Bonifazio Lupi: Richards, *Altichiero*.
122. *Gli Uffizi. Catalogo Generale* (Florence, 1979), p. 286: Plate 691; M. Boskovits, *La pittura fiorentina alla vigilia del Rinascimento, 1300–1400* (Florence, 1975); L. Marcucci, *I dipinti toscani del secolo XIV. Le gallerie nazionali di Firenze* (Rome, 1965), n. 70. Brasioli, 'Una collezione', p. 30 suggests that both these pictures were inherited by the hospital rather than being commissioned, though without providing any source for her assertion.
123. Deimling, 'Tradition and Innovation', pp. 140–1, based on Boskovits, *La pittura fiorentina*, pp. 104–5, 229 n. 90 bis; it is suggested that the polyptych was painted in 1386.
124. Cf. D. Franklin, *Rosso in Italy. The Italian Career of Rosso Fiorentino* (New Haven and London, 1994), pp. 35–53, esp. pp. 35–8.
125. See E. Lombardi, *Messer Bonifacio Lupi*, pp. 188–9, 208–10.
126. These included the chapter-houses of S. Francesco in Pisa and Prato, the sacristy of S. Croce in Florence and then a Passion cycle for the church of the Brigittine Order founded near Florence at Bardino by Antonio degli Alberti: F. Antal, *Florentine Painting and its Social Background* (Cambridge, Mass., and London, 1986), pp. 210–13.
127. Marcucci, *I dipinti toscani*, pp. 111–12.
128. SM 108, ff. 1r–14r (two undated inventories; the first is dated by Lucas-Lybor, 'The Spedale di S. Matteo', as c.1409), SM 328, ff. 302v–305r (1454). See also discussion in Lucas-Lybor, 'The Spedale di S. Matteo', pp. 194–214.
129. SM 328, f. 20r: 1.xi.1441: 'Frate Bartolomeo di Giovanni di Gierichese [Zurich] della Magna Bassa ... se obligha ... ogni in dì per l'avenire dire ... una messa nello spedale o dove gli paresse e a presso de'aiutare chantare la messa grande agli altri preti e altri ufici quando paresse alo spedalingho e spezialmente il vespro el mattutino in chiesa.'
130. SM 184, f. 45v: 'E a dì detto per xviiii lib. onze ii di chandele per dare a 38 preti e frati e chierici di più luoghi e di Sto. Marcho e acciendo in chiesa intorno al choro e agli altari e altre parte d'intorno.' (See discussion of her funeral below, Chapter 5.)

'E a dì ix si disse 13 messe e feciessi uno bello ossequio per l'anima sua dettesi a detti preti e chierici tra lla vigilia e le messe £6 e sol. xv, sicchè tra ciere e paghamento di preti e cherichi fanno in tutto £17 e sol. 6.'
131. SM 108, f. 4r: 'Una tavola colla figura di San Macteo bellissima et anticha, la quale tavola fu dell'Arte del Cambio et truovasi che lla tavola quando la detta Arte la fece fare, gostò fior. CXX vel circa. Et la detta tavola stava in Orto San Michele al pilastro della detta Arte, et quando per capitani d'Orto San Michele feceno levare de'pilastri

della chiesa tucte le tavole di tucte l'Arti allora fu levata questa et fu recata nella detta Arte. Et dipoi per la detta Arte la detta tavola fu donata a detti spedali.' For further discussion of this altarpiece see Lucas-Lybor, 'The Spedale di S. Matteo', pp. 203–8.
132. Henderson, *Piety and Charity*, p. 228.
133. See Marcucci, *I dipinti toscani*, pp. 79–80.
134. Antal, *Florentine Painting*, pp. 191–4.
135. According to the early eighteenth-century historian of the hospital: SMN 10, f. 8v: 'A dì xxvii d'agosto 1422 per detto Ser Michele spedalingo fu cominciato a fare edificare il chiostro primo del detto spedale e il cimitero delle ossa e il granaio al lato al cimiterio detto et il secondo cimiterio et il fondachetto et più altri muramenti di detto spedale, li quali furno per lui successivamente finiti.'
136. Filarete, *Trattato*, p. 309.
137. See Horden, 'A Non-Natural Environment'.
138. SM 328, f. 303r: 'Uno libro in su che è il testamento di Lelmo coperto d'asse e di cuoio, quasi bigie con più bullette grosse da ogni lato di fuori e così bullette di sopra e di sotto e dinanzi e di dietro.'
139. See the discussion in C. Gilchrist, *Gender and Material Culture: The Archaeology of Religious Women* (London, 1994). The main medical hospitals in Florence contained two cloisters, one for men and the other for women, with the possible exception of Messer Bonifazio. On S. Paolo see Goldthwaite and Rearick, 'Michelozzo', p. 279: 'it seems clear that the second cloister further to the west and the clutter of rooms around it also post-date the original fabric.'
140. The hospital's first surviving book of payments suggests that the cloister was being finished between 1325 and 1331 along with the women's ward, refectory and dormitory: SMN 4390, f. 28r: 30.v.1328: 'per ricoprire il tetto del chiostro, 20s.' Paatz, *Die Kirchen*, Vol. 4, pp. 12, 18 does not help with the dating of the cloister.
141. Access to the female complex at S. Maria Nuova was gained from the southern side of Piazza S. Egidio, through a couple of rooms described in the 1780 plan as being 'per vari usi', and past the refectory. At S. Matteo access was gained through the further end of the women's ward, after having passed through the loggia with the church and cemetery on the right.
142. SM 328, ff. 302v–305r; f. 303r: 'Nel chiostro degli uomini'; f. 303v: 'Nel chiostro tra lle donne' and 'In uno chassone nel chiostro [tra lle donne]'; f. 304r: 'Nel chassone del chiostro tra lle donne.'
143. For the most recent treatment see W. Hood, *Fra Angelico at San Marco* (New Haven and London, 1993), pp. 126–45.
144. Ibid., p. 124.
145. See ibid. generally.
146. SM 328, f. 303r: 'Una tavoletta di Nostra Donna picholina in uno tabernacoletto. Uno crocifisso picholo in uno tabernacoletto piccholo a due sporti.'
147. SM 188, f. 20r: see below. Cf. also Vasari-Milanesi, Vol. 2, p. 57n.
148. SM 188, f. 52r: 'Ogi questo dì 24 di maggio 1470 chome Messer Lucha, al presente nostro Spedalingho, ha alloghato a Stefano d'Antonio di Vanni dipintore a dipignere un'archetto sopra la porta di mezo che viene nel chiostro del nostro spedale chon patti che'l detto Stefano debba dipignere una nostra donna che abbia in grenbo el Nostro Signiore morto, chome di chostume nella Pietà. E dal chapo del nostro Signiore sia San Giovanni Vangelista e dappiè Sancta Maria Magdalena. El chanpo debba mettere d'oro fine e la chornice che getta intorno e chosì quella del chardinale debbe mettere d'oro fine e chosì in ogni altro luogho dove va oro debba mettere d'oro fine e lavorare di buoni cholori e dove va azuro vorssi oltramarino fine e ffare un fogliame sopra la chornice che paia stagato di marmo e nel chardinale della porta un fogliame chome sta quello della porte che va nello spedale delle donne e debbe mettere oro e cholori tutti di suo [spese]. E debba avere per paghamento di decto

lavorio lire 72 piccioli, el quale lavorio debba avere finito per tutto il mese di luglio proximo 1470.' Cf. also Vasari-Milanesi, Vol. 5, p. 57n.
149. Cf. Hood, *Fra Angelico at San Marco*, p. 158.
150. SM 326, f. 325v: 'per dipintura di due archetti à dipinti al detto spedale, cioè l'archetto che sopra la porta della chiesa di San Matteo nel quale dipinse San Matteo e l'archetto che sopra la porta dello Spedale delle Donne nel quale dipinse la fighura della Gloriosa Vergine Madonna e Santa Maria.' See also Vasari-Milanesi, Vol. 1, p. 611 n., Bellosi, ed., *Il Museo dello Spedale degli Innocenti*, p. 263 n. 248.
151. SM 326, f. 325v: 'nella prima porta a mano manca si entra nello spedale degli uomini.'
152. Hood, *Fra Angelico at San Marco*, p. 130.
153. SMN (1510–11), p. 183.
154. Paatz, *Die Kirchen*, Vol. 4, p. 27; Brasioli, 'Una collezione da riscoprire', p. 27; Richa, *Notizie*, Vol. 8, p. 195.
155. F.L. Del Migliore, *Firenze, città nobilissima illustrata* (Florence, 1684; anastatic edn, Bologna, 1976), p. 351; see also Richa, *Notizie*, Vol. 8, p. 195.
156. Richa, *Notizie*, Vol. 8, pp. 193–4.

Chapter 5

1. Alberti, *L'Architettura*, Vol. 1, pp. 367–8; Corsini, *La Morìa*, p. 34.
2. Cf. R. Meloncelli, 'Musica nell' "Arcispedale" di Santo Spirito', in V. Cappelletti and F. Tagliarini, eds, *L'antico Ospedale di Santo Spirito dall'istituzione papale alla sanità del terzo millenio* (Rome, 2001–2), Vol. 2, pp. 263–77.
3. See Henderson in Arrizabalaga, Henderson and French, *The Great Pox*, p. 177.
4. See Goldthwaite and Rearick, 'Michelozzo', p. 230: Plate 9.
5. Mori and Boffito, *Firenze nelle vedute e nelle piante*, pp. 12–21.
6. See Goldthwaite and Rearick, 'Michelozzo', pp. 232–3: Plates 8–11.
7. F. Brasioli and C. Lachi, 'Catalogo', in De Benedictis, ed., *Il patrimonio artistico*, pp. 230–1.
8. The most recent and comprehensive discussion of the evidence is by L. Baini, 'Ipotesi sull'origine della tipologia cruciforme per gli ospedali del XV secolo', in L. Giordano, ed., *Processi accumulativi, forme e funzioni. Saggi sull'architettura lombarda del Quattrocento* (Florence, 1996), pp. 59–102. See also L. Franchini, 'Introduzione', in L. Franchini, ed., *Ospedali Lombardi del Quattrocento. Fondazioni, trasformazioni, restauri* (Como, 1995), pp. 11–72, esp. pp. 6–8.
9. See J. Henderson, 'Peste, Mal Francese e gli Ospedali di Firenze nel Rinascimento', in A. Aleardi and L. Pieri, eds, *L'Ospedale e la città* (Florence, 2000), pp. 16–27.
10. Richa, *Notizie*, Vol. 8, p. 207. Cf. Passerini, *Storia*, p. 356; Pampaloni, *Lo Spedale di S. Maria Nuova*, p. 80 n. 47, based on SMN 1, ins. 3.
11. SMN 5046, c. 80; cf. Ciuccetti, 'Lo sviluppo architettonico dello Spedale di Santa Maria Nuova', p. 60 n. 45.
12. F. Leverotti, 'L'ospedale senese di S. Maria della Scala in una relazione del 1456', *Bulletino senese di storia patria*, 1984, pp. 276–91.
13. Ibid., pp. 280, 285; D. Gallavotti and A. Brogi, *Lo Spedale Grande di Siena. Fatti urbanistici e architettonici del Santa Maria della Scala. Ricerche, riflessioni, interrogativi* (Florence, 1987), p. 66: Plans VI.62–3.
14. L. Patetta, *L'architettura del Quattrocento a Milano* (Milan, 1987), p. 275; Welch, *Art and Authority*, p. 150.
15. M. Lazzaroni and A. Muñoz, *Filarete: scultore e architetto del secolo XV* (Rome, 1908), p. 186.
16. Patetta, *L'architettura*, p. 277: 25.vi.1456.
17. F. Leverotti, 'Ricerche sulle origini dell'Ospedale Maggiore di Milano', *Archivio Storico Lombardo*, 107 (1984), pp. 89, 65.

18. P. Foster, 'Per il disegno dell'Ospedale di Milano', *Arte Lombarda* (1973), pp. 7–8; A. Peroni, 'Il modello dell'ospedale cruciforme: il problema del rapporto tra l'Ospedale di Santa Maria Nuova di Firenze e gli ospedali lombardi', in S. Bertelli, N. Rubinstein and C.H. Smyth, eds, *Florence and Milan: Comparisons and Relations* (Florence, 1989), pp. 53–5.
19. Patetta, *L'architettura*, pp. 275–7; B. Pullan, *Rich and Poor in Renaissance Venice. The Social Institutions of a Catholic State to 1615* (Oxford, 1971), p. 204.
20. For this project see Ciuccetti, 'Un grandioso progetto di Bernardo Buontalenti', pp. 79–105.
21. The 1563 statutes of the Accademia del Disegno recount the various moves made by the artists' confraternity of S. Luca which still met at S. Maria Nuova in the early Cinquecento: BNCF, MSS II.I.359, cc. 1–8, printed in Z. Wazbinski, *L'Accademia Medicea del Disegno a Firenze nel Cinquecento: Idea e istituzione* (Florence, 1987), Vol. 2, p. 424.
22. 'Memoria della aggiunta dello Spedale deli huomini infermi di Santa Maria Nova': SMN 1286, c. 46: 'Adì 25 deto 1575 in venerdì, al giorno della Annunciazione della Santissima Vergine il Rev.mo don Vito Buonaccolti, monaco di Monte Oliveto, Spedalingo di detto spedale, messe la prima pietra intagliatavi sopra il santo nome di Giesù e scrittovi intorno "Santa Maria Nova, anno saluto 1575 addì XXV di marzo" e in due buche fatte in detta pietra drento a dua vasetti di piombo vi si messe l'appresso reliquie e prima più agnusdei benedetti dal santissimo Papa Pio V, uno ducato d'oro con l'impronta della Madonna e un aquila, scrittovi attorno "Federigo molto amico, tre grossi della Madonna scrittovi 'Virgo protege Pisa …' ", ma prima fatta la messa dello Spirito Santo, el detto Spedalingo nella nostra chiesa, di poi fatta la processione con tuta la nostra famiglia, maschi e femine, per la via della Pergola e entrati per la porta di dietro all'orto fatta per detta muraglia la Compagnia de' Bianchi, che si raguna accanto al nostro spedale, con un crocifisso di molta divozione, e lo Spedalingo, presso el legno della santissima croce riliquia della nostra casa, cantando el Tedeum e altri inni e orazioni appropriate a simili cirimonie.'
    Though this is a contemporary account, it was apparently misfiled before being found again on 15 June 1649. It was first published by P. Bagnesi, 'Alessandro Allori e lo Spedale di S. Maria Nuova', *Rivista d'arte*, 9 (1916–18), pp. 258–9, and then by Ciuccetti, 'Un grandioso progetto di Bernardo Buontalenti', pp. 81–2, though with minor errors of transcription which I have corrected.
23. SMN (1510–11), p. 181. This approximate calculation was made by applying the calculation of 0.83 metres per bed in the first three arms of the ward (i.e., the combined length of 82 metres divided by the number of patients) to the new extension, though allowing for some space for the new chapel.
24. Pampaloni, ed., *Lo Spedale di S. Maria Nuova*, ch. 4.
25. The longest was the original southern arm of 39 metres.
26. Chaney,' "Philanthropy in Italy" ', p. 91.
27. Pampaloni, ed., *Lo Spedale di S. Maria Nuova*, ch. 4.
28. See below, Chapter 8.
29. D. Mignani, 'Profilo storico-architettonico degli istituti Lorenesi dell'Accademia delle Belle Arti', in F. Falletti, ed., *L'Accademia, Michelangelo, L'Ottocento* (Livorno, 1997), pp. 17–18.
30. See the 1780 plans in ASF, SMN 24. The male ward of Messer Bonifazio was 50 metres long and 9.33 metres wide and of S. Paolo 52 by 10.33 metres.
31. See Rensi, 'L'Ospedale di S. Matteo', pp. 122, 95.
32. Calculated from the hospital's plans of 1780 in ASF, SMN 24.
33. The total number of beds in S. Matteo in 1454, according to the inventory of that year, included thirty for men and twenty-four for women: SM 328, f. 302v.
34. Saalman, *Filippo Brunelleschi*, pp. 36–64; cf. p. 54: Figure 2: 'Plan: state in 1449'.

35. For what follows see Goldthwaite and Rearick, 'Michelozzo'.
36. Zandri, Acidini Luchinat and Francolini, *Lo Spedale di Messer Bonifazio*, pp. 66–7.
37. See J.D. Thompson and G. Goldin, *The Hospital: A Social and Architectural History* (New Haven and London, 1975), pp. 15–22.
38. SM 123, f. 5r: 3.xii.1385: 'Ancora e detti maestri àno toltto a fare il tetto del sopradetto ispedalle sopra le sopradette mura e debono farvi dodici chavaletti al detto tetto a quella misura e altezza e grosezza di legniame e a quella ragione e modo sono quelli delo spedalle di S. Maria Nuova'; Rensi, 'L'Ospedale di San Matteo', p. 123.
39. SM 123, f. 5r: 3.xii.1385: 'insino al'alteza di bracia xviii in xviiii, chome piacerà al detto Lemmo'. He also laid down that the height of the male ward should be 'including the incline of the roof, *braccia* 20, *grosso* 1' (or 12 metres): SM 1, f. 27r: 'comprensuto il pendio del tetto braccia 20, grosso 1': Rensi, 'L'Ospedale di San Matteo', p. 132.
40. This was about double the height of the cloisters of the contiguous convent of S. Niccolò next to the female ward, according to Lemmo's instructions of two years later. The male ward would probably therefore have been built to the same height. 'In prima debono fare il muro che chiude il circhuito del chiostro già principiato, il quale deb'essere alto bracia otto': SM 123, f. 7r.
41. Cf. Provv. Reg. 35, f. 133v.
42. Richa, *Notizie*, Vol. 7, p. 82, cited by Rensi, 'L'Ospedale di San Matteo', p. 84.
43. M. Ficino, *Consilio contro la pestilenzia*, ed. E. Musacchio (Bologna, 1983), p. 55.
44. A. Courbin, *The Foul and the Fragrant. Odor and the French Social Imagination* (Cambridge, Mass., 1986), pp. 3–4; see also pp. 52–3, 106–7.
45. G. Targioni Tozzetti, *Notizie degli aggrandamenti delle scienze fisiche in Toscana* (Florence, 1780).
46. Ficino, *Consilio contro la pestilenzia*, p. 63.
47. Thompson and Goldin, *The Hospital*, p. 31.
48. SMN (1510–11), pp. 181–2.
49. 'Consiglio di Tommaso del Garbo Fiorentino contro la Pestilentia', in M. Ficino, *Contro alla peste* (Florence, 1576), p. 82.
50. For example, the Convento of S. Maria del Carmine, 1391, and the Badia Fiesolana, 1461: Schiaparelli, *La casa fiorentina*, pp. 125–7.
51. SMN 4474, f. 126r: 27.viii.1420: 'A Francescho di Giovanni e Bernardo di Francescho fanno finestre di vetro ... per reto di fl. 51.17s a oro per uno occhio di vetro per la chiesa che fue br. 14 1/5 ... e per la finestra di vetro di decta chiesa di verso il cimiterio fu br. 10 ... e per la rete di br. 14 £13 per la finestra di qua di verso il chiostro totale: fl. 46. s. 11d.'
52. Schiaparelli, *La casa fiorentina*, pp. 124–33.
53. England: personal communication of 6 Jan. 2000 from Roberta Gilchrist; France: Thompson and Goldin, *The Hospital*, pp. 21–2.
54. SMN 4471, f. 97r; 4468, f. 23v: 'A Niccholò di Piero maestro di finestre di vetro a dì xx di marzo [1414/15] per una finestra di vetro al lato alla cappella dello spedale degli uomini £32.15s. e per una finestra di vetro dirimpetto al crocifisso dello spedale: £33.'
55. SMN 4390, f. 13r: 22.i.1327: 'in dodici pezi d'assi per le finestre delo spedale di là dele femine: £13'; 13r: 31.i.1327: 'in bandelle e aghuti per le finestre ... dele femine: £7.18'; f. 13v: 18.ii.1327: 'in funi per le finestre'; f. 19r: 1.vii.1327: 'per funi per le finestre delo spedale nuovo £29.8s e in carucole per le femine del detto spedale: £10.10s.'
56. Payments by S. Maria Nuova in Jan. 1327 for planks of wood and nails 'for the windows' may have been for such shutters: SMN 4390, f. 13r: 'in dodici pezi d'assi per le finestre delo spedale di là dele femine: £13' (22.i.1327); 'in bandelle e aghuti per le finestre ... dele femine: £7.18' (31.i.27).
57. Del Migliore, *Firenze*, pp. 349–50.
58. Mignani, 'Profilo storico-architettonico', pp. 17–18.
59. On S. Maria della Scala see Gallavotti Cavallero, *Lo Spedale di Santa Maria della Scala*.

A useful introductory guide to the frescoes is A. Orlandini, *Gettatelli, pellegrini. Gli affreschi nella Sala del Pellegrino dell'Ospedale di Santa Maria della Scala di Siena* (Siena, 1997).
It was not actually set in the Pellegrinaio since the room was being worked on at the time, but rather in the contiguous male ward which had been built in 1379: Gallavotti Cavallero, *Lo Spedale*, p. 160.

60. SMN (1374), p. 63; see also the statutes of the hospital of Messer Bonifazio based extensively on the founder's will: Wellcome Institute Library, London, MS no. 453, ff. 8v–9v; the testament is discussed in detail by E. Lombardi, *Messer Bonifazio Lupi*, ch. 25.
61. From at least 1330 S. Maria Nuova had specialised in treating the sick poor; nobody who was not sick was allowed to stay for longer than three days.
62. SMN (1374), pp. 63–4.
63. SMN (1510–11), p. 181.
64. On this series of illuminations see most recently A. Kolega, 'Un capolavoro poco noto della miniatura trecentesca. Il "Liber Regulae" dell'Ordine degli Ospitalieri di Santo Spirito', in Cappelletti and Tagliarini, eds, *L'antico Ospedale di Santo Spirito*, Vol. 2, pp. 203–24.
65. SM 328, f. 302v.
66. SMN (1510–11), p. 181.
67. Ibid.
68. Ibid.
69. Bonifazio statutes, ff. 4v–5r; SMN 4390, f. 11r: purchases in 1325 of 'panno bigio' and 'panno romagnolo'; see also ibid., f. 5v purchases of slippers. SP 661 under 1347: purchase of 'panno virgato'.
70. In general see P. Thornton, *The Italian Renaissance Interior, 1400–1600* (London, 1991), pp. 111–67.
71. J.R. Spencer, ed., *Filarete's Treatise on Architecture, Being the Treatise by Antonio di Piero Averlino, Known as Filarete* (New Haven and London, 1965), p. 144.
72. SM 328, f. 302v.
73. Ibid.
74. Ibid.
75. For example, SM 108, f. 3r.
76. Thornton, *The Italian Renaissance Interior*, pp. 154–7.
77. SMN 4390, f. 9r (1326); 4428, ff. 30r, 132r, 181r (1375–9). See also S. Paolo's 1452 payment of 14 lire 4s to Antonio di Jacopo and Giovanni di Guccio *dipintori* 'to paint twenty-four beds': SP 644, f. 50v.
78. SM 108, f. 3r: listed in the hospital's first surviving inventory.
79. SMN 5076, c. 207 right: 2.iv.1490: 'Davitt di Tommaso dipintore … per richolorare et oro di lo tabernacholo di Nostra Donna ch'è sopra il lettuccio dello spedale dove si ponghono assedere gl'infermi quando venghono allo spedale.' I am grateful to Andrew Blume for this reference.
80. Ciuccetti, 'Profilo architettonico', pp. 10–15.
81. SMN 5107, f. 53v: payments to Allori; ff. 44v–45r for building the ward chapel.
82. Ibid. See also C. Avery, *Giambologna: The Complete Sculpture* (Oxford, 1987) and A. Fara, ed., *Bernardo Buontalenti e Firenze: architettura e disegno dal 1576 al 1607* (Florence, 1998).
83. Chaney, ' "Philanthropy in Italy" ', pp. 183–217.
84. See *Nuovo Osservatore*, 3 (1885), pp. 23–4; 4 (1885), p. 29; Siren in U. Thieme and F. Becker, *Allgemeines Lexicon der Bildenden Künstler von der Antike bis zur Gegenwart*, Vol. 13 (Leipzig, 1920), p. 465. All summarised by Paatz, *Die Kirchen*, Vol. 4, pp. 22, 28, 56 nn. 89, 132.
85. Antal, *Florentine Painting and its Social Background*, pp. 210–11.

NOTES TO PAGES 171–3

86. See L. Marcucci, *Gallerie Nazionali di Firenze*, Vol. 1: *Catalogo dei dipinti del secolo XIV* (Rome, 1965), no. 76a; discussed by Henderson, *Piety and Charity*, p. 162.
87. ASF, SMN 4465, f. 80r: 'A Niccholò di Piero dipintore a dì decto [23.xi.1414] per le infrascritte dipinture fatte dal lato delle donne:
    Prima per la storia della Neve coll'adornamento dintorno fior. viii.
    E per la storia della Natività di Christo coll'adornamento fior. x e di Sancta Lucia e di Sancta Angnesa e di Santa Cicilia fior. viiii e del frontespizio sopra a la sepoltura fior. ii e di S. Lisabetta fior. ii; e della storia di xii apostoli fior. viiii, e della faccia sopra a l'altare e colla finestra fior. x; e per tutto l'archo con due profeti e adornamenti fior. vi, e più le iiii sotto l'archo San Giorgio, Sancta Margherita, Sancta Barbera e San Giovanni Batista fior. vii; ed anche la Piatà nella faccia del pozzo dello spedale di là fior. ii; e per la dipintura di sopra alla porta dello spedale di là fior. xii. Somma fior. 77 lire 2 di grossi, di sol. 80 per fiorino.'
    This document was first published in *Nuovo Osservatore*, 4 (1885), p. 29, and republished in Brasioli and Lachi, 'Catalogo', pp. 230–1, with a commentary, though containing minor errors of transcription and omissions which I have corrected.
88. Brasioli and Lachi, 'Catalogo', pp. 230–1
89. SMN 4465, f. 28r: 'A Francesco di Giovanni di Lapo maestro di finestre de vetro adì xxviii di novembre per una finestra di vetro per la cappella dello spedale delle donne e fue br.v q.iii: £34.12s.'
90. Ciuccetti, 'Lo Spedale di Santa Maria Nuova', p. 24.
91. See payments recorded in SMN 4465.
92. Jacobus de Voragine, *The Golden Legend*, Vol. 2, pp. 318ff., and 202ff.
93. SMN 4424, f. 3r: 'paghamo decto dì (8.ix.1368) al Tuccio dipintore per la storia di Santa Lisabetta che dipinse nelo spedale da lato delle donne fior. 50 d'oro.'
94. It has been suggested that a large altarpiece commissioned by the hospital in about 1414 from Mariotto di Nardo took the place of Orcagna's *S. Matteo* in the hospital church some time before 1420 (R. Offner, *A Corpus of Florentine Painting*, Vol. 3. iv, p. 22; discussed by Lucas-Lybor, 'The Spedale di S. Matteo', pp. 208–11). However, this is incorrect: a payment to Mariotto in March 1414 specifically states that it was intended for the altar of a ward, probably the men's (SM 251, f. 59r: 'tavola dell'altare dello spedale': 13.iii.1414, as also noted by Lucas-Lybor, 'The Spedale di S. Matteo', p. 210). The subject may very well have been St Nicholas, reflecting his status as the hospital's joint patron with St Matthew. The association between the male ward and S. Niccolò is underlined by a payment of 14 gold florins in 1412 to Lorenzo the painter – probably Lorenzo Monaco – to include the price of 'gold and of colours', for 'a lunette painted above the door of the men's ward in which he painted the figure of the glorious confessor Messer Santo Nicholaio' (SM 326, f. 326r: 'Lorenzo di … dipintore' paid 14 gold florins in 1412 'per dipintura a ogni sua spesa d'oro e di cholori d'uno archetto dipinse sopra la porta dello spedale degli uomini nel quale dipinse la fighura del glorioso chonfessoro Messer Santo Nicholaio'). If this assumption is correct, Mariotto's predella of scenes from the life of St Nicholas of Bari, now in the Uffizi, would also have been intended for the male ward and not for the church, as is usually suggested (Cf. Paatz, *Die Kirchen*, Vol. 4, p. 153 while Offner, *Corpus of Florentine Painting*, Vol. 3, p. 22 rejects the idea that the predella could have been intended for Orcagna's *S. Matteo*). The subject of St Nicholas is hardly surprising for a hospital. In a general sense he was always associated with charitable acts given that he had used his parents' wealth to help the poor. More specifically Nicholas had for some time been associated with this site through the previous owners, the Monastery of S. Niccolò, which still occupied the southern half of the site (Rensi, 'L'Ospedale di San Matteo', p. 84).
95. Accademia, Inv. 1890, nn. 3162 and 3164. Discussed by Lucas-Lybor, 'The Spedale di S. Matteo', pp. 211–13, where she identifies the subject of the picture as the *Coronation of the Virgin*.

96. SM 328, f. 302v: 'Una altare maggiore con una tavola dipinta da ogni lato con uno crocifisso di sopra da ogni lato convale da ogni lato.'
97. SM 1.A, f. 31r: 'Chome ogi adì soprascritto Gerolamo Priore delo Spedale di Santo Matheo, cioè da Monte Chatino, e Ser Simone capellano del detto luogo e Monna Nanna la magiore delo spedale dele donne del detto spedale alugono e danno a fare una tavola dell'altare dele donne soprascritte, cioè che Mariotto di Cristofano dipintore ch'el detto Mariotto abi ordinare e logare a maestro di legname e el detto Mariotto abi dipingnere la detta tavola e ne mettere in seghuitione al meglio saprà e potrà. E la detta tavola a' esser dipinta dinanzi e di drietto e nela parte dinanti la Nostra Donna con questi santi, cioè [blank], e dela parte didrietto la Resuretione del Nostro Signor Yhesu Cristo… Et è contento soprascritto Mariotto dela dipintura loro colori e ogni altra cosa pertinente al maesterio suo, chome sarà giudicato per li soprascritti giudicatori.' As in Lucas-Lybor, 'The Spedale di S. Matteo', p. 212 n. 1; I have corrected some minor errors of transcription.
98. The contract of 6 Dec. 1445 stipulated that it was they who would provide the basic ideas: SM 1, f. 31r; Lucas-Lybor, 'The Spedale di S. Matteo', p. 212 n. 1.
99. S. Haskins, *Mary Magdalene. Myth and Metaphor* (London and New York, 1993), pp. 185–7.
100. As calculated by Lucas-Lybor, 'The Spedale di S. Matteo', p. 212.
101. SM 328, f. 302v.
102. Ibid.; SM 36, f. 6r.
103. SM 36, f. 6r: 'i testa di Sto Antonino.'
104. SM 328, f. 302v; 36, f. 6r: 1591 inventory. For the Spedale di S. Fina in San Gimignano see *Una farmacia preindustriale*, p. 34: inventory of 1495: 'Nel pellegrinaio delli homini: uno crocifixo grande.'
105. Presumably the sacristy: SM 302, f. 304r.
106. SMN 4428, f. 254r, 1374: 'A Andreuzzo dipintore adì 19 di luglio per disegnare la tavola di Santo Lucha nello spedale degl'uomini, fior. 2 d'oro'; f. 255r: 'per disegnare la tavola della chappella di sancto Lucha dal lato delgl'uomini all'Andreuzzo dipintore'; f. 255v: two further payments to Andreuzzo of 1 florin. Cf. Vasari–Milanesi, Vol. 1, p. 675, who says it was commissioned from Niccolò di Pietro Gerini in 1383.
107. Vasari-Milanesi, Vol. 1, p. 675; Paatz, *Die Kirchen*, Vol. 4, pp. 24, 51 n. 96a. I have taken this passage to mean that everybody is shown kneeling, though the wording is slightly unclear: 'e nella predella, da un lato gli uomini della Compagnia, e dall'altro tutte le donne ginocchioni.'
108. BNCF, MSS II.I.399: Wazbinski, *L'Accademia Medicea*, Vol. 2, p. 424. On the regular meetings of lay confraternities in this period see Henderson, *Piety and Charity*, chs 2, 3. From as early as October 1339 there were expenses in the hospital's account books for advertising the festival, 'per bandire la festa di Sancto Luca': SMN 4392, f. 42v. ASF, Accademia del Disegno 1, f. 2v: Wazbinski, *L'Accademia Medicea*, Vol. 2, p. 419.
109. The devotional activities of the company of S. Luca were complementary to those of the male ward, for this type of occupational confraternity met much less frequently than, for example, Laudesi companies whose members sang lauds together every evening: see Henderson, *Piety and Charity*, ch. 3.
110. SMN (1330), p. 58; also SMN (1374), pp. 69, 73. The 1510–11 'Ordinances' indicate the time of the Mass in the wards: SMN (1510–11), p. 180.
111. SMN (1510–11), p. 180.
112. Confessors who spoke French, Spanish and German: SMN 5075, c. 37.
113. Cf. A. Marquand, *Luca della Robbia* (Princeton, 1914), p. 65; J. Pope-Hennessey, *Luca della Robbia* (Oxford, 1980), pp. 234–5; Padoa Rizzo, 'Luca della Robbia e Verrocchio'; A. Butterfield, *The Sculptures of Andrea del Verrocchio* (New Haven and London, 1997), pp. 125, 220–1: no. 18.

114. For payments to Rossellino and Ghiberti see the hospital's 'quaderno di cassa' for 1449–52: SMN 5064, cc. 18r, 30r, 36r; and for 1448–50: SMN 5063, c.187. These extracts from the hospital's records were published by G. Poggi, 'Il ciborio di Bernardino Rossellino nella chiesa di S. Egidio', *Miscellanea d'arte*, 1 (1903), pp. 105–7. Cf. also R. Krautheimer, *Lorenzo Ghiberti* (Princeton, 1982), pp. 204, 207; A. Markham Schulz, *The Sculpture of Bernardino Rossellino and his Workshop* (Princeton, 1977), pp. 52–8, 160–1. For the tabernacle in the male ward see Padoa Rizzo, 'Luca della Robbia e Verrocchio', pp. 48–68.
115. Markham Schulz, *The Sculpture of Bernardino Rossellino*, pp. 160–1; M.P. Vignoli in *Lorenzo Ghiberti: materia e ragionamenti*, exh. cat. (Florence, 1978), pp. 426–7. The prototype for this design is Desiderio da Settignano's S. Lorenzo tabernacle.
116. Markham Schulz, *The Sculpture of Bernardino Rossellino*, p. 106.
117. SMN (1510–11), p. 183.
118. In 1289, 1334 and 1358: SMN 10, f. 13r; Del Migliore, *Firenze*, pp. 345–6.
119. SMN 10, f. 13r. Also described by Del Migliore, *Firenze*, pp. 345–6, and Richa, *Notizie*, Vol. 8, p. 191.
120. On tomb types and the *avello* in particular see A. Butterfield, 'Monument and Memory in Early Renaissance Florence', in G. Ciappelli and P. Lee Rubin, eds, *Art, Memory and Family in Renaissance Florence* (Cambridge, 2000), pp. 135–160, esp. pp. 143–5.
121. Horster, *Andrea del Castagno*, p. 189.
122. Del Migliore, *Firenze*, p. 345; Richa, *Notizie*, Vol. 8, p. 190, both cited by Paatz, *Die Kirchen*, Vol. 4, p. 29 n. 136, and Horster, *Andrea del Castagno*, p. 189. The painting is presumed to have been executed when Castagno was living at S. Maria Nuova and working on the *Last Supper* fresco in the male refectory and the fresco-cycle in S. Egidio. Indeed, the main subject of the Annunciation was linked closely to the theme of the cycle of the *Life of the Virgin* in the Cappella Maggiore of the hospital church rededicated to the Virgin: Horster, *Andrea del Castagno*, p. 205: doct. 11 publishes the terms of the agreement between S. Maria Nuova and Castagno which established that, in addition to a payment of 100 gold florins, he was to receive free board and lodging. He was to have 'una chamera nella fermeria': from SMN 36, f. 468r.
123. SMN 10, f.14r.
124. SM 125 under 24.vii.1415: 'una lanpana istà accesa di dì e di notte dinanzi alla fighura della Trinità posta nello spedale da lato delle donne.'
125. SM 23, f. 225r.
126. ASF, Accademia del Disegno 1, f. 2v: Wazbinski, *L'Accademia Medicea del Disegno a Firenze*, Vol. 2, p. 419.
127. Henderson, *Piety and Charity*, ch. 5.
128. ASF, Accademia del Disegno 1, f. 2r.
129. SMN 10, f. 13r: 'La cappella dello spedale da lato degli huomini, secondo che si vede per lettere intagliate nella pietra la quale è posta dal lato dinanzi all'altar' di detta cappella, fu edificata e fatta del mese di maggio 1369, al tempo di Ser Guido spedalingo e rettore di detto spedale.' SMN 1, f. 3v: ins. 3: 'nella testata della corsia era l'altare, quale era posto sotto una cupoletta, però coperto di legname e embrici.' SMN 4424, f. 16v: 'Paghamo adì xvi di maggio [1369] a Zanobi di Vinci per 10 cavretti de' quali mandamo tre a Messer lo vescovo quando facemo consegnare l'altare di Messer Sta Lucha.'
130. SMN 5107, ff. 96v–97v.
131. Ibid.
132. Cf. Henderson, *Piety and Charity*, ch. 3.

Chapter 6

1. M. Villani, *Cronica*, I.7.
2. Luther, *Table Talk*, p. 296.
3. Exceptions include Redon, 'Autour de l'Hôpital S. Maria della Scala à Sienne au XIIIe siècle' and Benvenuti-Papi, '*In Castro Poenitentiae*', pp. 647–8.
4. 1520: SM 198, ff. 258r–v: 'Ricordo come Monna Ginevra figlia fu di Sandro d'Antonio del Pescaia e al presente serva di Monna Gostanza donna fu di Bononcino Baroncini ci à dato in diposito flor. 17 lb. d'oro e Lire 1 … sia tenuto a riceptala sempre in tutte le sue infermità e tractarla a uso di comessa, come si fussi una delle nostre di casa. E quando detta Monna Ginevra pervenissi al'età di 60 anni in modo non potessi durare più fatica, che oggi secondo intendiamo è di età d'anni 33 in circa, detto spedale solvigla riceptarla qui in casa dargli vita e vestito.'
5. See the excellent discussion of this phenomenon in B. Harvey, *Living and Dying in England, 1100–1540. The Monastic Experience* (Oxford, 1993), ch. 6, and S. Beccaria, 'I conversi nel Medioevo. Un problema storico e storiografico', *Quaderni storici*, 46 (1998), pp. 120–56.
6. J.H. Mundy, 'Charity and Social Work in Toulouse, 1100–1250', *Traditio*, 22 (1966), pp. 203–87, esp. pp. 267–70; D.J. Osheim, 'Conversion, *Conversi*, and the Christian Life in Late Medieval Tuscany', *Speculum*, 58:2 (1983), pp. 368–90; G.G. Merlo, ed., *Esperienze religiose e opere assistenziali nei secoli XII e XIII* (Turin, 1987); F.-O. Touati, 'Les groupes des laïcs dans les hôpitaux et les léproseries au moyen-âge', in *Les mouvances laïques des ordres religieux* (Saint-Étienne, 1996), pp. 150–6; Brodman, *Charity and Welfare*, pp. 50–60.
7. SMN (1374), p. 65. Cf. SMN (1330), p. 54 and SMN (1510–11), pp. 177–8, 180. It should be stressed that from the very beginning S. Maria Nuova had both male and female nurses. This is contrary to the still strong local tradition that insists that Folco's servant, Monna Tessa, later founded the female *converse*, despite the lack of evidence and the convincing dismissal of these claims over 150 years ago by Luigi Passerini! See A. Lucarella, *Le oblate di S. Maria Nuova di Firenze* (Bari, 1985), p. 20; C.C. Calzolai, *Lo spirito di un servizio secolare*, in *Il VII centenario dell'Ospedale di S. Maria Nuova* (Barberino di Mugello, 1988), pp. 10–11; Passerini, *Storia*, pp. 286–7.
8. F. Dal Pino, 'Oblati e oblate conventuali presso i mendicanti "minori" nei secoli XIII–XIV', in *Uomini e donne in comunità. Quaderni di storia religiosa* (1994), Vol. 1, pp. 33–67.
9. For the hospital's early history see Passerini, *Storia*, pp. 163–88; R. Franci, 'L'Ospedale di San Paolo in Firenze e i Terziari Francescani'; G.G. Meersseman, *Ordo fraternitatis: confraternite e pietà dei laici nel Medioevo* (Rome, 1977); Benvenuti-Papi, '*In Castro Poenitentiae*', pp. 647–8.
10. For example, the control of the Portinari family over the inner workings of S. Maria Nuova was eroded by successive *spedalinghi* with the support of the Florentine bishop. In 1324 the Portinari had restricted the number of *conversi* to six, the family reserving to itself the right to approve the candidates chosen by the *spedalingo*: SMN 1, f. 4v. Then in 1346 the limit on *conversi* was abolished and ten years later the *spedalingo* obtained a free hand in their election and no longer were the Portinari able to remove officials from office, including the *spedalingo* himself. See SMN 10, f. 7r (22.iii.1345/6), f. 7v (16.viii.1356); SMN (1376), pp. 64–5; SMN (1510–11), p. 176; Passerini, *Storia*, pp. 290–3.
11. The Arte dei Giudici e Notai were appointed as the patrons and governors of S. Paolo in 1403. See the hospital's statutes: SP 976 (fragments of 1325); SP 912 (1572) as well as the hospital's own history written by the *spedalingo* in 1762: SP 616. Messer Bonifazio, S. Matteo and the Innocenti were under the patronage of the Calimala, Cambio and Seta guilds: Passerini, *Storia*, pp. 224–5 (Bonifazio); p. 155 (S. Matteo); Innocenti: Gavitt, *Charity and Children*, pp. 150–1.

NOTES TO PAGES 188–92   397

12. See Brodman, *Charity and Welfare*, ch. 4; Passerini, *Storia*, p. 663.
13. Passerini, *Storia*, pp. 142, 137.
14. L. Banchi, ed., *Statuti senesi scritti in volgare ne'secoli XIII e XIV* (Bologna, 1877), Vol. 3, p. 61. The records of the hospital also listed 'familiari', 'conversi' and 'oblati', though clearly in some cases these titles were interchangeable: *Statuti senesi*, Vol. 3, p. 12; Redon, 'Autour de l'Hôpital S. Maria', pp. 17–34, esp. p. 26.
15. For example, the staff at the hospital of S. Matteo between 1495 and 1499 included Salvestro di Piero di Salvestro, who was described as 'nostro servo e commesso': SM 193, f. 28v.
16. Rawcliffe, 'Hospital Nurses and their Work', p. 62.
17. SP 677, under 10.viii.1358; 675, under 31.v.1370; 644, f. 27r (15.ix.1442).
18. The same terms, *commesso* and *commessa*, were used by Messer Bonifazio Lupi, Lemmo Balducci and Francesco Datini. On Messer Bonifazio see E. Lombardi, *Messer Bonifacio Lupi*, pp. 232–6, 238; on S. Matteo see discussion of contracts below in this chapter and Passerini, *Storia*, p. 156; for the Innocenti see Gavitt, *Charity and Children*, pp. 173–9.
19. SM 197, f. 193v: 'Perché il detto Bartholomeo non è molto sano noi ci siamo convenuti seco che lui s'abbi esercitare intorno agl'infermi in quel modo che lui sapeva e potrà, con questo inteso che lui non sia tenuto a ffare la ghuardia agl'infermi la notte perché, come è detto, non è molto sano ... conosciamo che lui è venuto qui per vivere e morire e salvare l'anima sua ad essere amorevole degl'infermi e de' sani ... e avrebbe gran desiderio di guarire interamente per potersi esercitare il dì e la notte a fare ancora la guardia intorno agl'infermi.'
20. See also Kate Lowe's recent discussion of the election and admission of abbesses: 'Elections of Abbesses and Notions of Identity in Fifteenth- and Sixteenth-Century Italy, with Special Reference to Venice', *Renaissance Quarterly*, 54:2 (2001), pp. 389–429.
21. Passerini, *Storia*, p. 667 based his description on 'un libro antichissimo appartenuto al Brefotrofio; libro in pergamena, scritto nei primi anni del secolo XIV' in the Innocenti archive, though there is no trace of it now.
22. See Calzolai, 'Lo spirito di un servizio secolare', pp. 23–33, esp. p. 36. This manuscript has had a chequered history. Though it is allegedly in the Biblioteca Nazionale Centrale di Firenze (Fondo Manoscritti), recent attempts to locate its whereabouts have been in vain. Carlo Calzolai consulted a photocopy of the manuscript kept by the Suore Oblate in their library in Careggi, but even the photocopy has disappeared in the interim!
23. Calzolai, 'Lo spirito di un servizio secolare', p. 32.
24. Cf. also Messer Bonifazio Statutes, ff. 5v–6r; E. Lombardi, *Messer Bonifacio Lupi*, pp. 193–4.
25. On the habits of *conversi* see Beccaria, 'I conversi'.
26. SMN (1510–11), p. 177; the 1330 statutes merely say of the habits: those that 'usuato nel detto spedale': SMN (1330), p. 54.
27. Also true in other parts of Europe: cf. Rawcliffe on England: 'Hospital Nurses', p. 48.
28. Cf. Passerini, *Storia*, pp. 286–7.
29. Levi-D'Ancona, *Miniatura*, pp. 325–6, on Mariano del Buono.
30. BON Statutes, ff. 4v–5r, cited in Passerini, *Storia*, p. 225.
31. SMN 1, f. 2v (1329); cf. also SMN (1330), p. 55; SMN (1510–11), p. 179, no. 11.
32. For Messer Bonifazio see E. Lombardi, *Messer Bonifacio Lupi*, p. 194.
33. Gavitt, *Charity and Children*, pp. 174–9.
34. Goldthwaite and Rearick, 'Michelozzo', pp. 252–8.
35. Outlined by Passerini, *Storia*, pp. 163–76, and summarised in Goldthwaite and Rearick, 'Michelozzo', pp. 227–30.
36. Cf. Rawcliffe, 'Hospital Nurses', p. 48, commenting on hospitals like St Leonard's in York, which followed the Augustinian rule.

37. SMN (1330), p. 57: twice a year: 'le femine non possano andare a confessione fuori del detto spedale, ma nel detto spedale, cioè in chiesa e chapella'; SMN (1374), pp. 71–2; (1510–11), p. 179: confession three times a year; communion twice a year.
38. SMN (1330), p. 58; (1374), p. 73.
39. SMN (1374), p. 73.
40. Summarised in G. Zarri, 'Gender, Religious Institutions and Social Discipline: The Reform of the Regulars', in J.C. Brown and R.C. Davis, eds, *Gender and Society in Renaissance Italy* (London, 1998), pp. 193–212.
41. Rawcliffe, 'Hospital Nurses', pp. 48–9.
42. SMN (1510–11), pp. 187: no. 31.
43. Ibid., pp. 186–7.
44. Ibid., p. 186.
45. Ibid., p. 185; see also SMN (1330), p. 59; (1374), pp. 72, 74. Cf. Henderson, *Piety and Charity*, chs 2–3;
46. SMN (1510–11), pp. 185–6.
47. SMN (1374), pp. 65, 75.
48. SMN (1510–11), p. 179; see also SMN (1374), p. 73.
49. SMN (1330), p. 56: in the hospital's cemetery; SMN (1374), p. 70.
50. SM 184, f. 45v: 'Poi fu morta fu vestita vedovilmente e messa in uno chataletto nel mezzo dello spedale, cioé dalla medicheria inverso la porta in uno chataletto schoperto con molte panche intorno e le donne di chasa cholle mantelle in dosso e chosì le sue parenti … parte stettono in su dette panche e a chapo e appie di detto chataletto erano due chandellieri grandi con torchietti di lb. 6 acciesi. E sepellissi nell'avello allato alla porta che va nella Via del Chochomero.'
51. SM 196, f. 140r: 'noi siamo tenuti quando passa di questa vita vestirla di bigio col cordiglio a uso di Monaca del Terzo Ordine di San Francesco.'
52. Burial in hospital cemetery: SMN (1330), p. 56; SMN (1374), p. 70.
53. SP 644, f. 32r: 1445.
54. SM 195, ff. 155r–156r: 'Essendo oggi questo infrascritto dì xxiiii d'aghosto 1506, che fu la sera a ore 2 di notte, passò di questa vita la buona memoria di Messer Fenzio di Bertoldo Cicioni da San Miniato al Tedescho suto nostro spedalingho, presente frati di Sa(n) Marcho e servittori e donne delle nostre di chasa, cioé Monna Tomasa priora del nostro spedale chon altre sue chonpagnie e altri di chasa, che mancherebe a tuti rispetto lui esser stato di buona vita e di buono esempio che Dio l'abi ricevuto in pacie.
Dipoi che fu mortto aprimo la sua chasetta et essaminamo la sua scarsella, presente Fra Giovan Domenicho, lo Priore del Chonvento di San Marcho, e Ser Simone di Filippo da Montte Lupo nostro chappellano, e Messer Tomaso Spini el schrivano nel nostro spedale … Di poi l'altro dì che fu lunedì adì xxv di deto messe d'aghosto si fecie lo suo ofizio et onoranze di deto Messer Fenzio, che fu invitato tuti e preti di S. Maria del Fiore e frati di San Marcho tuti in buon numero, e più venono e nostri Signori Chonsoli chon tuto el chorpo dell'Artte e venono per onorare el sopradito. Esendo in Firenze uno Girolamo de' Cicioni chonsorto del sopradito messer Fenzio et nostri signori chonsoli lo invitorono e cholloro insieme venono a tale honoranza essendo tutti nella logia a sedere, entrò in perghamo et predichò Marsino … frate de' Servi. Et più venono tutti gli spedalinghi quali venono chollloro chapellani et servi e ciascheduno arechò 4 doppieri e andò dipoi tuti a prociessione in sulla Piaza di San Marcho et per lla via Largha tornorono de San Nicholò. Et tutti entrono in San Matteo e quivi lo sotterorono nella sipoltura degli spedalinghi chon gra[n] numero di ciera intorno e tuta la chiesa et più chandellieri picholi e grandi et tuti e preti ebono uno torchietto e tutto suo chorppo fu messo in una chassa et messosi in deta sepoltura e tuto quello si spenderà apare in questo libro a carta 20, havessi la ciera dal'Agnolo Rafaello.'

NOTES TO PAGES 196–200

55. For a detailed discussion of funerals and commemoration in this period see S.T. Strocchia, *Death and Ritual in Renaissance Florence* (Baltimore and London, 1992).
56. A. Tenenti, *Il senso della morte e l'amore della vita nel Rinascimento* (Turin, 1989), ch. 3.
57. SMN (1374), pp. 63–4, 78; (1510–11), pp. 176, 180.
58. SM 195, f. 155r; 190, f. 41v: 'Monna Maria di Michele Baldacci, maggiore delle nostre donne.'
59. SMN (1510–11), p. 186.
60. Catasto 291, f. 34r; 185.II, f. 606v; Passerini, *Storia*, pp. 302, 305. This would suggest that in a smaller hospital patients might have received more personal attention given that the staff–patient ratio was higher, but one has to exercise caution given that it is not known either what proportion of the staff worked in the ward or how many would have been on duty at any one time. It also has to be remembered that the number of patients varied according to various exogenous factors since hospitals would become flooded with patients during outbreaks of plague, other epidemics and famine: See below, Chapter 8. The same problem with determining the ratio between patients and nursing staff is evident from studies of hospitals elsewhere. For example, one of a comparable scale was the Hôtel-Dieu in Paris, which by the late fifteenth century treated up to five hundred people at any one time. Here the nursing staff consisted of 40 sisters, 28 'filles blanches' or novices, 4 female servants and 14 brothers with financial, legal and spiritual roles, together with a good number of male servants, but once again how many were specifically available to serve the sick at any one time is unknown: Saunier, '*Le pauvre malade*', pp. 79–80, 120–1; cf. also Rawcliffe, 'Hospital Nurses', pp. 43–4.
61. SMN (1510–11), p. 181.
62. Ibid., p. 186.
63. Saunier, '*Le pauvre malade*', p. 132.
64. Cf. Rawcliffe, 'Hospital Nurses', pp. 58–9.
65. SMN (1510–11), p. 183.
66. The fresco, which measures 102 × 163 cm, bears little resemblance to any surviving frescoes found in hospitals in Florence or elsewhere in Italy. They were usually on a much larger scale in the form of narrative cycles of lives of saints that covered whole walls. Pontormo's small fresco was, moreover, in monochrome rather than full colour and was therefore less costly, as in the almost contemporary fresco-cycle for the company of the Scalzo.
67. It is not entirely clear how far we are to believe that the columns were supposed to be part of the ward. It is possible that this was supposed to have been a view into the ward from outside. This would of course have meant a leap of imagination involving the removal of the intervening wall so that the interior of the ward would have been viewed from the contiguous loggia, whose Corinthian columns are reflected here in this elegant arcade. This suggests that the washing of the feet took place in the courtyard rather than in the ward, underlining the more public nature of the event since access to the female ward was restricted. An important feature that this fresco fails to reflect is the height of the ward beyond the arcade, since it is not possible to see properly into the space beyond the beds.
68. Little has been written about this fresco, even though it is mentioned in all the standard works on Pontormo. Most recently see P. Costamagna, *Pontormo* (Milan, 1994), pp. 113–14. See also F.M. Clapp, *Jacopo Carrucci da Pontormo* (New Haven, 1916), p. 115; L. Berti, *Pontormo* (Florence, 1966), esp. p. viii, with bibliography; J. Cox Rearick, *The Drawings of Pontormo* (Cambridge, Mass., 1964), Vol. 1, p. 100; *Frescoes from Florence* (London, 1969), pp. 198–9. The choice of the artist may have been made on the recommendation of the *spedalingo*, Alberto di Piero Bettini, from whose family Pontormo had received another commission: Costamagna, *Pontormo*, p. 113.

69. See, for example, at the Spedale degli Incurabili in Venice at Easter 1524: Henderson in Arrizabalaga, Henderson and French, *The Great Pox*, p. 167.
70. Lucrezia Tornabuoni, *La istoria della casta Susanna*, ed. O. Casazza and P. Orvieto (Bergamo, 1992), pp. 19–21. I am grateful to Judith Bryce for this reference.
71. From a record dated 14–16 Aug. 1402 listing the building work done to date at S. Matteo, it is possible to confirm that the positions of the female refectory and the kitchen in the early fifteenth century corresponded to those shown on the 1780 plan: SM I.A, ff. 21r–v (cf. Plate 3.12).
72. SMN (1510–11), p. 184.
73. Meals: SMN (1330), p. 56; SMN (1374), p. 69; SMN (1510–11), pp. 183–4.
74. He was to have 'una chamera nella fermeria': from SMN 36, f. 468r. Horster, *Andrea del Castagno*, p. 205, doct. 11 publishes the terms of this agreement between S. Maria Nuova and Castagno which established that in addition to a payment of 100 gold florins he was to receive free board and lodging.
75. They rarely mention the presence of frescoes since they normally only listed portable objects. An exception is the following rather cryptic note in S. Matteo's 1454 inventory: 'E'l dipinto della faticha [?] delle donne, costò fiorini 36 dipintura': SM 328, f. 303v.
76. SM 328, f. 303v: 'una crocie di legno con una grillanda di fiori di seta; uno libretto di santi padri comprarono le donne, coperto di sciughatoio; uno messale bello coverto di panno rosato, nuovo.'

    S. Matteo's first inventory also records in the refectory 'due predelle da altari negli spedali'. Evidently the predellas of the altarpieces in the main wards had been detached and displayed in the refectory (SM 108, f. 7v). Why this should have happened is not clear, though it was evidently only a temporary measure since the predellas were no longer listed in their 1454 inventory (SM 328, f. 303r).
77. For S. Paolo see Goldthwaite and Rearick, 'Michelozzo', p. 257. S. Maria Nuova's building accounts confirm that in 1423 it was located on the first floor 'above the cloister of the cemetery', that is, the Chiostro delle Ossa to the left of S. Egidio (Figure 1.1: 4). Payments to the stonemason Maso di Cecchino provide two additional pieces of information about this area: SMN 4474, f. 58v: 'A Maso di Cecchino maestro di scarpello per xiv finestre per le camere ed androne sopra al chiostro del cimiterio e da lato di figliuolo di Francesco Bettini … e per la finestra grande del dormentorio e per una finestra grande che vene sopra all'orto nostro.' The second payment was for the purchase of 5,840 tiles for the roof above 'the rooms of the dormitory', a series of more private single bedrooms in addition to the communal sleeping area: SMN 4474, f. 57r: 24.iii.1423: 'per 5,840 pianelle per lo tetto delle camere del dormentorio sopra al chiostro del cimiterio.'
78. SMN, 1376 inventory, pp. 28–30.
79. SM 108, ff. 9v, 12r; 328, f. 305r (1454 inventory).
80. SM 328, f. 305r: 'la tavola di Nostra Donna in capo di detto dormentorio.'
81. SMN (1510–11), p. 186.
82. For what follows see ibid.
83. Again SM I.A, f. 21r confirms that the position of the kitchen at S. Matteo in 1402 was the same as in 1780.
84. SMN (1510–11), p.186. The same was true at S. Matteo; SM I.A, f. 22r lists 'La casa de'lavatoi e de' fare il pane'.
85. See SMN 24: Plate 2.6 above: the 1780 plan of S. Maria Nuova describes these hatches as the 'Ruote where the nuns place the food for the men'.
86. SMN (1510–11), pp. 184–5.
87. Ibid., p. 183.
88. Ibid.
89. SM 328, ff. 304v–305r. S. Maria Nuova's 1376 inventory (pp. 35–6) surprisingly only contains a brief account.

90. SMN, 1376 inventory, pp. 36–7.
91. SMN (1510–11), p. 187.
92. Ibid., p. 185.
93. See SMN 24, Plan no. 15.
94. Varchi, *Storia fiorentina*, Book 9, p. 101.
95. SMN 4426, ff. 243r–v; cf. above, Chapter 2: Table 2.2.
96. SMN (1510–11), p. 186.
97. Cited by Grieco, 'Il vitto di un ospedale', p. 89.
98. SMN (1510–11), p. 187.
99. Grieco, 'Il vitto di un ospedale', pp. 88–9 on the Innocenti's garden, and more generally on diet at the hospital, a topic that would repay detailed research.
100. The boundaries of S. Matteo consisted of: the hospital buildings themselves, Via della Sapienza on the north, the back of the buildings fronting on to Piazza SS. Annunziata on the east and the convent of S. Niccolò on the south. A smaller area of garden appears to have been under cultivation behind the women's section in 1780 than had been the case in the late sixteenth century.
101. SMN (1510–11), p. 185.
102. Ibid., p. 184.
103. SM 328, ff. 302v–305r.
104. Gavitt, *Charity and Children*, p. 250.
105. The names of the Tertiaries of S. Paolo in the first half of the Trecento are listed in SP 977 and for more information on the hospital's *pinzochere* see Passerini, *Storia*, pp. 170, 173–4, 176. The names of the *conversi* and *converse* of S. Matteo are listed in SM 193, ff. 4r–46r, 123v–29v.
106. Based on SM 193.
107. The names of husband and father were always supplied in the cases of women who either were or had been married.
108. Herlihy and Klapisch-Zuber, *Tuscans and their Families*, p. 216: Table 7.3.
109. This also reflected their relatively high proportion in the adult male population of Florence (48 per cent): ibid.
110. Cf. F. Edler de Roover, *Glossary of Medieval Terms of Business: Italian Series, 1200–1600* (Cambridge, Mass., 1934).
111. SM 125, ff. 9r–v, 12r, 15v, 13r–15r.
112. BON 4, f. 117r: 1470.
113. SM 196, f. 143v: 2.v.1509.
114. SMN 82, f. 215r: 'Inventario delle cose che rimasono di Giovanni Anguilla nostro commesso el quale morì ... dì marzo 1527/8 in camera seconda salito le scale nel dormentorio di Frati di sotto, le quale cose sono queste, cioè in prima: dua saioni di panno mormorino, uno foderato di pelle l'altro di panno fiandrescho foderato di rovescio; una gabbanella di pannolane senza maniche a uso d'Ibernia, uno mantello di panno S. Martino; uno paio di lenzuola con più tovaglie e tovaglinini; sei camice da homo; quattro sciugatoi; sei grembiuli; dieci fodere da guanciali nuove e con ruggine; uno paio di coltegli con maniche d'avorio e con puntali d'argento ed una forchetta perchè detto Giovanni disse in confessione haverla perduta e con un paio di forbicine; dua corniole legate in oro una di ducati tre, l'altra di ducati uno e mezo.'
115. SMN 5792: 'Libro dei chomessi', 1541–87. See also for other books of commessi: 5793: Testamenti e lasciti; 5794: 1504–10; 5795: 1510–19 (incomplete); 5796: 1519–25; 5797: 1485–8; 5798: 1591–5.
116. SMN (1510–11), pp. 179, 177.
117. See Henderson, *Piety and Charity*, pp. 385–7 on the clientele of Orsanmichele, and pp. 393–5 on the Buonomini di S. Martino.
118. Herlihy and Klapisch-Zuber, *Tuscans and their Families*, p. 129: Table 4.8.
119. SMN 5792, c.96: 'Sandra figluola fu di Paghola di Menichuccio da Cerreto Guidi, già serva di Monna Maria di Portinari.'

120. Though nine of those admitted to Messer Bonifazio between 1405 and 1412 were from outside Florence, including one from Cologne and another from Albania: BON 387, ff. 21r–82r.
121. SM 190, f. 132r. See also the case of Monna Lucia di Piero *pinzochera*, who in 1488 gave S. Matteo 27 florins and in return was provided with two bushels of good-quality *grano* each year. As in other cases of contracts with *commesse*, Monna Lucia remained living in her house: 1488: SM 190, f. 134r.
122. SM 125, f. 21r.
123. Ibid., ff. 5v–6r.
124. SM 197, f. 193v: 'Ricordo come questo dì 19 d'agosto 1517 Bartholomeo di Bastiano di Michele da San Piero Gattolini è venuto a stare nel nostro spedale di San Matteo per servigiale e à donato a' poveri nel nostro spedale fior. 40 li d'oro'. See page 397 note 19.

'E per fede del verso io p. Alberto Bettino spedalingho ò fatto questo ricordo di mia propria mano e perchè il detto Bartholomeo non sa scrivere vole ed è contento si io scrivi per lui.'
125. SM 196, f. 131r: 1507: 'Ricordo come oggi questo dì 24 di diciembre 1506 Chorso di Stefano di Chorso da Luchulena di Valdarno di Sopra essendo d'anni settantotto in circha e avendo la quartana e volendosi commettere nel nostro spedale per la salute e quiete dell'anima sua e chorpo à dipositato nel nostro spedale flor. 10 d'oro in oro.' He was accepted on 10 May 1507.
126. SM 192, f. 145r: Bartolomeo di Tommaso Sassetti gave 50 gold florins. In return S. Matteo gave 'le spese del suo vivere durante la sua vita nel modo si dà a' chapellani e agli altri chomessi. E darli una chamera per suo uso che abbia aquaio e necessario e chamino dove possa fare fuocho ne' tempi bisognevoli cho[n] legna dello spedale e chon uno letto fornito. Quando Bartolomeo volessi mangiare in chamera li sia dati la separati a sua posta e quando volessi comprare più una chosa o l'altra lo debba fare di sue danari propri e lo spedale glie debbe fare quocere.

'Nel tempo della Quaresima perché lui à d'età d'anni 80 e non ci è obrighato nè potrebbe farle debba lo spedale darli il bisogno suo chostumatamente.

'In chaso di morìa sia lecito a Bartolomeo andare dove li pare ello spedale lo debba provedere delle ispese credito [?] di buono huomo.

'A Bartolomeo sia lecito d'usare il barbiere dello ispedale e per lo simile li debba essere inbianchati i panni per suo uso.

'Item in chaso d'infermità debb'essere ghovernato chon amore perché è questi la prima chagione perché lui si chometi nello spedale e quando anchora lui volessi altro medicho lo debba paghare lui de' sui propri danari.

'Quando lui volessi andare a starssi cho' figliuoli e con altri non debba lo spedale in quel tempo darli alchuna chosa. La sspesa de suoi vestiti se le debba fare lui de's-suoi proprii danari sichè lo spedale non abbi fornire nulla. E lle sue massarizie e panni possa sempre fornire la sua voluntà.'
127. Rawcliffe, 'Hospital Nurses'.
128. SM 198, f. 265v: 'Monna Piera di … d'Aranga d'anni 40 in circha la quale essendo alquanto malata nel nostro spedale e essendoci ancora la nostra casiera di Fibiana parlando fra loro insieme finalmente venie in questa conclusione che la detta Monna Piera ci dia e doni flor. 50 d'oro per la sua commissione inanzi venga per habitare in detto spedale … concordisi che detta Monna Piera non possi venire per stare stantialmente in detto spedale o ne sua siti se none passati e finiti sette anni da ogi. E questo si fa per dua cagione: primo, perché di lei al presente non ci è di bisogno, e secundario perché a Fibiana dove noi facciamo pensiero che sia e luogho suo per casiera come ne siano d'accordo ci pare per ancora troppa govane e però habiamo per lo detto tempo se già non fussi malata ese in detto tempo amalassi overo mancassi…

Ma passati detti sette anni comportandosi bene come intendiamo s'è portata per infino a questo dì vogliamo possa venire e avere la tornata in detto luogo o di fuora per casiera e avere victo e vestito come anno l'altre nostre commesse di casa durante la sua vita.'

On the widow's right of *tornata* see Klapisch-Zuber, *Women, Family and Ritual in Renaissance Italy*, pp. 122–4.

129. Redon, 'Autour'; Henderson, 'The Hospitals', p. 80.
130. Saunier, '*Le pauvre malade*', pp. 122–3.
131. Rawcliffe, 'Hospital Nurses', pp. 48–9.
132. D. Herlihy, 'Growing Old in the Quattrocento', in P. Stearns, ed., *Old Age in Pre-Industrial Society* (New York, 1982), p. 104.
133. SM 198, ff. 258r–v: 'Ricordo come Monna Ginevra figlia fu di Sandro d'Antonio del Pescaia e al presente serva di Monna Gostanza donna fu di Bononcino Baroncini ci à dato in diposito flor. 17 lb. d'oro e Lire 1 ... sia tenuto a riceptala sempre in tutte le sue infermità e tractarla a uso di comessa, come si fussi una delle nostre di casa. E quando detta Monna Ginevra pervenissi all'età di 60 anni in modo non potessi durare più fatica, che oggi secondo intendiamo è di età d'anni 33 in circa, detto spedale solvigla riceptarla qui in casa dargli vita e vestito.'
134. SM 188, f. 72v: 22.vii.1471: 'El quale Michele è stato amalato di grave infermità et perchè el padre è ciecho e va achattando et non sappendo che fare di questo suo figliuolo, da hora loda e dona al nostro spedale per stare perpetuo in detto spedale a servire infermi e tanto fare quanto gli farà commesso da me e da miei successori e chosì disse el fanciullo essere confinato e obblighasi quando sia la volontà di detto Baronc suo padre.'
135. SM 193, ff. 113v–114r (1496).
136. SM 190, f. 133r. The date of this entry, 24.i.1488, records the deposit of the dowry and the agreement with the Buonomini di S. Martino, and refers to the fact that Ginevra was already living in the hospital. See also the example of Monna Lisa and Monna Mea, 'sorelle e fi[glie] che furono di Nicholaio di Pippo Falcieri', whose gift of 80 gold florins enabled them to stay in the hospital: SM 193, f. 121r: 14.xi.1497.
137. See Henderson, *Piety and Charity*, ch. 8, pp. 394–5.
138. SM 191, f. 145r: 29.xi.1490.
139. SM 125 f. 10v.
140. Ibid., ff. 16r–v; continues on ff. 18r–20r.
141. Examples of agreements between couples and S. Matteo include: SM 189, f. 121r (1486); 190, f. 136r (1488); 190, ff. 139v, 141r (1489); 191, f. 146r (1491) ('casa sua'); 191, f. 155r (1493); 193, ff. 115v, 116v (1496); f. 150r (1510); f. 195v (1516).
142. SM 197, ff. 195v–196r.
143. Barcelona: Brodman, *Charity and Welfare*, p. 58; Paris: Saunier, '*Le pauvre malade*', pp. 119–22; York: P. Cullum, *Cremetts and Corrodies: Care of the Poor and Sick at St. Leonard's Hospital, York, in the Middle Ages* (York, 1991), pp. 26–7.
144. Quoted in Gavitt, *Charity and Children*, p. 155.

Chapter 7

1. (Basle, 1565), col. 905. Cited in J.J. Bylebyl, 'The School of Padua: Humanistic Medicine in the Sixteenth Century', in C. Webster, ed., *Health, Medicine and Mortality in the Sixteenth Century* (Cambridge, 1979), p. 348.
2. For what follows see ibid., pp. 335–70.
3. Ibid., p. 348.
4. R. French, 'The Medical Ethics of Gabriele de' Zerbi', in A. Wear, J. Geyer-Kordesch and R.K. French, eds, *Doctors and Ethics: The Earlier Historical Setting of Professional Ethics*, in *Clio Medica*, 24 (1993), pp. 74, 83.

5. G. Zerbus, *Opus utile de cautelis medicorum* (Padua, 1495), p. 57; cited by Park, *Doctors*, p. 68.
6. See Park, *Doctors*, pp. 66–72. On the medical marketplace and medical pluralism see D. Gentilcore, *Healers and Healing in Early Modern Italy* (Manchester, 1998); Pomata, *Contracting a Cure*.
7. R. Ciasca, ed., *Statuti dell'Arte dei medici e speziali di Firenze* (Florence, 1922), p. 23.
8. Catasto 81, f. 171r: Park, *Doctors*, p. 104 n. 59.
9. These figures may not be complete since not all the records of the main medical hospitals have survived from the fourteenth and fifteenth centuries. However, I have consulted all surviving documentation up to 1500 for Messer Bonifazio, S. Matteo and S. Paolo. Given the size of its archive, I have not examined all the financial records of S. Maria Nuova, but instead its 'Creditori e Debitori', which summarise all other ledgers, and, where this was not possible, its 'Entrata e Uscita'.
10. On S. Gallo see G. Pinto, 'Forme di conduzione e rendita fondiaria nel contado fiorentino: le terre dell'Ospedale di San Gallo', in *La Toscana nel tardo medioevo* (Florence, 1982), pp. 247–329. On the Innocenti see Gavitt, *Charity and Children*; Sandri, ed., *Gli Innocenti a Firenze nei secoli*.
11. They were Maestro Filippo, 'che medicha degli ochi', and Maestro Falconi del Maestro Rinuccio da Montalbino, 'medicus ocularis': SMN 4390, ff. 7v, 23v, 34v; SMN 4392, f. 20r; SMN 398, f. 43v.
12. SP 661: Jan. 1348 (under date: unpaginated).
13. SP 676: Feb. 1359; SMN 30: 15.iv.1362.
14. AIOF, ser. II, no. 5 (45), ff. 44r–48r.
15. Cited by Park, *Doctors*, p. 80.
16. BON 5, f. 12r and BON 6, f. 26v; SMN 5876, c. 109; SM 188, f. 39r. Even well-known local practitioners such as Maestro Lodovicho di Maestro Piero di Maestro Domenicho when employed by S. Maria Nuova could also be listed simply as 'nostro medicho nello spedale', whereas he was recorded elsewhere as a physician. He came from the Toscanelli family which had a long tradition of service as hospital physicians and of prominence in the guild and College of Physicians: SMN 5876, cc. 143, 644. See Park, *Doctors*, p. 32.
17. SMN 4477, ff. 38r, 39r: 1423–8; SMN 5817, c. 90: 1441, 1443–51; SMN 5818: 1443–51. See also Park, *Doctors*, pp. 67–8, 105n, 156n, 249.
18. SM 188, f. 32v; BON 4, f. 69v. This may be the same 'Maestro Batista medicho' who worked for S. Maria Nuova in 1465: SMN 5069, f. 124v.
19. Gavitt, *Charity and Children*, pp. 156–7.
20. Doctors supplying medicines from their workshops: 1325–6: Maestro Duccio, Maestro Durante medico, Maestro Dino (SMN 4390: ff. 2r, 11r, 46v; see also a payment in 1351 to 'Frate Antonio per pillole': SMN 4398, f. 44v).
21. SMN 4437, f. 42r: 'un libro di medicina per lo maestro di casa che si chiama Silogisme.'
22. Park, *Doctors*, pp. 28–30.
23. Ibid., pp. 163 n. 34; Park, 'The Readers at the Florentine Studio according to Communal Fiscal Records (1357–1380, 1413–1446)', *Rinascimento*, 2nd ser. 20 (1980), pp. 290, 294, 301, 302. Employed by S. Matteo: SM 186, f. 207r; 328, ff. 187r, 262r.
24. Park, *Doctors*, p. 75: Table 2.2.
25. Ibid., pp. 37, 75–8.
26. Cf. ibid., p. 75: Table 2.2: Classes of Doctors in City Tax Roles; in 1451 physicians and surgeons represented 73 per cent compared with 66 per cent a hundred years earlier.
27. SM 328, f. 92r: 'Maestro Donato d'Aghostino Bartolini medicho di fisicho e di cierusicho questo dì 9 d'aprile 1445 è stato d'achordo chon Girolamo d'Antonio nostro spedalingo di venire al nostro spedale per medicho a medichare qualunche bisognio

ochorresse a qualunche infermo di chasa o degli spedali infermi chosì da lato degli uomini chome da lato delle donne.'
28. As in the case of Maestro Domenicho di Piero employed by S. Maria Nuova in 1443: SMN 4477, c.33, or Maestro Antonio di Gianotto, whom S. Maria Nuova employed in 1401 as 'nostro medicho' who 'helps to [provide] treatment in the house': SMN 4453, f. 47r: 30.xi.1401.
29. For the Innocenti, see Gavitt, *Charity and Children*, pp. 154–7; and on monasteries, Park, *Doctors*, pp. 99–101.
30. Mencacci, 'L'assistenza sanitaria nello Spedale di Altopascio', pp. 130–2.
31. For what follows see SMN (1510–11), p. 182.
32. Ibid.
33. Ibid.
34. Ibid.
35. SMN 193, no. 67: 'Maestro Lorenzo di Michele Poggini, medico fisico in Firenze e dottorato a Pisa, già circha iv anni sono, debba per sei mesi attendere a medicare in Santa Maria Nuova e non possa fuori pigliare cure, ma si bene trovarsi in compagnia d'altri medici pratichi a vedere le loro ordinationi et cure.'
36. SMN 4453, ff. 44v, 47r.
37. Catasto 49, f. 55r.
38. BON 387, f. 15r. Cf. also Park, *Doctors*, p. 104 n. 61.
39. Cf. Goldthwaite, *The Building*, pp. 348–9 for wages and pp. 430, 436–9 for the changing value of the florin and wages in the fifteenth century.
40. For these figures see Park, *Doctors*, pp. 110, 113.
41. Ibid., p. 141.
42. See ibid., p. 104 n. 61; G. Pinto, 'Il personale, le balie e i salariati dell'Ospedale di San Gallo di Firenze negli anni 1395–1406: Note per la storia del salariato nelle città medievale', *Ricerche storiche*, n.s. 2 (1974), p. 91.
43. BON 5, f. 12r; BON 7, ff. 5r, 2v–13r; SM 335, f. 69r; SMN 5880, f. 208v; cf. also Park, *Doctors*, pp. 50–1, 53, 100 n. 49; 113–14n, 197n, 235–6.
44. On the Innocenti see Gavitt, *Charity and Children*, pp. 154–7.
45. See 'Ricordanze di Maestro Baccio di Lodovicho Alberighi cerusico, 1516–1551', AOIF, ser. 144. 22, ff. 1r, 3r, 6r–v, 7v, 8r, 11v ('per cavare sangue e altre apartenenze da lato delle donne').
46. BON 6, f. 12r.
47. Gavitt, *Charity and Children*, pp. 155–6.
48. Cited in ibid., p. 155 from the Innocenti's records: AOIF, Ricordanze A (XII,1), f. 3v: 8.iii.1445.
49. MAP XXXV.924: cited in Park, *Doctors*, p. 141 n. 71.
50. SMN (1510–11), p. 182.
51. Ibid., p. 186.
52. SMN, 'Ricettario' (see below, Chapter 9), ff. 66v ('Pillole di Benedetta'); f. 44r ('Unguento da capi rotti … il quale unguento lo facieva Monna Caterina'); f. 44v ('Unguento da capi rotti … da Monna Francesca e Monna Caterina'); f. 74r ('Lattovaro di Benedetta'); f. 190v ('Unguento nero il quale fa Maestra Caterina medicha di casa').
53. Ibid., f. 44v.
54. Ibid., f. 190v: 'Unghuento nero fine il quale fa maestra Caterina medicha di casa et ène buono a dolglie et a fferite et a talgliature e a capo ropto che ssia percosso o a qualunque altro male e si pone mirabilmente ad opera al capo rotto.'
55. BON 387, ff. 15r–16r.
56. Ibid., ff. 36r, 81r.
57. SM 186, f. 206v.
58. His contract is in SM 188, ff. 71r–v.

59. Ibid., f. 71v: 'et promette servire a qualunque tempo, chosì a tempo di pestilentia la quale Iddio piacessi chome a qualunque altro tempo, et debba fare prima residentia nel nostro spedale di dì e di notte.'
60. SM 328, f. 92r. For price of wheat see Goldthwaite, 'I prezzi', p. 33, and for the soldi-florin exchange rate Goldthwaite, *The Building*, p. 430. For Maestro Donato see Park, *Doctors*, p. 129 and n. 37; A. Gherardi, ed., *Statuti della università e studio fiorentino dell'anno 1387* (Florence, 1881), p. 414; Park, 'The Readers at the Florentine Studio', pp. 288, 290, 295.
61. SM 186, f. 206v: 20.vii.1468: 'Richordo chome oggi questo dì 20 di luglio 1468 Messer Lucha di ... nostro spedalingho è rimaso d'achordo chon Maestro Fruosino d'Andrea barbiere ch'el decto Maestro Fruosino debbe venire o mandare e sua gharzoni a radere e ghovernare tutta la famiglia di chasa chosì gli infermi, chome e servi, bene e diligentemente di 15 dì una volta a tempo d'inverno e a tempo d'estate ogni dì una volta. E oltre a questo el detto Maestro Fruosini s'obligha venire personalmente ogni mattina, lui ol suo chonpagno, per un'ora o per quello bisognierà, a stare alla nostra medicheria e medichare e churare bene e diligentemente tutti e nostri infermi o inferme avessimo nel nostro spedale e simile la famiglia di chasa, eziandio tutti quegli che venissino di fuori per medichamessi de' loro bisogni. E più s'obbligha el detto Fruosino di trarre sanghue e denti e reparare chome s'achadesse al bisogno a tutti e nostri infermi e inferme e famiglia di detto spedale. E tutte queste chose s'obligha di fare el detto Maestro Fruosino per un'anno, chominciato detto dì sopradetto e finito adì 19 di luglio 1469. E tutto questo fa per pregio e prezzo di fiorini 40 piccioli.'

  See also the contract with the barber Giovanni di Martino on 1 April 1442 for similar conditions.
62. SM 328, f. 15r: 1.iv.1442.
63. Ibid., f. 15r; SM 188, f. 72v.
64. Incurabili statutes, as discussed further by Henderson in Arrizabalaga, Henderson and French, *The Great Pox*, chs 7–8.
65. SM 328, f. 15r.
66. SM 196, f. 154v: Maestro Nicholò di Gianghano di Nicholò was employed in May 1511 for the 'consolatione di tutti i feriti e piaghati che verranno a essere curati in questo spedale.' In the same year the discussion of the role of surgery in S. Maria Nuova's 'Ordinances' was confined to a comment about treatment of 'sores and other minor illnesses' in their Medicheria. Cf. SMN 4424, f. 16r: 'Uno lastrone grande che bisongniò per la bottegha della medicheria: lire 1 1s' (8.v.1369).
67. SMN 4390, ff. 7v, 23v, 34v; his place as 'medici oculares' was taken in the early 1350s by Maestro Falconi di Maestro Rinuccio da Montalbino.
68. SMN 4458, f. 103v; SMN 4468, f. 29r; cf. Park, *Doctors*, pp. 67–8 n. 66.
69. SMN 4483, f. 44v.
70. SMN 59, f. 81r; cf. Park, *Doctors*, p. 69.
71. SM 186, f. 206v: 20.vii.1468.
72. SM 328, f. 302v (1454); 196, f. 137r (1508).
73. SMN 84, ff. 5r–v: 'Inventario de ferri della medicheria di Santa Maria Nuova, i quali stanno nel primo, quarto, terzo armadio:

  '*Il primo armadio ha stanze tre*:
  Nella prima sono dua argani da rassettare gambe; Sei ferri da dar fuoco a fistole
  Una carriola
  '*Nel secondo armadio*:
  Quattro speculi; 24 ferri da cavar palle extra
  5 scatole che sono nel quinto armadio le quali conoscono da numeri
    la prima ha dieci bruschi alla moderna
    tre zappette alla moderna
    5 gambautti in una guaina

2 ferri a uso di lime
   4 coltelli da sparare
   '*Seconda scatola* ha un mulinello alla moderna cioè:
   4 nespole; 12 lunette alla moderna; 9 bruschi doppi antichi; 1 lenticula; 4 lieve;
   1 tappetta; 1 martellino di piombo
   '*Quarta scatola*
   1 mulinello alla moderna; 5 lunette alla moderna; 5 poponcini; 2 lengticule;
   7 bruschi alla moderna; 2 serpentine; 8 nespole alla moderna
   1 tappetta; 5 lieve alla moderna
   '*La quinta scatola* ha ferri alla antica cioè:
   2 siringhe; 2 ferri da fuoco alle fistole; 1 ferro a rottorio acompagniato
   1 ottoncino fatto atromba; 1 allacciatoio accompagniato; 1 ferro da tagliare e dare fuoco
   1 ferro da tagliare la vergha; 3 ferri piccoli da dar fuoco
   '*Il terzo armadio* ve ferri da fuoco quali ferri sono di più sorte ma tutti alla moderna et sono in tutti:
   6 seghe cattive; 3 ferri da norcini; 1 segha buona; 1 chiave da rettor; 1 morse doppia da fistole
   '*Robe della medicheria che si adoperano giornalmente*:
   2 cassette grande per tenere al bancho di ottone
   2 cassette pichole per andare alle letta
   7 bacini tra grandi e picholi; 2 padellini grandi; 1 padellino picholino
   1 calderotto per distrugere cerotti; 3 calderotti per gli impiastri
   1 catinella di rame per mettere la farinata
   3 caldani di rame; 1 caldano per scaldare ferri
   3 padellini per li unguenti; 2 padellini per scaldare l'olio; 2 ferri per tenere caldani
   1 manticino; 1 caldano per mettere in caldo.'
74. The copy in Italian that belonged to S. Maria Nuova is listed in S. de Ricci, *Census of Medieval and Renaissance Manuscripts in the US and Canada* (New York, 1937), Vol. 2, pp. 1311–12. I am grateful to Peter Murray Jones for this reference.
75. SMN 84, ff. 5r–v.
76. Park, *Doctors*, pp. 42–3.
77. Ibid., pp. 42–5.
78. For the size of these places in 1427 see Herlihy and Klapisch-Zuber, *Tuscans and their Families*, p. 34; p. 58: Table 2.2.
79. Park, *Doctors*, pp. 79–80.
80. See BON 387, f. 16r.
81. Employed by S. Maria Nuova in 1476–8: see SMN 5875.
82. This number represented less than a third of the thirty-seven medical practitioners recorded as having submitted a return in Florence. Park, *Doctors*, Appendix III: pp. 249–52.
83. Herlihy and Klapisch-Zuber, *Tuscans and their Families*, p. 129: Table 7.8.
84. On Maestro Lionardo see Park, *Doctors*, pp. 181–2, 251. At the time of the Catasto of 1427 he was aged fifty-four. He was paid a salary by S. Maria Nuova in March 1415: SMN 4468, f. 29r; and is recorded as having received money the previous December related to a property transaction: SMN 5047, f. 141r: 26.xii.1414.
85. On Maestro Domenicho di Piero see Park, *Doctors*, pp. 32, 168, 172–3, 249. On his wealth see Catasto 67, ff. 92v–6v: Park, *Doctors*, p. 156n. He is recorded as working for S. Maria Nuova in 1443: SMN 5818, c.33.
86. On his 1427 Catasto return see Park, *Doctors*; pp. 169, 195, 250. He worked for the hospital of S. Matteo in 1409 and 1413: SM 326, f. 90r; 180, ff. 120v, 124r.
87. Franceschi di Nolo was employed by S. Maria Nuova from 1349 to 1353: SMN 4398, ff. 3v, 4r, 42v; 4400, f. 11r. According to Park (personal communication), he was

matriculated in the Arte in 1345/6 and appeared in the household tax of the Sega in 1351–2. Luca di Cecho was employed by S. Maria Nuova between 1373 and 1378: SMN 4426, ff. 258r–60r: 1373–4; 4428, f. xxxvb: 1374–8. According to Park (personal communication), he was matriculated in the Arte in 1363 and was cancelled as *miserabilis* in the Prestanze of 1369/70.

88. SMN 4437, f. 94r.
89. He was elected consul in 1383, 1388 and 1392; I am grateful to Katharine Park for this information.
90. Park, *Doctors*, pp. 45, 162, 169, 182n, 183n, 185. He was elected Prior in 1377 and 1390.
91. Bonifazio: 1405, 1425: BON 387, f. 15r: paid 6 gold florins a year and recorded as having died in 1425, when he was on the staff there; S. Paolo (1425): Park, *Doctors*, p. 104 n. 61; S. Gallo: Pinto, 'Il personale', p. 91: Maestro Cristofano, 1395–1406. His will is in Not. Antecos. F. 299 [1422–3].
92. On his social origins and political career see Park, *Doctors*, pp. 163, 169–70, 173–4, 177.
93. Brucker, *The Civic World of Early Renaissance Florence*, p. 269; Park, *Doctors*, pp. 182–4.
94. Park, *Doctors*, pp. 98, 116, 141.
95. Ibid., p. 163 n. 34; for employment by S. Matteo see SM 186, f. 207r; 328, ff. 187r, 262r.
96. See Park, *Doctors*, p. 32 for a family tree. On Domenicho see Park, *Doctors*, pp. 156n, 168, 172–3; on S. Maria Nuova see SMN 5818, c. 33. On Piero see Park, *Doctors*, pp. 29, 32, 54, 55n, 134n, 168n, 176, 182n, 183n, 185n; and on his involvement with S. Maria Nuova: SMN 4483, f. 49v; 5818, c. 209; 5876, c. 538. On Lodovicho see Park, *Doctors*, p. 32; and on his employment by S. Maria Nuova see SMN 5876, cc. 143, 644.
97. See *The Letters of Marsilio Ficino*, trans. School of Economic Science, London (London, 1978), Vol. 1, pp. 126–7 for his comments on his father.
98. On his social origins see Park, *Doctors*, pp. 114, 196n: he was listed in the Catasto of 1451 and 1458, and died in 1476–7. He was the Medici house doctor for Piero de' Medici: G. Pieraccini, *La Stirpe de' Medici di Cafaggiolo* (Florence, 1986), Vol. 1, pp. 29–33, 57–68, 87–92, 128–33. He was also doctor to Giovanni Rucellai's daughter-in-law: F.W. Kent, 'The Making of a Renaissance Patron of the Arts', in F.W. Kent, A. Perosa, B. Preyer, P. Sanpaolesi and R. Salvini, *Giovanni Rucellai ed il suo zibaldone*, Vol. 2. *A Florentine Patrician and his Palace* (London, 1981), p. 66 n. 5. He was also a member of the College in 1467 (thanks to Jonathan Davies for this reference). Hospitals: S. Maria Nuova: 1470–6: 'medicho [fisicho] nello spedale': SMN 5818, c. 210; SMN 5875 under 1476; Innocenti: from 1445 (Gavitt, *Charity and Children*, p. 155). See SMN 75, f. 353v for the books he donated to S. Maria Nuova.
99. Those hospital doctors who have also been identified as members of the College include Maestro Francesco di Messer Niccolò da Choltegrana, Maestro Cristofano di Giorgio Brandaglini, Maestro Domenicho di Maestro Giovanni di Maestro Ciuccio da Orvieto, Maestro Bartolomeo di Chambio, Maestro Ugholino di Piero da Pisa, Maestro Piero di Domenicho di Niccholò dal Pozzo Toscanelli, Maestro Lodovicho di Maestro Piero di Maestro Domenicho dal Pozzo Toscanelli, Maestro Mariotto di Niccholò di Gerino Gerini, Maestro Bandino di Maestro Giovanni Banducci da Prato, Maestro Lorenzo di Francesco di Domenico Marchi da Firenze, and Maestro Simone di Cinozzo di Giovanni Cini. I am most grateful to Jonathan Davies for the information on these physicians' membership of the College.
100. Park, *Doctors*, p. 39.
101. On these three physicians see Park, *Doctors*, pp. 105n, 141n, 156, 175, 182n, 249.
102. Park, 'The Readers', pp. 249–52.
103. See H. Rashdall, *The Universities of Europe in the Middle Ages*, 2nd edn, ed. F.M.

Powicke and A.B. Emden (Oxford, 1936), Vol. 2, pp. 47–8, and, more recently, Park, 'The Readers', pp. 249–310.
104. S. Matteo: SM 180, ff. 120v, 124r: 'Maestro Tomaxo d'Arezzo'; Maestro Lorenzo da Bibbiena: SMN 5818 (under 1474); I am grateful to Jonathan Davies for the dates of graduation. For Ficino's father see P.O. Kristeller, *Marsilio Ficino and his Work after Five Hundred Years* (Florence, 1987), p. 157. Employment by S. Maria Nuova in 1454: SMN 4497, f. 86r; 1474, 1476–7: 'Maestro Fecino d'Angnolo da Figline medichò e oggi medicha qui nello spedale': SMN 5818, c. 227; 'Maestro Fecino d'Angnolo medicho cierusicho': 1476–8: SMN 5875. Also by the hospital of S. Matteo: 'condotto a medichare': 1464: SM 186, f. 63r ('Maestro Fecino medicho cierusicho'): paid 8 gold florins p.a.
105. Kristeller, *Marsilio Ficino*, p. 157. He was employed by the hospital of Messer Bonifazio between 1444 and 1450: BON 398, ff. 50v–51r.
106. Maestro Bartholomeo di Nicholò Babachari da Lucha: on his teaching at the Studio see Park, 'The Readers', pp. 264–6; and for S. Matteo: 1409: SM 326, ff. 90r, 311v; 1410: SM 180, f. 52r. According to his tax declaration of 1427, he had a net wealth of 758 gold florins.
107. Maestro Bartolomeo di Chambio, 'medicho di fisico et di cierusicho': for his 1427 Catasto return see Park, *Doctors*, p. 249; he taught surgery at the Studio in 1419–20: Park, 'The Readers', p. 278. For his association with hospitals see S. Matteo: 'nostro medicho di fisico et di cierusicho': 1438: SM 254, f. 145r; 1442: SM 328, f. 59r; also employed by Messer Bonifazio in 1425: BON 392, f. 181r (Park, *Doctors*, pp. 156 n. 11, 249). Evidently also associated with S. Maria Nuova: he received money, though not described as a salary, on 13.vii.1415: SMN 5047 (under date).
108. See Park, *Doctors*, p. 129; Park, 'The Readers', pp. 288, 290, 295; Gherardi, *Statuti*, p. 414. He appears in both the Catasto of 1430 and that of 1450. For S. Matteo see SM 328, f. 92r.
109. Maestro Simone di Cinozzo's contracts with S. Matteo ran from 1442 to 1448, 1449 to 1450 and 1455 to 1468. For his connection with the Studio see Park, 'The Readers', pp. 290, 294, 301, 302; and for his employment by hospitals see SM 186, f. 207r: 1442–8; SM 328, ff. 187r, 262r: 1449–50, 1455, 1468. He was also an employee of the Badia Fiorentina: Park, *Doctors*, p. 100 n. 51.
110. My thanks to Jonathan Davies for supplying data about his role in the College.
111. For example, Lucarella, *Storia dell'arcispedale di Santa Maria Nuova di Firenze*, p. 131; E. Panconesi, 'S. Maria Nuova nella storia della medicina e del suo insegnamento', in *Santa Maria Nuova in Firenze: memorie, testimonianze, prospettive* (Florence, 1991), pp. 55–9; F. Marchi and G. Zambaldi, 'La scuola medica di Santa Maria Nuova', in ibid., p. 213; P. Luzzi and F. Fabbri, 'Tre orti botanici di Firenze', in S. Ferri and F. Vannozzi, eds, *I giardini dei semplici e gli orti botanici della Toscana* (Perugia, 1993), pp. 241–4. In general see E. Coturri, 'Vi furono, nella Toscana settentrionale, nell'alto medioevo, scuole nelle quali si insegnò la medicina?' in M. Santoro, ed., *Atti della IV biennale della Marca per la storia della medicina* (Fermo, 1961), pp. 339–51.
112. SMN (1510–11), p. 182.
113. See G. Fioravanti, 'La Filosofia e la medicina (1343–1543)', in E. Amatori, ed., *Storia dell'Università di Pisa* (Pisa, 1993), Vol. 1, pp. 267ff.
114. Park, *Doctors*, p. 61.
115. Ibid.
116. Ibid., pp. 38–9, 60–1, C.D. O'Malley and J.B. de C.M. Saunders, *Leonardo da Vinci on the Human Body: The Anatomical, Physiological, and Embryological Drawings of Leonardo da Vinci* (New York, 1952; 1982), p. 10.
117. K.D. Keele and C. Pedretti, *Leonardo da Vinci. Corpus of Anatomical Studies in the Collection of Her Majesty the Queen at Windsor Castle* (London and New York, 1979–80), vol. 2, pp. 205–6. See also: M. Azzolini, 'Leonardo in Context: Medical

Ideas and Practices in Renaissance Milan' (unpublished PhD thesis, University of Cambridge, 2001).
118. A. Benivieni, *De abditis nonnullis ac mirandis morborum et sanationum causis*, ed. G. Weber (Florence, 1994).
119. N. Siraisi, *The Clock and the Mirror. Girolamo Cardano and Renaissance Medicine* (Princeton, 1997), pp. 98–9.
120. As printed in K.-E. Barzman, *The Florentine Academy and the Early Modern State. The Discipline of Disegno* (Cambridge, 2000), p. 233; see also ibid., pp. 30, 56, 163–72.
121. Park, *Doctors*, p. 53.

Chapter 8

1. *Prediche del Beato Fra Giordano da Rivalto*, Vol. 1, p. 55.
2. Landino, *Scritti critici e teorici*, Vol. 1, p. 116.
3. Del Migliore, *Firenze*.
4. To Lorenzo degli Strozzi in Bruges, 25 Aug. 1461: *Lettere di una gentildonna fiorentina del secolo XV ai figliuoli esuli*, ed. C. Guasti (Florence, 1877), p. 249.
5. SMN (1510–11), p. 181.
6. For what follows see ibid., p. 182.
7. Ibid., p. 181.
8. In the case of the first and fourth hospitals I shall summarise studies by Lucia Sandri and Bernice Trexler, with additional analysis to address further questions raised by the material.
9. Park, 'Healing the Poor'; G.B. Ravenni, 'I libri dei morti dell'ospedale di Santa Maria Nuova di Firenze come fonti per lo studio della mortalità durante le crisi di sussistenza', in *La popolazione italiana nel Settecento* (Bologna, 1980); Sandri, 'Ospedali e utenti dell'assistenza'.
10. See above, Chapter 2.
11. A. Conti, G. Conti and P. Pirillo, eds, *Lo Spedale Serristori di Figline. Documenti e arredi* (Florence, 1982), pp. 21–33.
12. Trexler, 'Hospital Patients', pp. 50–1.
13. See, for example, SMN 733: 'Libro dei morti dei maschi'; cf. Chaney,' "Philanthropy in Italy" ', p. 191.
14. Pampaloni, ed., *Lo Spedale di S. Maria Nuova*, ch. 4.
15. Passerini, *Storia*, pp. 359–63.
16. An approximate idea can be obtained by extrapolating from the known totals of patients dying, an annual average of thirty in the period 1413 to 1456: Sandri, 'Ospedali e utenti', p. 68; Table 2.
17. Paolucci and Pinto, 'Gli "infermi" ', p. 127.
18. Trexler, 'Hospital Patients', p. 43. The admission books have not survived for female patients, but if we assume the same occupancy rate for the women's fifteen beds as for the men's twenty beds, 273 women would have been admitted.
19. Landino, *Scritti critici e teorici*, Vol. 1, p. 116.
20. As suggested by Park, 'Healing the Poor'.
21. For rates of real wages of unskilled labourers in Florence in this period see Goldthwaite, *The Building*, pp. 438–9.
22. Cf. Goldthwaite, *The Building*, Appendix; A. Corradi, *Annali delle epidemie occorse in Italia dalle prime memorie fino al 1850* (Bologna, 1865–9; repr. 1973), under years.
23. Studies of Sandri, 'Ospedali e utenti', pp. 63–8, esp. p. 68: Table 2; and Paolucci and Pinto, 'Gli "infermi" ', pp. 124–9, esp. p. 126: Table 4.
24. Main mortality peaks are summarised from the city's 'Books of the Dead' in Carmichael, *Plague and the Poor*, p. 36: Table 23.

25. For a more detailed analysis of mortality in these plague years see Carmichael, *Plague and the Poor*, ch. 3.
26. See discussion above, Chapter 3.5, on the role of hospitals as lazzarettos in the Quattrocento.
27. For further discussion of this see Paolucci and Pinto, 'Gli "infermi" ', pp. 127–9
28. Although the actual sex ratio of patients is not known in this period, when S. Matteo was founded each ward contained the same number of beds (twenty-three): SM 108, ff. 9r, 11v. An inventory of 1454 lists another seven beds for men and another one for women: SM 328, f. 302v.
29. Given that both the annual totals of admissions and deaths at S. Maria Nuova are known, it is possible to calculate the mortality rate of patients, although analysis over a long period is limited to males since information about admissions is rarely provided in the case of females. This figure is in line with mortality in the previous decade as calculated by Park, 'Healing the Poor', p. 34.
30. Trexler, 'Hospital Patients', p. 54 calculated a rate of 3.5 per cent for 1567–8, while Park, 'Healing the Poor', p. 35 gives a higher figure of 5.2 per cent for the years 1554–61.
31. Paolucci and Pinto, 'Gli "infermi" ', p. 127.
32. Herlihy and Klapisch-Zuber, *Tuscans and their Families*, p. 270.
33. While one can calculate the maximum number of males admitted in any one year, this is not possible on a monthly basis.
34. The annual ratio of male to female deaths for 1519–29 is: 1.27, 1.03, 1.19, 1.17, 1.33, 1.42, 1.19, 1.13, 1.34, 0.97, 1.34, 1.39. Data are missing for females in two months in 1518 and four months in 1530.
35. Luca Landucci, *Diario fiorentino dal 1450 al 1516*, ed. I. Del Badia (Florence, 1883), p. 338.
36. Summarised in Corradi, *Annali delle epidemie*, under years.
37. Goldthwaite, *The Building*, p. 439.
38. Goldthwaite, 'I prezzi', p. 36.
39. ASF, Signori e Collegi, Deliberazioni, ordinaria autorità 131, f. 36v: 'Et perché molti di decti poveri sono e truovonsi malati per le vie per la debolezza della fame di potere mandare decti poveri così malati alli spedali di S. Maria Nuova, Lelmo, San Pagolo et Bonifazio di Firenze ... e prefati excellentissimi Signori comandono alli spedalinghi di decti spedali ... ricevere e acceptare [tali poveri infermi] in decti loro spedali come gli altri poveri infermi sotto pena della loro indigniatione.'
40. See above, Chapter 3; Varchi, *Storia*, Book 3, p. 31; and Passerini, *Storia*, pp. 340–1.
41. Paolucci and Pinto, 'Gli "infermi" ', pp. 123–7, esp. p. 124: Table 3.
42. BON 5, f. 7v: 24.i.1475: 'Richordo chome questo dì 24 di gennaio e Chonsoli dell'Arte de Marchatanti insieme chon due proveditori dallo spedale per loro partito tutti d'achordo diliborano che da qui inanzi non si debba ne possa riccettare alchuna persona, chosì maschi chome femine, nello spedale di Messer Bonifazio per più tempo che da dì quindici ... Eccetto quei infermi e malati di febbre che rimanissino allo spedale ... infino che fussi di bisogno.'
43. The figures for male and female patients confirm Katharine Park's analysis of the years 1518–19: see Park, 'Healing the Poor', p. 43 n. 41.
44. Ibid., p. 35.
45. As suggested by Park, ibid., p. 36.
46. Herlihy and Klapisch-Zuber, *Tuscans and their Families*, ch. 7.
47. See Henderson, *Piety and Charity*, chs 7, 8.
48. Park, 'Healing the Poor', p. 36.
49. Only 5–6 per cent of the three thousand patients recorded in the Misericordia's fifteenth-century admission books mention illness: Paolucci and Pinto, 'Gli "infermi" ', pp. 120–3.

50. BNCF, Magl. XV.92, ff. 27r–192r, and a brief discussion by Park and Henderson in the introduction to SMN (1510–11), p. 174.
51. Trexler, 'Hospital Patients', pp. 41–59.
52. Paolucci and Pinto, 'Gli "infermi" ', pp. 120–3.
53. Sandri, 'L'assistenza', pp. 91–6.
54. SM 186, f. 92r: 'Ricordo oggi questo dì 25 d'aghosto 1464 che chon ciò sia chosa che Piero di Giovanni ferraio delgli Sciatesi popolo di Sancto Lorenzo di Firenze fussi rechato infino adì 8 di maggio 1464 infermo nel nostro spedale in pochi dì per la gratia di Dio lui guarì di febre, fu licienziato dallo spedale e dallo infermieri chome è d'usanza in simili spedali. Di che lui vedendosi vecchio e non potere esercitare più la persona fammi preghare a più persone e a suo parenti che io dovessi tenere per l'amor di Dio chome povero in detto spedale e per, chosì chomosso a passione, veduto la sua miseria lo ritenni vedutolo vechio, malsano solo chome lupo parla.'
55. SM 186, f. 92r.
56. SMN (1510–11), pp. 181, 183.
57. Ibid., p. 183.
58. Cf. ibid., p. 183 n. 54 and the mid-sixteenth-century description of the hospital made for Emperor Ferdinand in Passerini, *Storia*, p. 868.
59. SM 252, c. 93; 329, c. 67, as cited in Sandri, 'Assistenza', p. 92.
60. See G. Magherini and V. Biotti, *L'isola delle Stinche e i percorsi della follia a Firenze nei secoli XIV–XVIII* (Florence, 1992), pp. 160–8.
61. Trexler, 'Hospital Patients', p. 46: Chart A.
62. SMN 733, f. 137v: 'morì d'uno schopieto.'
63. Ibid., f. 195v: 'Uno fanciulo che non poteva favelare, vene a dì 13 di maggio 1527 e morì adì detto.'
64. Ibid., f. 16r: 'vene a letucio fedito da uno pazo di chasa adì 10 di luglio 1520 e morì alora che giu[n]se.'
65. Ibid., f. 179r: 'servo di chasa et morì adì 2 di marzo 1515 e amazosi da se' chon uno choltello che si schannosi una notte nel leto.'
66. Sandri, 'Assistenza', pp. 93–4.
67. It was not just a question of recording practices since all other entries contained both the admission and exit dates of patients who died.
68. See discussion in Trexler, 'Hospital Patients', p. 45.
69. Ibid., pp. 42–3.
70. For what follows see ibid., pp. 45–50 and esp. p. 49: Chart A.
71. SP 889, f. 110r.
72. Ibid., f. 113r.
73. Ibid., f. 122v.
74. See Henderson in Arrizabalaga, Henderson and French, *The Great Pox*, chs 2, 7, 8.
75. Trexler, 'Hospital Patients', pp. 50–1.
76. Herlihy and Klapisch-Zuber, *Tuscans and their Families*, p. 276: Table 9.5 analyses the years 1424–30, and Carmichael, *Plague and the Poor*, p. 37: Table 2.3: 1424–57.
77. Paolucci and Pinto, 'Gli "infermi" ', pp. 115–19.
78. Sandri, 'L'assistenza', pp. 74–6, esp. Table 7.
79. For a more detailed discussion of this phenomenon see Henderson, *Piety and Charity*.
80. Sandri, 'Assistenza', pp. 77–83, esp. Tables 8, 9.
81. SM 178, f. 37r: 'certi suoi stracci di panni di pocha valuta.'
82. SMN 62: ff. 91r: 18.xii.1370: 'I gonella di panno romagnola da huomo rotta; I farsetto cattivo; I cioppa di huomo rotta; I mantellucccio da homo romagnolo; I mantelo e capperone chattivo; II stracci di panno romagnolo chattivi; I gonnelluccia da femina di panno nero; I straccio di panno cilestro; I straccio di panno mescholato.'

The most detailed analysis of patients' clothes is in my discussion of S. Giacomo in Rome: Henderson in Arrizabalaga, Henderson and French, *The Great Pox*, ch. 8.

83. SMN 733, f. 186r.
84. Ibid., f. 70v.
85. SMN (1510–11), ch. 21: p. 182.
86. SMN 733, ff. 186r, 167v, 156v, 149v.
87. SMN (1510–11), p. 183.
88. Herlihy and Klapisch-Zuber, *Tuscans and their Families*, p. 128: Table 4.7.
89. Ibid.
90. SMN (1510–11), p. 183.
91. See A. Molho, *Marriage Alliance in Late Medieval Florence* (Cambridge, Mass., 1994), pp. 365–75: App. 3.
92. Biblioteca Casanatense, Rome, cod. 4201, f. 4r: 'nello spedale di San Matteo detto di Lemmo della casa de' Balducci. In quest' luogo nelle stanze che prima servivano per lo spedalingo nel tempo che di sopra se è detto [2 June 1536] nacque il Ser. Alessandro.'
93. Cf. Herlihy and Kaplish-Zuber, *Tuscans and their Families*, p. 124.
94. Park, 'Healing the Poor', p. 44 n. 44, although it should be pointed out that these results may have been skewed by the higher levels of mortality in the city as a whole in this year.
95. *Lo Spedale Serristori di Figline*, pp. 24–27: average stay 1586–95 for men was twelve or thirteen days and a week longer for women.
96. According to the 1427 Catasto: Herlihy and Klapisch-Zuber, *Tuscans and their Families*, p. 216: 25 per cent. The less complete Catasto of 1480 suggests that in the intervening period there may have been a reduction in the proportion of widows in the population. However, this may have been less true of the poorer levels of society to whom the majority of S. Maria Nuova's patients belonged, since many would have been exempt and not appeared in the tax records (see the discussion in Molho, *Marriage Alliance*, pp. 215–18 and p. 218 n. 56). Cf. Sandri, 'L'assistenza', p. 73: Table 5, who analyses the marital status of female patients of S. Matteo and S. Maria Nuova in the fifteenth century and records roughly the same proportion of married women.
97. Cf. for a discussion of pressures on the family economy of the poor in the fifteenth century see Henderson, *Piety and Charity*, ch. 8.
98. SMN (1510–11), p. 181.
99. Identification of the exact geographical origins of a patient is not always straightforward, hence the 8 per cent 'unknown' in Table 8.7. Sometimes it proved impossible to trace the names of small communities or otherwise the information provided was too inexact, as in the case of S. Casciano where there is more than one place in Tuscany with the same name, the best-known of which are in the Valdelsa and in the Valdipesa. (These cases are in the 'Tuscany' category in Table 8.10 rather than in the *contado*.) A wider problem is to determine how long an individual might have been resident in the city and whether the declared place of origin was that of the family or of the individual patient. (Cf. Herlihy and Klapisch-Zuber, *Tuscans and their Families*, p. 110; Cohn, *The Laboring Classes*, p. 96.)
100. This includes entries where the location is either illegible or not given. Comparable figures for the Misericordia in Prato were higher: between 13 and 32 per cent of patients did not have a declared provenance and 1.4 to 2.4 per cent were not identified (Paolucci and Pinto, 'Gli "infermi" ', p. 113: Table 1). In the case of S. Matteo in Florence, 8 to 10 per cent were without provenance, as were 17 per cent of male patients and 31 per cent of females dying at S. Maria Nuova in the last quarter of the fifteenth century (Sandri, 'L'assistenza', pp. 70–1: Tables 3 and 4).
101. Paolucci and Pinto, 'Gli "infermi" ', p. 115; *Lo Spedale Serristori di Figline*, pp. 24–7.
102. I have followed E. Conti, *La formazione della struttura agraria moderna nel contado fiorentino* III, Parte 2a, *Monografie e tavole statistiche (secoli XV–XIX)* (Rome, 1965) in adopting modern administrative divisions for Tuscany and the *contado*.

103. In general see Goldthwaite, *The Building*, and pp. 243–9 on Lombard masons; cf. also Pinto, *La Toscana nel medioevo*, pp. 428–42 on Lombard masons employed in the building industry in fifteenth-century Siena.
104. F. Franceschi, *Oltre il 'Tumulto'. I lavoratori fiorentini dell'Arte della Lana fra Tre e Quattrocento* (Florence, 1993), p. 120: Table 15.
105. Cohn, *The Laboring Classes*, pp. 102–3; H. Hoshino, *L'Arte della Lana in Firenze nel basso medioevo. Il commercio della lana e il mercato dei panni fiorentini nei secoli XIII–XV* (Florence, 1980), ch. 5.
106. Cohn, *The Laboring Classes*, p. 103.
107. Sandri, 'L'assistenza', pp. 69–71; Paolucci and Pinto, 'Gli "infermi" ', p. 114.
108. Conti, *La formazione*, Vol. 2, pp. 240–1; C. Klapisch-Zuber, *Una carta del popolamento toscano negli anni 1427–1430* (Milan, 1983).
109. See Klapisch-Zuber, *Una carta* for divisions of the Florentine territory.
110. In the case of Barberino di Mugello I have added 117 patients who declared their origins as simply 'from the Mugello' and two as 'from the Sieve'.
111. Gavitt, *Charity and Children*, pp. 206–7, though the geographical origins of the foundlings need more detailed analysis before any significant comparisons can be made.
112. SMN (1374), p. 63.
113. G.G. Gilino, *La relazione ai deputati dell'Ospedale Grande di Milano* (1508), ed. S. Spinelli (Milan, 1937); cf. Albini, *Città e ospedali*, pp. 103–9.
114. Piccinni, 'L'Ospedale di Santa Maria della Scala di Siena', pp. 303–4.
115. See Henderson in Arrizabalaga, Henderson and French, *The Great Pox*, ch. 8.
116. See ibid., pp. 194–200.
117. Brodman, *Charity and Welfare*, pp. 67, 95–6, summarising J. Danon, *Visió històrica de l'Hospital General de Santa Cru de Barcelona* (Barcelona, 1978).
118. B. Geremek, *The Margins of Society in Late Medieval Paris*, trans. J. Birrell (Cambridge, 1987), p. 175. See also Saunier, 'Le pauvre malade', pp. 195–203 on mortality at a series of maisons-Dieu in northern France.
119. On Norwich see Rawcliffe, *Medicine for the Soul*, ch. 6; Cullum, *Cremetts and Corrodies*.

Chapter 9

1. SM 196, f. 135r: 1.xii.1507: 'Ricordo oggi questo dì primo di dicembre [1507] habbiamo tolto per nostro spetiale e infermiere Girolamo di Ser Nicholaio di Neri, il quale s'obligha di fare tutto quello s'apartiene fare nella spetieria e fare le medicine e sciloppi che achadranno fare a nostri infermi e aiutare a servi a tempi si dà a mangiare a nostri infermi e havere chura non si facci errori al tempo che la febre fussi in aughamento e così in ogni altra necessità. Con questo non sia tenuto affare la guardia la notte più che si voglia perchè non si torna al vitto ne albergho nel nostro spedale senone tanto quanto fussi di bisognio.'
2. Cf. above, Chapter 8.
3. SM 190, f. 136v: 18.xi.1488: Maestro Giovanni di Marcho Nuti.
4. SM 193, f. 115r: 27.ix.1496.
5. SMN (1510–11), p. 182.
6. Archivio di Stato di Prato, Spedali delle Misericordia e Dolce 1877, ff. 1r–30r: 1492–1502.
7. SMN 4390, ff. 1r, 9r, 13r, 20v; cf. SMN (1510–11), p. 181.
8. SMN 4398, ff. 43v–45r. Physicians were also named sources for the purchase of medicines, as in the payment 'to the shop of Maestro Silvestro for the syrups and medicines and other things, £5 14s'. See also: 'to the shop of Maestro Durante, doc-

tor, 12s.'; 'to the shop of Maestro Dino for medicines, 9s 4d': SMN 4390, ff. 11r, 33r, 46r.
9. R. Ciasca, *L'arte dei medici e speziali nella storia e nel commercio fiorentino dal secolo XII al XV* (Florence, 1927), pp. 314–15; Park, *Doctors*, pp. 29–30, 108–9. A medical practitioner could also own the workshop or a share in it, an arrangement suggested by these examples from S. Maria Nuova and from the hospital of S. Paolo when it began in-house treatment of the sick in the 1340s: SP, ff. 1r–2v.
10. In general see Park, *Doctors*, pp. 28–32.
11. SMN 5875, cc. 219, 248, 375.
12. SMN 4398, f. 44r: 'Item paghamo decto dì [3.vi.1352] per erbe per fare medicine s. 4 e per una mezzetta di vino biancho per gl'infermi s.3 6d; f. 44v: Item paghamo decto dì [15.vi.1352] a Frate Antonio per pillole, s.5; f. 45r: Item paghamo decto dì [25.vi.1352] per chose da fare unguenti per gl'infermi s.15.'
13. SMN 4426, ff. 248r–v: 'Paghamo a Ugholino di Bonsi e chonpagni dì iiii di novembre 1373 fior. 100 d'oro, i quali danari ebbe per parte di paghamento di zuchero e polvere di zuchero, confetti, trementina, chassia, miele, pillole, incenso, anici, zafferano, penniti, cera, candele, torchi e torchietti, folgli di banbagia, gesso, piombo, e altra spezeria ch'abbiamo avuto dalloro ... dal xvii d'aprile adì 8 di dicembre 1373.'
14. A. Astorri, 'Appunti sull'esercizio dello Speziale a Firenze nel Quattrocento', *ASI*, 147 (1989), p. 33.
15. SMN, 1376 inventory, pp. 13–22.
16. SMN 4437, f. 35r. No salary was recorded as having been paid to an apothecary in the account books from Nov. 1373 to July 1378: SMN 4426, 4428. Cf. SMN (1374).
17. SM 180, ff. 6v–8r: for S. Matteo's purchases of medicines in 1409–10. See also the discussion of these entries in Sandri, 'Ospedali e utenti', pp. 86–9; the earliest reference to Messer Bonifazio employing an apothecary and buying medicines was in 1408: BON 387, f. 46r.
18. Girolamo di Ser Nicholaio di Neri was paid 96 lire or 14 gold florins a year in 1507 (SM 196, f. 135r: 1.xii.1507), Maestro Giovanni di Marcho Nuti was paid 50 lire or 8 gold florins, including free board and lodging (SM 190, f. 136v: 18.xi.1488).
19. BON 387, ff. 46r: 31.x.1408; f. 84r: 17.xii.1412: 'Angniolo di Luca da Cortona vene a stare con esso noi per spetiale e infermieri nello spedale adì 17 di dicembre 1412 ... e de'avere l'anno per suo salario fior. 15 acominciando dì decto.'
20. SM 188, ff. 71r–v.
21. Herlihy and Klapisch-Zuber, *Tuscans and their Families*, p. 129: Table 4.8; p. 95.
22. BON 387, f. 84r; Goldthwaite, *The Building*, pp. 348, 436. Of course, these figures are only a rough guide given that labourers would rarely have found work for as many as 365 days a year.
23. SM 196, f. 135r: 1.xii.1507; Goldthwaite, *The Building*, p. 437; and ibid., p. 430 for the value of the florin.
24. Lorenzo di Brandino (Cora, *Storia della maiolica di Firenze e del contado*, p. 238) and Domenicho d'Antonio (SMN 5817, f. 51r). The figures for their Catasto returns are to be found in the Catasto printout. I am grateful to Sam Cohn for supplying me with this information.
25. SMN 4477, f. 51r (1427). For Pagolo di Ser Giovanni Mini see Catasto, Campioni 80, f. 143v: cited in Astorri, 'Appunti', p. 40.
26. SMN (1510–11), p. 180.
27. Gavitt, *Charity and Children*, p. 156.
28. *Nuovo riceptario composto dal famossimo chollegio degli eximii doctori della arte et medicina della inclita cipta di Firenze*, ed. A.M. Carmona i Cornet (Florence, 1499; facs. edn Barcelona, 1992), pp. xxv, I, doct. i.
29. Hospital statutes provide little information about pharmacies, simply mentioning the distribution of syrups, confections and medicines to patients: SMN (1374), f. 25v: p. 78.

30. The same principle of accessibility governed the positioning of pharmacies in other Florentine hospitals, as at S. Matteo, where the pharmacy was listed in the 1454 inventory immediately after the male ward and *medicheria* and identified by the image of 'Our Lady with child made from glazed plaster, above the door to the apothecary's shop, in a little tabernacle' (SM 328, f. 302v: 'Ia nostra donna di giesso invetriata, col fanciullo sopra l'uscio della spezieria, in tabernacholetto'). The apothecary's shop was still in the same position in 1780 (Plate 3.13: 'M'), for in this way, as at S. Maria Nuova, it could be easily reached by the public through the left, northern end of the loggia.
31. Cited by M. Franchi, in *Una farmacia preindustriale*, p. 123. Cf. also the hospital of the Knights of St John of Jerusalem in Altopascio: *L'ospitalità in Altopascio*, p. 135.
32. SMN 4479, ff. 56r–v, 119r–120v; 4480, f. 31v; cf. Cora, *Storia della maiolica di Firenze*, pp. 273, 231.
33. The classic study is A. Castiglioni, 'La bottega dello speziale', in A. Castiglioni, *Il volto di Ippocrate* (Milan, 1925), pp. 75–99.
34. SM 36, f. 5r; *Una farmacia preindustriale*, p. 43 n. 30.
35. See Park, *Doctors*, pp. 29–30.
36. SMN, 1376 inventory, p. 14.
37. P.A. Mattioli, *I discorsi di M. Pietro Andrea Matthioli Medico Sanese nei sei libri della materia medicinale di Pedacio Dioscoride Anazarbeo* (Venice, 1557; facs. edn, Bologna, 1984), p. 7.
38. SMN, 1376 inventory, pp. 13–14.
39. SMN 4480, f. 31v: 'Adì XXI di luglio per più alberelli e orciuoli e altri vaselli dati per la nuova spezieria, al memoriale segnato F a c. 170 lire dugientonove levati dal quaderno segnato a c. 4 … e più ebbe fl. due nuovi … somma fl. 2 £210.' See Cora, *Storia della maiolica di Firenze*, Vol. 1, pp. 55–7, 272–5, 231, 273; Wilson, *Ceramic Art of the Italian Renaissance*, p. 32.
40. SMN 4483, f. 30r: 'a dì v di gennaio [1435]: e per cc alberellini smalti £I, e per ii alberelli grandi di quarto £I e per tre alberelini bianchi £II.'
41. Cf. *Nuovo Riceptario*, p. 63.
42. It has been suggested by Cora, *Storia della maiolica di Firenze*, Vol. 1, pp. 55–7, 272–5, that this together with other examples of relief-blue jars found scattered in collections throughout the world can be associated with the order placed by S. Maria Nuova with Giunta di Tugio in 1430–1. More recently doubt has been thrown on this assumption: J.E. Poole, *Italian Maiolica and Incised Slipware in the Fitzwilliam Museum, Cambridge* (Cambridge, 1995), p. 98.
43. *Una farmacia preindustriale*, p. 41, pp. 59–106 for a detailed discussion of the collection of the hospital's maiolica pharmacy jars in the Museo Civico of San Gimignano.
44. Poole, *Italian Maiolica*, p. 98.
45. SMN, 1376 inventory, pp. 13–15; *Una farmacia preindustriale*, ch. 2.
46. SMN, 1376 inventory, pp. 13–15.
47. *Una farmacia preindustriale*, p. 43 n. 29.
48. As suggested by its 1507 inventory: *ibid.*, p. 40.
49. SMN (1510–11), p. 182.
50. SMN, 1376 inventory, pp. 13–22.
51. Ibid., pp. 13–14; SM 328, f. 302v; cf. also 196, f. 138r.
52. S. Maria Nuova also owned two sets of scales, the larger of which would have been used in the workshop to weigh the simples to be treated with heat or other methods. The second and smaller scales were probably used in the apothecary's shop to make up compound medicines according to the recipes of the hospital doctors.
53. SMN, 1376 inventory, pp. 13–14.
54. I am grateful to James Shaw for this point. Mattioli, *I discorsi*, p. 744.
55. SMN, 1376 inventory, p. 13.

56. SM 196, f. 138r.
57. Mattioli, *I discorsi*, p. 744.
58. SMN (1510–11), p. 182. The number of these instruments continued to increase: see the inventory of 1.vi.1588 in SMN 83, ff. 3v–5v.
59. BNCF, Magl. XV.92, ff. 27r–192r. In total there were 1,035 recipes, including a few that were repeated.
60. For example, while its 1456 inventory did not include a recipe collection, by 1507 S. Matteo possessed both '1 recipe book bound in parchment and strips of linen and with covers' and '1 new recipe book bound in wooden boards', though neither survives.
61. SMN, *Ricettario*, f. 1r: 'Iscripto per me Hectorre di Lionello di Francesco Baldovinecti ad petizione di Maestro Pagholo medicho, oggi questo dì xvii d'ottobre MDXV.'
62. SMN 5876, c. 50 for 1485–7. Neither of the extant account books covering this period records payments in 1515 to either the scribe or the physician: SMN 5089, 'Quadernuccio', 1513–16; 5886, 'Libro Maestro', 1513–16.
63. *Nuovo riceptario*, p. A ii. The most recent detailed study of the *Ricettario fiorentino* is M. T. Huguet Hermes, 'Aproximación histórico-farmacológica y estudio comparativo de los códigos más representativos de las primeras tendencias a la oficialización en el contexto de la terapia preparacelsiana en Europa (unpublished Ph.D. thesis, University of Barcelona, 1998).
64. See ASF, Arte dei Medici e Speziali, Collegio dei Medici.
65. *Una farmacia preindustriale*, p. 48,
66. SMN, *Ricettario*, f. 1r: 'Et di poi seguita uno libro universale di più chose, tucte riciette isperimentate et provate aute et cavate pure di Sancta Maria Nuova.'
67. SMN, *Ricettario*, f. 49r: 'Lattovaro che ffu fatto per Francesco nostro camarlingho secondo uno riciatta che lui mi diè per la vista per lui'; f. 181r: 'maravigliosamente libera la donna di quello che patisce di suffocatione, sichome io viddi et questo è ne provato.' I thank James Shaw for these references.
68. SMN, *Ricettario*, f. 189r: 'lascia secchare chom'io dissi di sopra.'
69. Archivio di Stato di Prato, Spedali delle Misericordia e Dolce 1877, ff. 2v–6r:
Per una bambina
R: Zuchero biancho: 1oncia
Fanne polvere sottilissima per usare secondo el modo dato
Item olio di cologne 1oncia
Per ugnere lo stomacho
Per uno vecchio di chasa
R. Locheo [di Mesué] sano et experto 2oncie
Per tenere in bocha a ogni hora
Per Stephano
R. Olio di spigho: 1oncia
Per ugnere lo stomacho sera e mattina inanzi pasto
Per Frate Antonio
R. Regolitia rasa: 3oncie
Passule di corinto: 3oncie
Sebesten n. viii
Prune: n. vi
Gugole: n. xx
Orzo modo se comuni: m. 1
Per fare aqua pettorale
Per La Maria
R. Syropo di endiva composto
Acetoso semplice
Aqua di lupoli: 2oncie

Capelvenere: 2oncie
Viole: 2oncie
Mestola per ii preste
Per Giovanni infermieri
R. Cerotto da percosse: iiii oncie
Per sopra porre alla percossa.

70. SMN 4477, under date 4.ii.1427.
71. SMN, *Ricettario*, f. 1r: 'Et prima è uno tractato fatto et ordinato da Maestro Piero Ispano chiamato "Tesoro di Poveri". Il quale libro sebbe di Sancta Maria Nuova.'
72. SP 662 under 9.ii.1349.
73. Cf. Huguet Hermes, 'Aproximación histórico-farmacológica', pp. 101–2; Table 3.
74. Park, *Doctors*, pp. 169–70, 173–4 (prior), 177.
75. *Nuovo riceptario*, p. 33v.
76. Huguet Hermes, 'Aproximación histórico-farmacológica', p. 80 n. 194.
77. Eighty-three of the 136 recipes were by a 'medico della casa.'
78. SMN, *Ricettario*, ff. 26v, 75r, 102v, 106v.
79. SMN, *Ricettario*, f. 55r; see also ff. 34v, 40v, 56r, 190r; SM 186, f. 206v for Maestro Fruosino's contract with S. Matteo to 'medichare et churare.'
80. See above, Chapter 4.
81. See *The Letters of Marsilio Ficino*, Vol. 1, pp. 126–7.
82. Park, *Doctors and Medicine*, pp. 160n, 166–7, 173, 182n.
83. See *Nuovo riceptario*.
84. *The Letters of Marsilio Ficino*, Vol. 1, p. 126.
85. Masino, *Voci di spezieria dei secoli XIV–XVIII*, p. 130.
86. Ibid., p. 144.
87. For example, SMN, *Ricettario*, ff. 27v, 34v, 51v, 168r.
88. Ibid., ff. 55r, 179r.
89. Ibid., ff. 39v, 53v.
90. For a useful general guide to these theories see N.G. Siraisi, *Medieval and Early Renaissance Medicine. An Introduction to Knowledge and Practice* (Chicago and London, 1990), pp. 100–6.
91. N.G. Siraisi, *Taddeo Alderotti and his Pupils. Two Generations of Italian Medical Tradition* (Princeton, 1981), p. 281; Mattioli, *I discorsi*, at end of section entitled 'Tavola e delli Rimedi di tutti i Morbi del corpo humano' (unpaginated).
92. Petrus Hispanus, *Thesaurus pauperum* (Florence, c.1497), p. 2.
93. Siraisi, *Medieval and Early Renaissance Medicine*, pp. 131–2.
94. See R. Palmer, 'Medical Botany in Northern Italy in the Renaissance', *Journal of the Royal Society of Medicine*, 78 (1985), pp. 149–57.
95. While 872 symptoms or body parts are mentioned in the *Ricettario*, they appear in only 737 recipes since some were for multiple uses, treating more than one condition.
96. Listed in Mattioli, *I discorsi*, immediately after the index at the beginning of the book, 'Tavola di tutte le cose che si contengono nel presente volume.'
97. M.R. McVaugh, 'The Nature of Limits of Medical Certitude at Early Fourteenth-Century Montpellier', in M.R. McVaugh and N.G. Siraisi, eds, *Renaissance Medical Learning: Evolution of a Tradition*, in *Osiris*, 6 (1990), pp. 62–84.
98. See Arrizabalaga, Henderson and French, *The Great Pox*, chs 4, 5, 10.
99. SMN, *Ricettario*, f. 127v: 'Polvere da pistolenzia secondo Alberto Mangnio.'
100. Ficino, *Consilio contro la pestilenzia*, p. 66.
101. SMN, *Ricettario*, ff. 36v, 138r: 'Lattovaro o vero pillole per la pistolenza, ma ssono molte calde.'
102. SMN, *Ricettario*: pills: ff. 36v, 72v, 152v–153r; cf. Mattioli, *I discorsi*, aloe: pp. 344–5; Armenian bole: p. 640; myrrh: p. 66; saffron: p. 640.
103. SMN, *Ricettario*, f. 127v; Mattioli, *I discorsi*, pp. 640 (bole), 44 (sandalwood), 335 (dittamo), 272 (endive), 80 (camphor).

104. Ficino, *Consilio contro la pestilenzia*, p. 67.
105. Much has been written on fevers, but see for a useful discussion the collection of essays edited by W.F. Bynum and V. Nutton, *Theories of Fever from Antiquity to the Enlightenment*, in *Medical History*, Supplement No. 1 (London, 1981).
106. I.M. Lonie, 'Fever Pathology in the Sixteenth Century: Tradition and Innovation', in Bynum and Nutton, eds, *Theories of Fever*, pp. 20–1.
107. SMN, *Ricettario*, f. 36v.
108. Mattioli, *I discorsi*, pp. 503–4, 697–8, 492–3.
109. Ibid., pp. 68–9, 272.
110. SMN, *Ricettario*, f. 36v.
111. F. Baldasseroni and G. Degli Azzi, 'Consiglio medico di maestr'Ugolino da Montecatini ad Averardo de'Medici', *ASI*, 5th ser., 38 (1906), p. 142.
112. Mattioli, *I discorsi*, p. 345.
113. SMN, *Ricettario*, ff. 94r–v.
114. Ibid., f. 61r: 'A cchi fusse flematicho avendo pena nel petto overo nel petto o nella boccha dello istomacho abbi a usare la mattina a buona ora aromaticho rosato et per volta tanto quanto una buona fava et digiunarlo ò una ò dua ore et questo è ne provato.'
115. Mattioli, *I discorsi*, p. 119.
116. Baldasseroni and Degli Azzi, 'Consiglio medico di maestr'Ugolino da Montecatini', p. 142.
117. See M. Laharie, *La folie au moyen âge, XIe–XIIIe siècles* (Paris, 1991), ch. 7.
118. On epilepsy see O. Temkin, *The Falling Sickness*, 2nd edn (Baltimore and London, 1971).
119. Mattioli, *I discorsi*, pp. 387–9: 'parlano fuor di proposito.'
120. Ibid., pp. 297, 525.
121. Ibid., pp. 452–3.
122. SMN, *Ricettario*, f. 2v.
123. Ibid.
124. Laharie, *La folie*, pp. 129–31.
125. SMN, *Ricettario*, ff. 51r, 86v; Mattioli, *I discorsi*, pp. 556–7.
126. SMN, *Ricettario*, ff. 43r–v.
127. Mattioli, *I discorsi*, pp. 584–5 (*polipodio*); pp. 321–2 (*agharico*); pp. 552–3 (*elebero nero*); pp. 350–1 (lavender).
128. SMN (1510–11), p. 183.
129. Laharie, *La folie*, p. 201; see also the 'Ordinances' of S. Maria Nuova prepared for the emperor Ferdinand: Passerini, *Storia*, p. 868.
130. Laharie, *La folie*, p. 127.
131. SMN, *Ricettario*, f. 55r
132. Mattioli, *I discorsi*, pp. 577, 579.
133. On madness see L.P. Conrad et al., *The Western Medical Tradition, 800 BC to AD 1800* (Cambridge, 1985), pp. 183ff. See also S. Maria Nuova's 'Ordinances', where a separate room for madmen is described (SMN, 1510–11, p. 183), and more generally Margherini and Biotti, *L'isola delle Stinche*.
134. SMN, *Ricettario*, f. 55r: 'Cose da mettere inn uno pollo overo inn uno polmone di castro per metterlo in su uno capo el capo vuole essere raso che lli chuopra tutto il capo per far dormire uno pazzo.'
135. Laharie, *La folie*, p. 221.
136. Mattioli, *I discorsi*, pp. 493–4, 337, 262.
137. SMN, *Ricettario*, f. 159r.
138. Ibid., f. 92v.
139. Mattioli, *I discorsi*, pp. 390–1, 356–7, 160–2.
140. SMN, *Ricettario*, ff. 142r, 190r.

141. Mattioli, *I discorsi*, p. 397.
142. SMN, *Ricettario*, f. 29v.
143. Ibid., ff.156r–v.
144. Ibid., f. 67v.
145. Ibid., f. 155r; Mattioli, *I discorsi*, pp. 124–5.
146. SMN, *Ricettario*, f. 156v; Mattioli, *I discorsi*, p. 834.
147. SMN, *Ricettario*, f. 156r; Mattioli, *I discorsi*, p. 291.
148. SMN, *Ricettario*, f. 156v; Mattioli, *I discorsi*, pp. 378–9.
149. SMN, *Ricettario*, f. 58v; Mattioli, *I discorsi*, p. 248.
150. SMN, *Ricettario*, ff. 68v, 121v.
151. Mattioli, *I discorsi*, p. 697.
152. SMN, *Ricettario*, f. 40r.
153. Mattioli, *I discorsi*, pp. 493–4.
154. Ibid., pp. 362–3, 69, 72–4.
155. Ibid., pp. 33–5, 50.
156. SMN, *Ricettario*, f. 44v: 'Unghuento da capi rotti viene a essere verde il quale unghuento avemo da Mona Francesca et Mona Caterina mediche di casa et da lloro avemo la ricietta di mirabile operatione.'
157. Mattioli, *I discorsi*, pp. 56–7: laurel oil; ibid., p. 74: pine resin.
158. As recommended by Mattioli, ibid., p. 220.
159. Ibid., pp. 462, 356–7, 389–90.
160. Ibid., pp. 462, 356, 389–90, 452–3.
161. SMN, *Ricettario*, f. 61v: 'Impiastro da capi rotti la chui ricietta avemo da maestro Ficino medicho di casa et è di mirabile operatione, ebbela Neri di Gino Capponi da Maestro Michele.'
162. Mattioli, *I discorsi*, pp. 219–20 provides a guide to the methods for preparing various types of animal fats.
163. Ibid., pp. 219, 186–7.
164. Ibid., p. 66.
165. Ibid., p. 71.
166. Ibid., p. 633.
167. See M.R. McVaugh, 'Quantified Medical Theory and Practice at 14th-Century Montpellier', *Bulletin of the History of Medicine*, 43 (1969), pp. 397–413.
168. On eyes see L.M. Eldredge, 'The Anatomy of the Eye in the Thirteenth Century. The Transmission of Theory and the Extent of Medical Knowledge', *Micrologus. Nature, Sciences and Medieval Societies*, 5 (1997), pp. 145–60.
169. SMN, *Ricettario*, ff. 111v–112r.
170. Ibid., f. 104v: 'Impiastro da rottura di carne d'occhi.'
171. Mattioli, *I discorsi*, p. 136.
172. Ibid., p. 125.
173. Ibid., p. 264.
174. SMN, *Ricettario*, f. 42r.
175. Ibid., f. 154b.
176. Ibid., ff. 27v, 42r, 65r, 67v, 100r, 162v, 163v.
177. Ibid., f. 55r.
178. Mattioli, *I discorsi*, pp. 646–7.
179. Ibid., p. 623.
180. Ibid.
181. SMN, *Ricettario*, f. 142v: 'A dolglia di denti.'
182. Mattioli, *I discorsi*, pp. 491–2, 380, 389, 292.
183. SMN, *Ricettario*, f. 142v; Mattioli, *I discorsi*, p. 557.
184. SMN, *Ricettario*, f. 155r; Mattioli, *I discorsi*, pp. 397–8.
185. SMN, *Ricettario*, f. 156v; Mattioli, *I discorsi*, pp. 203–5.

186. SMN, *Ricettario*, f. 154v: 'A Trarre denti.'
187. Jacobus de Voragine, *The Golden Legend*, trans. W. Granger Ryan (Princeton, 1993) Vol. 1, p. 268; *Butler's Lives of the Saints*, Vol. 1, p. 286.
188. For a general description of the system see *Galen on the Usefulness of the Parts of the Body*, trans. and intro. by M. Tallmadge May (Ithaca, NY, 1968), Vol. 1, pp. 44–64; Siraisi, *Medieval and Early Renaissance Medicine*, pp. 105–7.
189. *De conservatione sanitatis di Maestro Benedetto da Norcia*, ed. F. Lombardi, *Scientia Veterum*, 32 (Genoa, 1962), p. 23.
190. A useful general discussion is: A. Wear, 'Medicine in Early Modern Europe, 1500–1700' in L. Conrad, M. Neve, V. Nutton and R. Porter, *The Western Medical Tradition* (Cambridge, 1995), pp. 325–6.
191. SMN, *Ricettario*, f. 108v.
192. Ibid., f. 62v.
193. Mattioli, *I discorsi*, p. 102.
194. SMN, *Ricettario*, f. 87v.
195. Mattioli, *I discorsi*, p. 21.
196. SMN, *Ricettario*, f. 34r.
197. Ibid., f. 155v.
198. Ibid., f. 92r; Mattioli, *I discorsi*, p. 173.
199. SMN, *Ricettario*, f. 155r.
200. Ibid., ff. 179v–180r: 'Al male della milza.'
201. *The Diseases of Women by Trotula of Salerno*, trans. E. Mason-Hohl (Los Angeles, 1940), pp. 1–2.
202. *The Diseases of Women*, Prologue, pp. 1–2; also on women see Rawcliffe, *Medicine and Society*, ch. 8.
203. *The Diseases of Women*, p. 8.
204. SMN, *Ricettario*, f. 37r.
205. Ibid., ff. 37r, 178v.
206. Mattioli, *I discorsi*, pp. 483–4.
207. Ibid., p. 484.
208. SMN, *Ricettario*, ff. 37r, 41v, 60r.
209. Ibid., ff. 115r–v.
210. *The Diseases of Women*, ch. 7, pp. 13–14.
211. SMN, *Ricettario*, ff. 115r–v.
212. *The Diseases of Women*, p. 13.
213. Ibid., ch. 4: pp. 10–11.
214. Ibid.
215. Ibid., p. 11; Mattioli, *I discorsi*, pp. 92–3, 398, 370, 186.
216. SMN, *Ricettario*, f. 181r.
217. Mattioli, *I discorsi*, pp. 517–18, 371.
218. SMN, *Ricettario*, f. 181r; Mattioli, *I discorsi*, pp. 726, 297, 290–1. The 'I' is not identified, but may have either been the scribe or more likely the unnamed doctor who provided him with the recipe.
219. SMN, *Ricettario*, f. 35v.
220. Mattioli, *I discorsi*, pp. 138, 136–7, 45, 344–5, 40–1, 235.
221. SMN, *Ricettario*, ff. 155v–156r: 'Medicina se alchuno huomo o femina fussino affaturati che non potessino husare insieme.'
222. Mattioli, *I discorsi*, pp. 476–7.
223. See Henderson in Arrizabalaga, Henderson and French, *The Great Pox*, ch. 2.
224. SMN, *Ricettario*, f. 37r: 'A lividore di menbra'; for *sugho d'assenzio* see Mattioli, *I discorsi*, pp. 346–8, where he describes its hot and drying qualities.
225. SMN, *Ricettario*, f. 155v; for *mandorle amare* see Mattioli, *I discorsi*, pp. 154–5; it heats and dries and provokes menses.

226. SMN, *Ricettario*, f. 157r.
227. Ibid., f. 125v.
228. Ibid., f. 39r.
229. Mattioli, *I discorsi*, pp. 245, 246, 437, 244, 367, 221, 575.
230. Masino, *Voci*, p. 90.
231. SMN, *Ricettario*, f. 128v.
232. SMN, *Ricettario*, f. 88r: 'Lattovaro detto del Ducha dal Ducha Ruberto Ghulglielmo.'
233. Ibid., f. 95v; Mattioli, *I discorsi*, p. 665.
234. SMN, *Ricettario*, ff. 77r–v; 137v–138r.
235. Masino, *Voci*, p. 79.
236. Mattioli, *I discorsi*, pp. 375, 37–8, 227, 322.
237. On cicadas see Mattioli, *I discorsi*, p. 198; for the qualities of the blood of various animals, including that of goats, p. 224; clove leaves, p. 297; cinnamon, pp. 35–7.
238. McVaugh, *Medicine before the Plague*, p. 155.

Bibliography

Primary Sources (Manuscript)

Archivio dell'Ospedale degli Innocenti di Firenze

Series II
Series III
Series CXLIV
Ricordanze

Archivio di Stato di Firenze

Accademia del Disegno
Arte del Cambio
Arte della Seta
Bigallo
Capitoli
Catasto
Compagnie Religiose Soppresse
Decima della Repubblica
Diplomatico
Guardaroba
Magistrato Supremo
Mediceo Avanti il Principato (MAP)
Mediceo del Principato
Monastero di S. Maria e S. Niccolò del Ceppo
Monastero di S. Caterina
Monte Comune
Notarile Antecosimiano
Ospedale degli Incurabili
Ospedale di Messer Bonifazio
Ospedale di S. Eusebio
Ospedale di S. Matteo detto di Lemmo Balducci
Ospedale di S. Maria Nuova
Ospedale di S. Paolo dei Convalescenti
Otto di Guardia e Balìa, Periodo della Repubblica
Provvisioni Duplicati
Provvisioni Registri
Senato dei Quarantotto
Signori e Collegi, Deliberazioni, Ordinaria Autorità

Archivio di Stato di Prato

Spedali delle Misericordia e Dolce

Archivio di Stato di Roma

Ospedale di S. Spirito

Biblioteca Nazionale Centrale di Firenze

Conventi Soppressi
Magliabechiano
MSS II
Nuovi Acquisti

Museo Nazionale del Bargello

MSS

Wellcome Institute Library, London

Wellcome Western MSS

Primary Sources (Printed)

L.B. Alberti, *L'Architettura* (*De re aedificatoria*), ed. G. Orlandi and P. Portoghesi (Milan, 1966), 2 vols.

L.B. Alberti, *On the Art of Building in Ten Books*, trans. J. Rykwert, N. Leach and R. Tavernor (Cambridge, Mass., and London, 1988).

Antonio Averlino detto il Filarete. Trattato di architettura, ed. A.M. Finioli and L. Grassi (Milan, 1972), 2 vols.

F. Baldasseroni and G. Degli Azzi, 'Consiglio medico di maestr'Ugolino da Montecatini ad Averardo de'Medici', *ASI*, 5th ser., 38 (1906), pp. 140–52.

L. Banchi, ed., *Statuti senesi scritti in volgare ne'secoli XIII e XIV* (Bologna, 1877).

A. Benivieni, *De abditis nonnullis ac mirandis morborum et sanationum causis*, ed. G. Weber (Florence, 1994).

Butler's Lives of the Saints, ed. H. Thurston and D. Attwater (London, 1956), 5 vols.

Domenico Cavalca, *Lo Specchio della Croce*, ed. Tito Sante Centi (Bologna, 1992).

A.M. Cherubino, ed., *Bullarium Romanum a B. Leone Magno usque as S.D.N. Clementem X* (Lyon, 1892).

L. Chiappelli and A. Corsini, 'Un antico inventario dello Spedale di Santa Maria Nuova in Firenze (a.1376)', *Rivista delle Biblioteche e degli Archivi*, 32 (1921), pp. 13–22.

R. Ciasca, ed., *Statuti dell'Arte dei medici e speziali di Firenze* (Florence, 1922).

'Consiglio di Tommaso del Garbo Fiorentino contro la Pestilentia', in M. Ficino, *Contro alla peste* (Florence, 1576).

Cronica di Giovanni Villani: a miglior lezione ridotta coll'aiuto de'testi a penna (Florence, 1823; repr. Rome, 1980), 8 vols.

Cronica di Matteo e Filippo Villani: a miglior lezione ridotta coll'aiuto de'testi a penna (Florence, 1825–6; repr. Rome, 1980), 4 vols.

G. Da Monte, *Consultationum* (Basle, 1565).

G. Dati, *Istoria di Firenze*, ed. L. Pratesi (Florence, 1904).

De conservatione sanitatis di Maestro Benedetto da Norcia, ed. F. Lombardi, *Scientia Veterum*, 32 (Genoa, 1962).

Jacques de Vitry, *'Histoire Occidentale'. Historia occidentalis*, trans. and ed. G. Duchey-Suchaux and J. Longère (Paris, 1997).

Jacobus de Voragine, *The Golden Legend. Readings on the Saints*, trans. W. Granger Ryan (Princeton, 1993), 2 vols.

'Diario Fiorentino di Bartolommeo di Michele del Corazza, anni 1405–1438', ed. G.O. Corazzini, *Archivio storico italiano*, 5th series, 14 (1894), pp. 233–98.

The Diseases of Women by Trotula of Salerno, trans. E. Mason-Hohl (Hollywood, Ca., 1940).

P. Fanfani, ed., *Capitoli della Compagnia dei Portatori o S. Giovanni Decollato* (Bologna, 1858).

M. Ficino, *Consilio contro la pestilenzia*, ed. E. Musacchio (Bologna, 1983).

Galen on the Usefulness of the Parts of the Body, trans. and intro. by M. Tallmadge May (Ithaca, NY, 1968).

A. Gherardi, ed., *Statuti della università e studio fiorentino dell'anno 1387* (Florence, 1881).

G.G. Gilino, *La relazione ai deputati dell'Ospedale Grande di Milano, 1508*, ed. S. Spinelli (Milan, 1937).

Giordano da Pisa, *Prediche inedite (dal MS. Laurenziano, Acquisti e Doni 290)*, ed. C. Iannella (Pisa, 1997).

P. Giusti and P. Guidi, eds, *Rationes Decimarum Italiae nei secoli XIII e XIV. Tuscia* (Città di Vaticano, 1932–42).

C. Landino, *Scritti critici e teorici*, ed. R. Cardini (Rome, 1974).

L. Landucci, *Diario fiorentino dal 1450 al 1516*, ed. I. Del Badia (Florence, 1883; repr. 1985).

Lettere di una gentildonna fiorentina del secolo XV ai figliuoli esuli, ed. C. Guasti (Florence, 1877).

The Letters of Marsilio Ficino, trans. School of Economic Science, London (London, 1978), 2 vols.

Il libro di Antonio Billi, ed. F. Benedettucci (Rome, 1991).

Marchionne di Coppo Stefani, *Cronaca fiorentina*, ed. N. Rodolico, *Rerum Italicarum Scriptores*, n.s. 31:1 (Città di Castello, 1903).

Martin Luther, *Table Talk*, in *Luther's Works*, ed. and trans. T.G. Tappert (Philadelphia, 1967), vol. 54.

P.A. Mattioli, *I discorsi di M. Pietro Andrea Matthioli Medico Sanese nei sei libri della materia medicinale di Pedacio Dioscoride Anazarbeo* (Venice, 1557; facs. edn Bologna, 1984).

J. Nardi, *Istorie della città di Firenze*, ed. L. Arbib (Florence, 1842).

Nuovo riceptario composto dal famosissimo chollegio degli eximii doctori della arte et medicina della inclita cipta di Firenze, ed. A.M. Carmona i Cornet (Florence, 1499; facs. edn Barcelona, 1992).

S. Orlandi, ed., *'Necrologio' di Santa Maria Novella* (Florence, 1955).

G. Pinto, ed., *Il libro del Biadaiolo. Carestie e annona a Firenze dalla metà del '200 al 1348* (Florence, 1978).

Prediche del Beato Fra Giordano da Rivalto dell'Ordine dei Predicatori recitate in Firenze dal MCCCIII al MCCCVI, ed. D. Moreni (Florence, 1831), 2 vols.

Il regio arcispedale di S. Maria Nuova. I suoi benefattori, sue antiche memorie, Florence, 1888 (the statutes of S. Maria Nuova from 1330 to 1374).

J.R. Spencer, ed., *Filarete's Treatise on Architecture. Being the Treatise by Antonio di Piero Averlino, Known as Filarete* (New Haven and London, 1965).

Statuti della Repubblica Fiorentina, ed. R. Caggese, Vol. 2: *Statuto del Podestà dell'anno 1325*, new edn (Florence, 1999).

N.P. Tanner, ed., *Decrees of the Ecumenical Councils*, Vol. 1: *Nicaea I to Lateran V* (London and Georgetown, 1990).

L. Tornabuoni, *La istoria della casta Susanna*, ed. P. Orvieto (Bergamo, 1992).

B. Varchi, *Storia fiorentina*, ed. L. Arbib (Florence, 1839–41), Vol. 2.

G. Vasari, *Le vite de più eccellenti pittori, scultori e archittetori*, in *Le opere di Giorgio Vasari*, ed. G. Milanesi (Florence, 1906; 1973), 9 vols.

G. Zerbus, *Opus utile de cautelis medicorum* (Padua, 1495).

Secondary sources

B. Aikema and D. Meijers, eds, *Nel regno dei poveri. Arte e storia dei grandi ospedali veneziani in età moderna, 1474–1799* (Venice, 1989).

G. Albini, *Guerra, fame, peste. Crisi di mortalità e sistema sanitario nella Lombardia tardo-medioevale* (Milan, 1982).

G. Albini, *Città e ospedali nella Lombardia medievale* (Bologna, 1993).

J.J.G. Alexander, ed., *The Painted Page. Italian Renaissance Book Illumination, 1450–1550* (London and Munich, 1994).

F. Ames-Lewis, 'Domenico Veneziano and the Medici', *Jahrbuch der Berliner Museen*, 21 (1979), pp. 67–90.

O. Andreucci, *Il Fiorentino istruito nella chiesa della Nunziata di Firenze. Memoria storica* (Florence, 1857).

F. Antal, *Florentine Painting and its Social Background: The Bourgeois Republic before Cosimo de' Medici's Advent to Power: XIV and Early XV Centuries* (Cambridge, Mass., and London, 1986).

R. Arbesmann, 'The Concept of "Christus Medicus" in St. Augustine', *Traditio*, 10 (1954), pp. 1–28.

C. Arrigoni, *Istituti di beneficenza fiorentini* (Florence/Rome, 1882).

J. Arrizabalaga, J. Henderson and R. French, *The Great Pox: The French Disease in Renaissance Europe* (New Haven and London, 1997).

Assistenza e ospitalità nella Marca medievale: atti del XXVI Convegno di studi maceratesi, San Ginesio, 17–18 novembre 1990 (Macerata, 1990).

A. Astorri, 'Appunti sull'esercizio dello speziale a Firenze nel Quattrocento', *ASI*, 147 (1989), pp. 31–62.

C. Avery, *Giambologna: The Complete Sculpture* (Oxford, 1987).

S. Avery-Quash, in G. Finaldi, *The Image of Christ. The Catalogue of the Exhibition Seeing Salvation* (London, 2000), entry no. 68, pp. 176–7.

M. Azzolini, 'Leonardo in Context: medical ideas and practices in Renaissance Milan' (unpublished Ph.D. thesis, University of Cambridge, 2001).

P. Bagnesi, 'Alessandro Allori e lo Spedale di S. Maria Nuova', *Rivista d'arte*, 9 (1916–18), pp. 253–72.

L. Baini, 'Ipotesi sull'origine della tipologia cruciforme per gli ospedali del XV secolo', in L. Giordano, ed., *Processi accumulativi, forme e funzioni. Saggi sull'architettura lombarda del Quattrocento* (Florence, 1996), pp. 59–102.

D. Balestracci and G. Piccinni, 'L'Ospedale e la città', in D. Gallavotti Cavallero, ed., *Lo Spedale di Santa Maria della Scala in Siena. Vicenda di una committenza artistica* (Siena, 1985), pp. 19–39.

K.-E. Barzman, *The Florentine Academy and the Early Modern State. The Discipline of Disegno* (Cambridge, 2000).

G.C. Bascapé, 'L'assistenza e la beneficenza a Milano dall'alto medioevo alla fine della dinastia sforzesca', in Fondazione G. Treccani degli Alfieri, *Storia di Milano* (Milan, 1957), Vol. 8, pp. 387–419.

S. Beccaria, 'I conversi nel Medioevo. Un problema storico e storiografico', *Quaderni storici*, 46 (1998), pp. 120–56.

J.H. Beck, 'Masaccio's Early Career as a Sculptor', *Art Bulletin*, 53:2 (1971), pp. 177–95.

M. Becker, 'Aspects of Lay Piety in Renaissance Florence', in C. Trinkaus and H. Oberman, eds, *The Pursuit of Holiness* (Leiden, 1974), pp. 177–99.

L. Bellosi, ed., *Il museo dello Spedale degli Innocenti* (Milan, 1977).

N. Bemporad and D. Mignani Galli, *Ex-ospedale di San Matteo – la loggia. Restauro dell'aula di scenografia nell'Accademia di Belle Arti* (Florence, 1979).

A. Benvenuti Papi, *'In Castro Poenitentiae.' Santità e società femminile nell'Italia medievale* (Rome, 1990).

L. Berti, *Pontormo* (Florence, 1964).

P. Biller and J. Ziegler, eds, *Religion and Medicine in the Middle Ages* (York, 2001).
E. Borsook, 'Cults and Imagery at Sant'Ambrogio in Florence', *MKIF*, 25 (1981), pp. 147–202.
M. Boskovits, *La pittura fiorentina alla vigilia del Rinascimento, 1370–1400* (Florence, 1975).
W.M. Bowsky, 'The Confraternity of Priests and San Lorenzo of Florence: A Church, a Parish and a Clerical Brotherhood', *Ricerche storiche*, 27 (1997), pp. 53–92.
F. Brasioli, 'Una Collezione da Riscoprire e Rivalutare', in F. Brasioli and L. Cinuccetti, *Santa Maria Nuova. Il tesoro dell'arte nell'antico ospedale fiorentino* (Florence, 1989).
F. Brasioli and L. Ciuccetti, *S. Maria Nuova. Il tesoro dell'arte nell'antico ospedale fiorentino* (Florence, 1989).
F. Brasioli and C. Lachi, 'Catalogo', in C. De Benedictis, ed., *Il patrimonio artistico dell'Ospedale Santa Maria Nuova di Firenze. Episodi di commitenza*, pp. 227–86.
C. Bresnahan Menning, *The Monte di Pietà of Florence. Charity and the State in Late Renaissance Italy* (Ithaca and London, 1993).
E. Bressan, 'Storia ospedaliera e storia della carità. Alle origini del CISO', *Sanità, scienza e storia*, 2 (1990–1), pp. 27–43.
L. Brockliss and C. Jones, *The Medical World of Early Modern France* (Oxford, 1997).
J.W. Brodman, *Charity and Welfare: Hospitals and the Poor in Medieval Catalonia* (Philadelphia, 1998).
G.A. Brucker, *Florentine Politics and Society, 1343–1378* (Princeton, 1962).
G.A. Brucker, *The Civic World of Early Renaissance Florence* (Princeton, 1977).
G.A. Brucker, 'Urban Parishes and their Clergy in Quattrocento Florence: A Preliminary "Sondage" ', in A. Morrogh et al., eds, *Renaissance Studies in Honor of Hugh Craig Smyth* (Florence, 1985), Vol. 1, pp. 17–28.
B. Buhler Walsh, 'The Fresco Painting of Bicci di Lorenzo' (unpublished Ph.D. thesis, Indiana University, 1981).
A. Butterfield, 'Monument and Memory in Early Renaissance Florence', in G. Ciappelli and P. Lee Rubin, eds, *Art, Memory and Family in Renaissance Florence* (Cambridge, 2000), pp. 135–60
A. Butterfield, *The Sculptures of Andrea del Verrocchio* (New Haven and London, 1997).
H.C. Butters, *Governors and Government in Early Sixteenth-Century Florence, 1502–1519* (Oxford, 1985).
J.J. Bylebyl, 'The School of Padua: Humanistic Medicine in the Sixteenth Century', in C. Webster, ed., *Health, Medicine and Mortality in the Sixteenth Century* (Cambridge, 1979), pp. 335–70.
W.F. Bynum and V. Nutton, eds, *Theories of Fever from Antiquity to the Enlightenment*, in *Medical History*, Supplement No. 1 (London, 1981).
W.F. Bynum and R. Porter, eds, *Companion Encyclopaedia of the History of Medicine* (London, 1993), 2 vols.
C.C. Calzolai, 'Lo spirito di un servizio secolare', in *Il VII centenario dell'Ospedale di S. Maria Nuova* (Barberino di Mugello, 1988).
V. Cappelletti and F. Tagliarini, eds, *L'antico Ospedale di Santo Spirito dall'istituzione papale alla sanità del terzo millenio* (Rome, 2001–2), 2 vols.
A.G. Carmichael, *Plague and the Poor in Renaissance Florence* (Cambridge, 1986).
F. Carrara, 'Ospedale di S. Maria Nuova. Analisi delle fasi di crescita dello Spedale' (unpublished plans).
F. Carrara and M.P. Mannini, *Lo Spedale della Misericordia e Dolce di Prato. Storia e collezioni* (Prato, 1993).
F. Carrara, L. Sebregondi and U. Tramonti, *Gli Istituti di beneficenza a Firenze. Storia e architettura* (Florence, 1999).
A. Castiglioni, 'La bottega dello speziale', in A. Castiglione, *Il volto di Ippocrate* (Milan, 1925), pp. 75–99.
S. Cavallo, *Charity and Power in Early Modern Italy. Benefactors and their Motives in Turin, 1541–1789* (Cambridge, 1995).

A. Cavaterra, 'L'Ospedalità a Roma nell'età moderna. Il caso di San Giacomo (1585–1605)', *Sanità, scienza e storia*, 2, 1986, pp. 87–123.
L. Cavazzini, 'Dipinti e sculture nelle chiese dell'Ospedale', in L. Sandri, ed., *Gli Innocenti e Firenze nei secoli. Un ospedale, un archivio, una città* (Florence, 1996), pp. 112–50.
A. Cenci, ed., *L'ospitalità in Altopascio. Storia e funzioni di un grande centro ospitaliero. Il cibo, la medicina e il controllo della strada* (Lucca, 1996).
E. Chaney, ' "Philanthropy in Italy": English Observations on Italian Hospitals, 1545–1789', in T. Riis, ed., *Aspects of Poverty in Early Modern Europe* (Stuttgart, 1981), pp. 183–217.
J. Chiffoleau, *La comptabilité de l'au-delà. Les hommes, la mort et la religion dans la région d'Avignon à la fin du moyen-âge (vers 1320–vers 1480)* (Rome, 1980).
K. Christiansen, 'The View from Italy', in M.A. Ainsworth and K. Christiansen, eds, *From Van Eyck to Breugel: Early Netherlandish Painting in the Metropolitan Museum of Art*, exh. cat., Metropolitan Museum of Art (New York, 1998), pp. 39–62.
G. Ciappelli and P. Lee Rubin, eds, *Art, Memory and Family in Renaissance Florence* (Cambridge, 2000).
R. Ciasca, *L'arte dei medici e speziali nella storia e nel commercio fiorentino dal secolo XII al XV* (Florence, 1927; repr. 1977).
C.M. Cipolla, *Public Health and the Medical Profession in the Renaissance* (Cambridge, 1976).
L. Ciuccetti, 'Profilo architettonico del complesso di S. Maria Nuova', in F. Brasioli and L. Ciuccetti, eds, *S. Maria Nuova. Il tesoro dell'arte nell'antico ospedale fiorentino* (Florence, 1989), pp. 9–17.
L. Ciuccetti, 'Un grandioso progetto di Bernardo Buontalenti: scoperte, ipotesi e conferme', in De Benedictis, ed., *Il patrimonio artistico*, pp. 79–106.
L. Ciuccetti, 'Lo Spedale di Santa Maria Nuova e la sua evoluzione attraverso settecento anni di storia', in De Benedictis, ed., *Il patrimonio artistico*, pp. 13–46.
L. Ciuccetti, 'Lo sviluppo architettonico dello Spedale di Santa Maria Nuova dalla sua fondazione al XV secolo', in De Benedictis, ed., *Il patrimonio artistico*, pp. 47–62.
F.M. Clapp, *Jacopo Carrucci da Pontormo* (New Haven, 1916).
S. Cohen, *The Evolution of Women's Asylums since 1500. From Refuges for Ex-Prostitutes to Shelters for Battered Women* (New York and Oxford, 1992).
S.K. Cohn Jr, *The Laboring Classes in Renaissance Florence* (New York and London, 1980).
S.K. Cohn Jr, *Death and Property in Siena, 1205–1800* (Baltimore, 1988).
S.K. Cohn Jr, *The Cult of Remembrance and the Black Death* (Baltimore and London, 1992).
L.P. Conrad et al., *The Western Medical Tradition, 800 BC to AD 1800* (Cambridge, 1985).
A. Conti, G. Conti and P. Pirillo, eds, *Lo Spedale Serristori di Figline. Documenti e arredi* (Florence, 1982).
E. Conti, *La formazione della struttura agraria moderna nel contado fiorentino*, III, Parte 2ᵉ, *Monografie e tavole statistiche (secoli XV–XIX)* (Rome, 1965).
Contributi per la storia dello Spedale del Ceppo a Pistoia (Pistoia, 1977).
G. Cora, *Storia della maiolica di Firenze e del contado: secoli XIV e XV* (Florence, 1973).
C. Corghi, 'Il CISO tra passato e futuro. Introduzione ai lavori', *Sanità, scienza e storia*, 1 (1989), pp. 59–65.
A. Corradi, *Annali delle epidemie occorse in Italia dalle prime memorie fino al 1850* (Bologna, 1865–9; repr. 1973).
A. Corsini, *La Morìa del 1464 in Toscana e l'istituzione dei primi Lazzaretti in Firenze ed in Pisa* (Florence, 1911).
G. Cosmacini, *La Cà Grande dei Milanesi: Storia dell'Ospedale Maggiore* (Rome and Bari, 1999).
G. Cosmacini and P. Pasini, eds, *Il bene e il bello. I luoghi della cura-cinquemila anni di storia* (Milan, 2000).
P. Costamagna, *Pontormo* (Milan, 1994).
E. Coturri, 'L'ospedale cosidetto "di Bonifazio" in Firenze', *Pagine di storia della medicina*, 3:2 (1959), pp. 73–8.

E. Coturri, 'Vi furono, nella Toscana settentrionale, nell'alto medioevo, scuole nelle quali si insegnò la medicina?', in M. Santoro, ed., *Atti della IV biennale della Marca per la storia della medicina* (Fermo, 1961), pp. 339–51.

A. Courbin, *The Foul and the Fragrant. Odor and the French Social Imagination* (Cambridge, Mass., 1986).

J. Cox Rearick, *The Drawings of Pontormo* (Cambridge, Mass., 1964).

R. Crotti, *Il sistema caritativo-assistenziale nella Lombardia medievale. Il caso pavese* (Pavia, 2002).

R.J. Crum, 'Facing the Closed Doors to Reception? Speculations on Foreign Exchange, Liturgical Diversity and the "Failure" of the Portinari Altarpiece', *Art Journal*, 57 (1998), pp. 5–13.

P. Cullum, *Cremetts and Corrodies: Care of the Poor and Sick at St. Leonard's Hospital, York, in the Middle Ages* (York, 1991).

G.L. Daccò and M. Rossetto, eds, *L'Ospedale di Cremona: medicina, arte, storia* (Milan, 2001).

A. D'Addario, 'Burocrazia, economia e finanze dello Stato Fiorentino alla metà del Cinquecento', *ASI*, 121 (1963), pp. 385–456.

A. D'Addario, *Aspetti della Controriforma a Firenze* (Rome, 1972).

A. D'Addario, 'Testimonianze archivistiche, cronistiche e bibliografiche', in *La comunità cristiana fiorentina e toscana nella dialettica religiosa del Cinquecento* (Florence, 1980), pp. 23–194.

F. Dal Pino, 'Oblati e oblate conventuali presso i mendicanti "minori" nei secoli XIII–XIV', in *Uomini e donne in comunità, Quaderni di storia religiosa*, Vol. 1 (1994), pp. 33–67.

J. Danon, *Visió històrica de l'Hospital General de Santa Cru de Barcelona* (Barcelona, 1978).

R. Davidsohn, *Forschungen zur älteren Geschichte von Florenz* (Berlin, 1896–1908), 4 vols.

R. Davidsohn, *Storia di Firenze*, trans. G.B. Klein (Florence, 1972–3), 8 vols.

P. De Angelis, *L'Ospedale di S. Spirito in Sassia* (Rome, 1960–2), 2 vols.

C. De Benedictis, 'Vicende e trasformazioni dell'Ospedale di Santa Maria di Orbatello', *Antichità viva*, 26 (1987), pp. 28–34.

C. De Benedictis, ed., *Il patrimonio artistico dell'Ospedale Santa Maria Nuova di Firenze. Episodi di commitenza* (Florence, 2002).

B. Deimling, 'Tommaso del Mazza (Master of Santa Verdiana)', in S. Pasquinucci and B. Deimling, 'Tradition and Innovation in Florentine Trecento Painting: Giovanni Bondi-Tommaso del Mazza', in M. Boskovits, ed., *A Corpus of Florentine Painting*, section IV (Florence, 2000), Vol. 8, pp. 228–9.

C.-M. de La Roncière, 'Indirect Taxes or "Gabelles" at Florence', in N. Rubinstein, ed., *Florentine Studies: Politics and Society in Renaissance Florence* (London, 1968), pp. 140–92.

C.-M. de La Roncière, 'Pauvres et pauvreté à Florence au xive siècle', in M. Mollat, ed., *Etudes sur l'histoire de la pauvreté* (Paris, 1974), pp. 661–745.

C.-M. de La Roncière, *Prix et salaires à Florence au xive siècle, 1280–1380* (Rome, 1982).

F. L. Del Migliore, *Firenze, città nobilissima illustrata* (Florence, 1684, facs. edn Bologna, 1976).

S. De Ricci, *Census of Medieval and Renaissance Manuscripts in the US and Canada* (New York, 1937).

R. De Roover, *The Rise and Decline of the Medici Bank* (Cambridge, Mass., 1963).

E. Dhanens, *Hugo van der Goes* (Antwerp 1998).

E. Diana, *San Matteo e San Giovanni di Dio: due ospedali nella storia fiorentina. Struttura nosocomiale, patrimonio fondiario e assistenza nella Firenze dei secoli XV–XVIII* (Florence, 1999).

F. Diaz, *Il Granducato di Toscana. I Medici* (Turin, 1976).

S. Edgington, 'Medical Care in the Hospital of Jerusalem', in *The Military Orders*, Vol. 2: *Welfare and Warfare*, ed. H. Nicholson (Aldershot, 1998), pp. 3–26.

F. Edler De Roover, *Glossary of Medieval Terms of Business: Italian Series, 1200–1600* (Cambridge, Mass., 1934).

M. Eisenberg, *Lorenzo Monaco* (Princeton, 1989).

L.M. Eldredge, 'The Anatomy of the Eye in the Thirteenth Century. The Transmission of Theory and the Extent of Medical Knowledge', *Micrologus. Nature, Sciences and Medieval Societies*, 5 (1997), pp. 145–60.

S.R. Epstein, *Alle origini della fattoria toscana. L'Ospedale della Scala di Siena e le sue terre (metà '200–metà '400)* (Florence, 1986).

A. Esposito, 'Gli ospedali romani tra iniziative laicali e politica pontificia (secc. XIII–XV)', in A.J. Grieco and L. Sandri, eds, *Ospedali e città. L'Italia del Centro-Nord, XIII–XVI* (Florence, 1997), pp. 233–51.

G. Fanelli, *Firenze. Le città nella storia d'Italia* (Rome and Bari, 1981).

O. Fantozzi Micali and P. Roselli, *Le soppressioni dei conventi a Firenze. Riuso e trasformazioni dal sec. XVIII in poi* (Florence, 1980).

A. Fara, ed., *Bernardo Buontalenti e Firenze: architettura e disegno dal 1576 al 1607* (Florence, 1998).

Una farmacia preindustriale in Valdelsa. La spezieria e lo spedale di Santa Fina nella città di San Gimignano, secc. XIV–XVIII (San Gimignano, 1981).

A. Feigenbaum, 'Early History of Cataract and the Ancient Operation for Cataract', *American Journal of Opthamology*, 49 (1960), pp. 305–26.

G. Finaldi, ed., *The Image of Christ. The Catalogue of the Exhibition Seeing Salvation* (London, 2000).

G. Fioravanti, 'La Filosofia e la medicina (1343–1543)', in E. Amatori, ed., *Storia dell'Università di Pisa* (Pisa, 1993).

E. Fiumi, 'La demografia fiorentina nelle pagine di Giovanni Villani', *ASI*, 108 (1950), pp. 105–18.

E. Fiumi, 'Fioritura e decadenza dell'economia fiorentina', *ASI*, 115 (1957), pp. 385–439; 116 (1958), pp. 443–510; 117 (1959), pp. 427–502.

A. Foa, 'Il nuovo e il vecchio: l'insorgere della sifilide (1494–1530)', *Quaderni storici*, 19 (1984), pp. 11–34.

P. Foster, 'Per il disegno dell'Ospedale di Milano', *Arte Lombarda*, 38–9 (1973), pp. 1–22.

F. Franceschi, *Oltre il 'Tumulto'. I lavoratori fiorentini dell'Arte della Lana fra Tre e Quattrocento* (Florence, 1993).

L. Franchini, 'Introduzione', in L. Franchini, ed., *Ospedali Lombardi del Quattrocento. Fondazioni, trasformazioni, restauri* (Como, 1995), pp. 11–72.

R. Franci, 'L'Ospedale di S. Paolo in Firenze e i Terziari Francescani', *VII centenario del Terz'Ordine Francescano, Studi francescani*, n.s. 7 (18) (1921), pp. 52–70.

T. Frangenberg, 'Choreographies of Florence. The Use of City Views and Plans in the 16th Century', *Imago Mundi*, 46 (1994), pp. 41–64.

D. Franklin, *Rosso in Italy. The Italian Career of Rosso Fiorentino* (New Haven and London, 1994).

R. French, 'The Medical Ethics of Gabriele de' Zerbi', in A. Wear, J. Geyer-Kordesch and R.K. French, eds, *Doctors and Ethics: The Earlier Historical Setting of Professional Ethics*, in *Clio Medica*, 24 (1993), pp. 72–97.

Frescoes from Florence (London, 1969).

R. Friedenthal, *Luther: His Life and Times* (London, 1970).

D. Gallavotti Cavallero, ed., *Lo Spedale di Santa Maria della Scala in Siena. Vicenda di una committenza artistica* (Siena, 1985).

D. Gallavotti Cavallero and A. Brogi, *Lo Spedale Grande di Siena. Fatti urbanistici e architettonici del Santa Maria della Scala. Ricerche, riflessioni, interrogativi* (Florence, 1987).

M. Garbellotti, 'Ospedali e storia nell'Italia moderna: percorsi di ricerca', in J. Henderson and A. Pastore, eds, *Medicina dell'anima, medicina del corpo: l'Ospedale in Europa tra Medio Evo ed Età Moderna, Medicina e storia*, 6 (2004), pp. 115–38.

J. Gardner, 'Altars, Altarpieces, and Art History: Legislation and Usage', in E. Borsook and F. Superbi Gioffredi, eds, *Italian Altarpieces, 1250–1550. Function and Design* (Oxford, 1994), pp. 5–40.

E. Garin, 'La cité idéale de la renaissance italienne', in *Les utopies à la renaissance* (Brussels and Paris, 1963), pp. 13–37.

P. Gavitt, *Charity and Children in Renaissance Florence. The Ospedale degli Innocenti, 1410–1536* (Ann Arbor, 1990).

P. Gavitt, ' "Perché non avea chi la governasse." Cultural Values, Family Resources and Abandonment in the Florence of Lorenzo de'Medici, 1467–85', in J. Henderson and R. Wall, eds, *Poor Women and Children in the European Past* (London, 1994), pp. 65–93.

D. Gentilcore, *From Bishop to Witch: the system of the sacred in early modern Terra d'Otranto* (Manchester, 1992).

D. Gentilcore, *Healers and Healing in Early Modern Italy* (Manchester, 1998).

B. Geremek, 'Il pauperismo nell'età preindustriale (secc. XIV–XVIII)', in *Storia d'Italia*, Vol. 5: *I documenti* (Turin, 1973), pp. 678–84.

B. Geremek, *The Margins of Society in Late Medieval Paris*, trans. J. Birrell (Cambridge, 1987).

C. Gilbert, 'The Earliest Guide to Florentine Architecture', *MKIF*, 14 (1969–70), pp. 33–46.

C. Gilchrist, *Gender and Material Culture: The Archaeology of Religious Women* (London, 1994).

G. Giordanengo, 'Les hôpitaux arlésiens du xiie au xive^e siècle', *Assistance et charité* (Cahiers de Fanjeaux, 13) (Toulouse, 1978), pp. 189–212.

L. Giordano, ed., *Processi accumulativi, forme e funzioni. Saggi sull'architettura lombarda del Quattrocento* (Florence, 1996).

S. Giovannini and G. Mancini, *La farmacia di Santa Maria Novella* (Florence, 1987).

R.A. Goldthwaite, 'I prezzi del grano a Firenze dal XIV al XVI secolo', *Quaderni storici*, 28 (1975), pp. 5–36.

R.A. Goldthwaite, *The Building of Renaissance Florence. An Economic and Social History* (Baltimore and London, 1980).

R.A. Goldthwaite, 'Local Banking in Renaissance Florence', *Journal of European Economic History*, 14 (1985), pp. 5–55.

R.A. Goldthwaite, 'Michelozzo and the Ospedale di San Paolo in Florence: Addendum', *MKIF*, 44 (2000), pp. 338–9.

R.A. Goldthwaite and W.R. Rearick, 'Michelozzo and the Ospedale di San Paolo in Florence', *MKIF*, 21 (1977), pp. 221–306.

A.J. Grieco, 'Il vitto di un ospedale: pratica, distinzioni sociali e teorie mediche alla metà del Quattrocento', in L. Sandri, ed., *Gli Innocenti e Firenze nei secoli: un ospedale, un archivio, una città* (Florence, 1996), pp. 85–92.

A. Grieco and L. Sandri, eds, *Ospedali e città. L'Italia del Centro-Nord, XIII–XVI secolo* (Florence, 1997)

F. Gurrieri, 'L'architettura dello "Spedale di S. Maria Nuova", 1288–1988', in *Lo Spedale di S. Maria Nuova, 1288–1988* (Florence, 1988), pp. 29–46.

F. Gurrieri and A. Amendola, *Il Fregio robbiano dell'Ospedale del Ceppo a Pistoia* (Pistoia, 1982).

B. Harvey, *Living and Dying in England, 1100–1540. The Monastic Experience* (Oxford, 1993).

S. Haskins, *Mary Magdalene. Myth and Metaphor* (London and New York, 1993).

R. Hatfield, *The Wealth of Michelangelo* (Rome, 2002).

B. Hatfield Strens, 'L'arrivo del Trittico Portinari a Firenze', *Commentari. Rivista di critica e storia dell'arte*, 19 (1968), pp. 315–19.

A. Hayum, *The Isenheim Altarpiece. God's Medicine and the Painter's Vision* (Princeton, 1989).

J. Henderson, 'Epidemie nella Firenze del Rinascimento: teoria sanitaria e provvedimenti governativi', in A. Pastore and P. Sorcinelli, eds, *Sanità e Società. Emilia Romagna, Toscana, Marche, Umbria, Lazio, secoli XVI–XX* (Udine, 1987), pp. 49–60.

J. Henderson, ed., 'Charity and the Poor in Medieval and Renaissance Europe', *Continuity and Change*, 3:2 (1988).

J. Henderson, 'Charity in Late-Medieval Florence: The Role of the Religious Confraternities', in S. Bertelli, N. Rubinstein and C.H. Smyth, eds, *Florence and Milan. Acts of Two Conferences at Villa I Tatti, Florence* (Florence, 1988), Vol. 2, pp. 147–63.

J. Henderson, 'The Parish and the Poor in Florence at the Time of the Black Death: The Case of S. Frediano', in J. Henderson, ed., *Charity and the Poor in Medieval and Renaissance Europe*, in *Continuity and Change*, 3:2 (1988), pp. 247–72.

J. Henderson, 'The Hospitals of Late Medieval and Renaissance Florence: A Preliminary Survey', in L. Granshaw and R. Porter, eds, *The Hospital in History* (London, 1989), pp. 63–92.

J. Henderson, *Piety and Charity in Late Medieval Florence* (Oxford, 1994, Chicago, 1997).

J. Henderson, ' "Splendide case di cura." Spedali, medicina ed assistenza a Firenze nel Trecento', in A.J. Grieco and L. Sandri, eds, *Ospedali e città. L'Italia del centro-Nord, XIII–XVI secolo* (Florence, 1997), pp. 15–50.

J. Henderson, 'Charity and Welfare in Sixteenth-Century Tuscany', in A. Cunningham and O. Grell, eds, *Charity and Medicine in Southern Europe* (London, 1999), pp. 56–86.

J. Henderson, 'The Mal Francese in Sixteenth-Century Rome: The Ospedale di San Giacomo in Augusta and the "Incurabili" ', in E. Sonnino, ed., *La popolazione di Roma dal medioevo all' età contemporanea. Fonti, problemi di ricerca, risultati* (Rome, 1999), pp. 483–523.

J. Henderson, 'Peste, Mal Francese e gli Ospedali di Firenze nel Rinascimento', in A. Aleardi and L. Pieri, eds, *L'Ospedale e la città* (Florence, 2000), pp. 16–27.

J. Henderson, 'Healing the Body and Healing the Soul: Hospitals in Renaissance Florence', *Renaissance Studies*, 2001, pp. 188–216.

J. Henderson and A. Pastore, eds, *Medicina dell'Anima, Medicina del Corpo: l'Ospedale in Europa tra Medio Evo ed Età Moderna, Medicina e storia*, 6 (2004).

J. Henderson and R. Wall, eds, *Poor Women and Children in the European Past* (London, 1994).

D. Herlihy, *Medieval and Renaissance Pistoia. The Social History of an Italian Town* (New Haven, 1967).

D. Herlihy, 'Growing Old in the Quattrocento', in P.N. Stearns, ed., *Old Age in Pre-Industrial Society* (New York, 1982), pp. 104–18.

D. Herlihy and C. Klapisch-Zuber, *Tuscans and their Families: A Study of the Florentine Catasto of 1427* (New Haven and London, 1985).

L.H. Heydenreich, *Architecture in Italy, 1400–1500* (Harmondsworth, 1974; New Haven and London, 1996).

M. Holmes, 'Disrobing the Virgin. The *Madonna Lactans* in Fifteenth-Century Florentine Art', in G. Johnson and S. Matthews Grieco, eds, *Picturing Women in Renaissance and Baroque Italy* (Cambridge, 1997), pp. 167–95.

M. Holmes, *Fra Filippo Lippi. The Carmelite Painter* (New Haven and London, 1999).

M. Holmes, 'Giovanni Benci's Patronage of the Nunnery Le Murate', in P. Rubin and G. Ciappelli, eds, *Art, Memory and Family in Rennaissance Florence* (Cambridge, 2000), pp. 114–34.

W. Hood, *Fra Angelico at San Marco* (New Haven and London, 1993).

J. Hook, *Siena: A City and its History* (London, 1978).

P. Horden, ' "A Discipline of Relevance": The Historiography of the Later Medieval Hospital', *Social History of Medicine* (1988), pp. 359–74.

P. Horden, 'A Non-Natural Environment: Medicine without Doctors and the Medieval European Hospital', in B. Bowers, ed., *The Medieval Hospital and Medical Practice* (Aldershot, forthcoming).

P. Horden and R. Smith, eds, *The Locus of Care* (London, 1998).

M. Horster, *Andrea del Castagno* (Oxford, 1980).

H. Hoshino, *L'arte della lana in Firenze nel basso medioevo. Il commercio della lana e il mercato dei panni fiorentini nei secoli XIII–XV* (Florence, 1980).

E. Howe, *The Hospital of Santo Spirito in Sassia* (New York, 1978).

M.T. Huguet Hermes, 'Aproximación histórico-farmacológica y estudio comparativo de los códigos más representativos de las primeras tendencias a la oficialización en el contexto de la terapia preparacelsiana en Europa (unpublished Ph.D. thesis, University of Barcelona, 1998).

J. Imbert, *Histoire des hôpitaux en France* (Toulouse, 1982).

M.A. Jack Ward, 'The Accademia del Disegno in 16th-Century Florence. A Study of an Artists' Institution' (unpublished Ph.D. thesis, University of Chicago, 1972).

D. Jacquart, *Le milieu médical en France du XIIe au XVe siècle* (Geneva, 1981).

D. Jacquart, 'Medical Practice in Paris in the First Half of the Fourteenth Century', in L. Garcia-Ballester et al, eds, *Practical Medicine from Salerno to the Black Death* (Cambridge, 1994), pp. 186–210.

D. Jetter, *Das europäische Hospital von der Spätantike bis 1800* (Cologne, 1986).

D. Jetter, *Santiago, Toledo, Granada: drei spanische Kreuzhallenspitaler und ihr Nachhall in aller Welt* (Stuttgart, 1987).

C. Jones, 'The Construction of the Hospital Patient in Early Modern France', in N. Finzsch and R. Jütte, eds, *Institutions of Confinement: Hospitals, Asylums and Prisons in Western Europe and North America, 1500–1950* (Cambridge, 1996), pp. 55–74.

L.B. Kanter et al., *Painting and Illumination in Early Renaissance Florence, 1300–1450* (New York, 1994), pp. 287–293.

B.Z. Kedar, 'A Twelfth-Century Description of the Jerusalem Hospital', in *The Military Orders*, Vol. 2: *Welfare and Warfare*, ed. H. Nicholson (Aldershot, 1998), pp. 3–26.

K.D. Keele and C. Pedretti, *Leonardo da Vinci. Corpus of Anatomical Studies in the Collection of Her Majesty the Queen at Windsor Castle* (London and New York, 1979–80), 2 vols.

F.W. Kent, 'The Rucellai Family and its Loggia', *JWCI*, 35 (1972), pp. 397–401.

D. Kent, *Cosimo de' Medici and the Florentine Renaissance* (New Haven and London, 2000).

F.W. Kent, 'The Making of a Renaissance Patron of the Arts', in F.W. Kent, A. Perosa, B. Preyer, P. Sanpaolesi and R. Salvini, *Giovanni Rucellai ed il suo zibaldone, II. A Florentine Patrician and his Palace* (London, 1981), pp. 9–95.

C. Klapisch-Zuber, *Una carta del popolamento toscano negli anni 1427–1430* (Milan, 1983).

C. Klapisch-Zuber, *Women, Family and Ritual in Renaissance Italy* (Chicago and London, 1985).

C. Knorr, 'The Coming of the Shepherds', *Art Bulletin*, 78 (1996), pp. 370–1.

R.A. Koch, 'Flower Symbolism in the Portinari Altarpiece', *Art Bulletin*, 46 (1964), pp. 76–7.

A. Kolega, 'Un capolavoro poco noto della miniatura trecentesca. Il "Liber Regulae" dell'Ordine degli Ospitalieri di Santo Spirito', in Cappelletti and Tagliarini, eds, *L'antico Ospedale di Santo Spirito*, Vol. 2, pp. 203–24.

R. Krautheimer, *Lorenzo Ghiberti* (Princeton, 1982).

P.O. Kristeller, *Marsilio Ficino and his Work after Five Hundred Years* (Florence, 1987).

M. Laharie, *La folie au moyen-âge, XIe–XIIIe siècles* (Paris, 1991).

P. La Porta, ed., *Spezieria di Santa Fina* (Siena, 2000).

S. La Sorsa, *La compagnia d'Or San Michele, ovvero una pagina della beneficenza in Toscana nel secolo XIV* (Trani, 1902).

M. Lazzaroni and A. Muñoz, *Filarete: scultore e architetto del secolo XV* (Rome, 1908).

M. Levi-D'Acona, *Miniatura e miniatori a Firenze dal XIV al XVI secolo: Documenti per la storia della miniatura* (Florence, 1962).

G. Leoncini, 'L'Arcispedale di Santa Maria Nuova e la sua storia architettonica', in De Benedictis, ed., *Il patrimonio artistico*, pp. 107–18.

F. Leverotti, 'L'ospedale senese di S. Maria della Scala in una relazione del 1456', *Bulletino senese di storia patria*, 1984, pp. 276–91.

F. Leverotti, 'Ricerche sulle origini dell'Ospedale Maggiore di Milano', *Archivio Storico*

Lombardo, 107 (1984), pp. 77–113.
B. Licata, 'Il problema del grano e delle carestie', in G. Spini, ed., *Architettura e politica da Cosimo I a Ferdinando I* (Florence, 1976), pp. 331–419.
D. Lombardi, 'Poveri a Firenze. Programmi e realizzazioni della politica assistenziale dei Medici tra cinque e seicento', in G. Politi, M. Rosa and F. Della Peruta, eds, *Timore e carità. I poveri nell'Italia moderna* (Cremona, 1982), pp. 165–84.
D. Lombardi, *Povertà maschile, povertà femminile. L'Ospedale dei mendicanti nella Firenze dei Medici* (Bologna, 1988).
D. Lombardi, 'L'ondata di pauperismo', *Il XVII secolo: la dinamica di una crisi*, in R. Romano, ed., *Storia d'Italia* (Milan, 1989), pp. 169–92.
E. Lombardi, *Messer Bonifacio Lupi da Parma e la sua fondazione in Via San Gallo in Firenze* (Florence, 1992).
I.M. Lonie, 'Fever Pathology in the Sixteenth Century: Tradition and Innovation', in W.F. Bynum and V. Nutton, eds, *Theories of Fever from Antiquity to the Enlightenment, Medical History*, Supplement No. 1 (London, 1981), pp. 19–44.
M.T. López Díaz, 'La botica del Hospital del Amor de Dios de Sevilla', *Boletín de la Sociedad española de historia de la farmacia*, 37 (1986) pp. 171–88.
M.T. López Díaz, *Estudio histórico-farmacéutico del Hospital del Amor de Dios de Sevilla (1655–1755)* (Seville, 1987).
K.P. Lowe, 'Elections of Abbesses and Notions of Identity in Fifteenth- and Sixteenth-Century Italy, with Special Reference to Venice', *Renaissance Quarterly*, 54:2 (2001), pp. 389–429.
A. Lucarella, *Le oblate di S. Maria Nuova di Firenze* (Bari, 1985).
A. Lucarella, *Storia dell'arcispedale di Santa Maria Nuova di Firenze* (Bari, 1986).
E. Lucas-Lybor, 'The Spedale di S. Matteo in Florence' (unpublished Ph.D. thesis, University of Essex, 1988).
P. Luzzi and F. Fabbri, 'Tre orti botanici di Firenze', in S. Ferri and F. Vannozzi, eds, *I giardini dei semplici e gli orti botanici della Toscana* (Perugia, 1993), pp. 241–4.
M.R. McVaugh, 'Quantified Medical Theory and Practice at 14th-Century Montpellier', *Bulletin of the History of Medicine*, 43 (1969), pp. 397–413.
M.R. McVaugh, 'The Nature and Limits of Medical Certitude at Early Fourteenth-Century Montpellier', in *Renaissance Medical Learning: Evolution of a Tradition*, ed. M.R. McVaugh and N.G. Siraisi, in *Osiris*, 6 (1990), pp. 62–84.
M.R. McVaugh, *Medicine before the Plague. Practitioners and their Patients in the Crown of Aragon, 1285–1345* (Cambridge, 1993).
G. Magherini and V. Biotti, *L'isola delle Stinche e i percorsi della follia a Firenze nei secoli XIV–XVIII* (Florence, 1992).
A. Malamani, 'Notizie sul Mal Francese e gli spedali degli incurabili in età moderna', *Critica storica*, 15 (1978), pp. 193–216.
C. Marchesini and G. Sperati, *Ospedali genovesi nel medioevo. Atti della società ligure di storia patria*, n.s. 21 (1981).
F. Marchi and G. Zambaldi, 'La Scuola Medica di Santa Maria Nuova', in *Santa Maria Nuova in Firenze: memorie, testimonianze, prospettive* (Florence, 1991).
L. Marcucci, *I dipinti toscani del secolo XIV. Le gallerie nazionali di Firenze* (Rome, 1965).
L. Marcucci, *Gallerie Nazionali di Firenze*, Vol. 1: *Catalogo dei dipinti del secolo XIV* (Rome, 1965).
A. Markham Schulz, *The Sculpture of Bernardino Rossellino and his Workshop* (Princeton, 1977).
A. Marquand, *Luca della Robbia* (Princeton, 1914).
J.J. Martin, 'Introduction: The Renaissance: Between Myth and History', in J.J. Martin, ed., *The Renaissance. Italy and Abroad* (London, 2003), pp. 1–23.
C. Massino, *Voci di spezieria dei secoli XIV–XVIII*, ed. D. Talmelli and G. Maggioni (Padua, 1988).

U. Mayer and R. Steffens, *Die Spätmittelalterlichen Urbare des Heiliggeist-Spitals in Mainz* (Stuttgart, 1992).
M.S. Mazzi, 'La peste a Firenze nel Quattrocento', in R. Comba, G. Piccinni and G. Pinto, eds, *Strutture familiari, epidemie, migrazioni nell'Italia medievale* (Naples, 1984), pp. 125–42.
G.G. Meersseman, *Dossier de l'Ordre de la Pénitence au XIIIe siècle* (Freiburg, 1961).
G.G. Meersseman, *Ordo fraternitatis: confraternite e pietà dei laici nel Medioevo* (Rome, 1977).
M. Meiss, *Painting in Florence and Siena after the Black Death* (New York and London, 1973).
R. Meloncelli, 'Musica nell'Arcispedale di Santo Spirito', in V. Cappelletti and F. Tagliarini, eds, *L'antico Ospedale di Santo Spirito* (Rome, 2001–2), Vol. 2, pp. 263–77.
L. Mencacci, 'L'assistenza sanitaria nello spedale di Altopascio', in A. Cenci, ed., *L'ospitalità in Altopascio. Storia e funzioni di un grande centro ospitaliero. Il cibo, la medicina e il controllo della strada* (Lucca, 1996), pp. 130–48.
G.G. Merlo, ed., *Esperienze religiose e opere assistenziali nei secoli XII e XIII* (Turin, 1987).
U. Middeldorf, 'Dello Delli and *The Man of Sorrows* in the Victoria and Albert Museum', *Burlington Magazine*, 456, vol. 78 (March 1941), pp. 77–8.
D. Mignani, 'Profilo storico-architettonico degli istituti lorenesi dell'Accademia delle Belle Arti', in F. Falletti, ed., *L'Accademia, Michelangelo, L'Ottocento* (Livorno, 1997), pp. 16–27.
J.I. Miller, 'Miraculous Childbirth and the Portinari Altarpiece', *Art Bulletin*, 77:2 (1995), pp. 249–61.
A. Molho, *Marriage Alliance in Late Medieval Florence* (Cambridge, Mass., 1994).
M. Mollat, 'La vie quotidienne dans les hôpitaux medievaux', in J. Imbert, ed., *Histoire des hôpitaux* (Toulouse, 1982).
A. Mori and G. Boffito, *Firenze nelle vedute e piante. Studio storico cartografico* (Florence, 1926).
R.W. Muncey, *A History of the Consecration of Churches and Churchyards* (Cambridge, 1930).
J.H. Mundy, 'Charity and Social Work in Toulouse, 1100–1250', *Traditio*, 22 (1966), pp. 203–87.
P. Murray, 'Art Historians and Art Critics: 4.14. Uomini Singhularii in Firenze', *Burlington Magazine*, no. 655, vol. 99 (1957), pp. 330–6.
I. Naso, *Medici e strutture sanitarie nella società tardo-medievale. Il Piemonte dei secoli XIV e XV* (Milan, 1982).
F. Niccolai, ed., *La Misericordia di Firenze: memorie, curiosità, tradizioni* (Florence, 1984).
Nuovo Osservatore, 3 (1885), pp. 23–4; 4 (1885), p. 29.
P. Nuttall, 'Early Netherlandish Painting in Florence: Acquisition, Ownership and Influence, c.1435–1500' (unpublished Ph.D. thesis, University of London, 1990).
V. Nutton, 'Continuity or Rediscovery? The City Physician in Classical Antiquity and Medieval Italy', in A.W. Russell, ed., *The Town and State Physician in Europe from the Middle Ages to the Enlightenment* (Wolfenbüttel, 1981), pp. 9–46.
C. O'Boyle, 'Surgical Texts and Social Contexts: Physicians and Surgeons in Paris, c.1270 to 1430', in L. Garcia-Ballester et al., eds, *Practical Medicine from Salerno to the Black Death* (Cambridge, 1994), pp. 156–85.
R. Offner, *A Critical and Historical Corpus of Florentine Painting* (Florence, 1986), III.4.
C.D. O'Malley and J.B. de C.M. Saunders, *Leonardo da Vinci on the Human Body: The Anatomical, Physiological, and Embryological Drawings of Leonardo da Vinci* (New York, 1952; 1983).
S. Orlandi, *Fra Angelico* (Florence, 1964).
A. Orlandini, *Gettatelli, pellegrini. Gli affreschi nella Sala del Pellegrino dell'Ospedale di Santa Maria della Scala di Siena* (Siena, 1997).
N. Orme and M. Webster, *The English Hospital, 1070–1570* (New Haven and London, 1995).
D.J. Osheim, 'Conversion, *Conversi*, and the Christian Life in Late Medieval Tuscany', *Speculum*, 58:2 (1983), pp. 368–90.
W. and E. Paatz, *Die Kirchen von Florenz* (Frankfurt-am-Main, 1940–55), 6 vols.

A. Padoa Rizzo, 'Cenni di Francesco', in *Dizionario biografico degli Italiani* (Rome, 1979), Vol. 23, p. 536.
A. Padoa Rizzo, 'Luca della Robbia e Verrocchio. Un nuovo documento e una nuova interpretazione iconografica del tabernacolo di Peretola', *MKIF*, 38 (1994), pp. 48–67.
R.J. Palmer, 'L'azione della Repubblica di Venezia nel controllo della peste. Lo sviluppo della politica governativa', in *Venezia e la peste, 1348–1797* (Venice, 1979), pp. 103–10.
R. Palmer, 'Medical Botany in Northern Italy in the Renaissance', *Journal of the Royal Society of Medicine*, 78 (1985), pp. 149–57.
G. Pampaloni, ed., *Lo Spedale di S. Maria Nuova e la costruzione del loggiato di Bernardo Buontalenti ora completata dalla Cassa di Risparmio di Firenze* (Florence, 1961).
E. Panconesi, 'S. Maria Nuova nella storia della medicina e del suo insegnamento', in *Santa Maria Nuova in Firenze: memorie, testimonianze, prospettive* (Florence, 1991), pp. 55–9.
E. Panofsky, *Early Netherlandish Painting: Its Origins and Character* (Cambridge, Mass., 1953).
G. Paolucci and G. Pinto, 'Gli "infermi" della Misericordia di Prato', in G. Pinto, ed., *La società del bisogno* (Florence, 1989), pp. 101–29.
G. Parenti, *Prezzi e mercato del grano a Siena (1546–1765)* (Florence, 1942).
K. Park, *Doctors and Medicine in Early Renaissance Florence* (Princeton, 1985).
K. Park, 'Healing the Poor: Hospitals and Medical Assistance in Renaissance Florence', in J. Barry and C. Jones, eds, *Medicine and Charity before the Welfare State* (London, 1991), pp. 26–45.
K. Park, 'The Readers at the Florentine Studio according to Communal Fiscal Records (1357–1380, 1413–1446)', *Rinascimento*, 2nd ser., 20 (1980), pp. 249–310.
K. Park and J. Henderson, ' "The First Hospital among Christians": The Ospedale di Santa Maria Nuova in Early Sixteenth-Century Florence', *Medical History*, 35 (1991), pp. 164–88.
L. Passerini, *Storia degli stabilimenti di beneficenza e d'istruzione elementare gratuita della città di Firenze* (Florence, 1853).
A. Pastore, 'Strutture assistenziali fra Chiesa e Stati nell'Italia della Controriforma', in G. Chittolini and G. Miccoli, eds, *La chiesa e il potere politico*, in *Storia d'Italia. Annali*, 9 (Turin, 1986), pp. 431–65.
A. Pastore et al, eds, *L'Ospedale e la città. Cinquecento anni d'arte a Verona* (Verona, 1996).
A. Patetta, 'Gli Ospedali a Pisa nel Medioevo', in *Strutture Sanitarie a Pisa. Contributi alla storia di una città, secc. XIII–XIX* (Pisa, 1986).
L. Patetta, *L'architettura del Quattrocento a Milano* (Milan, 1987).
A. Patetta, *La storia dell'Ospedale di S. Chiara in Pisa: dalle origini fino al 1771* (Pisa, 1994).
M. Pelling and F. White, *Medical Conflicts in Early Modern London. Patronage, physicians and irregular practitioners, 1550–1640* (Oxford, 2003).
A. Peroni, 'Il modello dell'ospedale cruciforme: il problema del rapporto tra l'Ospedale di Santa Maria Nuova di Firenze e gli ospedali lombardi', in S. Bertelli, N. Rubinstein and C.H. Smyth, eds, *Florence and Milan: Comparisons and Relations* (Florence, 1989), pp. 53–65.
G. Piccinni, 'L'Ospedale di S. Maria Scala della di Siena. Note sulle origini dell'assistenza sanitaria in Toscana (XIV–XV secolo)', in *Città e servizi sociali nell'Italia dei secoli XII–XV* (Pistoia, 1990), pp. 297–324.
G. Piccinni and L. Travaini, *Il libro del Pellegrino (Siena, 1382–1446). Affari, uomini, monete nell'Ospedale di Santa Maria della Scala* (Naples, 2003).
G. Piccinni and L. Vigni, 'Modelli di assistenza ospedaliera tra Medioevo ed Età Moderna. Quotidianità, amministrazione, conflitti nell'Ospedale di S. Maria della Scala di Siena', in G. Pinto, ed., *La società del bisogno. Povertà e assistenza nella Toscana medievale* (Florence, 1989), pp. 131–74.
G. Pieraccini, *La Stirpe de' Medici di Cafaggiolo* (Florence, 1986).
G. Pinto, 'Il personale, le balie e i salariati dell'Ospedale di San Gallo di Firenze negli anni

1395–1406: note per la storia del salariato nelle città medievale', *Ricerche storiche*, n.s. 2 (1974), pp. 113–68.
G. Pinto, *La Toscana nel tardo Medioevo. Ambiente, economia rurale, società* (Florence, 1982).
G. Pinto and G. Paolucci, 'Gli "infermi" della Misericordia di Prato (1401–1491)', in G. Pinto, ed., *La società del bisogno. Povertà e assistenza nella Toscana medievale* (Florence, 1989), pp. 101–29.
G. Poggi, 'Il ciborio di Bernardino Rossellino nella chiesa di S. Egidio', *Miscellanea d'arte*, 1 (1903), pp. 105–7.
L. Polizzotto, *The Elect Nation. The Savonarolan Movement in Florence, 1494–1545* (Oxford, 1994).
G. Pomata, *Contracting a Cure. Patients, Healers and the Law in Early Modern Bologna* (Baltimore and London, 1998).
J.E. Poole, *Italian Maiolica and Incised Slipware in the Fitzwilliam Museum, Cambridge* (Cambridge, 1995).
J. Pope-Hennessey, *Catalogue of Italian Sculpture in the Victoria and Albert Museum* (London, 1964).
J. Pope-Hennessey, *Fra Angelico* (London, 1974).
J. Pope-Hennessey, *Luca della Robbia* (Oxford, 1980).
B. Pullan, 'The Famine of Venice and the New Poor Law, 1527–1529', *Bollettino dell'Istituto di Storia della Società e dello Stato Veneziano*, 5–6 (1963–4), pp. 141–202.
B. Pullan, *Rich and Poor in Renaissance Venice. The Social Institutions of a Catholic State to 1615* (Oxford, 1971).
B. Pullan, 'Support and Redeem: Charity and Poor Relief in Italian Cities from the Fourteenth to the Seventeenth Century', in J. Henderson, ed., *Charity and the Poor in Medieval and Renaissance Europe*, in *Continuity and Change*, 3:2 (1988), pp. 177–208.
B. Rano, 'Ospitalieri di Santo Spirito', in G. Pelliccia and G. Rocca, eds, *Dizionario degli Istituti di Perfezione* (Rome, 1974–88), Vol. 6, pp. 994–1006.
H. Rashdall, *The Universities of Europe in the Middle Ages*, 2nd edn, ed. F.M. Powicke and A.B. Emden (Oxford, 1936).
G.B. Ravenni, 'I libri dei morti dell'ospedale di Santa Maria Nuova di Firenze come fonti per lo studio della mortalità durante le crisi di sussistenza', in *La popolazione italiana nel Settecento* (Bologna, 1980).
C. Rawcliffe, *The Hospitals of Medieval Norwich* (Norwich, 1995).
C. Rawcliffe, 'Hospital Nurses and their Work', in R. Britnell, ed., *Daily Life in the Late Middle Ages* (Stroud, 1998), pp. 43–64, 202–6.
C. Rawcliffe, *Medicine for the Soul. The Life, Death and Resurrection of an English Medieval Hospital* (Stroud, 1999).
C. Rawcliffe, 'Medicine for the Soul: The Medieval English Hospital and the Quest for Spiritual Health', in J. Hinnells and R. Porter, eds, *Religion, Health and Suffering* (London, 1999), pp. 316–38.
O. Redon, 'Autour de l'Hôpital S. Maria della Scala à Sienne au XIIIe siècle', *Ricerche storiche*, 15:1 (1985), pp. 17–34.
A. Rensi, 'L'Ospedale di San Matteo a Firenze', *Rivista d'arte*, 39 (1987), pp. 83–145.
A. Rensi, 'Interventi architettonici del primo Quattrocento nello Spedale di Santa Maria Nuova', in C. De Benedictis, ed., *Il patrimonio artistico dell'Ospedale Santa Maria Nuova di Firenze. Episodi di commitenza* (Florence, 2002), pp. 63–78.
G. Richa, *Notizie istoriche delle chiese fiorentine divise nei quartieri* (Florence, 1754), 10 vols.
J. Richards, *Altichiero. An Artist and his Patrons in the Trecento* (Cambridge, 2000).
G.C. Romby, 'Le vicende architettoniche nei secoli', in L. Sandri, ed., *Gli Innocenti e Firenze nei secoli* (Florence, 1996), pp. 21–32.
C. Roth, *The Last Florentine Republic* (London, 1925).
E.P. Rothrauff, 'Charity in a Medieval Community: Politics, Piety and Poor-relief in Pisa,

1257–1312' (unpublished Ph.D. thesis, University of California at Berkeley, 1994).
M. Rubin, *Corpus Christ: The Eucharist in Late Medieval Culture* (Cambridge, 1991).
N. Rubinstein, *The Government of Florence under the Medici, 1434–1492* (Oxford, 1966).
A. Rubio Vela, *Podreza, enfermedad y asistencia hospitaria en la Valencia del siglo XIV* (Valencia, 1984).
I. Ruffino, 'Canonici regolari di Sant'Agostino di Sant'Antonio di Vienne', *Diz. Ist. Perf.*, Vol. 2, pp. 134–41.
N.S. Rushton, 'Monastic Charitable Provision in Tudor England: Quantifying and Qualifying Poor Relief in the Early Sixteenth Century', *Continuity and Change*, 16:1 (2001), pp. 9–44.
H. Saalman, *The Bigallo: The Oratory and Residence of the Compagnia del Bigallo e della Misericordia in Florence* (New York, 1969).
H. Saalman, *Filippo Brunelleschi. The Buildings* (London, 1993).
L. Sandri, 'Ospedali e utenti dell'assistenza nella Firenze del Quattrocento', in G. Pinto, ed., *La società del bisogno. Povertà e assistenza nella Toscana medievale* (Florence, 1989), pp. 61–100.
L. Sandri, 'Aspetti dell'assistenza ospedaliera a Firenze nel xv secolo', in Centro Italiano di Studi e d'Arte, Pistoia, *Città e servizi nell'Italia dei secoli XII–XV* (Pistoia, 1990), pp. 241–6.
L. Sandri, ed., *L'archivio dell'Ospedale di San Giovanni di Dio di Firenze (1604–1890)* (Milan, 1991).
L. Sandri, ed., *Gli Innocenti e Firenze nei secoli. Un ospedale, un archivio, una città* (Florence, 1996).
L. Sandri, 'La gestione dell'assistenza a Firenze nel XV secolo', in *La Toscana al tempo di Lorenzo il Magnifico. Politica, economia, cultura, arte* (Pisa, 1996), Vol. 3, pp. 1363–80.
Santa Maria Nuova in Firenze. Memorie, testimonianze, prospettive (Florence, 1991).
P. Sanpaolesi, 'Alcuni documenti sull'Ospedale di San Matteo in Firenze', *Belle arti*, 2 (1946–8), pp. 76–87.
P. Saulnier, *De capite sacri ordinis* (Rome, 1649).
A. Saunier, *'Le pauvre malade' dans le cadre hospitalier médiéval. France du nord, vers 1300–1500* (Paris, 1993).
F. Scharf, *Der Freskenzyklus des Pellegrinaios in S. Maria della Scala zu Siena: Historienmalerei und Wirklichkeit in einem Hospital der Frührenaissance* (Hildersheim, 2001).
A. Schiaparelli, *La casa fiorentina e i suoi arredi nei secoli XIV e XV* (Florence, 1908).
C. Seymour Jr, *Sculpture in Italy: 1400–1500* (Harmondsworth, 1966).
M. Sichi, *Un'istituzione di beneficenza fiorentina: Il Bigallo* (Naples, 1927).
G. Silini, *Umori e farmaci. Terapia medica tardo-medievale* (Bergamo, 2001).
N.G. Siraisi, *Taddeo Alderotti and his Pupils. Two Generations of Italian Medical Tradition* (Princeton, 1981).
N.G. Siraisi, *Medieval and Early Renaissance Medicine. An Introduction to Knowledge and Practice* (Chicago and London, 1990).
N.G. Siraisi, *The Clock and the Mirror. Girolamo Cardano and Renaissance Medicine* (Princeton, 1997).
P. Skinner, *Health and Medicine in Early Medieval Southern Italy* (Leiden, 1997).
J.R. Spencer, 'Two New Documents on the Ospedale Maggiore, Milan and Filarete', *Arte lombarda*, 16 (1971), pp. 114–16.
J.R. Spencer, *Andrea del Castagno and his Patrons* (Durham, NC, and London, 1991).
J.T. Spike, *Fra Angelico* (New York and London, 1997).
P. Spilner, ' "Ut Civitas Amplietur." Studies in Florentine Urban Development, 1282–1400' (unpublished Ph.D. thesis, Columbia University, 1987).
J.N. Stephens, *The Fall of the Florentine Republic, 1512–1530* (Oxford, 1983).
C. Stevenson, *Medicine and Magnificence. British Hospital and Asylum Architecture, 1660–1815* (New Haven and London, 2000).

R. Stopani ed., *Firenze e i primi Giubilei. Un momento di storia fiorentina della solidarietà* (Florence, 1999).
S.T. Strocchia, *Death and Ritual in Renaissance Florence* (Baltimore and London, 1992).
F. Sznura, *L'espansione urbana di Firenze nel Duegento* (Florence, 1975).
G. Targioni Tozzetti, *Notizie deglí aggrandimenti delle scienze fisiche accaduti in Toscana nel corso di anni 60 del secolo XVII* (Florence, 1780).
O. Temkin, *The Falling Sickness*, 2nd edn (Baltimore and London, 1971).
A. Tenenti, *Il senso della morte e l'amore della vita nel Rinascimento* (Turin, 1989).
N. Terpstra, 'Competing Visions of the State and Social Welfare: The Medici Dukes, the Bigallo Magistrates and Local Hospitals in Sixteenth-Century Tuscany', *Renaissance Quarterly*, 54 (2001), pp. 1319–55.
U. Thieme and F. Becker, *Allgemeines Lexicon der Bildenden Künstler von der Antike bis zur Gegenwart* (Leipzig, 1920), Vol. 13.
J.D. Thompson and G. Goldin, *The Hospital: A Social and Architectural History* (New Haven and London, 1975).
P. Thornton, *The Italian Renaissance Interior, 1400–1600* (London, 1991).
F.-O. Touati, 'Les groupes des laïcs dans les hôpitaux et les léproseries au moyen âge', in *Les mouvances laïques des ordres religieux* (Saint-Étienne, 1996), pp. 137–62.
B.J. Trexler, 'Hospital Patients in Florence, San Paolo, 1567–68', *Bulletin of the History of Medicine*, 48 (1974), pp. 41–59.
R.C. Trexler, 'Death and Testament in the Episcopal Constitutions of Florence (1327)', in A. Molho and J.A. Tedeschi, eds, *Renaissance Studies in Honor of Hans Baron* (Florence, 1971), pp. 31–74.
R.C. Trexler, '"Florence by the Grace of the Lord Pope ..."', *Studies in Medieval and Renaissance History*, 9 (1972), pp. 116–215.
R.C. Trexler, 'The Foundlings of Florence: New Sources and First Results', *History of Childhood Quarterly*, 1 (1974), pp. 259–84.
R.C. Trexler, *Public Life in Renaissance Florence* (New York, 1980).
R.C. Trexler, 'A Widows' Asylum of the Renaissance: The Orbatello of Florence', in P.N. Stearns, ed., *Old Age in Pre-Industrial Society* (New York, 1982), pp. 119–49.
Gli Uffizi. Catalogo Generale (Florence, 1979).
V. Vannucci, *Istituzioni fiorentine* (Florence, 1902).
H.W. van Os, *Vecchietta and the Sacristy of the Siena Hospital Church. A Study in Renaissance Symbolism* (Maarssen, 1974).
T. Verdon and J. Henderson, eds, *Christianity and the Renaissance* (Syracuse, 1990).
V. Vestri, *Malati, medici e terapie all'Ospedale della Misericordia di Prato nel secolo XIV* (Prato, 1998).
M.P. Vignoli in *Lorenzo Ghiberti: materia e ragionamenti*, exh. cat. (Florence, 1978), pp. 426–7.
L.A. Waldman, 'New Documents for Memling's Portinari Portraits in the Metropolitan Museum of Art', *Apollo*, Feb. 2001, pp. 28–33.
M. Warner, *Alone of All her Sex. The Myth and Cult of the Virgin Mary* (London, 1978).
Z. Wazbinski, *L'Accademia Medicea del Disegno a Firenze nel Cinquecento: Idea e istituzione* (Florence, 1987).
A. Wear, 'Medicine in Early Modern Europe, 1500–1700' in L. Conrad, M. Neve, V. Nutton and R. Porter, *The Western Medical Tradition* (Cambridge, 1995), pp 207–361.
E.S. Welch, *Art and Authority in Renaissance Milan* (New Haven and London, 1995).
A. Whitley, 'Concepts of ill health and pestilence in fifteenth-century Siena' (unpublished Ph.D. thesis, University of London, 2004).
T. Wilson, *Ceramic Art of the Italian Renaissance* (London, 1987).
H. Wohl, *The Paintings of Domenico Veneziano, ca. 1410–1461. A Study of Florentine Art of the Early Renaissance* (Oxford, 1980).
S. Woolf, *The Poor in Western Europe in the Eighteenth and Nineteenth Centuries* (London, 1986).

S. Woolf, ed., *Domestic Strategies : Work and Family in France and Italy, 1600–1800* (Cambridge, 1991).

A.M. Zandri, C. Acidini Luchinat and S. Francolini, *Lo Spedale di Messer Bonifazio* (Florence, 1989).

G. Zarri, 'Gender, Religious Institutions and Social Discipline: The Reform of the Regulars', in J.C. Brown and R.C. Davis, eds, *Gender and Society in Renaissance Italy* (London, 1998), pp. 193–212.

J. Ziegler, *Medicine and Religion, c.1300. The Case of Arnau de Vilanova* (Oxford, 1998).

Index

Note: Page references in *italic* indicate illustrations.

Agnes, St 175
Agostino, Maestro 304, 313, 316, 324
Agnolo di Luca da Cortona, *speziale* 289
Agnolo, Maestro 229
ailments 264–7
   chronic 45, 216, 264, 280, 281–2
air, and transmission of disease 28, 95, 158–60, 339
albarelli 130–1, 292, 293–4
Alberighi, Maestro Baccio di Lodovico 234
Alberti, Leon Battista xxv, xxxiv, 69, 70, 77, 89–90, 109, 338, 340
Albertinelli, Mariotto (with Bartolommeo della Porta, Fra), *The Last Judgement* *143*, 145
Albertus Magnus 307–8, 311
Alderotti, Taddeo 304
Allori, Alessandro 168, 172
alms, charitable 9, 25–6, 32, 50, 57
aloe, in medicines 311, 312
altarpieces 339
   Messer Bonifazio hospital *134*, 136–7
   S. Egidio church 119–20, 123–6, *124*, 128–30, *129*, 132
   S. Matteo hospital 138–40, 145, 173–6, *174*
   ward chapels 58, 169–70, 180
Altopascio, hospital 9, 32, 230–1
Ambruogio di Giovanni, Maestro 233
anatomy, teaching 247–8
Andrea di Cione (Orcagna) 138–40, *139*
Andreuzza (painter) 58, 176
Angelico, Fra
   Annalena Altarpiece 384 n.65
   Coronation of the Virgin 124, 125–6, 132

Marriage of the Virgin 123
Virgin and Child with Saints 384 n.65
Antoninus, Archbishop of Florence 68, 133
   Summa theologia 88
Antonio, medico da Norcia 239
Antonio da Urbino 151
Antonio di Gianotto da Castelfranco, Maestro 233
Antonite Order 19
apothecaries xxxiii, 26, 56–7, 85, 86, 286–90
   and doctors 226, 229–30, 231–2, 253
   as infirmarers 287, 289–90
   payment 52, 287, 289–90
   and physicians 287, 288
   workshops *see* pharmacies
Arcangelo Michele e dei Broccardi hospital (Florence) 44, 107, 110, 348, 361 n.42
architecture 69, 121–3, 184
   and beauty and utility xxvi, xxxii, xxxiv, 71–81, 251, 338, 340
   and classicism xxxiv
   cruciform ward design 82, 147, 151–5, 157
   monastic model 86–7
   and scale and organisation 81–8
   and specialisation of function 89–90
   see also cloisters; façades; loggia
Arnold of Villanova 307, 311
art, hospital xxvi, xxxi–xxxii, 339
Arte dei Guidici e Notai 52, 67, 170, 396 n.11
Arte dei Medici e Speziali 27, 28, 226, 227–8, 230, 241–3, 244–6
Arte del Cambio 396 n.11

and S. Matteo 52, 85, 138–40, 170, 196–7, 220
Arte di Calimala 396 n.11
  and Messer Bonifazio 137, 262
  and S. Eusebio 12–13, 29, 30–1, 52
Arte di Por S. Maria della Seta 17, 25, 30, 46, 52, 68, 76, 105, 170, 296 n.11
artisans, and hospices 15–16, 44–5
Augustine of Hippo, St 113–14
avello tombs 180, *181*
Avicenna (Ibn Sina) 301, 303, 308, 318, 333, 334

babies, abandoned 17–18, 32, 43, 46
Babachari, Bartholomeo di Nicholò da Lucha, Maestro 246
Baccio d'Arezzo, Maestro Tomaso di 246
Baldovinetti, Alesso, *Life of the Virgin* frescoes 123, 126, 127, 132
Baldovinetti, Hectorre di Lionello 297
Balducci, Lemmo 50–1, 75, 84–5, 117, 137, 157–8, 396 n.18
banking, Florentine 6–7
Bandino di Maestro Banducci da Prato, Maestro 246
Barbara, St 172, 181–2
barbers 26, 36–7, 47, 52, 57
  numbers 230
  payment 27, 237
  and surgeons 228, 229, 238
Bardi, Messer Girolamo di Bernardo di 384 n.62
Bartholomeus Anglicus 314
Bartolini, Maestro Donato d'Agostino 230, 237–8, 246, 250
Bartolommeo della Porta, Fra (with Mariotto Albertinelli), *The Last Judgement* 143, 145
Bartolomeo di Chambio, Maestro 246, 249
beds and bedding 56, 65, 88, 165–7, 203, 217
  bed numbers 41, 43–4, 53, 58, 254, 280
  bed occupancy 254
  see also laundries
beggars
  attitudes to 71, 90, 106, 108–9, 268
  hostels xxxi, 338
  and Mal Francese 93, 98, *99*
bellezza xxvi, xxxii, 70, 71–81, 86, 91, 140, 338, 339, 340
Benedetta, Monna, 'medica di casa' (S. Maria Nuova) 302

Benedetto di Miniato, *speziale* 298–9
Benivieni, Antonio di Ser Pagholo, Maestro 234, 248
Benvenuti, Vezzano di Giovanni, Maestro 229
bequests to hospitals 35, 40, 45, 92
  and commemoration 51, 135
  Orsanmichele 37–8
  S. Maria della Scala 29, 52
  S. Maria Nuova 34, 36, 37–8, 55, 57, 68, 88, 181
  S. Matteo 377 n.63
Bergamo, hospitals 152
Bernardo di Maestro Nicholo da Migliazi, Maestro 234
Bettino da Imola 151
Bianchi (penitential movement, 1400) 52, 154
Bibbiena, Messer Lorenzo di Jacopo da (*spedalingo*) 21, 151
Bicci di Lorenzo 144
  Pope Martin Confirming the Consecration of S. Egidio xxvi–xxviii, *xxvii*, 58, 72, 114–17, *114*, 125, 159, 189–90
  and S. Egidio church 118, 122, 126–7
Bigallo confraternity 17, 38, 43, 65, 77
  loggia 76, *76*
  symbol *19*
  wealth 60
bile 56, 311, 323
Black Death 34–6
  economic impact 34–5
  impact on S. Maria Nuova 36–8, 88, 151, 186
  and specialisation of charity 27–8, 35
blood-letting 26, 36, 47, 52, 237, 238–9, 304
Boncompagno da Signa xxv, 9–10
bone doctors 229, 237, 239, 242, 303
Boniface VIII, Pope 11, 19
Bonini, Bonino d'Antonio di Maso (*spedalingo*) *78*, 79, 95–6, 135, 151, 304, 324
Bonsignori, Stefano 150, *150*, 154, 168, 206–9, *208*
Borromei, Margherita 107–8
Botti, Giovan Battista 108
Brandaglini, Maestro Cristofano di Giorgio 224–5, 233, 244–5, 246, 249, 300–1
Brasioli, F. 387 n.122
Brescia, hospitals 152
Bresnahan Menning, C. 105, 379 n.144

Broccardi hospital (Florence) 44, 107, 110, 348, 361 n.42
Brunelleschi, Filippo 41, 73, 75, 77
Buffalmacco, Buonamico 18
Buonaccolti, Don Vito (*spedalingo*) 153–4, 182–3
Buonafede, Lionardo di Giovanni 79
Buonamico hospital (Florence) 9, 18, 345
Buonomini del Bigallo 106–7, 108
Buonomini di S. Martino 106, 176, 219
Buontalenti, Bernardo 82, 153, 154, 168, *170*, 182
Burckhardt, Jacob xxviii
burial
  of patients 179, 182–3
  of staff 138, 195

Callisto da Piacenza, Don 98–9
Calza hospital (Florence) 5, 42–4, *42*, 350
Cambio guild *see* Arte del Cambio
Capocchi, **Fra** Alessandro 108
Cappella di S. Maria del Fiori hospital (Florence) 44
Capponi, Neri di Gino 317–18
Cardano, Girolamo 248
care and treatment of patients 57–8, 88–93, 287
Carrara, Francesca 375 n.27
Castagno, Andrea di Bartolomeo di
  Annunciation 180
  The Last Supper 201
  Life of the Virgin frescoes 127, 140, 201, 383 n.58
cataracts, removal 27, 239, 319
catarrh, treatment 311–12
Caterina, Monna, 'medica di casa' (S. Maria Nuova) 236, 302, 316–17
Catasto tax returns
  and apothecaries 289–90
  and doctors 243
  and hospital buildings 48–9
  and hospital finances 43–6, 60, 63–6, 90, 92, 371 n.156
  and occupations 270
  and widows 413 n.96
Catherine of Alexandria, St 138, 173–5, *174*
Cavalca, Fra Domenico, *Lo specchio della croce* 115
Cenni di Francesco di Ser Cenni 386 n.120
Ceppo delle Sette Opere della Misericordia hospital (Florence) 44, 107, 352
Ceppo hospital (Pistoia) 165, 207, 235
  and bed numbering 165, *165*

façade 79, *79*, 226–7, *227*
finances 60, 63
miraculous bed 166, 167, *167*
ceremonies, public 68, 80–1, 182–4
Chambio, Maestro Bartolomeo di 246, 249–50
charity
  centralisation 71, 90–1, 104–9, 337
  specialisation xxx, 4, 14–25, *14*, 39, 45, 52, 88, 337
chicken soup (S. Maria Nuova) 36, 93, 204, 294–5, 308
childbirth, Virgin Mary and St Margaret as patrons 130, 173
children, abandoned 17–18, 32, 43, 46–7, 106–8; *see also* orphans
choler, treatment 311, 312
Christ the Pilgrim 58, 162, 184
Christ Showing His Wound 72, 114–15, *114*
Christus Medicus 113–17, 135, 234, 335
Church and State
  and control of hospitals 66–7, 68, 104–5
  and poor relief xxxi, 28–31
Cinozzo, Maestro Simone di Cinozzo di Giovanni 229–30, 245, 246, 249
Circle of the Master of the S. Giorgio Codex
  Chaplains Confess Patients 163
  Corpse of a Patient 180
  Death and Burial of a Patient 180
  Nurses Delouse Patients and Wash their Feet 163
  Receiving the Poor at the Hospital Door 252
Ciuccio da Orvieto, Maestro 229
Clement VII, Pope 104
cloisters 140–6, *141*, *143*
  decoration 142–5
  female 84, 142, 200, 209
  male 84, *84*, *141*, 142
  see also S. Maria Nuova
clothing 49, 56, 65, 199, 200, 268–9
  nursing staff 164, 187, 189–91, 200
  see also laundries
Cluny, monastic infirmary 157
Codice Rustici 23, *24*, 48, *48*, 82, 121
Cohn, Samuel 38
College of Physicians 226, 230, 233, 245–7, 249
  Nuovo riceptario (*Ricettario fiorentino*) (1499) 290, 297, 300–2
commemoration, and role of hospital churches xxxi, 57, 117, 135–40,

179–80
commesse and *commessi* xxxii, 187–8, 263
  death and burial 195
  discipline 194–5
  food preparation 203–6
  habits 164, 187, 189–91, 200
  and herb cultivation 199, 207
  medical role 236
  religious observance 192–3
Commissioners for the Poor 102, 260
confession
  of nursing staff 192, 194
  of patients 163, 176–7, 253
confraternities 6, 19, 40, 58, 337, 361 n.42
  clientele 35, 268
  commemorative role 182
  increase in numbers 7
  and ward chapels 170, 176
  Buonomini di S. Martino 106, 176, 219
  Divine Love 98, 99–100
  Gesù Pellegrino 171
  Laudesi di S. Agnese 45
  Laudesi di S. Spirito 66
  S. Luca 120, 153, 170, 176, 182
  see also Bigallo confraternity; Misericordia confraternity; Orsanmichele
conservatories for girls 107–8, 110
construction industry 40, 211, 275
contado
  hospital property in 61
  immigration from 5–7, 15, 25
  nursing staff from 215
  patients from 97, 274–9, 277, *278*
contracts
  apothecaries 286–7, 289
  medical staff 27, 228–9, 230, 233, 237–9, 242
  nursing staff 187, 210–20, 221
converse and *conversi* xxviii, xxxii, 52, 119, 187, 190–1, 193
  see also nursing staff
convertite (reformed prostitutes) 5, 110
Cora, G. 416 n.42
Corazza, Bartolommeo di Michele del xxvii, 80, 121–3
corrodians *see converse* and *conversi*
corruption, by hospital officials 37, 66–7
Counter-Reformation xxx, 108, 110, 183, 193, 203, 338–9
Cremona, hospitals 152
crutch, as symbol of S. Maria Nuova xxviii, 123, 149, 151, 189, 190, 293

D'Addario, Arnaldo 105
Da Monte, Gianbattista 225, 226, 247, 248
Dati, Gregorio 780
Datini, Francesco di Marco 50, 51–2, 117, 396 n.18
death and burial 138, 145, 161, 179, 182–3, 195–7, 339
Del Migliore, Ferdinando 145, 161, 180
Della Robbia, Andrea 77–9, *78*
Della Robbia, Giovanni di Andrea's workshop 79, *79*, 207
  Care of the Sick 165, 226–7, *227*, 235, 239
Della Robbia, Luca 177
Delli, Dello
  Christ Showing His Wound 114–15, *114*
  Coronation of the Virgin 72, 115–16, *116*, 125, 132
  and S. Egidio 122, 125, 132
Devote della Vergine Maria hospital (Florence) 45, 47, 351–2
devote and *devoti* xxxii, 187
diagnosis 227, 231, 253
diet, in treatment of the sick xxx, 56, 65, 88, 287–8
digestion, aids to 324–5
Dino del Garbo 300, 301
Dioscorides, *Materia medica* 226, 291–3, 305, 318, 322, 334
Diotifeci d'Agnolo da Figline *see under* Ficino
disease
  categories 306–7
  incurable 89, 91, 98–100, 104, 267, 307
  and poverty 14, 52, 71
  and sin 113
  transmission 158–9
  see also epidemics; fevers; humoral theory; Mal Francese; plague
distillation, in preparation of medicines 56, 295–6
doctors xxxiii, 225–50
  and apothecaries 226, 229–30, 231–2
  and charity 234
  contracts 228–9, 230, 233, 237–9, 242
  geographical origins 241–4, *241*, *242*, 245
  junior (*adstantes*) 231–3
  and medicalisation 228–9, 286
  numbers 228
  professional networks 244–8, 249
  social status 241–4
  training xxvi, 27, 225–6
  variety 227–8, *228*
  see also physicians; surgeons

Domenico di Bartolo
  Care of the Sick 161, *162*, 163–4, 165, 188
  'Confession of a Dying Patient' *165*, 166, 177
  'The Physician' 231, *232*
  'Sala di San Piero' *155*, 160
  'A Semi-Clad Man' *252*, 268
  'Surgeon with Pincers' *232*, 236, 239
  'A Crippled Beggar' *252*
  'Wounded Male Patient' *235*
  Feeding the Poor 10, *10*
Domenico di Maestro Ciuccio da Orvieto, Maestro 246
Domenico di Maestro Giovanni dell'ossa, Maestro 229, 239
Domenico Veneziano, *Life of the Virgin* frescoes 126–7, 140
Dominican Order
  and founding of hospitals 9
  friary of S. Maria Novella 78, 80, 143
Donati, Francesco 58
Donnucce hospital (Donne Spagnole; Florence) 44, 45, 61, 353
dowries, provision 35, 219
drug jars 130–1, *292*, 293–4

Eisenheim Altarpiece (Grünewald) 114, 128, 131
electuaries 56, 297–8, 300, 303–4, 324, 326, 332–3
Elizabeth of Hungary, St 172–3, 175, 191, *191*
empirics 227, 230, 243, 319
epidemics
  economic effects 6–7, 24, 28, 34–5, 93, 268
  and hospitals 48–9, 71, 91–7, 100, 336–8
  and siege of Florence 102
  see also Mal Francese; plague
epilepsy (*mal caduco*), treatment 306, 312
eyes
  symptoms *319*
  treatments for 126, 239, 319–20

façades xxvi, 86, 146, 149
  Ceppo (Pistoia) 79, *79*, 226–7, *227*
  Innocenti 73–4, *73*, 75, 77–8, 151
  Messer Bonifazio 159
  S. Maria Nuova xxvi–xxviii, 72, 74, *75*, 149
  S. Matteo 74, 75
  S. Paolo 74, *74*, 76–7, 159

S. Piero Novello *41*
  see also loggias
famiglia of hospitals 36, 47, 52, 154, 176, 192
  see also nursing staff
famine 6–7, 29, 91, 93, 96–7, 102, 107, 259–60, 268
Fantoni, Lapo 17
feast-days and festivals 31, 49, 66, 68, 119, 132–3, 145, 176
febbre di spedale 159
fevers 266
  and sin 12
  treatment 287, 307, 308–9
Ficino, Diotifeci d'Agnolo da Figline 245, 246, 301–3, *302*, 315, 316–19, 330
Ficino, Marsilio 159, 301, 302–3, 307–8
Fieschi, St Caterina 98
Filarete, Antonio Averlino 69, 77, 89, 141, 152, 159, 166
Filippo, Maestro (bone doctor) 239
Fitzwilliam Museum, Cambridge *292*, 294
Florence
  city walls 7–9, 16, 20–1, 49
  and civic pride 3–4, 28, 69, 89–90, 92, 110, 135, 336–8
  economy 6, 7–8, 24–5, 28, 34–5, 93
  flood of 1333 43
  hospitals *see* hospitals *and under individual hospitals*
  immigrant labour 5–7, 15, 25
  Ordinances of Justice (1293) 13, 28
  Piviere di S. Giovanni 273, 276
  Republic 13, 67, 103, 105
  welfare system 70–1, 88–93, 103–9, 336–8
  see also contado; feast-days and festivals; Monte Comune; population; Sanità; siege of Florence; Signoria
flowers
  medicinal use 131
  symbolism 130
food xxv, 9, 49, 88
  expenditure on 63–5, *64*
  growing 206–9
  poultry 36, 207
  preparation 203–6
  provision 36, 49, 56, 102, 186
  shortages 6–7, 91, 93, 96–7, 102, 259–60, 335
Foucault, Michel xxx–xxxi, 109, 261, 339

foundling hospitals 46–7, 52, 61, 89, 92
  see also Innocenti; S. Gallo; S. Maria della Scala
Francesca, Monna, 'medica di casa' (S. Maria Nuova) 236, 302, 316–17
Francescho di Nolo, Maestro 243
Francesco di Gerino, *speziale* 288
Francesco di Domenico, Maestro 234
Franciscan Order
  Observant 90, 137, 143
  Tertiaries 20, 25–6, 52, 66–7, 78, 137, 187–8, 192
Fratellani, Maestro Giovanni, Maestro
Frati Saccati 21, 85, 136
French disease *see* Mal Francese
frescoes 339
  cloister 142–5
  S. Maria Nuova xxvi–xxviii, *xxvii*, 72, 77, 80–9, 170–2
  ward 170–2, 176
Fruosino, Bartolommeo di 119, 123, 288
Fruosino d'Andrea, Maestro 237–9, 301, 321
Fruosino di Cino della Fioraia, Maestro 228
Fruosino, Piero di Giovanni, *speziale* 288

gabelles 55, 68, 92, 104
Galen
  recipes 301, 307, 308, 311, 312, 315–16, 318, 322, 334
  and stomach, liver and spleen 309, 323, 326
  and theory of humours xxix, 248, 320, 326
Gamborta, Violante 251
gardens and gardeners 49, 206–9, 317–18
Gavitt, Philip 277
Gerini, Lorenzo di Niccolò, *Madonna Lactans* 392 n.28
Gerini, Maestro Mariotto di Niccholò di Gerino da Castiglione Aretino 245
Gerini, Niccolò di Pietro 170–1, 176
  The Adoration of the Magi 171, 172
  Crucifixion with Saints 136–8, 140
  The Last Judgement 171, 172–3
Gesù Pellegrino, Compagnia dei Pretoni hospital (Florence) *16*, 17, 31, 66, 347–8
Ghiberti, Lorenzo 178, *178*
Ghirlandaio, Davide di Tommaso 167
Giambologna 168, *170*

Giamboni hospital (Florence) 346
Gilini, Giovanni Giacomo 280
Giordano da Rivalto, Fra 11, 12, 251
Giorgio da Capri, Maestro 229
Giovanni, Maestro 229
Giovanni di Giusto da Castel S. Niccolò, Maestro 244
Giovanni di Maestro Ciuccio da Orvieto, Maestro (bone doctor) 239
Giovanni di Martino, Maestro (barber-surgeon, Piazza S. Giovanni) 238
Giovanni Battista, Maestro 229
Giovanni di Miniato, Gherardo and Monte di
  Annunciation 141, *141*
  Celebration of Mass 116, 120
  Commesse Praying 193
  Friar Preaching to S. Maria Nuova's Commesse 176, *177*
  The Funeral of S. Egidio 197
  Martin V Greeted by the Spedalingo of S. Maria Nuova 72, 80–1, *81*
  Pope Martin V Blessing the Altar 121–3, *122*
  service book illumination 119, 133, *134*, 190
Giovanni di Ser Bartolo di Maestro Giovanni da Radda 243
Giovanni di Vigo 317
girls, hostels for 107–8, 110
Girolamo di Messer Niccolò da Parma, Maestro 242
Girolomo di Ser Nicholaio di Neri, *speziale a S. Matteo* 286–7
Great Pox *see* Mal Francese
Gregory IX, Pope 230
Gregory X, Pope 21
Grünewald (Matthis Neithardt-Gothardt), *Eisenheim Altarpiece* 114, 128, 131
Guaiacum wood (drug) xxx, 110, 238, 267
Guerriero di Michelotto da Pescia, Maestro 237
Guidalotto di Volto dall'Orco 11–12, 29–30
guilds
  and administration of hospitals 12–13, 17, 30–1, 52, 188
  and feast-days 49, 68
  medical *see* Arte dei Medici e Speziali
  see also under names of individual Arte

Hallé, Jean-Noël 158
Hayum, André xxix
head problems

INDEX

eyes 126, 129, 319–20
headaches 314–15
insomnia 315–16
mental disturbance 265, 312–14
mouth 320–3
symptoms 309–10, *310*
treatment 309–23, *310*
wounds 227, 236, 239, 302–3, 316–19
Henry VII of England, King xxvi, 280
herbs
  cultivation 199, 207
  use in medicines 288, 317–18, 326–7
Herlihy, David 60
Hoby, Thomas xxvi
Hospice of the Orbatello (Florence) 35, 46, 350–1, 367 n.43
hospices
  artisans 15–16, 44–5
  façades xxvi–xxviii, 72–3
  pilgrims 10, 17, 32, 44, 131, *155*, 337
hospital churches and chapels xxxi, 23, 44, 58, 86, 117–46, 339
  and commemoration xxxi, 57, 117, 135–40
  and cure of the soul 117–35
  S. Maria Nuova 156
  S. Matteo 84, 86
  see also S. Egidio church; ward chapels
hospitals 3–5, *4*, *5*, *6*, *7*, 9–10, 14, 38–54, *39*, *50*, *53*, *70*, *90*
  administration *see* guilds; *spedalingo*
  centralisation of resources 71, 90–1, 106–7, 109
  convalescent 105
  distribution 8–10, 16–19, 39, 40
  expansion 40–1, 337–9
  finances 54–67, 92–3, 103–6
  foundation 5–6, 7, 8, 9, 14, 15, 38–54, *39*
  isolation *see* lazzarettos
  kitchens 205–6
  length of stay 44, 53, 56–7, 262–4
  list 341–55
  liturgical life xxxi, 58, 119–20, 145, 192–3
  location 13–14, 16–17, 40, 41–2
  monastic infirmaries 5, 8–9
  property 11, 13, 29–31, 55, 60–1, 103, 187
  religious role xxix, xxxi–xxxii, 12, 34–69, 70, 86–8, 110, 113
  and Renaissance medicine 225–6
  size 44, 46, 53–4, 254, 337
  standard of care 57–8, 88–93, 251, 336

see also architecture; bequests to hospitals; foundling hospitals; Incurabili hospitals; medicalisation of hospitals; mortality rates; nursing staff; specialisation of hospitals
hostels
  for beggars xxxi, 338
  monastic 9
  for pilgrims 9, 10–11, 15, 20, 32, 44–5, 53, 61, 90–1
  for reformed prostitutes 5, 228
humanism, medical 225–6, 243
humoral theory xxix, 12, 159, 248
  and balance of non-naturals 304, 311
  and blood-letting 238–9, 304
  evidenced in recipes 308, 309, 313, 318, 322, 323–6, 332
  and treatment of plague 308
hysteria 306, 329–30

iconography:
  of Christ 114–15, *114*
  and sick poor 131–2
  and Virgin Mary 115–17, *116*, 125, 130
illness
  chronic 45, 216, 264, 280, 281–2
  incurable 71, 98–100, 104, 267
  mental 265, 312–14
incense, in medicines 303, 316, 318
Incurabili hospitals xxx, 71, 104, 267, 307, 338
  S. Giacomo (Rome) 98, *99*, 281
  SS. Trinita 89, 91, 98–100, 101, 110, 267, 354–5
indulgences 30, 31, 132, 136
infirmarers 198–9, 201, 204, 231–2, 253
  apothecaries as 287, 289–90
Innocent III, Pope 32
Innocent IV, Pope 30
Innocenti hospital 4, 68
  architecture 41, 73–5, *73*, 77
  cellars 206
  decoration 77–8, *78*
  expansion 92, 157
  façade 73–4, *73*, 75, 77–8, 151, 184
  finances 63, 93, 103, 104–5, 373 n.188
  food provision 207
  foundation 35, 51–2
  foundlings 18, 46, 89, 92–3, 280
  garden 208–9
  geographical origins of foundlings 277–8
  hospital church 118

loggia *73*, 73–4, *74*, 77, 148
  and laundry 209
  medical staff 47, 221, 228, 229, 234, 245–6, 249
  nursing staff 192
  and state control 105
insomnia, treatment 315–16
Issogne, Valle d'Aosta *xvi*, 291, *292*

Jacopo di Cione *138–40, 139*
Jacopo di Coluccino da Lucca, Maestro 233

Knights Hospitallers:
  and Altopascio 9, 32, 231
  and S. Giovanni di Gerusalemme 9, 32, 42–3, 188
  and S. Sepulcro hospital 9, 18
Knights Templar 42, 344

La Riva, Bonsevin de 54
laicisation 31
land, availability 19, 21, 23–4, 40–1, 85–6
Landino, Cristoforo 88–90, 251, 255
Landucci, Luca 98, 258, 288
Lanfranc of Milan 227
Lateran Council, Fourth, 1215 120, 192
laundries 209–10
lazzarettos xxxi, 69, 71, 93, 100, 158, 336, 338
  S. Bastiano 91, 94–5, 96–7, 101, 110
  and S. Maria della Scala 96
  and S. Maria Nuova 94–7, 256, 257, 260
Leo X, Pope xxvi, 99
Leonardo da Vinci 247–8, 340
Leoniceno, Niccolò 225
leprosaria 12–13, *48*, 49–50, 52
lettiera (litter) 165–6, 203
Lionardo di Maestro Angnolo di Ser Tignoso da Bibbiena 243
Lippi, Fra Filippo, *Scenes of Early Carmelites* 143
liver, problems 309, 323, 325–7, *325*
loggias 147, 184
  Ceppo (Pistoia) 79, *79*
  function 76–7, 146
  Innocenti 73–4, *73*, 77, 148
  Messer Bonifazio 74–5, 128
  S. Antonio 75
  S. Giovanni Evangelista 73
  S. Guiliano a Colombaia 43
  S. Lorenzo 73
  S. Maria della Scala 18
  S. Maria Nuova 74, *75*, 86

S. Matteo 74–5, *74*, *76*, 77, 83–4, 149, 158
S. Paolo 74, *74*, 76–7
London, Savoy Hospital xxvi, 218
Lorenzo di Bicci, *Madonna of Humility and Saints* 140, 386 n.120
Lucca, Maestro Iacopo di Coluccino da 233
Lucca di Ceccho, Maestro 243
lunettes, decorated 72, 77–8, *78*, 114–17, *114*, 125, 137, 143–5, 291
Lupi, Messer Bonifazio 36, 50, 117, 136–8, 191, 369 n.88, 396 n.18
Luther, Martin xxvi, xxxiii, 88, 186, 270

Machi, Giovanni di Francesco, Maestro 237, 289
Mal Francese xxx, 91, 331
  and Incurabili hospitals 71, 89, 97–101, *99*, 266–7, 338
  mortality rates 93
  treatment 238, 240, 307
Mal Persiano (St Anthony's Fire) 19
Malmaritate 108
'Man of Sorrows' 72, 114–17, *114*
mandrake oil 308–9
Mantua, hospitals 152
Marescalchi, Francesco, of Ferrara 302–3
Mariano del Buono di Jacopo 191, *191*
Marini, Benedetto di Lozo, *infermiere* at S. Paolo 266
Mariotto di Cristofano 173–6, *174*
Mariotto di Niccolò, Maestro 234
Martin V, Pope xxvi–xxviii, 67, 68, 80–1, 132, 190
Mary, iconography 115–17, *116*, 125, 130, 133
Masaccio (Tommaso di Ser Giovanni di Mone Cassai)
  Sagra 143
  The Tribute Money 160
Massaio, Piero del, *Veduta di Firenze* 3–5, *3*, 72, 149, 376 n.42
Masses
  commemorative xxxi, 57, 117, 135–40, 182
  and ward chapels 23, 147–9, 156, 160, 169–70, 175–6, 185, 192
Master of S. Verdiana (Tommaso del Mazza)
  SS. John the Baptist and Anthony of Padua 134, 136, 137
  SS. John the Evangelist and Louis of Toulouse 134, 136, 137
Mattioli, Pietro Andrea 291–3, 295–6, *296*,

INDEX

297
and treatment of illness 304, 305–6, 309, 311–12, 313, 314–18, 320–2, 326, 329, 331, 334
medicalisation of hospitals xxix, xxx, 11, 14, 25–8, 32–3, 53, 71, 282
and doctors 228–9, 286
and effects of Black Death 35, 47, 228–9
medicheria (hospital surgery) 85, 239–40
Medici, Alessandro de' 103, 105, 271
Medici, Averardo de' 309, 311
Medici, Benardetto de' 127
Medici, Cardinal Guilio de' 98–100
Medici, Cosimo di Giovanni de' 152, 245, 301
and S. Egidio church 118, 126–7
Medici dukes and grand dukes of Tuscany
Cosimo I de' 103, 104–7, 109, 337
Cosimo II de' 156, 254
and artistic patronage 140
and reform of welfare system 71, 103–9, 337
and S. Maria Nuova 133–4
and siege of Florence 102
Ferdinando I 104–5
Ferdinando II 254–5
Francesco I 82, 154
Medici, Giovanni de' 135, 152
Medici, Lorenzo de' 234
Medici, Manetto di Neri de' 211
Medici, Monna Chaterina de' 127
Medici, Piero de' 245
medicine
modern studies xxix–xxxi
preventative xxix, 238–9
professionalisation 28, 36, 226, 286–90
spiritual and secular xxix, xxxi–xxxii, 12, 34–69, 70, 86–8, 143, 147–9, 166, 335, 339; and bequests to hospitals 35, 36–7, 51, 57; and commemoration xxxi, 57, 117, 135–40, 179–83, 666; and founding of hospitals 50–1; and redemptive charity 110, 338; and religious imagery 58, 77–8, 115–35, 136–40; *see also* hospital churches and chapels; ward chapels; wards
teaching and learning 225–6, 245–9
medicines
costs 56, 65
preparation 294–6
storage 56, 131, 291–4, *292*
see also apothecaries; electuaries; pills; plasters; poultices; recipes; simples;
unguents
melancholy, treatment 306, 311, 312–13
men
and length of hospital stay *262*, 263
and mortality rates 257–8, *257*, *259*, *260*, 263
and sexual problems 331–2, *332*
Mendicant friars 78
and Third Orders 19–20
Mendicanti hospital (Florence) xxxi, 109, 338
menstruation 176, 327–9
Messer Bonifazio hospital 4, 87, 159, 351
apothecaries 52, 287, 289
architecture 74–5, *74*, 82
expansion 157
finances 60, 63, *64*, 65, 68
foundation 35, 41
gardens 209
hospital church 118, 136, 170
length of patient stay 262
medical staff 229, 233–4, 237, 242, 244, 249
nursing staff 52, 191–2, 198, 211, 401 n.120
and plague victims 96
religious and medical roles 52, 66
and segregation of patients 86
and sick poor 50, 102
size 53, 254
wards 149, 156, 390 n.30
Mesué, Yuhanna ibn Masawayh 301, 303, 311, 313
Michelangelo Buonarotti 62
Michele di Fruosino, *spedalingo* of S. Maria Nuova 288
Michele di Maestro Michele da Pescia, 301–3, 324
Michele di Mariano, Maestro 301
Michelozzi, Girolomo 108
Michelozzo Michelozzi 74, 77, 157
midwives 199
migraine, treatment 314–15
Milan
Brolo hospital 32, 54
hospitals 53–4
lazzaretto 96
Ospedale Maggiore xxvi, 77, 90, 101, 141, 152–3, 159, 166, 248, 280, 337
Milanesi, Gaetano 131
Mini, Lucca di Nanni, *speziale* 290
Misericordia confraternity 34, 38, 60, 62, 71, 97, 101, 106

450 INDEX

Misericordia hospital (Prato)
  geographical origins of patients 413 n.100
  length of patient stay 262
  mortality rates 257–8, *257*
  patient admissions 255–6, *255*, 264
  recipes 298
  socio-economic status of patients 267–9
mithraditum (drug) 307–8
Molho, Anthony 271
Monaco, Lorenzo 292 n.94
  Adoration of the Magi 123–4, 131, 132
  as illuminator 119, *124*, 125, 140
  Pietà 145
  St Nicholas 145
monasteries
  and foundation of hospitals 5, 8–9
  and infirmaries 9, 157, 184
Monastero del Ceppo 44, 107
Monastero delle Fanciulle Abbandonate della Pietà 108
Monastero di S. Caterina 108
Monastero di S Maria e S Niccolò 107–8
Montaigne, Michel de xxvi
Monte Comune 61, 94–5, 127, 220
Monte di Pietà 104, 105
Morrison, Fynes xxvi
mortality rates 339
  female 102, 156, *257*, 258, *259*, *260*, 263, 272, *272*
  and food shortages 102, 259, 260–1
  and length of patient stay 262–3, *262*
  male 102, 257–8, *257*, *259*, *260*, 263
  and patient admissions 255–6, *255*, *256*, 281
  and plague 37, 101–2, 256–7, 259–60
mouth
  symptoms *320*
  treatments for 301, 320–3

Nardi, Jacopo 97
Nardo, Mariotto di 144–5, 393 n.94
Neri, Girolamo di Ser Nicholaio di 286, 289
Niccolò da Parma, Maestro (bone doctor) 237, 242
Nicholò di Ghianghano di Nicholò, Maestro 239
Noli, Francesco, Maestro 288
non-naturals xxix–xxx, 142, 247, 304, 311
  see also diet
nursing staff xxxii, 36, 52–3, 69, 83, 162, 175, 186–221, 339

  age 217–18
  contracts 187, 210–20, 221
  discipline 192–5, 220
  dormitories 21, 58, 201–3
  female 209, 210–11
  food cultivation 206–9
  food preparation 203–6
  habits 164, 187, 189–91, 200
  investiture ceremony 189
  laundries 209–10
  male 236
  medical role 236
  numbers 198, 203
  physical and spiritual roles 200
  refectories 200–1, 203, 217
  socio-economic status 212–13, *213–14*
  types 187–8
Giovanni di Marcho Nuti, Maestro 287

oculus *16*, 17, 23, 149, 159–60
ointments 175, 308–9, 324, 331
opium 309, 316, 321–2
Orbatello hospital (Florence) 35, 46, 350–1, 367 n.43
Orcagna (Andrea di Cione) 138–40, *139*, 145, 393 n.94
orcioli *292*, 293–4
Orco, Guidalotto di Volto dall' 29–30
Ordinances of S. Maria Nuova (1510–11) xxvi, 89, 280
  and ailments treated 264–5
  and apothecaries and pharmacy 287, 294–5
  and death of patients 179
  and female surgeons 83
  and hospital food 206, 207
  and medical staff 231–2, 236, 241, 243, 247
  and nursing staff 83, 186, 197–9, 204, 209
  and reception of patients 162–5, 253–4, 272
  and socio-economic status of patients 270–1
organs, ward 147–9
Orlandi, Stefano 384 n.62
orphanages 4, 17–18, 46–7
orphans
  increase in numbers 92–3
  and poor relief 35, 219
Orsanmichele, Company of 139
  bequests to 37–8, 62
  corruption allegations 37

legal privileges 29
  and poor relief 34, 35, 53, 337
  wealth 60, 67
Ortolani, Giovanni 168–70, *169*
Ospizio del Servante (Florence) 346
Ospizio delle vedove di Sant'Agnese (Florence) 45, 47, 351–2
Ospizio delle vedove in Via Chiara 63, 353

Padua, University and teaching of medicine 225, 242
Pagholo di Maestro Giovanbatista, Maestro 297
Pagolo di Pagolo, barber from Piazza S. Giovanni 237
Panofsky, Erwin 130
Parigi, Giulio il Vecchio 74
Paris, Hôtel-Dieu 33, 281
Park, Katharine 263
Parte Guelfa 46, 80, 228
Passerini, Luigi 96, 105
patients 251–85, 340
  admission to wards 161–4, 199, 253–6
  ailments 264–7
  clothing 164, 199, 200
  and confession 163, 176–7, 253
  death and burial 145, 161, 179, 182–3
  expulsion 13
  female 271–2
  food 36, 56, 204
  geographical origins 272–9, *272*, **273**, *277*, *278*, 283–5
  length of stay in hospital 44, 53, 56–7, 262–4
  modern studies xxix–xxx, xxxiii
  numbering 164–5, 253, 287
  numbers 53, 92, 254–6, 280
  from outside Florence 254
  physical care 57–8, 88–93, 161–8, 185
  segregation 82–3, 85–6, 89, 95, 142
  socio-economic status 267–72, 279–80, 282–3
  spiritual care 147, 149, 168–84
patron saints 130, 172–5, 393 n.94
patronage
  artistic xxviii, xxxi–xxxii, xxxiv, 81, 117, 120, 140, 170
  financial 25, 52, 61, 68, 91, 118, 133–5, 140, 149
  and rights 30
  see also commemoration
Pavia, hospitals, S. Matteo xxv, 153
pediments, *pietra serena* 16, 17

Penitenti, Franciscan 20, 26
pestle and mortar, in preparation of medicines 295
Peter of Spain, *Thesaurus pauperum 235*, 239–40
  and *Ricettario* of S. Maria Nuova 299, 301–2, 304, 312, 320, 334
pharmacies xxxiii, 32, 226, 229, 290–6, 339
  appearance 291, *292*, 294
  cucina 294–5
  location 291
  Messer Bonifazio 52
  and out-patients 56, 85, 291
  and physicians 291
  preparation of medicines 294–5
  S. Maria Nuova 56, 65, 66, 229, 289, 291–6
  S. Matteo 5, 85, 295–6
  storage of medicines 56, 131, 291–4, *292*
  see also medicines
pharmacists *see* apothecaries
phlegm 311, 312, 313, 324
physicians 32, 36–7, 47, 52
  and apothecaries 287, 288
  Arab 226, 299, 301, 303
  and divine physician 113–14
  geographical origins 242–3, *242*
  income 27, 57, 233–4, 237–8, 243–4
  number 229, 230
  and pharmacies 291
  prestige 28, 231–3, 234
  professional networks 244, 249
  professionalisation 28, 227
  role 230–4
  and the Studio 230, 245–6
  ward rounds 231–2, 253, 287
Pieratti, Giovanni Battista 99–100, 161
Piero della Francesco, *Life of the Virgin* frescoes 126–7
Piero di Puccio, Maestro 229
Piero, Maestro, 'doctor of the house' (S. Maria Nuova) 307
Pierozzi da S. Casciano, Orlando di (*spedalingo*) 23, 38, 151
Piers, Henry 156, 254
Pietro Leopoldo of Lorraine, Grand Duke of Tuscany 5, 17, 90
pilgrims
  accommodation 9, 10–11, 15, 20, 32, 39, 43–4, 53, 61, 90–1
  female 44, 45
pills 56, 303, 308, 311, 324
Pinto, Giuliano 61

Pirillo, Paolo 254
Pisa, hospitals 53
Pistoia *see* Ceppo hospital
plague xxx, 34–6, 52, 91–7, 101
   and lazzarettos xxxi, 69, 71, 91, 94–6, 256, 260, 336, 338
   and location of hospitals 14, 158
   and mortality rates 101–2, 256–7, 259–60
   and specialisation of charity 27–8, 35, 337–8
   treatments 306–8
plasters 298, 316, 324–5, 326
Poggini, Maestro Lorenzo di Michele 233
Pollini, Cione di Lapo di Gherardo 17, 52
Pontormo, Jacopo, *Scenes in a Ward* 164, *198*, 199–200
poor
   and economic crises 6–7, 34–5, 102
   and foundation of hospitals 10–11, 15, 21, 25–6, 50–2
   and monastic alms 9, 25–6, 32, 50, 57
   in paintings 131
   and the plague xxx, 36–8
   standard of care 57–8, 88–93
   temporary accommodation 39, 89
   worthy and unworthy 71, 106, 268–9, 279–80, 340
poor relief xxvi, 35
   and Church and State xxxi, 28–31
   institutionalisation 71
   outdoor relief 25–6, 27, 53, 96
   and social control xxx–xxxi, 71, 90, 338
Pope-Hennessy, John 383 n.56
population, Florentine:
   decline 40, 91
   growth 5–6, 7, 9, 15, 27–8, 71, 91
Portinari, Accerito 57, 180
Portinari, Antonio 131
Portinari, Bernardo 304
Portinari, Falganaccio 180
Portinari family
   coat of arms *181*
   and S. Egidio 120, 123, 126, 127–8, 135
   and S. Maria Nuova xxviii, 26, 30, 57, 58, 61, 85, 104–5, 118, 133, 180, 396 n.10
Portinari, Folco d'Adoardo 118, 127, 136
Portinari, Folco di Ricovero 21, 25, 30, 57, 117, 127, 135–6, 180, *181*
Portinari, Francesco xxvi, 89
Portinari, Manetto 57, 180
Portinari, Pigello 126, 127–8
Portinari, Tommaso di Folco 126, 128, 131, 137
poultices 302–3, 319–20, 329, 330, 332
poultry 36, 65, 207
poverty
   and disease 14, 52, 71
   and economic crises 28, 34–5
   types 267–72
powders, medicinal 324
Prato
   Spedale del Ceppo 51, 62
   see also Misericordia hospital
prescriptions xxxiii, 297
professionalisation of medicine 28, 36, 226, 286–90
prostitutes, reformed 5, 110, 338
public health
   and location of hospitals 13–14
   and medicalisation of hospitals 28, 36, 69, 71, 282
   and plague measures 101
Pullan, Brian 110
purgation 56, 239, 311, 313, 334

Rawcliffe, Carole xxix, 188
recipes xxxiii, 236, 239
   beauty treatments 304, 334–5
   for eye treatments 126, 319–20
   named authors *299–300*, 300–1, 309, 315–16
   S. Maria Nuova xxxiii, 126, 236, 237, 239, 297–304
Redon, Odile 218
refectories 21, 85, 200–1, 203
Reguardati, Maestro Benedetto da Norcia 324–5
relics 68, 120–1, 154
Renaissance
   continuity and innovation xxviii–xxix
   and laicisation 31
Rhazes (Razi Abü Bakr Muhammad ibn Zakarïya') 301, 303, 304, 324
Ricettario of S. Maria Nuova xxxiii, 264, 297–304, *299–300*
   abdominal problems 323–34, *333*
   beauty treatments 304, 334–5
   eye conditions 126, 319–20
   fevers 308–9
   head problems 309–23, *310*, *323*
   head wounds 236, 239, 303, 316–19
   named authors 239, 299–303, *299–300*, *302*, 309, 315; women 199, 236, 302, 316–17
   plagues and pestilences 306–8

INDEX

symptoms *305*, 306
urogenital infections 239, *326*, 327–34, *332*, 335
Richa, Giuseppe 145–6, 151, 158, 180
Rome, hospitals, S. Giacomo in Augusta 98, 99, 281
see also S. Spirito
roofs, 'a cavaletti' 159
rose-water, use in medicines 56, 288, 311
Rosselli, Francesco, *Veduta di Firenze* 11–12, *12*, 84, *84*, 149
Rossellino, Bernardo 152, 178, *178*
Rosso, Giovanni Battista (Rosso Florentino), *Virgin and Child Enthroned* 137
roundels
  Innocenti 77–8
  S. Paolo *78*, 79
Rustici, Marco di Bartolommeo 23, *24*, 82, 121

St Anthony's Fire 4, 19, 25, 48, 131, 307
S. Agniolo della Povertà dei Chapponi hospital, Florence 354
S. Antonio hospital (Florence) 4, 19, 48–9, *48*, 68, 75, 131, 188, 349
S. Bartolomeo al Mugnone hospital (Florence) 25, 347
S. Bastiano degli ammorbati hospital (Florence) 91, 94–5, 96–7, 101, 110, 353
S. Bernardino degli Uberti hospital (Florence) 347, 361 n.45
S. Candida hospital (Florence) 346
S. Caterina dei Talani hospital (Florence) 99, 107, 350, 367 n.43
S. Dionisio hospital (Florence) 355
S. Egidio church (S. Maria Nuova) 72, 77, 82, *122*
  architecture 121–3
  Cappella Maggiore 118, 120, 121, 125, 131; *Life of the Virgin* frescoes 123, 126–8, 132
  choir screen (Tramezzo) 125, 383–4 n.56
  and *commesse* 191, *191*
  decoration 117, 120–32
  dedication and rededication xxvi–xxvii, 68, 80–1, 119–21, 126, 132
  devotional objects 119–20, 133
  feast-days 119, 132–3
  financial patronage 118, 133–5
  ground-plan 118, 121
  inventory (1376) 118–20
and investiture of nursing staff 189
main altar 120, 123–30, 132
and relics 119–21, 126
remodelling xxvi, 65, 82, 121
role 131–2, 136
service books 80, 119, 123, 133
size 118
tombs 180
vestments 119
S. Eusebio hospital (S. Jacopo a San Eusebio, Spedale di S. Sebio) *48*, 49–50, 52, 343, 367 n.38
  and Calimala 12–13, 29, 30–1, 52
  Campoluccio site 49
  finances 63, *64*
  location 12, 14
  May Day celebrations 31
  medical staff 49
  religious and medical roles 66
S. Fina hospital, S. Gimignano 291, 294, 297
S. Gallo hospital *12*, 344
  and Church and State 29–30
  demolition 103
  expansion 12–13, 14, 228
  finances 60, 61, 63–5, 93
  and guilds 30
  location 9, 11–12
  medical staff 47, 228–9, 233–4, 244, 249
  and orphans 4, 46, 47, 93
  and pilgrims 11
  property 11, 13, 61
  and sick poor 47
S. Giorgio dello Spirito Santo hospital (Florence) 345
S. Giovanni hospital (Florence) 354
S. Giovanni Battista Decollato hospital (Florence) 16–17, 44, 347
S. Giovanni Battista della Calza hospital (Florence) 5, 42–4, *42*, 350
S. Giovanni Evangelista hospital (Florence) xxv, 8, 9–10, 24, 73, 342
S. Giovanni fra l'Arcora hospital (Florence) 18, 103, 188, 348
S. Giuliano hospital (Florence) 90–1, 354
S. Giuliano a Colombaia de'Vettori hospital (Florence) *42*, 43, 350
S. Giuliano in Verzaia hospital (Florence) 44, 352
S. Jacopo in Campo Corbolini hospital (Florence) 25, 347
S. Lò hospital (SS. Eligio e Lorenzo dei

454   INDEX

maniscalchi; Florence) 44, 350
S. Lodovicho hospital (Florence) 354
S. Lorenzo hospital (Florence) 73, 343, 351
S. Lorenzo a S. Pier Gattolino hospital (Florence) 351
S. Lucia de'Magnoli hospital (Florence) 43–4, 61, 345–6
S. Maria de Laudibus ('Pigeon') hospital (Florence) 17, *18*
S. Maria degli Angioli dei battilani hospital (Florence) 90, 353–4
S. Maria degli Innocenti hospital (Florence) *see* Innocenti hospital
S. Maria del Bigallo hospital (Florence) 65, 354
S. Maria della Scala (Florence) 4, 348
  bequests 29, 52
  finances 68
  foundation 17
  as foundling hospital 17–18, 46–7
  infirmary 160
  loggia *20*, 74
  medical staff 228
  and plague victims 96
  wards 152
S. Maria della Scala (Siena) xxv, 68, 275
  and art xxxi, 77, 101
  bequests to 62
  as foundling hospital 32, 101
  frescoes *155*, 161, *162*
  nursing staff 218
  as pilgrim hospice 10, 17, 32, 131, *155*, 337
  relics 68, 121
  and St Catherine of Siena 126
  and sick poor 101, 280
  and Tertiaries 188
  wards 153
S. Maria delle Stinche hospital (Florence) 53, 349, 367 n.43
S. Maria dell'Umiltà hospital (Florence) 43–4, 351
S. Maria e S. Niccolò hospital (Florence) 107–8
S. Maria Nuova 4, 5, 22, *24*, 59, 150, 202, 346
  apothecaries 287–90
  architecture xxv–xxvi, xxviii, 23–4, 72, 74, *75*, 78–9, 82
  bequests to 34, 36, 37–8, 55, 57, 68, 88, 181
  'Books of the Dead' 253–4, 255, 264, 267
  and Catasto returns 367 n.43
  cellars 202, 206
  Chiostro delle Medicherie xxviii, 65, 72, 140, *141*
  Chiostro delle Oblate 23
  Chiostro delle Ossa xxviii, 21, 65, 115, 117, 123, 145, 179
  and Church and State 29–30, 104–5
  conditions treated 265–6
  cruciform wards 23, 147, 151–5
  crutch symbol xxviii, 123, 149, 151, 189, 190, 293
  decoration 77, 114
  devotional life 58
  and dissection 247–8
  expansion 21–4, 27, 35, 41, 57–8, 65–7, 82, 85, 228
  famiglia 36, 52, 154, 176
  female cloister 142, *143*, 209
  female ward *155*; building work *21–3, 58, 66, 82*; chapel *23, 156, 181*; decoration *130*; exterior *150,* 150; fresco-cycle 170–3; nursing staff 83; open plan 155–7; overcrowding 156, 254–5; possessions 211–12; tabernacle 178–9, *178*; upper terrace *208*; windows 156, 160, 172
  festivals 66, 119, 132, 176
  finances 54–60, *55*, 61–2, 63, *64*, 65–6, 92, 103–4, 261, 373 n.188
  financial patronage 133–5
  food 36, 56, 203–6
  foundation 14, 19, 21
  frescoes xxvi–xxviii, *xxvii*, 72, 77, 80–1, 114–17
  gardens and gardeners 206–7
  impact of Black Death 36–8, 88, 151, 186
  and infirmarers 287
  infirmary 58, 159
  kitchen 206
  lazzaretto 94–7, 100, 256, 257
  legal privileges 29, 68
  liturgical life 58, 119–20, 145, 192–3
  male cloister 72, 142, 144
  male ward 72, 149, *169*; chapel 58, 120, 136, 168–70, 176, 182–3; cruciform shape 23, 151, 153–5; extension 21, 23, 82, 92; tabernacles 177–8; windows xxviii, 72, 149, 159
  medical school 247
  medical staff 26–7, 36, 57, 229, 231–4, 244–6, 249
  and medicalisation 25, 26–7, 228

INDEX

medicheria (hospital surgery) 240, 265
medicines 56
mortality rates 37, 102, 156, *256*, 257–61, *259*, *260*, *262*, 263, 281
nursing staff 36, 83, 105, 186, 187, 189–92, 193–5, 197–8; contracts 212–15, *213–14*; dormitories 21, 58, 201–3; and food preparation 203–6; refectories 21, 200–1, *202*, 203
patients xxxiii, 254–6, *256*; geographical origins 273–9, *273*, *274*, *278*, 283–5; length of stay 44, 56–7, *262*, *263*; marital status *272*; number 92, 280; socio-economic status 268–71, *270*, *271*
pharmacy 56, 65, 66, 229, 289, 291–6
and plague victims 93–7, 100, 307
priests 177, 269–70
private rooms 88, 251, 270–1
reputation 36
Sapientia 88, 186, 270
and sick poor 26–7, 69, 102, 280, 337, 391 n.61
size 53, 254
standards of care 88, 91
see also Ordinances of S. Maria Nuova; *Ricettario*; S. Egidio church; *spedalingo*
S. Maria in Via Chiara hospital (Florence) 63, 353
S. Matteo hospital 4, *83*, 202, 351
apothecary 85, 286–7, 289
architecture 74–5, *74*, *76*, 77, 83–5
and Arte del Cambio 52, 85, 138–40, 170, 196–7, 220
bequests to 377 n.63
and children 218–19
decoration 77, 138–40, *139*, 166–7, 199–200
expansion 41
female cloister 84, 142, 200, 209
female ward 84, 85–6, *139*, 147, 156–8, 161, 173–4, 181, 199–200
finances 60, 62–5, *64*, 94, 371 n.156
foundation 35, 50–1
garden 207–9
hospital church 118
kitchen 205
loggia 74–5, *74*, *76*, 77; and oculus 83–4, 149, 158
male cloister 84, *84*, *141*, 142, 143
male ward 84, 85–6, *139*, 149, 166, 257
medical staff 229–30, 234, 237–9, 245–6, 249, 250

medicheria (hospital surgery) 85, 240
mortality rates 256–7
nursing staff 52, 175, 188–9, 192, 195, 198, 209; contracts 210–13, 215–20; dormitories 203; refectories 85, 200–1, 217
and patients: conditions treated 264–5; numbers 255; sick poor 69; socio-economic status 268–9, 282–3
pharmacy 5, 295–6
and plague 94, 96
recipes 416–17 n.61
religious and medical role 52, 66
salaries 63
size 53, 254
tax privileges 377 nn. 63, 64
ward chapels 86, 173–7
and widows 272
S. Miniato del Ponte hospital (Spedale di Folco, Florence) 9, 343, 360 n.17
S. Niccolò hospital, Borgo di S. Maria Novella (Florence) 344
S. Niccolò hospital, near Porta La Croce (Florence) 352
S. Niccolò della Badia Fiorentina hospital 8, 9, 342
S. Niccolò della Misericordia hospital (Florence) 17, *19*, 349
S. Onofrio hospital (S. Nofri de' Tintori, Florence) 66, 345
S. Pancrazio hospital (Florence) 9, 344
S. Paolo dei Convalescenti hospital 87, 343–4
and apothecaries 290
architecture 74, *74*, 76–7
and Church and State 66–7, 104–5
as convalescent home 267
decoration 78–9, *78*
expansion 4, 14, 19–20, 25, 35, 40, 228
famiglia 52
female cloister 209
finances 60, 66–7, 105
hospital church 118
location 9, 19
medical staff 26, 37, 233, 244, 246, 249
and medicalisation 25, 53, 228
mortality rates 257, 263
nursing staff 52–3, 106, 187–8, 192
patients: conditions treated 265, 266–7, *266*; numbers 255; segregation 86; socio-economic status 269
and recipes 299
refectories 200

remodelling 74, 157
and sick poor 25–6, 27, 37, 53, 66, 102, 106, 269, 337
size 53, 254
wards 149, 156
S. Paolo a Pinti hospital (Spedale di Pinti/Spedale di S. Pier Maggiore, Florence) 8, 9, 342, 367 n.43
S. Pier Gattolino hospital (Florence) 345
S. Piero Novello dei Ridolfi hospital (Florence) 41–2, *41*, 349–50
S. Rocco hospital (Florence) 91, 99, 354
S. Salvadore hospital (Florence) 44, 61, 352
S. Sebastiano degli ammorbati *see* S. Bastiano degli ammorbati hospital
S. Sepolcro al Ponte Vecchio hospital (Florence) 9, 18, 42, 343
S. Spirito della Madonna Santa Maria del Piccione hospital (Florence) 17, *20*, 25, 66, 346, 348–9
S. Spirito hospital (Rome) xxvi, xxxi
Corsia Sistina 147, *148*, 160
Liber regulae 32, 58, 163–4, 179, *180*, 267
patients treated 253, 280–1
as pilgrim hospice 10, 337
S. Stefano e S. Martino hospital (Florence) 353
S. Trinita dei Calzolai hospital (Florence) 349, 367 n.43
S. Trinita hospital (Florence) 9, 345
safe-deposit boxes 61–2
salaries 27, 52, 57, 63, 233–4, 237–8, 287, 289–90
salt 92
Sanità (health board) 71, 97, 101
secularisation theories xxxi
segregation
of patients 82–3, 85–6, 89, 95, 142
of staff 85, 193–4
Senato dei Quarantotto 100, 104, 107
Serviti hospital (Florence) 344–5
sexual problems, treatment 330–1
Sforza, Francesco, Duke of Milan 134, 152–3, 324
siege of Florence (1529–30) 11, 18, 71, 91, 101, 105, 361 n.50
and hospital mortality rates 102, 160–1
Siena *see* S. Maria della Scala (Siena)
Signoria xxvii, 68, 92–3, 94, 96, 216, 245, 336
silk guild *see* Arte di Por S. Maria della Seta
simples 291, 298, 305, 316–21, 324, 334
plant-based 65, 131, 295, 308–9, 315, 326–7, 332
purchase 52, 264
in treatment of madness 313–14
sin, and disease 12, 113
Siraisi, Nancy 248
skin complaints 303
sleep, inducing 309, 313–14, 315–16
smallpox 307
specialisation of hospitals xxx, 4, 14–25, *14*, 39, 45, 88, 337
and architecture 89–90
and contagious disease 89–90, 93–101
foundling hospitals 46–7, 52, 61, 89
and plague 27–8, 35, 307, 337–8
Spedale dei Preti hospital (Florence) 63
spedalingo 86
age 218
and apothecaries 287
and Orsanmichele 37
and S. Bastiano 95–7
corruption 9, 37, 66–7, 68
death and burial 57, 182–3, 195–7
and disciplining of staff 194
elections 103–4
Innocenti 105
mealtimes 200–1
right of presentation 30
S. Maria della Scala 68
S. Maria Nuova 29–30, 59, 68, 82, 103–5, 127–8, 137, 176; Bonini, Bonino d'Antonio di Maso (*spedalingo*) 78, 79, 95–6, 135, 151, 304, 324; Buonaccolti, Vito 153–4, 182–3; Buonafede, Lionardo di Giovanni 79; Lorenzo di Jacopo da Bibbiena, 21, 151; Michele di Fruosino 288; Pierozzi, Orlando, da San Casciano 23, 38, 151; Ricasoli, Filippo 161
S. Matteo 94, 173, 195–7, 287, 399 n.68
salaries 43–4
Solosmsei, Maestro Giovanni di Maestro Ambrogio 244
speziali see apothecaries
SS. Gherardo e Clemente hospital (Florence) 349, 361 n.42
SS. Jacopo e Filippo della Porcellana e dei Michi hospital (Florence) 61, 347, 361 n.45
SS. Maria e Niccolò hospital (Florence) 107
SS. Salvi e Michele hospital (Florence) 353
SS. Trinita degli Incurabili hospital (Florence) 89, 91, 98–100, 101, 110, 267, 354–5

staff xxxii, xxxiii, 25–7, 47, 49
　salaries 27, 52, 57, 63, 233–4, 237–8, 287, 289–90
standard of living
　decline in 6, 28, 71, 91, 102
　rise in 50, 256
Stinche hospital *see* S. Maria delle Stinche hospital
stomach, problems with 324–5
Strozzi, Lorenzo 253
Studio Fiorentino (University) 226, 230, 245–8, 249
sub-infirmarer 163–4, 199, 205, 272
surgeons 26, 27, 32, 37, 57, 227, 235–41
　and barbers 228, 229, 238
　as dentists 238, 239
　geographical origins 242
　income 237, 243, 244
　instruments 240
　numbers 230
　prestige 28, 228, 236
　professional networks 244
　and the Studio 246
　women as 236
syrups 303, 324, 334

Targioni Tozzetti, Giovanni 158–9
taxation
　Decima 13, 90
　exemptions 29, 43, 68, 92, 94
　gabelle 55, 68, 92, 104
　imposition 103
　Prestanza 243, 244
　see also Catasto tax returns
teeth
　extraction 319, 322–3
　problems with 320–1
Templar hospital (Florence) 344
Tertiaries 69, 137
　and S. Paolo 25–6, 52, 66–7, 78, 187–8
textile workers 47, 211, 213, 268, 269–70, 275–6, 280
theriac (drug) 292, 307, 326–7, 330
Third Orders 19–20
　see also Tertiaries
Thomas of Cantimpré 314
Tomaso di Baccio d'Arezzo, Maestro 246
Tommaso del Garbo 159
Tommaso del Mazza *see* Master of S. Verdiana
Toscanelli, Domenico di Piero, Maestro 243, 245
Toscanelli, Paolo di Piero 243
Toscanelli, Piero del Maestro Domenico di Piero, Maestro 245
travellers, accommodation 39, 43–4, 50, 89, 90–1
Trexler, Bernice 254
Trotula of Salerno 327–30

Uccello, Paolo, *Creation Scenes* 143
Ugholino di Bonsi, *speziale* 288
Ugholino di Piero da Pisa, Maestro 246
Ugolino da Montecatini, Maestro 309, 311–2
unguents 175, 236, 302–3, 316–17
Urban VI, Pope 51, 136
urine, as aid to diagnosis 227, 231
usury, and patronage of hospitals 25, 50–1

Van der Goes, Hugo 140
　Adoration of the Shepherds 120, 128–32, *129*, 132, 137, 179
　Annunciation 129, 130
Vanni, Francesco di 120
Vanni, Stefano d'Antonio di 144
Varchi, Benedetto, *Storia fiorentina* 39, 60, 89, 92, 103, 206, 280, 336
Vasari, Giorgio 18, 125, 127, 131–2, 176, 383 n.47
Vecchietta 121
Venice, lazzaretto 94
Vernazza, Ettore 98, 99
Verrocchio, Andrea 177–8
Vienne, Council (1311–12) 29
Villani, Giovanni, *Cronica* 13, 24, 337
Villani, Matteo, *Cronica* 34, 36–7, 50, 53, 55, 88–9, 186
Virgin Mary, coronation 115–17, *116*

ward chapels 23, 168, 339
　altarpieces 58, 169–70, 173–5
　and celebration of Mass 23, 86, 147–9, 156, 160, 169–70, 175–6, 185, 192
　commemorative role 57, 135–6, 179–83
　and confraternities 120
wards 147–85
　admission of patients 161–4, 199, 253–6
　cruciform 23, 147, 151–5, 157, 184–5
　and death of patients 179
　exteriors 149–50, *150*
　height xxviii, 149, 157–61
　interiors 151–61
　open 21–3, 155–7
　and physical care 147, 149, 161–8
　and spiritual care 147, 149, 168–84

surgical treatment 239
windows xxviii, 72, 149, 159–61, 172
see also beds and bedding
wet-nurses 17, 46–7, 92
widows
  as nurses xxxii, 210–11, 212, 215–16, 218
  and poor relief 35, 39, 45–6, 91, 272
William of Saliceto 240
windows, and air circulation 159–61
wine, for patients xxv, 9, 56, 204, 206, 288
women
  and food preparation 203–6
  hospitals for 39, 45–6, 108, 110
  and laundry 209–10
  and length of hospital stay *262*, 263, 272
  marital status 272
  medical roles 199, 236, 302, 316–19
  and mortality rates 156, *257*, 258, *259*, *260*, 263, 272, *272*
  as pilgrims 44, 45
  and poor relief 26, 35
  treatment of urogenital symptoms 326–30, *326*
  see also nursing staff; widows

Zanchini, Giulio 108
Zerbi, Gabriele de' 225
Zocchi, Cosimo
  Veduta dell'Ospedale di Messer Bonifazio 74
  Veduta della Piazza di S. Maria Nuova 74, *75*